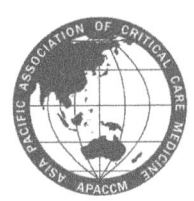

Evidence Based Core Topics in
CRITICAL CARE MEDICINE 2019

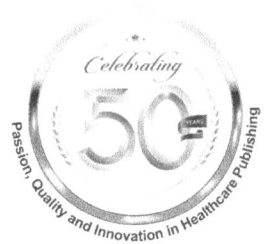

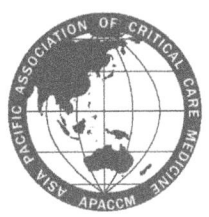

Evidence Based Core Topics in
CRITICAL CARE MEDICINE 2019

Ross Callum Freebairn
BHB MBChB Dip Obst FANZCA FRCP FJFICM FCICM
President, Asia Pacific Association of Critical Care Medicine (APACCM)
Consultant, Intensive Care Services, Hawke's Bay Hospital, Hastings, New Zealand
Associate Dean (Hawke's Bay)
University of Otago, Wellington, New Zealand
Adjunct Associate Professor, Chinese University of Hong Kong, Hong Kong

Atul Prabhakar Kulkarni
MD (Anesthesiology) PGDHHM FISCCM FICCM
Secretary General, Asia Pacific Association of Critical Care Medicine (APACCM)
Professor and Head
Division of Critical Care Medicine
Tata Memorial Hospital
Homi Bhabha National Institute
Mumbai, Maharashtra, India

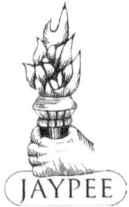

JAYPEE BROTHERS MEDICAL PUBLISHERS
The Health Sciences Publisher
New Delhi | London | Panama

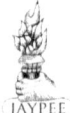

Jaypee Brothers Medical Publishers (P) Ltd

Headquarters
Jaypee Brothers Medical Publishers (P) Ltd
4838/24, Ansari Road, Daryaganj
New Delhi 110 002, India
Phone: +91-11-43574357
Fax: +91-11-43574314
Email: jaypee@jaypeebrothers.com

Overseas Offices

J.P. Medical Ltd
83 Victoria Street, London
SW1H 0HW (UK)
Phone: +44 20 3170 8910
Fax: +44 (0)20 3008 6180
Email: info@jpmedpub.com

Jaypee-Highlights Medical Publishers Inc
City of Knowledge, Bld. 235, 2nd Floor
Clayton, Panama City, Panama
Phone: +1 507-301-0496
Fax: +1 507-301-0499
Email: cservice@jphmedical.com

Jaypee Brothers Medical Publishers (P) Ltd
Bhotahity, Kathmandu, Nepal
Phone: +977-9741283608
Email: kathmandu@jaypeebrothers.com

Website: www.jaypeebrothers.com
Website: www.jaypeedigital.com

© 2019, Jaypee Brothers Medical Publishers

The views and opinions expressed in this book are solely those of the original contributor(s)/author(s) and do not necessarily represent those of editor(s) of the book.

All rights reserved. No part of this publication may be reproduced, stored or transmitted in any form or by any means, electronic, mechanical, photocopying, recording or otherwise, without the prior permission in writing of the publishers.

All brand names and product names used in this book are trade names, service marks, trademarks or registered trademarks of their respective owners. The publisher is not associated with any product or vendor mentioned in this book.

Medical knowledge and practice change constantly. This book is designed to provide accurate, authoritative information about the subject matter in question. However, readers are advised to check the most current information available on procedures included and check information from the manufacturer of each product to be administered, to verify the recommended dose, formula, method and duration of administration, adverse effects and contraindications. It is the responsibility of the practitioner to take all appropriate safety precautions. Neither the publisher nor the author(s)/editor(s) assume any liability for any injury and/or damage to persons or property arising from or related to use of material in this book.

This book is sold on the understanding that the publisher is not engaged in providing professional medical services. If such advice or services are required, the services of a competent medical professional should be sought.

Every effort has been made where necessary to contact holders of copyright to obtain permission to reproduce copyright material. If any have been inadvertently overlooked, the publisher will be pleased to make the necessary arrangements at the first opportunity. The **CD/DVD-ROM** (if any) provided in the sealed envelope with this book is complimentary and free of cost. **Not meant for sale.**

Inquiries for bulk sales may be solicited at: jaypee@jaypeebrothers.com

Evidence Based Core Topics in Critical Care Medicine 2019

First Edition: **2019**

ISBN 978-93-5270-906-9

Printed at

Dedicated to

All the hardworking, caring, and sincere souls who provide compassionate care to the critically ill in the Asia Pacific Region selflessly.

Contributors

Abdullah Al Shimemeri MBChB MD FRCPC
Consultant
Department of Pulmonary and Critical Care Medicine
Professor, College of Medicine
King Saud bin Abdulaziz University for Health Sciences
Riyadh, Saudi Arabia

Ajmer Singh MD
Director, Cardiac Anesthesia
Medanta Institute of Critical Care and Anesthesiology
Gurugram, Haryana, India

Alexis Kate Ford LLB (Hons) GDLP MBBS FRACGP
Medical Officer
Australian Defence Force
Australia

Alexis Tabah MD FCICM
Staff Specialist
Department of Intensive Care
Caboolture and Redcliffe Hospitals
Senior Lecturer, Department of Medicine
The University of Queensland
Brisbane, Queensland, Australia

Amarja Ashok Havaldar
MD (Anaesthesiology) FNB (Critical Care Medicine)
DM (Critical Care Medicine) EDIC
Assistant Professor
Department of Critical Care Medicine
St John's Medical College Hospital
Bengaluru, Karnataka, India

Amartya Mukhopadhyay MBBS MD MRCP FRCP EDIC MPH
Division of Respiratory and Critical Care
University Medicine Cluster
Department of Medicine
National University Health System and
National University of Singapore
Singapore

Amit Kansal MBBS MD (Anesthesia) FCICM
Consultant
Department of Intensive Care Medicine
Ng Teng Fong General Hospital
Singapore

Amit Madhukar Narkhede
MD DNB DM (Critical Care Medicine)
Specialist Senior Registrar
Division of Critical Care Medicine
Tata Memorial Hospital
Mumbai, Maharashtra, India

Amol Kothekar MD IDCC
Associate Professor
Division of Critical Care Medicine
Department of Anesthesiology, Critical Care and Pain
Tata Memorial Hospital
Homi Bhabha National Institute
Mumbai, Maharashtra, India

Andrew Li MBBS MRCP (UK) DFD (CAW)
Division of Respiratory and Critical Care
University Medicine Cluster
Department of Medicine
National University Health System and
National University of Singapore
Singapore

Anthony David Holley
BSc MBBCh DipPaeds DipDHM FACEM FCiCM
Senior Staff Specialist
Department of Intensive Care Medicine
Royal Brisbane and Women's Hospital
Brisbane, Queensland, Australia

Anthony S McLean MBBS MD FRACP FCICM FCSANZ
Professor and Head
Department of Intensive Care Medicine
Nepean Hospital
University of Sydney
Australia

Atul Prabhakar Kulkarni
MD (Anesthesiology) PGDHHM FISCCM FICCM
Secretary General
Asia Pacific Association of Critical Care Medicine (APACCM)
Professor and Head, Division of Critical Care Medicine
Tata Memorial Hospital
Homi Bhabha National Institute
Mumbai, Maharashtra, India

B Craig Ellis
MBChB FACEM Dip IMC (RCSEd) DipObs
Specialist Emergency Physician
St John New Zealand
Deputy Medical Director
Mount Wellington, Auckland, New Zealand

Bhuvana Krishna
MD (General Medicine) IDCCM IFCCM
Professor
Department of Critical Care Medicine
St John's Medical College and Hospital
Bengaluru, Karnataka, India

Brigitte Hollander
MBChB (Otago) PGDipOMG (Otago)
Senior Registrar
Intensive Care Services
Hawke's Bay Hospital
Hastings New Zealand

Carol D'silva
MD (Anesthesiology) FNB (Critical Care Medicine)
Assistant Professor
Department of Critical Care Medicine
St John's Medical College Hospital
Bengaluru, Karnataka, India

Catherine L Tacon
BSc (Med) MBBS FCICM MPH&TM PostGradCertAeromedRetrieval
Intensive Care Specialist
Cairns Hospital
Cairns, Queensland, Australia

Charudatt Vaity
MD (Med) DNB (Med) MRCP (UK) EDIC MFICM (UK)
Senior Consultant
Department of Critical Care
Fortis Hospital
Mumbai, Maharashtra, India

Chulananda Dias Goonasekera
MBBS FCAI FRCP (UK) PhD MPhil MD (Anesthesiology) DCH MRCPCH
Consultant Anesthetics
Department of Anesthesia
King's College Hospital, NHS Trust
London, England

Dhanvijay Shekhar Yadavrao
MBBS MD (Anesthesia) FCICM
Consultant
Department of Intensive care Medicine
Ng Teng Fong General Hospital
Singapore

Dhruva Chaudhry
MD (Med) DNB (Med) DM (PCCM)
Senior Professor and Head
Department of Pulmonary and Critical Care Medicine
Pt. BD Sharma PGIMS
Rohtak, Haryana, India

Elizabeth Jane Bennett MBBS FANZCA FCICM MPH
TM (Masters public health and tropical Medicine)
Coordinator
Department of Anesthesia and Intensive Care
School of Medical Science
College of Medicine, Nursing and Health Sciences
Fiji National University
Suva, Fiji Islands

Elizabeth Louise Trent FCICM FANZCA BHB MBChB DipObs
Intensivist
Department of Intensive Care Unit
Hawke's Bay Intensive Care Unit
Hawkes Bay District Health Board
Hastings, Hawke's Bay, New Zealand

Ganshyam Jagathkar MD FNB
Head
Department of Critical Care
Maxcure Hospital
Hyderabad, Telangana, India

Gentle Sunder Shrestha MD FACC EDIC FCCP
Assistant Professor
Department of Anesthesiology
Tribhuvan University Teaching Hospital
Maharajgunj, Kathmandu, Nepal

Hao Zheng Wong MBBS
ICU Senior registrar
Department of Intensive Care Unit
Royal Adelaide Hospital
Adelaide, Australia

Harish MM
MBBS MD DNB IDCCM DM (Critical Care Medicine) EDIC
Consultant and Incharge
Department of Critical Care Medicine
Narayana Hrudayalaya
Bengaluru, Karnataka, India

Jaikrit Bhutani
MD (Med) DNB (Med) DM (PCCM) PGMed 2nd year Intern
Internal Medicine
Pt BDS PGIMS
Rohtak, Haryana, India

Jane O'Donnell MN RN
Senior Research Scientist
Department of Respiratory and Acute Care
Fisher and Paykel Healthcare
Auckland, New Zealand

Jeffrey Lipman
MBBCh DA FFA FFA (Crit Care) FCICM MD (Research)
Senior Specialist, Department of Intensive Care Services
Royal Brisbane and Women's Hospital
Professor and Head
Department of Anesthesiology and Critical Care
The University of Queensland
Brisbane, Queensland, Australia

John Botha MBChB MMed FCP(SA) FCICM
Adjunct Clinical Professor
Monash University
Melbourne, Victoria, Australia

Juhi Chandwani
MD (Anesthesiology) DNB FFARCSI EDIC
Consultant
Department of Anesthesia and Intensive Care Unit
Royal Hospital
Muscat, Oman

Kate Barnett MBChB (Hon) MRCP (UK) FACEM FCICM
Consultant
Intensive Care Services
Hawke's Bay Hospital
Hastings, New Zealand

Khalid Ismail Khatib MD (Medicine)
Professor
Department of Medicine
SKN Medical College
Pune, Maharashtra, India

Lakshman Karalliedde DA FCA
Former Consultant
Department of Anesthesiology and Toxicology
Guy's and St Thomas' NHS Foundation Trust
London, England

Lalita Gouri Mitra DA MD DNB MNAMS
Associate Professor
Department of Critical Care
Institute of Liver and Biliary Sciences
New Delhi, India

Lata Bhattacharya MD (Anesthesiology)
Senior Consultant and Head
Department of Anesthesiology
Jawaharlal Nehru Cancer Hospital and Research Centre
Bhopal, Madhya Pradesh, India

Lounja Bouikhsaine
Diploma (Fine Arts) BSc (Psychology)
MSc (Neuropsychology & Speech and Language Therapy)
Medical Illustrator
Department of Pediatric Recovery
King's College Hospital, NHS Foundation Trust
London, England

Lyndal Russell MBBS FCICM FRACP
Consultant
Department of Intensive Care
Townsville Hospital
Townsville, Queensland, Australia

Madiha Hashmi FFARCSI
Assistant Professor
Department of Anesthesiology
Aga Khan University
Karachi, Pakistan

Maika Vuli Seru MBBS PGDA
Senior Registrar
Department of Anesthesia
Colonial War Memorial Hospital
Suva, Fiji, Islands

Matthew Edward Cove
MBChB BSc (Hons) FAMS FCCP
Senior Resident
Department of Respiratory and Critical Care Medicine
National University Hospital
Singapore

Michael AJ Park MBChB MRCP (UK) FCICM
Medical Director, Acute Medical Services
Intensive Care Services
Hawke's Bay Hospital
Hastings, New Zealand

Michael J O'Leary MD FRCA FCICM
Senior Staff Specialist
Department of Intensive Care Service
Royal Prince Alfred Hospital
Camperdown, Sydney, Australia
Co-State Medical Director-Organ and Tissue Donation Service

Michael Toolis MBBS BSc (Hons) GCertClinUS
Intensive Care Unit
Frankston Hospital
Melbourne, Victoria, Australia

Monika Gulati Kansal MBBS MD (Anesthesia) FCICM
Consultant
Department of Intensive Care Medicine
Ng Teng Fong General Hospital
Singapore

Muhammad Habibullah Rana MBBS MRCP EDIC
Resident Physician
Department of Intensive Care Medicine
Ng Teng Fong General Hospital
Singapore

Nattachai Srisawat
MD MSc EDIC (European Diploma Intensive Care Medicine)
Assistant Professor
Department of Medicine
Chulalongkorn University
Bangkok, Thailand

Nimita Deora MSc (Microbiology)
Clinical Research Coordinator
Department of Anesthesiology
Chirayu Medical College and Hospital
Bhopal, Madhya Pradesh, India

Nishanth Baliga DM (Critical Care Medicine)
Senior Resident
Department of Anesthesia, Critical Care and Pain
Tata Memorial Hospital
Mumbai, Maharashtra, India

Niteen D Karnik MD FICP
Professor and Head
Department of Medicine
LTMMC and LTMGH (Sion Hospital)
Mumbai, Maharashtra, India

Nupur N Karnik MD
Senior Resident
Department of Pathology
Tata Memorial Hospital
Mumbai, Maharashtra, India

Nuttha Lumlertgul MD MSc
Instructor
Department of Medicine
Chulalongkorn University
Bangkok, Thailand

Pradip Kumar Bhattacharya
MD (Anesthesiology) FICCM FCCCM MS
Director
Critical Care and Emergency Services
Head and Professor
Department of Anesthesiology
Chirayu Medical College and Hospital
Bhopal, Madhya Pradesh, India

Pradnya Atul Kulkarni MBBS DPB
Blood Transfusion Officer
Department of Pathology (Blood Bank)
KJ Somaiya Hospital and Research Center
Mumbai, Maharashtra, India

Pravin Amin MD FCCM
Head
Department of Critical Care Medicine
Bombay Hospital Institute of Medical Sciences
Mumbai, Maharashtra, India

Pravina Yande BHMS MBA
Medical Administrator
National Burns Centre
Navi Mumbai, Maharashtra, India

Priya Bhate MD
Assistant Professor
Department of Medicine
Seth GSMC and KEM Hospital
Mumbai, Maharashtra, India

Rahul Pandit
FCICM FJFICM EDIC FCCP FICCM DA
Director, Critical Care
Fortis Hospital
Mumbai, Maharashtra, India

Ravi N Mistry MBChB
Senior Registrar
Department of Intensive Care
Wellington Hospital
New Zealand

Ravindranath Tiruvoipati
MBBS MS FRCSEd MCh MSc FCICM EDIC
Consultant Intensivist and Director
Intensive Care Research, Intensive Care Medicine
Frankston Hospital
Frankston, Victoria, Australia

Rob Bevan
MBBS (Lond) BMedSci MRCP (UK) FRACP FCICM
Intensive Care Specialist
Critical Care Complex
Middlemore Hospital
Auckland, New Zealand

Ross C Freebairn
BHB MBChB DipObst FANZCA FRCP FJFICM FCICM
President
Asia Pacific Association of Critical Care Medicine (APACCM)
Consultant, Intensive Care Services
Hawke's Bay Hospital, Hastings, New Zealand
Associate Dean (Hawke's Bay)
University of Otago, Wellington, New Zealand
Adjunct Associate Professor, Chinese University of Hong Kong,
Hong Kong

Ruchira W Khasne
MBBS DA DNB IDCCM EDAIC EDIC
Consultant and Head
Department of Critical Care
Ashoka Medicover Hospital
Nashik, Maharashtra, India

Sadudee Peerapornratana MSc MD
Instructor
Department of Medicine
Chulalongkorn University
Bangkok, Thailand

Sandeep Kantor MD (Anesthesiology) FCCP FCCM FCCP
Consultant
Department of Anesthesia and Intensive Care Unit
Royal Hospital
Muscat, Oman

Sanya Chaudhry
MD (Med) DNB (Med) DM (PCCM) PGMed. 2nd year Intern
Internship
SGT Medical College
Gurugram, Haryana, India

Saurabh Pradhan MD (Anesthesiology) DM
Critical Care Medicine Resident
Department of Anesthesiology
Tribhuvan University Teaching Hospital
Maharajgunj, Kathmandu, Nepal

Sheetal Gaikwad MD
Assistant Professor
Department of Anesthesia, Critical Care and Pain
Tata Memorial Hospital
Mumbai, Maharashtra, India

Shruti Dutta MSc PhD
Senior Research Officer
Skin Bank and Research
National Burns Centre
Navi Mumbai, Maharashtra, India

Simon Smith MBChB FRACP DTM&H
Infectious Diseases Specialist
Department of Medicine, Cairns Hospital
Cairns, Queensland, Australia

Sing Chee Tan MBBS, MMed (ClinEpi) BMedSc
Registrar, Department of Intensive Care Unit
Austin Health
Victoria, Australia

Srinivas Samavedam
MD DNB FRCP FNB EDIC FICCCM DMLE MHA
Head, Department of Critical Care
Virinchi Hospital
Hyderabad, Telangana, India

Subhal Bhalchandra Dixit
MD (Medicine) IDCCM FCCM FICCM
President-Elect
Indian society of Critical Care Medicine
Consultant, Department of Critical Care
Director, Intensive Care Unit
Sanjeevan and MJM Hospitals
Pune, Maharashtra, India

Subhash Prasad Acharya MD (Anesthesiology)
Associate Professor
Department of Anesthesiology
Tribhuvan University Teaching Hospital
Maharajgunj, Kathmandu, Nepal

Sunil M Keswani MS MCh (Plastic Surgery)
Medical Director
National Burns Centre
Navi Mumbai, Maharashtra, India

Thomas A Doyle BA (Hon) MBBS MRCP (UK) FCICM
Intensive Care Specialist
Cairns Hospital
Cairns, Queensland, Australia

Timothy Martin Wilkinson MA DPhil (Oxon)
Professor
Department of Politics and International Relations
University of Auckland
Auckland, New Zealand

Valencia Lim
MBBS, MRCP
Senior Resident
Department of Respiratory and Critical Care Medicine
National University Hospital
Singapore

Vandana Saluja
MD PDCC Liver Transplant Anesthesia
Associate Professor
Department of Critical Care
Institute of Liver and Biliary Sciences
New Delhi, India

Vijaya Patil DA MD
Professor and Head
Division of Anesthesiology
Department of Clinical Anesthesia, Critical Care and Pain
Tata Memorial Hospital
Mumbai, Maharashtra, India

Vikas Bhagat
DO MD DM EDIC
Specialist Senior Resident
Department of Anesthesia, Critical Care and Pain
Tata Memorial Hospital
Mumbai, Maharashtra, India

Vinay Amin MBBS
Registrar, Department of Medicine
Bombay Hospital Institute of Medical Sciences
Mumbai, Maharashtra, India

Yatin Mehta
MD MNAMS FRCA FAMS FIACTA FICCM FTEE
President
Indian Society of Critical Care Medicine
Chairman
Medanta Institute of Critical Care and Anesthesiology
Gurugram, Haryana, India

Preface

As of Saturday, 5th January 2019, the estimated population of Asia is 4,565,540,460, equivalent to roughly 60% of the total world population.

In contrast to the population, compared to the western intensive care units, critical disease profile, information about the diagnosis, treatment and patient outcome of diseases suffered by patients of that population, the intensive care units in Asia and the Pacific regions reported in scientific journals reports and critical care educational texts are in significant minority. However, the organization of intensive care delivery in Asia Pacific region is rapidly evolving, and within over 50 countries that comprise the "Asia Pacific" region. There is an ever-increasing demand for services for critically ill and an increasing desire to have information relevant to intensive care medicine practice in this region.

This desire led the Asia Pacific Association of Critical Care Medicine (APACCM) to organize and sponsor this publication "Evidence Based Core Topics in Critical Care Medicine 2019" to assist dissemination of the available evidence in the field. The book has been exclusively written by 85 authors, who practice in the Asia Pacific regions intensive care environment, and as such provides a contemporary overview of the practice intensive care medicine in our region. In addition to sections of general assessment and organ support in critically ill, over half of the book is dedicated to organ dysfunction and specific critical illness syndromes (including the infectious diseases) that are prevalent in areas of the region.

We are grateful to many authors for their commitment and their expertise in producing this book, and to the publishers for their consideration and care in its production.

Ross Callum Freebairn
Atul Prabhakar Kulkarni

Acknowledgments

We wish to thank all contributors from all member countries of APACCM (Asia Pacific Association of Critical Care Medicine) for their efforts in contributing the chapters to the first ever book published by Asia Pacific Association of Critical Care Medicine. This book would not have been possible without their hard work, put in, in spite of their busy clinical schedule.

We would also like to extend our appreciation to Shri Jitendar P Vij (Group Chairman), Mr Ankit Vij (Group President), Ms Chetna Malhotra Vohra (Associate Director-Content Strategy), Ms Prerna Bajaj (Development Editor), and all the staff of M/s Jaypee Brothers Medical Publishers (P) Ltd, New Delhi, India, for their efforts and input enabling timely publication of the book.

Contents

SECTION 1: General Assessment and Support in Critically Ill

1. **Blood Pressure in Intensive Care Unit** — 3
   Charudatt Vaity, Rahul Pandit
   - Methods of Blood Pressure Monitoring in Intensive Care Unit 3
   - Mean Arterial Pressure 6
   - What is an Ideal Map? 7

2. **Adjunctive Therapies in Acute Myocardial Infarction** — 9
   Harish MM, Atul Prabhakar Kulkarni
   - Morphine 9

3. **Echocardiography in the Critical Care Unit** — 16
   Anthony S McLean
   - Competency Levels 16
   - Evaluation of Pathologies Commonly Encountered in Critically Ill Patients 17
   - Echocardiography in the Management of the Shock 21

4. **Assessment of Nutritional Status in Critically Ill** — 23
   Andrew Li, Amartya Mukhopadhyay
   - Provision of Energy in Critically Ill 23
   - Provision of Protein in Critically Ill 23
   - Nutritional Risk Assessment 24
   - Determining Energy Requirements 24
   - Feeding Strategies 24
   - Protein Intake 26
   - Total Parenteral Nutrition 26

5. **Prognosis and Risk Factors for Poor Outcome in Critically Ill Patients with Respiratory Illness** — 28
   Amit Kansal, Dhanvijay Shekhar Yadavrao
   - Prognosis and Risk Factors for Poor Outcome in Community-Acquired Pneumonia 28
   - Prognosis and Risk Factors for Poor Outcome in Hospital-Acquired Pneumonia and Ventilator-Associated Pneumonia 29
   - Prognosis and Risk Factors for Poor Outcome in Acute Respiratory Distress Syndrome 30
   - Prognosis Among Critically Ill Patients with Chronic Obstructive Pulmonary Disease 31

6. **Blood Transfusion in Critically Ill Patients** — 34
   Ruchira W Khasne, Pradnya Atul Kulkarni, Atul Prabhakar Kulkarni
   - Epidemiology 34
   - Transfusion Trigger 34
   - Impact of Blood Transfusion on Patient Outcomes 35
   - Association of Anemia in Intensive Care Unit and Blood Transfusion 35
   - Restrictive Transfusion Strategy 36
   - Association of Blood Transfusion with Mortality in Cardiac Patients 37
   - Storage Lesions 38
   - Role of Leukodepleted Blood 39
   - Current Evidence for the Use of Artificial Blood 40

7. **Antibiotics in Intensive Care Unit** — 42
   Alexis Tabah, Jeffrey Lipman
   - Rational Antibiotic Use 42
   - Other Important Aspects to Consider 44
   - Pharmacokinetic Principles 45
   - Main Antibiotic Classes 45
   - Practice Prescription 46

8. **Sedation in the Critically Ill** — 48
   Andrew Li, Amartya Mukhopadhyay
   - Commonly Used Sedatives and Analgesics in the Intensive Care Unit 48
   - The Pain, Agitation, and Delirium Syndrome in Intensive Care Unit 50
   - Use of Sedatives in Elderly 52

9. **Delirium: Prognosis and Outcome** — 54
   Ruchira W Khasne, Atul Prabhakar Kulkarni
   - Epidemiology 54
   - Subtypes of Delirium 54
   - Pathophysiology 54
   - Clinical Features 55
   - Risk Factors for Delirium 55
   - Delirium Monitoring Tools 55
   - Impact of Delirium on Patient's Outcome 56
   - Management 57

10. **Brain Death** 63
   Elizabeth Louise Trent, Timothy Martin Wilkinson
   - Biophilosophical Arguments Explained 63
   - Physiological and Biological Plausibility of Brain Death 64
   - Clinical Practice 65
   - Clinical Examination 66

11. **Organ Donation** 69
   Michael J O'Leary
   - Potential Donor Identification 69
   - Assessment of Potential Donor Suitability 71
   - Family Approach for Donation 71
   - Donor Management 72
   - Organ Donation and the Community 73

12. **Do-Not-Attempt Cardiopulmonary Resuscitation Decision-Making** 75
   Michael AJ Park, Kate Barnett, Ross C Freebairn
   - Definition 75
   - Principles 75
   - Discussion about Cardiopulmonary Resuscitation 76
   - Limited Resuscitation 78
   - Documentation 78
   - Is a DNACPR Status Permanent? 78
   - Conflict Resolution 78

Section 2: Organ Dysfunction

13. **Atrial Fibrillation in Intensive Care Unit** 83
   Muhammad Habibullah Rana, Monika Gulati Kansal, Hao Zheng Wong
   - Etiopathology 83
   - Diagnosis of Atrial Fibrillation 84
   - Classification 84
   - Impact of Atrial Fibrillation 84
   - Evidence 85
   - Management 85
   - Practice Prescriptions 88

14. **Cardiogenic Shock (with Intra-Aortic Balloon Pump)** 91
   Yatin Mehta, Ajmer Singh 91
   - Diagnosis 91
   - Etiology 91
   - Pathophysiology 92
   - Laboratory Evaluation 92
   - Management 92

15. **Asthma and Chronic Obstructive Pulmonary Disease** 96
   Sing Chee Tan, Amit Kansal
   - Epidemiology 96
   - Pathophysiology 96
   - Pharmacotherapy 96
   - Mechanical Ventilation and Oxygen Therapy 98
   - Intensive Care Unit Polyneuromyopathy 99
   - Nutritional Support 99
   - Prognosis 99

16. **Acute Pulmonary Embolism** 101
   Dhanvijay Shekhar Yadavrao, Monika Gulati Kansal, Amit Kansal
   - Classification of Pulmonary Embolism 101
   - Clinical Features 102
   - Investigations 102
   - Treatment 104

17. **Chest Trauma** 108
   Anthony David Holley, Alexis Kate Ford
   - Chest Wall 109
   - Pulmonary/Pleural Injury 109
   - Tracheobronchial Injuries 111

18. **Traumatic Brain Injury** 116
   Amit Madhukar Narkhede, Atul Prabhakar Kulkarni
   - Pathophysiology of Traumatic Brain Injury 117
   - Prognostic Prediction Models 120
   - Management 121
   - Potential Use of Biomarkers in Traumatic Brain Injury 123

19. **Encephalitis** 125
   Rob Bevan
   - Pathophysiology 125
   - Evidence 126
   - Practice Prescription 126

20. **Acute Liver Failure** 130
   Lalita Gouri Mitra, Vandana Saluja
   - Pathophysiology 131
   - Etiology and Outcomes 131
   - Diagnostic Approach 131
   - Management of Acute Liver Failure in Intensive Care Unit 132

21. **Diarrhea in Intensive Care Unit** 137
   Sheetal Gaikwad, Amol Kothekar, Vijaya Patil
   - Physiology of the Digestive System 137
   - Definition of Diarrhea 137
   - Classification of Diarrhea 137
   - Management of Diarrhea 141

22. **Gastric Stasis in Intensive Care Unit** 144
   Amol Kothekar, Nishanth Baliga, Vikas Bhagat
   - Incidence 144
   - Physiology of Gastric Emptying 144
   - Pathophysiology of Gastric Stasis 145
   - Treatment 146

23. **Mesenteric Ischemia** 151
   Subhal Bhalchandra Dixit, Khalid Ismail Khatib
   - Pathophysiology of Intestinal Ischemia 151
   - Intestinal Response to Ischemia 151

- Etiology of Mesenteric Ischemia 152
- Risk Factors for Mesenteric Ischemia 152
- Clinical Features 152
- Evidence 152

24. **Necrotizing Pancreatitis** 156
    Pravin Amin, Vinay Amin
    - Classification 156
    - Assessment of Severity 157
    - Etiology of Acute Pancreatitis 157
    - Clinical Manifestations of Acute Pancreatitis 157
    - Complications of Pancreatitis 158
    - Diagnosis 158
    - Course of the Disease 159
    - Management of Pancreatitis 159
    - Surgical Intervention 162

25. **Critical Care in Burns** 165
    Sunil M Keswani, Shruti Dutta, Pravina Yande
    - Classification of Burns 165
    - Pathophysiology of Burns 165
    - Criteria for Hospitalization 165
    - Burn Wound Assessment 166
    - Patient Evaluation after Burns Injury 167
    - Acute Burns Management 169
    - Debridement and Skin Grafting 169

26. **Necrotizing Soft Tissue Infections** 172
    Rob Bevan
    - Evidence 172
    - Practice Prescription 175

27. **Metabolic Acidosis** 178
    Michael AJ Park, Ross C Freebairn
    - Metabolic Acidosis Versus Acidemia 178
    - Gamblegram 178
    - Bicarbonate 179
    - Evaluating Metabolic Acidosis 179
    - Anion Gap Method 179
    - Normal Anion Gap Acidosis 180
    - Raised Anion Gap Acidosis 180
    - The Physiochemical or Net Unmeasured Ions (Strong Ion Gap) Method 180
    - Estimating NUI Using Anion Gap Corrected for Albumin and Lactate 181
    - What are the Net Unmeasured Ions (NUI)? 182
    - Why Measure NUI? 182
    - Management of Metabolic Acidosis. Is It H⁺ Or the Anion the Problem? 182
    - Effect of Fluids 182
    - Role of Sodium Bicarbonate 183

28. **Anaphylaxis** 185
    B Craig Ellis
    - Causes 186
    - Biochemical Mediators 186
    - Clinical Presentation 186
    - Management 187

29. **Organophosphate Poisoning** 190
    Amarja Ashok Havaldar, Carol D'silva, Bhuvana Krishna
    - History 190
    - Chemistry 190
    - Classification 191
    - Clinical Features 192
    - Diagnosis 192
    - Delayed Effects 193
    - Management 194
    - Supportive Therapies with No Proven Benefit As of Today 194
    - Definitive Therapy 195
    - Carbamate Poisoning 196
    - Treatment 197

30. **Snake Envenomation** 199
    Srinivas Samavedam, Ganshyam Jagathkar
    - Clinical Features 199
    - Management of Snakebite Envenomation 201
    - Assessment 201
    - Antisnake Venom 201
    - Scorpion Sting Envenomation 202
    - Bee Sting 204

31. **Toxidromes** 206
    Chulananda Dias Goonasekera, Lakshman Karalliedde, Lounja Bouikhsaine
    - Generic Principles of Therapy 207
    - Anticholinergic Toxidrome 208
    - Cholinergic Toxidrome 209
    - Sympathomimetic Toxidrome 211
    - Sympathoplegia Toxidrome 213
    - Neuromuscular Blockade 213
    - Opioid Toxidrome 214
    - Serotoninergic (Serotonergic) Toxidrome 215
    - Cyanide Toxidrome 215
    - Salicylate Toxidrome 217
    - Envenoming 217
    - Plant Toxidromes 219
    - Miscellaneous Drug Overdoses 220
    - Acetaminophen 220
    - Neuroleptic Malignant Syndrome 220

Section 3: Specific Syndromes

32. **Influenza in the Intensive Care Unit** 233
    Michael Toolis, John Botha
    - Transmission and Replication 233
    - Pathogenesis and Pathology 234
    - Clinical Manifestations 234
    - Diagnosis 235
    - Treatment 235

33. **Middle East Respiratory Syndrome Coronavirus** 238
    Sandeep Kantor, Juhi Chandwani
    - Epidemiology 238
    - Pathogenesis 240

- Clinical Features and Progress of the Disease 240
- Case Definitions 241
- Treatment and Prevention of Infection (Vaccine) 242

34. Tetanus 245
Gentle Sunder Shrestha, Saurabh Pradhan, Subhash Prasad Acharya, Jeffrey Lipman

- Biological Plausibility 245
- Evidence Base 248
- Practice Prescription 248

35. Intensive Care Management of Leptospirosis 251
Elizabeth Jane Bennett, Maika Vuli Seru

- Introduction: Epidemiology and Risk Factors 251
- Presentation: Assessment and Diagnosis 251
- Treatment Evidence and Practice Recommendations 252

36. Dengue in Intensive Care Unit 256
Madiha Hashmi 256

- Transmission 256
- Classification 256
- Clinical Presentations 257
- Laboratory Diagnosis 259
- Management 259
- Immunization 261
- Dengue in the Elderly 261
- Dengue in Pregnancy 261

37. Scrub Typhus 263
Dhruva Chaudhry, Jaikrit Bhutani, Sanya Chaudhry

- Epidemiology 263
- Etiopathogenesis 264
- Clinical Features 264
- Diagnosis 265
- Treatment 267
- Prevention 268

38. Malaria in the Intensive Care Unit 271
Niteen D Karnik, Priya Bhate, Nupur N Karnik

- Physiology 271
- Pathogenesis 272
- Severe Malaria 272
- Diagnosis 272
- Management 273
- Complications and Management 274

39. Tuberculosis in Intensive Care Unit 276
Pradip Kumar Bhattacharya, Lata Bhattacharya, Nimita Deora

- Reasons and Outcome for ICU Admission in Tuberculosis Patients 276
- Management of Patients with Tuberculosis in the ICU 276
- Diagnosis and Treatment of Tuberculosis Patients Coinfected with Human Immunodeficiency Virus 281
- Infection Prevention and Control Measures to Reduce Transmission 282

40. Melioidosis 285
Catherine L Tacon, Thomas A Doyle, Simon Smith

- Epidemiology 285
- Clinical Features 287
- Clinical Images 288
- Diagnosis 288
- Management 288

Section 4: Organ Support in Critical Care

41. Oxygen 295
Brigitte Hollander, Ross C Freebairn

- The Role of Oxygen 295
- Normal Physiological Adaptations 295
- Oxygen as a Drug 296
- Oxygen Cascade 296
- Dysoxia 298

42. Positive End-Expiratory Pressure 303
Ross C Freebairn, Ravi N Mistry, Michael AJ Park

- Definition 303
- History 303
- General Physiology 303
- Positive End-Expiratory Pressure Titration 304
- Gas Exchange: Oxygen Positive End-Expiratory Pressure Tables 304
- Gas Exchange: Carbon Dioxide 305
- Compliance 305
- Pressure–Volume Curve: Volume 306
- Stress Index 307
- Esophageal Manometry 307
- Lung Volume 307
- Imaging 308
- Summary and Recommendations 308

43. Driving Pressure in Acute Respiratory Distress Syndrome 311
Atul Prabhakar Kulkarni, Ruchira W Khasne

- What is Airway Driving Pressure (ΔP)? 311
- Physiology of ΔP 312
- Effect of ΔP on Mortality 312
- Mechanical Power As Applied to the Respiratory System 313
- Consequences of ΔP 313
- Transpulmonary Driving Pressure (ΔPL) 314
- Clinical Use of ΔP 314
- How to Adjust Ventilatory Parameters According to ΔP 315
- Limitations of ΔP 315

44. Weaning From Ventilation 317
Ravi N Mistry, Brigitte Hollander, Ross C Freebairn

- Physiology/Scientific Rationale/Biological Plausibility 317

- Routine Weaning 317
- Barriers and Challenges to a Spontaneous Breathing Trial and Weaning 319

45. High-Flow Nasal Cannula Respiratory Support 324
Jane O' Donnell

- Nasal High-flow Mechanisms of Action 324
- Therapeutic Efficacy—Clinical Outcomes 326
- Nasal High-flow Delivery 327
- Nasal High-flow Strategies for Clinical Applications 327
- Research Focus Areas 329

46. Evidence-Based Review of Noninvasive Ventilation 331
Abdullah Al Shimemeri

- Scientific Rationale of Noninvasive Ventilation 331
- Clinical Evidence in Support of Noninvasive Ventilation 332
- Practice Prescription 333

47. Extracorporeal Membrane Oxygenation 337
Lyndal Russell, Ross Callum Freebairn, Ravindranath Tiruvoipati

- Evidence 337
- Practice 338
- Conclusion and Recommendations 342

48. Extracorporeal Carbon Dioxide Removal 345
Valencia Lim, Matthew Edward Cove

- Principles of Extracorporeal Carbon Dioxide Removal 345
- $ECCO_2R$ in Clinical Practice 346
- Guidelines for $ECCO_2R$ Use 349

49. Continuous Renal Replacement Therapy: An Update 351
Nattachai Srisawat, Nuttha Lumlertgul, Sadudee Peerapornratana

- Optimal Timing of Continuous Renal Replacement Therapy 351

50. Extracorporeal Blood Purification Therapy for Sepsis 359
Nattachai Srisawat 359

- Extracorporeal Blood Purification for Sepsis 359

Index 367

SECTION 1

General Assessment and Support in Critically Ill

Outlines

1. Blood Pressure in Intensive Care Unit
2. Adjunctive Therapies in Acute Myocardial Infarction
3. Echocardiography in the Critical Care Unit
4. Assessment of Nutritional Status in Critically ill
5. Prognosis and Risk Factors for Poor Outcome in Critically Ill Patients with Respiratory Illness
6. Blood Transfusion in Critically Ill Patients
7. Antibiotics in Intensive Care Unit
8. Sedation in the Critically Ill
9. Delerium: Prognosis and Outcome
10. Brain Death
11. Organ Donation
12. Do-not-attempt Cardiopulmonary Resuscitation Decision-Making

CHAPTER 1

Blood Pressure in Intensive Care Unit

Charudatt Vaity, Rahul Pandit

INTRODUCTION

Both high and low blood pressure can cause organ dysfunction. Monitoring blood pressure remains a vital component of hemodynamic monitoring and management in intensive care unit (ICU). Blood pressure monitoring, in combination with other monitoring, has shown to detect more than 90% adverse events when used in anesthesia.[1] This chapter looks into different methods of blood pressure monitoring and which is preferred method, invasive or noninvasive. It also attempts to answer which is the better target mean or systolic blood pressure and if there is any ideal target.

METHODS OF BLOOD PRESSURE MONITORING IN INTENSIVE CARE UNIT

Blood pressure monitoring is an essential component of managing hemodynamically unstable patients in ICU. The methods of monitoring can be classified broadly into (1) noninvasive and (2) invasive.

Noninvasive Blood Pressure Monitoring

Noninvasive blood pressure monitoring can be intermittent or continuous. Intermittent noninvasive blood pressure (NIBP), measurements can further be classified into (1) manual and (2) automated.

Manual Noninvasive Blood Pressure Measurement

Manual NIBP can be measured using auscultatory technique. The auscultatory technique has been mainstay of clinical blood pressure recording for as long as blood pressure has been recorded but is now gradually replaced by automated versions.

The auscultatory method uses either mercury, aneroid, or hybrid sphygmomanometers. Korotkoff's technique, which is used for measuring blood pressure, has not changed for more than 100 years. A blood pressure cuff is placed around the arm and the cuff is inflated above the systolic pressure so that brachial artery is occluded. As the cuff is deflated the blood flow is re-established and is accompanied by sounds which can be heard by holding a stethoscope above the brachial artery just below the cuff. The sounds are thought to originate from turbulent flow and oscillations in the arterial wall. The Korotkoff technique tends to give lower systolic and higher diastolic blood pressure reading higher, than intra-arterial pressure.[2,3]

A mercury sphygmomanometer is regarded as the gold standard in clinical blood pressure measurement although it is gradually fading out due to the ban on use of mercury in some countries due to environmental reasons.[4] The simplistic design of the mercury devices makes less room for errors. Though this should not be any reason for being complacent, studies have found that a significant number of devices can be inaccurate due to technical reasons.[5,6]

Aneroid sphygmomanometers are devices with mechanical system of metal bellows that expand with the increase in cuff pressure and a series of levers record this pressure on a circular scale. The inaccuracies associated with aneroid devices can be as high as 44%; therefore, they need frequent recalibration.[5]

Hybrid sphygmomanometers combine features of both electronic and auscultatory devices. The mercury column is replaced by an electronic pressure gauge. Blood pressure is taken in the same manner as with mercury or aneroid using auscultatory technique. The cuff pressure can be displayed as simulated mercury column, simulated aneroid display, or digital display. The hybrid sphygmomanometer has the potential to replace mercury devices because it combines best features of mercury and automated devices.[7]

Automated Blood Pressure Measurement

The automated blood pressure recorder uses the oscillometric method. It has been demonstrated that when the oscillations of the pressure in the sphygmomanometer are recorded, the point of maximum oscillation corresponds to mean arterial pressure (MAP).[8,9] The oscillation starts before the true systolic blood pressure and continues beyond the true diastolic blood pressure. The manufactures use algorithm to detect the systolic and diastolic blood pressure. The algorithm used can vary between manufacturers. This can cause considerable variations between devices.[10] But overall it is seen that oscillatory technique compares well with intra-arterial and auscultatory method.[11]

Noninvasive Continuous Blood Pressure Measurement

Currently, there are two different techniques to record continuous NIBP.
1. Arterial applanation tonometry
2. Volume clamp method

Arterial applanation tonometry: An arterial pulse wave can be obtained by strapping a transducer to an artery with a bone underneath.[12] This technique has been refined and is now available. T-Line system is the device available, allowing automated radial artery applanation tonometry (Tensys Medical, San Diego, CA, USA).[13] MAP and diastolic arterial pressure (DAP) have been shown to correlate well when compared with intra-arterial measurements, but systolic arterial pressure (SAP) measurements need further improvement.[14]

Volume clamp method: It was developed by Penáz[15] on the principle of vascular unloading. It combines an inflatable cuff with a photodiode. The photodiode sensor measures the changes in the blood volume based on the amount of light transmitted through the finger. The cuff pressure closely follows the blood pressure changes in the finger arteries. This is then calculated beat to beat, after calibration with built-in oscillometric measurement and a real-time arterial pressure, waveform is displayed. Commercially available devices based on this technology are Infinity® CNAP™ SmartPod®-Drager and ClearSight—Edwards, USA.

This technology has been validated in different studies and is found to be comparable to invasive arterial blood pressure monitoring within limitations.[16,17]

The continuous noninvasive devices have an appeal in its noninvasiveness and can be used in situations where there is need to assess, document, and maintain hemodynamic stability, and arterial blood gas measurements are not required. On the other hand, it has its limitations, in cases with severe vasoconstriction, peripheral vascular disease, and distorted fingers due to arthritis where there may be difficulty in obtaining a proper waveform.

Invasive Blood Pressure Monitoring

Invasive blood pressure (IBP) is the gold standard in blood pressure measurement as it gives beat-to-beat information. It is useful when rapid changes in blood pressure are anticipated due to cardiovascular instability or when NIBP measurements are not possible or unreliable, e.g. obesity, arrhythmias, nonpulsatile flow on extracorporeal membrane oxygenation. It is also recommended when the patients are extremely sick and repetitive cuff inflations can cause localize tissue damage and when there is requirement of repeated blood gas analysis.

The Hemodynamic Monitoring System

The basic principle in any invasive pressure monitoring system is to provide a continuous column of liquid connecting the arterial blood to the transducer. The components required are as follows:
- Intra-arterial cannula
- Tubing
- Transducers
- Microprocessor and display screen

Intra-arterial Cannula

A short cannula is inserted into an artery. A 20-G cannula is generally used. Preferably a nonend artery is cannulated. A radial artery is the most commonly cannulated artery. The advantage of choosing a nonend artery is that, should thrombosis occur, arterial sufficiency is maintained via collateral supply. The collateral supply to the hand can be assessed by performing modified Allen's test although it is not 100% reliable.[18] If cannulation of nonend artery such as radial or dorsalis pedis is not feasible then brachial or femoral may be used with due monitoring of signs of distal insufficiency.

Tubing

Correct setup and maintenance of the tubing system and transducer are crucial to avoid erroneous readings. With improperly and inadequately prepared monitoring system, the hemodynamic indices measured will be inaccurate and invalidate patient's entire hemodynamic profile misleading the treatment. Three steps need to be followed to prepare the monitoring tubing to ensure accuracy: priming the tubing, leveling and zeroing, and dynamic response testing.

Priming the Pressure Tubing
An arterial catheter is connected to the monitoring system by fluid-filled tubing. The fluid column in the tubing carries the mechanical signal created by the arterial pressure wave to the diaphragm of the transducer. The transducer converts the mechanical signal into electrical signal.

Air transmits mechanical impulses differently than fluid. Air bubbles in the tubing are one of the most common sources of error in IBP monitoring. Air bubbles blunt or damp the propagation of the mechanical signal, causing erroneous readings.[19] Therefore air-free priming of the entire tubing is one of the most important steps to avoid error. The entire system should be flushed to achieve air-free priming.

Leveling and Zeroing
The zero reference point is set at the atmospheric pressure and this must be referenced to the level of the heart. This process is called leveling and zeroing. Leveling of the catheter system is achieved by aligning the air–fluid interface of the monitoring system with the external reference point of the heart. The external reference point is called the phlebostatic point, and the axis passing through this point is the phlebostatic axis. This can be located by finding the junction of two lines—the vertical line drawn from the fourth intercostal space and a horizontal line drawn through the midpoint of a line going from anterior to posterior side of chest.[20,21] Arterial blood pressure is the key determinant of organ prefusion, and the phlebostatic axis accurately reflects the level of the heart.

Zeroing is a simple but important process and is performed by opening the air–fluid interface to the atmosphere and then electronically zeroing the system. Zeroing establishes the atmospheric pressure as the zero reference point for the monitor.

Leveling and zeroing should be done every time after the air–fluid interface and reference point are changed to ensure accuracy and consistency. It is important to appreciate that small offsets from the phlebostatic axis and zero reference point can cause large errors, and this can lead to inappropriate treatment. Therefore once the reference point is identified, it should be marked.

Dynamic Response Testing
In order to ensure that the monitoring system accurately reproduces hemodynamic characteristics, it is important that the system is tested for its dynamic response. The dynamic response can be defined by its resonance and the damping coefficient.

Each system has its own natural oscillatory frequency or resonant frequency. If this resonant frequency of the monitoring system is the same as the frequency making up the arterial waveform then the subsequent signal will be distorted. It is therefore important that the natural frequency of the system is kept very high. If the frequency of the system is 25 Hz or higher, the system will mostly function properly. The natural frequency of the system can be increased by using a wide bore, high pressure tubing with low compliance, and its length limited to less than 122 cm.[19,22] Most systems available have natural frequency of around 200 Hz, but this is reduced by addition of three-way stopcocks, air-bubbles, clots, and additional length of tubing.

The resonance of the system can be measured by performing "Fast flush" test (Fig. 1.1).

The damping coefficient of the monitoring system is a reflection on how soon the oscillations excited by the shock of arterial pressure wave eventually come to rest.[19,22] Some degree of damping is intrinsic to the system and is essential. The damping coefficient can be measured by using the fast flush test (Fig. 1.2).

Based on the damping coefficient factors, the monitoring system can be as follows:
- *Optimally damped*: The monitoring system responds quickly to any change (damping coefficient of 0.7).
- *Critically damped*: No overshooting but system is slow to respond (damping coefficient 1.0).

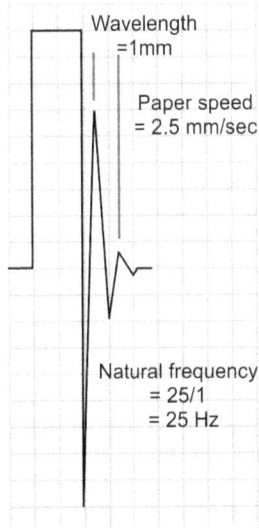

FIGURE 1.1: Fast flush test to calculate the resonance frequency.

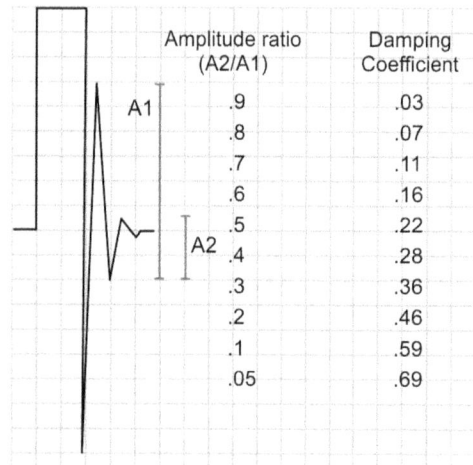

FIGURE 1.2: Fast flush test to calculate damping coefficient.

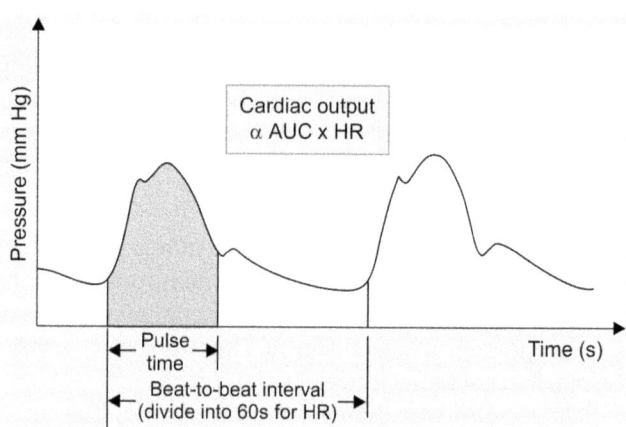

FIGURE 1.3: PICCO monitor (pulsion medical systems) uses the AUC to calculated the stroke volume. (AUC: area under the curve).

- *Under damped*: Due to occurrence of resonance, the overshooting is required (damping coefficient <0.7).
- *Over damped*: The signal takes long time to reach equilibrium and will not overshoot (damping coefficient >1.0).

The over damping can exist because of multiple factors, such as bubbles/clots in the system, severe vasospasm of the artery, narrow long soft tubing and kinks in the cannula/tubing. These may be major sources of erroneous recording of blood pressure. The systolic blood pressure is underread and the diastolic is overread. There is no much change to the mean blood pressure.

Under damping can also pose problems. There is an overshoot of pressure waves; therefore, the systolic readings are excessively high and diastolic readings are low.

Transducers

The pressure wave of the arterial impulse is transmitted via the fluid interface in the tubing to a transducer. There is a diaphragm that moves in the response to this pressure wave and the movement is converted into an electrical signal. The transducer uses the strain gauge to convert mechanical energy into electrical energy.

Microprocessor and Display Screen

A numerical and graphical display of the arterial blood pressure is provided on a beat-to-beat basis. This allows us to perform waveform analysis. Information regarding volume status and cardiac output (CO) can be determined by looking at the morphology, position of the dicrotic notch, and the "swing."

Some systems, such as PICCO, LiDCO, and FloTrac, use pulse contour analysis to derive stroke volume (SV), CO, and systemic vascular resistance (SVR) (Fig. 1.3).

MEAN ARTERIAL PRESSURE

Mean arterial pressure is a very important hemodynamic index. It has more influence on the blood flow regulation and organ perfusion. MAP can be calculated by direct and indirect measurement of arterial pressure. When measured by looking at the arterial pressure trace, due to the shape of the trace, the MAP value is more geometric mean then arithmetic average (Fig. 1.4).

It is important to understand the relationship between MAP, CO, and SVR. Cardiovascular system is a hydraulic circuit, and it follows the same principles that are defined by Ohm's law to define the equation between pressure, flow, and resistance.

According to Ohm's law:
Pressure = flow × resistance
This can be rewritten as follows for cardiovascular system:
MAP = CO × SVR
As CO can be derived by multiplying SV by heart rate (HR), the above equation can be further expanded as:

MAP = SV × HR × SVR

So as per the above derivation, MAP values are dependent on the interplay between the three parameters: SV, HR, and SVR (Fig. 1.5).

Mean or systolic, invasive, or NIBP measurements:

There is significant clinical difference in systolic blood pressure recordings by invasive and noninvasive methods. As discussed above, noninvasive oscillometric methods measure MAP and the systolic and diastolic recordings are estimated by algorithms. Lehman et al.[23] conducted a retrospective study, which looked into blood pressure

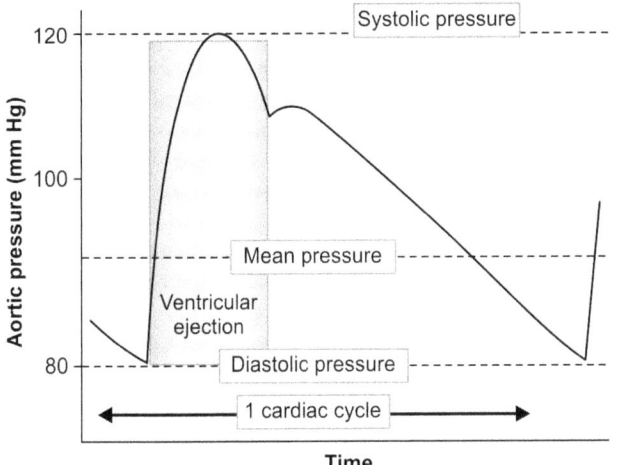

FIGURE 1.4: Mean arterial pressure—geometric average when derived from arterial pressure trace.

Note: MAP can also be calculated by using the formula: MAP = [(2 Diastolic BP) + systolic BP]/3

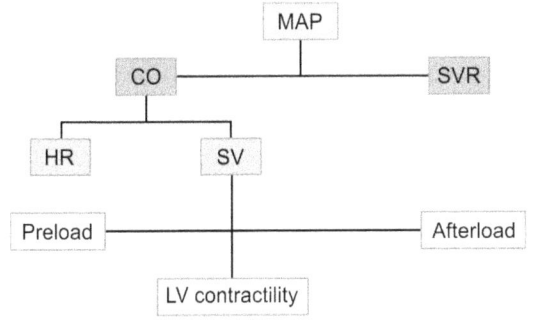

FIGURE 1.5: Factors determining MAP.

(MAP: mean arterial pressure; CO: cardiac output; SVR: system vascular resistance; HR: heart rate; SV: stroke volume; LV: left ventricular)

monitoring techniques in ICU and whether SAP or MAP should be targeted for therapeutic intervention. The study noted that MAP corresponds well between invasive and noninvasive methods; in comparison, the systolic pressure readings were discordant. The MAP value is a most consistent unit for recording blood pressure in ICU, and it does not vary with measurement modality. However, certain pathologies may still require recording of systolic and diastolic pressures (e.g. aneurysms and dissections, stroke, acute coronary syndromes, and valvular regurgitation).

Invasive blood pressure monitoring is preferred in critically ill patients as NIBP overestimates the systolic blood pressure in hypotensive and low flow states and vice versa. This can be clinically significant, hypotensive systolic NIBP values (<70 mm Hg) are associated with a higher rate of acute kidney injury (AKI) and mortality as compared to IBP of the same value.[23]

WHAT IS AN IDEAL MAP?

As important as this question is, there is no clear answer to define effective MAP. It is important to understand the physiological changes during hypotension. When the pressure drops below critical pressure (approximately 50 mm Hg), the blood flow to the brain which is maintained by cerebral autoregulation ceases, and as the pressure drops, so does the cerebral blood flow. The critical point of oxygen delivery varies hugely between different organs; gut is the first organ to get affected during shock state. In patients who are chronically hypertensive, the autoregulatory curve is shifted. Critical pressure is higher than what it is in normal individuals. With long-term treatment and blood pressure control, the autoregulatory curve also normalizes.

In a large, multicentered, randomized clinical trial,[24] which looked at high (80–85 mm Hg) versus low (65–70 mm Hg) MAP targets in septic patients found that there was no significant mortality difference between the two groups. The high MAP target group had less risk of developing AKI and need for renal replacement therapy in patients with known hypertension. It is also important here to remember how the MAP targets are achieved, either by preload optimization or vasopressors. Referring to the interplay between MAP, CO, and SVR, adequate fluid resuscitation is important; otherwise, excessive use of vasopressors without adequate fluid resuscitation increases the risk of kidney injury.

At the other end of the spectrum, in patients with traumatic brain injury, MAP needs to be maintained so that cerebral perfusion is adequate. Cerebral perfusion pressure (CPP) is defined as:

CPP = MAP − ICP

ICP is the intracranial pressure.

Cerebral perfusion pressure target should be maintained above 60 mm Hg to prevent secondary brain injury.

Therefore, there is no fixed value of MAP. The MAP target needs to be individualized depending on the circumstances of the patient.

In a recent retrospective analysis of patients with sepsis, Maheshwari et al. found that the risk for myocardial injury, ICU mortality, and AKI were present even at an MAP of 85 mm Hg. When MAP remained less than 65 mm Hg, it had relation to mortality. The longer the time spent below MAP 65 mm Hg, the higher the risk of renal and myocardial injury and mortality.[25] They suggested that MAP be maintained well above the usual threshold of 65 mm Hg.[25]

CONCLUSION

Invasive blood pressure monitoring remains the "gold standard" in ICU. Automated continuous blood pressure monitoring using oscillometric techniques have comparable MAP recordings with IBP monitoring, but their role probably remains limited for assessment and documentation in relative stable patients. Invasive monitoring with absolute numbers is preferred in patients with hemodynamic instability.

Although both invasive and noninvasive methods give SAP, DAP, and MAP, guidelines have often recommended systolic rather than mean as the target and which modality is used to monitor is usually not appreciated.[26-29] MAP is more relevant for organ prefusion, and it is more constant across measuring methods and should be preferred parameter to target therapy although having a single MAP target is difficult and therapy should be personalized to the patient.

REFERENCES

1. Webb RK, van der Walt JH, Runciman WB, et al. The Australian Incident Monitoring Study. Which monitor? An analysis of 2000 incident reports. Anaesth Intensive Care. 1993;21:529-42.
2. Roberts LN, Smiley JR, Manning GW. A comparison of direct and indirect blood-pressure determinations. Circulation. 1953;8:232-42.
3. Holland WW, Humerfelt S. Measurement of blood-pressure: comparison of intra-arterial and cuff values. Br Med J. 1964;2(5419):1241-3.
4. U.S. Environmental Protection Agency. Mercury study report to Congress. EPA-452/R-97-003. 1997. p. 1.
5. Mion D, Pierin AM. How accurate are sphygmomanometers? J Hum Hypertens. 1998;12:245-8.
6. Markandu ND, Whitcher F, Arnold A, et al. The mercury sphygmomanometer should be abandoned before it is proscribed. J Hum Hypertens. 2000;14:31-6.
7. Graves JW, Tibor M, Murtagh B, et al. The Accoson Greenlight 300TM, the first non-automated mercury-free blood pressure measurement device to pass the International Protocol for blood pressure measuring devices in adult. Blood Press Monit. 2004;9:13-7.
8. Yelderman M, Ream AK. Indirect measurement of mean blood pressure in the anesthetized patient. Anesthesiology. 1979;50:253-6.
9. Mauck GW, Smith CR, Geddes LA, et al. The meaning of the point of maximum oscillations in cuff pressure in the indirect measurement of blood pressure—Part II. J Biomech Eng. 1980;102:28-33.
10. Amoore JN, Scott DH. Can simulators evaluate systematic differences between oscillometric non-invasive blood-pressure monitors? Blood Press Monit. 2000;5:81-9.
11. Borow KM, Newburger JW. Noninvasive estimation of central aortic pressure using the oscillometric method for analyzing systemic artery pulsatile blood flow: comparative study of indirect systolic, diastolic, and mean brachial artery pressure with simultaneous direct ascending aortic pressure measurements. Am Heart J. 1982;103:879-86.
12. Pressman GL, Newgard PM. A transducer for the continuous external measurement of arterial blood pressure. IEEE Trans Biomed Eng. 1963;10:73-81.
13. Dueck R, Goedje O, Clopton P. Noninvasive continuous beat-to-beat radial artery pressure via TL-200 applanation tonometry. J Clin Monit Comput. 2012;26:75-83.
14. Meidert AS, Huber W, Müller JN, et al. Radial artery applanation tonometry for continuous non-invasive arterial pressure monitoring in intensive care unit patients: comparison with invasively assessed radial arterial pressure. Br J Anaesth. 2014;112:521-8.
15. Penáz J, Voigt A, Teichmann W. Contribution to the continuous indirect blood pressure measurement. Z Gesamte Inn Med. 1976;31:1030-3.
16. Jeleazcov C, Krajinovic L, Münster T, et al. Precision and accuracy of a new device (CNAPTM) for continuous non-invasive arterial pressure monitoring: assessment during general anaesthesia. Br J Anaesth. 2010;105:264-72.
17. Stover JF, Stocker R, Lenherr R, et al. Noninvasive cardiac output and blood pressure monitoring cannot replace an invasive monitoring system in critically ill patients. BMC Anesthesiol. 2009;9:6.
18. Romeu-Bordas Ó, Ballesteros-Peña S. Reliability and validity of the modified Allen test: a systematic review and metanalysis. Emergencias. 2017;29:126-35.
19. Gibbs NC, Gardner RM. Dynamics of invasive pressure monitoring systems: clinical and laboratory evaluation. Heart Lung. 1988;17:43-51.
20. Kee LL, Simonson JS, Stotts NA, et al. Echocardiographic determination of valid zero reference levels in supine and lateral positions. Am J Crit Care. 1993;2:72-80.
21. Winsor T, Burch GE. Phlebostatic axis and phlebostatic level, reference levels for venous pressure measurements in man. Exp Biol Med. 1945;58:165-9.
22. Bridges ME, Middleton R. Direct arterial vs oscillometric monitoring of blood pressure: stop comparing and pick one (a decision-making algorithm). Crit Care Nurse. 1997;17(58-66):68-72.
23. Li-wei Lehman H, Saeed M, Talmor D, et al. Methods of blood pressure measurement in the ICU. Crit Care Med. 2013;41:34-40.
24. Asfar P, Meziani F, Hamel J-F, et al. High versus low blood-pressure target in patients with septic shock. N Engl J Med. 2014;370:1583-93.
25. Maheshwari K, Nathanson BH, Munson SH, Khangulov V, Stevens M, Badani H, et. al. The relationship between ICU hypotension and in-hospital mortality and morbidity in septic patients. Intensive Care Med. 2018;44:857-67.
26. Rhodes A, Evans LE, Alhazzani W, et al. Surviving sepsis campaign: international guidelines for management of sepsis and septic shock: Intensive Care Med. 2017;43:304-77.
27. Gall J-R. A New Simplified Acute Physiology Score (SAPS II) based on a European/North American Multicenter Study. JAMA. 1993;270:2957-63.
28. LeGall JR, Loirat P, Alpérovitch A. APACHE II-A severity of disease classification system. Crit Care Med. 1986;14:754-5.
29. Chobanian AV, Bakris GL, Black HR, et al. Seventh report of the joint national committee on prevention, detection, evaluation, and treatment of high blood pressure. Hypertension. 2003;42:1206-52.

Adjunctive Therapies in Acute Myocardial Infarction

Harish MM, Atul Prabhakar Kulkarni

INTRODUCTION

Acute coronary syndrome (ACS) is one of the leading causes of death among global population. Approximately one in seven deaths is secondary to coronary heart disease.[1]

Diagnostic and therapeutic modalities for acute myocardial infarction have vastly evolved over the last decades. Since this disease entity was first reported by Herrick in 1912, adjuvant and pharmacological modalities for the management of ACS have changed greatly and resulted in better pain relief and decreased mortality.[1]

MORPHINE

Morphine has been used as agent of choice for symptomatic relief of patients with chest pain. Morphine is given as injection for to patients with ongoing symptoms of chest discomfort and it is usually titrated till pain is relieved as per the individual need.[2]

In the studies which showed benefits with morphine also received aspirin, heparin, clopidogrel, diagnostic coronary angiography, and percutaneous coronary intervention (PCI).[1]

Patients not treated with morphine did not received even other optimal medical treatment. Morphine use may be an indicator of severity of myocardial infarction because it is usually prescribed for patients with acute pulmonary edema or refractory pain. However, this presumption was also determined to be untrue in many studies, since the analgesic effects may mask the severity of angina and result in misinterpretation of signs and symptoms, hiding true severity of the problem. Studies showed that morphine is associated with delayed activity of antiplatelet agents in patients presenting with ST-segment elevation myocardial infarction (STEMI).[1]

Owing to these negative findings, morphine administration has been recommended to be class IIb indication in the American Heart Association/American College of Cardiology (AHA/ACC) guidelines.[1]

Value is placed on its ability to relieve pain and distress, understanding that the evidence for its supposed benefit is lacking. Further research is required whether morphine really causes harm or not, as per data mentioned in some of the registry.[3]

Oxygen

Oxygen should be initiated only if the patient has breathlessness, hypoxemia (SpO_2 <94%), or signs of heart failure or shock. The use of pulse oximetry may be very useful in guiding oxygen therapy. However, it is important to understand that recent data suggests hyperoxemia is potentially harmful in uncomplicated myocardial infarction. Oxygen may have a distinct indication in other emergency situations along with ACS (e.g. water accidents, gas embolism etc.).[2]

The oxygen therapy is assumed to increase oxygen delivery to the ischemic myocardium and thereby limit progression of infarct size and its subsequent complications. The rationale for this practice is limited to experimental in vitro data and small clinical studies.[4] However, high oxygen levels in the blood can cause coronary vasoconstriction and increase the production of reactive oxygen radicals, which can cause reperfusion injury.[5]

One of the most robust data pertaining to the use of oxygen is provided by the "Air Versus Oxygen in Myocardial Infarction" (AVOID) trial. This was a major multicenter, randomized controlled trial which compared the effects of the administration of oxygen (8 L/min) versus no supplemental oxygen in patients with STEMI and oxygen saturation more than or equal to 94% measured using a pulse oximeter. The primary endpoint was infarct size measured using troponin and cardiac enzyme assays. Secondary endpoints included recurrent myocardial infarction and cardiac arrhythmias. At 6-month follow-up the secondary endpoints were observed to be statistically significant favoring a no-oxygen strategy group. The overall incidence of in-hospital recurrent myocardial infarction and cardiac arrhythmias were more in the oxygen supplementation group (5.5% × 0.9%, P = 0.006 and 40.4% × 31.4%, P = 0.05).[6]

Recently, the "Determination of the Role of Oxygen in Suspected Acute Myocardial Infarction" ($DETO_2X$-AMI) trial included ACS patients with an oxygen saturation of more than or equal to 90% to receive oxygen supplementation versus inhalation of ambient air. The study showed no statistically significant difference in 1-year all-cause mortality observed among the groups. Non-ST-segment elevation myocardial infarction (NSTEMI) and STEMI AHA/ACC guidelines recommend the use of supplemental oxygen only when oxygen saturation is less than or equal to 90%.[7]

Nitrates

Intravenous or sublingual nitroglycerin administration was of probable useful only within 3 hours of the onset of symptoms in patients with infarction in the era prior to the advent of reperfusion therapy (based on extrapolation from other contexts). In the present situation no trial has specifically evaluated efficacy of nitrates in patients with acute myocardial infarction in the emergency department (ED) or prehospital settings. It is reasonable to consider the early administration of nitroglycerin only in selected group of patients without any contraindications, particularly if they have persistent pain even after antiplatelet and other anti-ischemic medications.[2]

However routine use of nitroglycerin is neither supported nor refuted by the evidence, may it be in the ED or prehospital setting in patients with a suspected ACS.

In specific situations like cocaine-associated chest pain lorazepam and nitroglycerin may be useful in the alleviation of chest pain.[8]

Aspirin

Aspirin is the single most important adjunctive therapy for ACS infarction. The major evidence for the efficacy of aspirin in decreasing mortality associated with ACS was demonstrated in the "Second International Study of Infarct Survival" (ISIS-2), in this patients were randomized to aspirin, streptokinase, a combination of the both, or placebo therapy. The mortality with use of aspirin was 23% in comparison with 25% for streptokinase and 41% for the combination of these agents relative to placebo. Aspirin acts by inhibiting platelet function by irreversible inactivation of platelet cyclo-oxygenase enzyme, which occurs within 15 minutes after a single 325-mg tablet has been chewed and swallowed. Aspirin-related allergy and thrombocytopenia are relative contraindications for its use. In patients with any of the relative contraindications, orally administered ticlopidine hydrochloride (250 mg twice a day) is a reasonable alternative agent, although no trials in acute infarction have been reported.[3,9] The use of enteric-coated aspirin is not suitable in the immediate treatment of acute myocardial infarction. Chewable aspirin should be the choice for all the patients with acute infarction or unstable angina except for those with the aforementioned contraindications.[9]

The early administration of aspirin as an antiplatelet dose of 300 mg is recommended in patients with suspected ACS when contraindications such as true anaphylaxis or bleeding disorder have been excluded. The patients should be advised to chew the tablet (which should not be enteric coated). Dissolvable aspirin is preferred at this acute condition.[9]

There is currently limited evidence to directly support the strategy of dispatcher directed or bystander administration of aspirin, however, it is considered to be a reasonable approach if the carer is able to exclude a history of true anaphylaxis or bleeding disorder.

Antiplatelet Agents

Clopidogrel: Clopidogrel is a thienopyridine group of drug that inhibits P2Y12 platelet receptor. The drug requires activation by a two stage biotransformation within the liver. This process is modulated by genetic polymorphisms, which results in variability in overall clinical effect. Benefit has been established when added to aspirin in non-ST elevation acute coronary syndrome (NSTEACS) patients, including those treated with PCI. Showed reductions in cardiovascular death, myocardial infarction and stroke but with an increase in major bleeding.[10] It should be considered that patients who have moderate to high risk

NSTEACS and STEMI should receive clopidogrel in addition to the standard care (aspirin, anticoagulation and/or a reperfusion). The ideal dose in elderly has not yet been determined. However, in patients under the age of 75 years the loading dose of clopidogrel is 600 mg if PCI is planned or 300 mg if a noninvasive strategy with fibrinolysis is the planned treatment option.[11]

Prasugrel: Prasugrel is a newer thienopyridine agent that produces more rapid and consistent platelet inhibition than clopidogrel. In the clopidogrel naïve patient, prasugrel (compared to clopidogrel) reduced the incidence of myocardial infarction in patients with moderate to high risk NSTEACS and patients with STEMI planned for primary PCI. Prasugrel has been associated with a higher rate of bleeding complications in patients older than 75 years of age, those with a history of stroke or transient ischemic attack and body weight less than 60 kg. Prasugrel should not be given to patients with STEMI who have already received fibrinolysis. It may be used as an alternative to clopidogrel in patients with STEMI of less than 12 hours duration where PPCI is planned.[12]

In patients with NSTEMI, prasugrel may be administered after angiography when the coronary anatomy is known and the plan is to proceed to PCI.

The advised dose of prasugrel is 60 mg in place of clopidogrel, particularly when they are not at high risk from bleeding.

Ticagrelor is a pyrimidine derivative, which binds reversibly to the P2Y12 receptor without any biotransformation. Like prasugrel, it has a more rapid and consistent onset of action compared with clopidogrel, but other added advantage is its quicker offset of action so that recovery of platelet function is faster.[13]

Ticagrelor has showed some benefits compared to clopidogrel in patients with moderate-to-high risk NSTEACS (treated conservatively or invasively) and patients with STEMI planned for primary PCI (PPCI) in terms of a reduction in death from vascular causes and myocardial infarction. Overall there was no increase in major bleeding observed but an increase in minor bleeding was seen.[13]

The adverse effects of ticagrelor are dyspnea, increased frequency of mostly asymptomatic ventricular pauses, and asymptomatic increase in uric acid.

Ticagrelor can be an option for patients at moderate-to-high risk of ischemic events (e.g. troponin positive ACS), regardless of initial planned treatment strategy and including those pretreated with clopidogrel. The initial dose is 180 mg (loading dose) and then 90 mg twice daily. Ticagrelor may be used then in place of clopidogrel in patients with ACS.[14]

The risks and benefits of combinations of the newer antiplatelet agents are not established completely. When planned for switch over, these newer agents should not be used as combination. But these can be used with aspirin as combination safely.

Prehospital administration of these newer agents in the setting of STEMI in recent studies has shown no mortality benefit or harm.[14]

Vorapaxar: It is one of the most recent addition to the arsenal of antiplatelet agents. A high-affinity oral antagonist that selectively inhibits thrombin from activating platelets through the protease-activated receptor. Vorapaxar is indicated for the reduction of thrombotic cardiovascular events in patients with a history of myocardial infarction or with peripheral arterial disease (PAD). This novel agent was approved by the FDA in 2014 based on the results of a large, phase III randomized controlled trial. This trial included 26,449 patients with a history of myocardial infarction, ischemic stroke, or PAD who were randomly assigned to receive vorapaxar (2.5 mg daily) or placebo in addition to standard antiplatelet therapy for a median time of 30 months.[15] Vorapaxar showed a 1.2% absolute risk reduction in the primary composite endpoint of death from cardiovascular causes, myocardial infarction, or stroke as compared with placebo (hazard ratio (HR), 0.87; 95% confidence interval (CI), 0.80–0.94; P = -0.001, NNT 84 patients). Moderate-to-severe bleeding was more common in the vorapaxar group as opposed to the placebo group (4.2 vs 2.5%; HR, 1.66; 95% CI, 1.43–1.93; P = -0.001, NNH 58 patients).[16]

The role of vorapaxar in the management of ACS has not been fully established, needs further studies on this newer drug in the coming years.

Beta-adrenergic Blocking Agents

Beta-adrenergic blocking agents are the second most important adjunctive drug (next to aspirin) for acute infarction and for the other ischemic syndromes. The mechanisms by which beta-adrenergic receptor blockers decrease mortality is by reduction in myocardial oxygen consumption, an antagonism of arrhythmogenic and toxic biochemical effects of catecholamines, a possible direct effect on myocardial ventricular fibrillation threshold, and a decrease in the incidence of cardiac rupture.[17]

Although most benefits from beta-adrenergic blocking agents are derived during the first week, the continued advantage of decreased mortality has been substantiated to at least 5 years. The beneficial effects of the beta-adrenergic blockers are similar to all agents without intrinsic sympathomimetic activity. Some contraindications to the administration of these agents are gross congestive heart failure or pulmonary edema, asthma or severe bronchospastic airways disease, hypotension, and heart block greater than first degree.[17]

The presence of a mild degree of left ventricular failure or known severe left ventricular dysfunction is not an absolute contraindication, in such a setting, a short-acting drug for example, esmolol hydrochloride administered in an intravenous bolus of 0.5 µg/kg followed by infusion at 50 µg/kg/min should be considered. This therapy can be terminated if congestive heart failure worsens.[18]

Preferably, beta blockers should be administered at the time of admission, although benefits have been confirmed with later in-hospital administration as well.[19] In patients with absolute contraindications to beta blockade and with no evidence of left ventricular failure, the calcium channel blocker verapamil hydrochloride has been shown to be effective in secondary prevention of death and recurrent infarction. This agent, however, should be avoided in patients with poor LV contractility (EF <30%). Can be considered for late administration (>7 days) after initial assessment, and is also more likely to produce higher grades of atrioventricular block than beta blockers.[18]

Angiotensin-converting Enzyme Inhibitors

Another adjunctive pharmacologic agent now definitely shown to decrease mortality after myocardial infarction is the angiotensin-converting enzyme (ACE) inhibitor. Near about eight randomized trials of ACE inhibitors, given either selectively to patients with reduced left ventricular function (less than 45% ejection fraction) or nonselectively, have been performed, seven of these trials showed a significant reduction in postinfarct mortality.[18]

In two large recent mega trials "Gruppo Italiano per 10 Studio della Sopravvivenza nell'lnfarto Miocardico" (GISSI-3)[20] and the "Fourth International Study of Infarct Survival" (ISIS-4)[21] approximately 77,000 patients were randomly assigned to the use of captopril (ISIS-4) or lisinopril (GISSI-3), administered within 24 hours after onset of symptoms, versus placebo. Both trials demonstrated a statistically significant reduction in mortality (absolute numbers of 4-5 lives saved per 1,000 patients treated). Although such a benefit can be expected from the universal administration of these agents to all the infarct survivors, a much larger impact is evident with the selective use of these drugs.[20,21]

In a recent trial (SMILE—Survival of Myocardial Infarction Long-Term Evaluation) in which early oral administration of zofenopril was restricted to patients with anterior wall infarction, which was not treated with thrombolytic agents, a decrease in mortality of 41 lives saved per 1,000 patients treated was achieved, this is as same as that similar in magnitude to that attainable with thrombolysis itself.[22] Administration of ACE inhibitors helps in decreasing the blood pressure and ventricular wall stress, it has also been shown to have a useful effect on reducing late ventricular remodeling, which may help preserve left ventricular function.[11]

In addition, in the Survival and Ventricular Enlargement trial, the overall incidence of reinfarction was decreased, which shows a possible direct vascular action. In GISSI-3, 5 mg of lisinopril was administered orally in the beginning, followed by 5 mg after 24 hours, 10 mg after 48 hours, and then 10 mg daily. If the systolic blood pressure was less than 120 mm Hg at the time of initial assessment or within the first 3 days, a lower dosage of 2.5 mg daily was used. If the blood pressure declined below 100 mm Hg, a lower daily maintenance dose of 5 mg and temporary reductions to 2.5 mg/day were allowed. Administration of the drug was discontinued when blood pressure was less than 90 mm Hg. Contraindications to the administration of ACE inhibitors include confirmed prior allergic reactions and hypotension, as previously described.[20]

The optimal duration of therapy with these agents after infarction is not clearly defined, but like aspirin and beta-adrenergic blockers, the therapy may be continued indefinitely, especially if the patient has severe left ventricular dysfunction (ejection fraction of <45%) or in patients with moderate to severe mitral regurgitation. Care must be taken to avoid hypotension (systolic blood pressure of <90-100 mm Hg).

Heparin

Heparin binds to naturally occurring anticoagulation that is antithrombin and induces a conformational change, causing rapid inhibition of factor IIa (thrombin), factor IXa, and factor Xa, thus it prevents further thrombus propagation. An intravenous bolus of 60 units/kg produces a time to peak of 5-10 minutes and a half-life of 30-60 minutes.[23]

Heparin can be reversed by using protamine sulfate (1 mg per 100 units of heparin). For ACS, it is given in a bolus of 60 units/kg not exceeding 4,000 units, followed by a continuous infusion of 12-15 units/kg/hour, with monitoring of the activated partial thromboplastin time every 6 hours with a goal value of 50-70 seconds or 1.5-2.5 times control value. Side effects of heparin include thrombocytopenia, heparin-induced thrombocytopenia (a distinct condition), and bleeding.[23]

The efficacy of unfractionated heparin was tested in ACS in the early 1990s. Oler et al. performed meta-analysis of six randomized trials and found a 33% lower rate of death in patients treated with heparin in addition to aspirin in ACS, as well less reported ischemic pain.[24,25]

Advantages of unfractionated heparin are that it has stood the test of time, rapid onset of action, is inexpensive, and can be rapidly reversed. The disadvantages are that it can have serious side effects, including heparin-induced thrombocytopenia, and is more likely to cause bleeding than the newer intravenous anticoagulants discussed below. Thus, its position as the main anticoagulant in ACS is being challenged in recent data.[15]

Enoxaparin (A Low-molecular-weight Heparin)

Enoxaparin is a low-molecular-weight heparin that inhibits factor IIa and factor Xa via antithrombin, roughly in a ratio of 1:3. It has a time to peak effect of 10 minutes when given intravenously and 3-5 hours when given subcutaneously. Its half-life is 4.5 hours, but it is longer in patients with renal dysfunction, requiring dose adjustments in this population.[24]

Its anticoagulant effect is partially reversible. If it is to be reversed between 0 hours and 8 hours after dosing, the recommended reversal regimen is 1 mg of protamine sulfate for every 1 mg of enoxaparin used. At 8-12 hours, it is 0.5 mg of protamine for every 1 mg of enoxaparin.

After 12 hours, no protamine is required. Compared with unfractionated heparin, enoxaparin has less plasma protein binding and a more consistent and predicted anticoagulant effect. Because of its high bioavailability, it can be administered as subcutaneous dosing also. Its greater anti-Xa activity inhibits thrombin generation more effectively, and it causes lower rates of thrombocytopenia and heparin-induced thrombocytopenia as compared to unfractionated heparin. de Lemos et al. found that, in ACS patients in whom an early conservative approach of medical management was planned, enoxaparin was more efficacious than unfractionated heparin and with a similar incidence of bleeding.[26]

A meta-analysis of 12 trials among 49,088 ACS patients, also found that enoxaparin had a net clinical benefit compared with unfractionated heparin in reducing rates of myocardial reinfarction and death despite of more bleeding.[27] The ESSENCE trial compared enoxaparin versus unfractionated heparin in 3,171 patients with ACS. It found fewer ischemic events with enoxaparin in the early phase, more minor bleeding, but no increase in major bleeding.[28]

Fondaparinux (A Factor Xa-inhibitor)

Fondaparinux is a synthetic pentasaccharide that indirectly inhibits factor Xa through the action of antithrombin. After a 2.5-mg subcutaneous dose, it has a time to peak concentration of 2 hours and a half-life of 17-21 hours.

The OASIS-5 (The Fifth Organization to Assess Strategies in Acute Ischemic Syndromes) trial compared fondaparinux and enoxaparin in 20,078 patients treated for NSTEACS. Although the rates of death, myocardial infarction, and refractory ischemia at 9 days were similar for both drugs, the fondaparinux group had a significantly (almost 50%) lower rate of bleeding at 30 days, translating into significantly fewer deaths at 30 days as compared enoxaparin. However, patients receiving fondaparinux who underwent PCI had a threefold higher rate of catheter-related thrombosis.[29]

The OASIS-6 trial compared fondaparinux versus usual care (placebo in those in whom unfractionated heparin was not indicated or unfractionated heparin was given for up to 48 hours followed by placebo for up to 8 days) among 12,092 patients with STEMI. There was a 1.5% absolute risk reduction in death and reinfarction without an increase in bleeding at 30 days, with trends persisting 6 months into the study. However, fondaparinux was not superior to heparin in the 3% of patients who underwent primary PCI.[30] As in OASIS-5, there was more catheter-related thrombosis in the fondaparinux group. Although the use of supplemental unfractionated heparin appears to have mitigated this risk, fondaparinux remains a less-than ideal option in the era of primary PCI for STEMI and has therefore found limited use in this group of patients.

It should, however, be considered in patients for whom a conservative strategy is planned, especially if bleeding risk is deemed to be high.

Oral Anticoagulants

Oral anticoagulants provide anti-ischemic benefit in selected patients with ACS—at the price of a higher risk of significant bleeding.

Warfarin

Warfarin was investigated in many trails like WARIS II, CARS, and CHAMP. WARIS II looked at the use of aspirin alone, warfarin alone, and aspirin and warfarin in combination. The rates of the primary endpoints of stroke, nonfatal infarction, and death were lower in the warfarin group.[31]

CARS trail found no difference in the rate of the primary endpoint of fatal infarction, nonfatal ischemic stroke, or cardiovascular death, with aspirin versus warfarin plus aspirin.[32]

CHAMP trail also saw similar trends, i.e. no difference in the rate of death, recurrent myocardial infarction, or stroke with warfarin plus aspirin versus aspirin alone.[33]

All three studies showed increases in major bleeding with warfarin use. Putting all these trials into context, the significant net clinical benefit of dual antiplatelet therapy in the current era compared with the significant bleeding and questionable conflicting evidence supporting benefit with warfarin has limited its use in ACS patients.

Rivaroxaban (An Oral Factor Xa-inhibitor)

Rivaroxaban is a novel oral direct reversible factor Xa-inhibitor. The ATLAS ACS 2-TIMI 51 trial found rivaroxaban 2.5 mg or 5 mg to yield a significantly lower rate of the primary outcome of cardiovascular death, myocardial infarction, ischemic stroke, and in-stent thrombosis compared with placebo. Unfortunately rivaroxaban had significantly more major non-CABG bleeding and intracranial hemorrhage as compared to placebo.[34]

The dose used in this trial was much lower than the dose used in trials investigating the role of this drug in stroke prophylaxis in nonvalvular atrial fibrillation.

Apixaban (An Oral Factor Xa-inhibitor)

Apixaban is another direct factor Xa-inhibitor. The APPRAISE-2 trial compared apixaban 5 mg twice daily versus placebo in ACS. There was no difference in the rate of cardiovascular death, myocardial infarction, or stroke, like rivaroxaban, apixaban also had significantly more bleeding, prompting early termination of this study.[35]

Dabigatran (An Oral Thrombin Inhibitor)

Dabigatran is an oral direct thrombin inhibitor. The RE-DEEM trial compared four doses of dabigatran (50, 75, 110, and 150 mg twice daily) and placebo in ACS patients. The dabigatran groups showed dose related increase in bleeding. In addition, the rates of ischemic endpoints were no lower with dabigatran, although this trial was not powered to show differences in clinical events.[36]

CONCLUSION

Adjunctive therapy for acute myocardial infarction should include aspirin, beta-adrenergic blocking agents, and, in most patients, consideration of the use of ACE inhibitors, especially if left ventricular function is reduced. Heparin has an important adjunctive role in enhancing early vessel patency in patients who receive tissue-type plasminogen activator and in decreasing the frequency of re-occlusion of an infarct-related artery during any thrombolytic therapy. Heparin must also be administered to all patients who undergo primary angioplasty. Intravenously administered nitroglycerin and orally administered nitrates are not indicated in all the patients, its routine use should be avoided.

Calcium channel blockers for most patients with acute myocardial infarction. Currently, in the management of patients with acute myocardial infarction, the immediate goals are relief of pain from ischemia, assessment and stabilization of the hemodynamic status, and administration of reperfusion therapy, in conjunction with either thrombolytic agents or, when available, urgent direct angioplasty of the occluded infarct-related artery.

In addition to strategies for reperfusion, adjunctive pharmacologic therapy retains an important role in reducing mortality and morbidity from acute infarction.

REFERENCES

1. Alencar Neto J. Morphine, oxygen, nitrates, and mortality reducing pharmacological treatment for acute coronary syndrome: an evidence-based review. Cureus. 2018;10(1): e2114.
2. ARC. (2012). ANZCOR Guideline 14.2—ACS: Initial Medical Therapy. [online]. Available from https://resus.org.au/wpfb-file/anzcor-guideline-14-2-jan16-pdf/ [Accessed December, 2018].
3. Reeder GS. Concise review for primary-care physicians: Adjunctive therapy in the management of patients with acute myocardial infarction. Mayo Clin Proc. 1995;70:464-8.
4. Syed FA, Bett JH, Walters DL. Anti-platelet therapy for acute coronary syndrome: a review of currently available agents and what the future holds. Cardiovasc Hematol Disord Drug Targets. 2011;11:79-86.
5. Nicolau JC, Cohen M, Montalescot G. Differences among low-molecular-weight heparins: evidence in patients with acute coronary syndromes. J Cardiovasc Pharmacol. 2009;53:440-5.
6. Morrow DA, Braunwald E, Bonaca MP, et al. Vorapaxar in the secondary prevention of atherothrombotic events. N Engl J Med. 2012;366:1404-13.
7. Ganetsky VS, Hadley DE, Thomas TF. Role of novel and emerging oral anticoagulants for secondary prevention of acute coronary syndromes. Pharmacotherapy. 2014;34:590-604.
8. Reeder GS, Gersh BJ. Modern management of acute myocardial infarction. Curr Probl Cardiol. 1993;18:81-155.
9. Hansen JF. Danish Study Group on Verapamil in Myocardial Infarction. Treatment with verapamil during and after an acute myocardial infarction: a review based on the Danish Verapamil Infarction Trials I and II. J Cardiovasc Pharmacol. 1991;18(Suppl 6):S20-S25.
10. GISSI-3: effects of lisinopril and transdermal glyceryl trinitrate singly and together on 6-week mortality and ventricular function after acute myocardial infarction. Gruppo Italiano per

lo Studio della Sopravvivenza nell'infarto Miocardico. Lancet. 1994; 343:11151-22.
11. ISIS-4 (Fourth International Study of Infarct Survival) Collaborative Group. Presentation at the American Heart Association Meeting; Atlanta (GA): 1993.
12. Aslam MS, Sundberg S, Sabri MN, et al. Pharmacokinetics of intravenous/subcutaneous enoxaparin in patients with acute coronary syndrome undergoing percutaneous coronary interventions. Catheter Cardiovasc Interv. 2002;57:187-90.
13. De Lemos JA, Blazing MA, Wiviott SD, et al. Enoxaparin versus unfractionated heparin in patients treated with tirofiban, aspirin and an early conservative initial management strategy: results from the A phase of the A-to-Z trial. Eur Heart J. 2004;25:1688-94.
14. Murphy SA, Gibson CM, Morrow DA, et al. Efficacy and safety of the low-molecular weight heparin enoxaparin compared with unfractionated heparin across the acute coronary syndrome spectrum: a meta-analysis. Eur Heart J. 2007;28:2077-86.
15. Cohen M, Demers C, Gurfinkel EP, et al. A comparison of low-molecular weight heparin with unfractionated heparin for unstable coronary artery disease. Efficacy and Safety of Subcutaneous Enoxaparin in Non-Q-Wave Coronary Events Study Group. N Engl J Med. 1997;337:447-52.
16. Fifth Organization to Assess Strategies in Acute Ischemic Syndromes Investigators; Yusuf S, Mehta SR, et al. Comparison of fondaparinux and enoxaparin in acute coronary syndromes. N Engl J Med. 2006;354:1464-76.
17. Yusuf S, Mehta SR, Chrolavicius S, et al. OASIS-6 Trial Group. Effects of fondaparinux on mortality and reinfarction in patients with acute ST segment elevation myocardial infarction: the OASIS-6 randomized trial. JAMA. 2006;295:1519-30.
18. Hurlen M, Abdelnoor M, Smith P, et al. Warfarin, aspirin, or both after myocardial infarction. N Engl J Med. 2002;347:969-74.
19. Randomised double-blind trial of fixed low-dose warfarin with aspirin after myocardial infarction. Coumadin Aspirin Reinfarction Study (CARS) Investigators. Lancet. 1997;350:389-96.
20. Fiore LD, Ezekowitz MD, Brophy MT, et al. Department of Veterans Affairs Cooperative Studies Program Clinical Trial comparing combined warfarin and aspirin with aspirin alone in survivors of acute myocardial infarction: primary results of the CHAMP study. Circulation. 2002;105:557-63.
21. Mega JL, Braunwald E, Wiviott SD, et al. Rivaroxaban in patients with a recent acute coronary syndrome. N Engl J Med. 2012;366:9-19.
22. Alexander JH, Lopes RD, James S, et al. Apixaban with antiplatelet therapy after acute coronary syndrome. N Engl J Med. 2011;365:699-708.
23. Oldgren J, Budaj A, Granger CB, et al. Dabigatran vs placebo in patients with acute coronary syndromes on dual antiplatelet therapy: a randomized, double-blind, phase II trial. Eur Heart J. 2011;32:2781-89.
24. Singh D, Gupta K, Vacek JL. Anticoagulation and antiplatelet therapy in acute coronary syndromes. Cleveland Clin J Med. 2014;81(2):103-14.
25. Oler A, Whooley MA, Oler J, et al. Adding heparin to aspirin reduces the incidence of myocardial infarction and death in patients with unstable angina. A meta-analysis. JAMA. 1996;276:811-5.
26. Meine TJ, Roe MT, Chen AY, et al. Association of intravenous morphine use and outcomes in acute coronary syndromes: results from the CRUSADE Quality Improvement Initiative. Am Heart J. 2005;149:1043-9.
27. Stub D, Smith K, Bernard S, et al. Air versus Oxygen in ST-Segment Elevation Myocardial Infarction. Circulation. 2015;131:2143-50.
28. Madias JE, Madias NE, Hood WB Jr. Precordial ST-segment mapping. 2. Effects of oxygen inhalation on ischemic injury in patients with acute myocardial infarction. Circulation. 1976;53:411-7.
29. Moradkhan R, Sinoway LI. Revisiting the role of oxygen therapy in cardiac patients. J Am Coll Cardiol. 2010;56:1013-6.
30. Hofmann R, James SK, Jernberg T, et al. Oxygen therapy in suspected acute myocardial infarction. N Engl J Med. 2017;377:1240-9.
31. Honderick T, Williams D, Seaberg D, Wears R. A prospective, randomized, controlled trial of benzodiazepines and nitroglycerine or nitroglycerine alone in the treatment of cocaine-associated acute coronary syndromes. Am J Emerg Med. 2003;21(1):39-42.
32. Yusuf S, Zhao F, Mehta SR, et al. Effects of clopidogrel in addition to aspirin in patients with acute coronary syndromes without ST-segment elevation. N Engl J Med. 2001;345:494-502.
33. Mehta SR, Bassand JP, Chrolavicius S, et al. Dose comparisons of clopidogrel and aspirin in acute coronary syndromes. N Engl J Med. 2010;363:930-42.
34. Nicolau JC, Cohen M, Montalescot G. Differences among low-molecular-weight heparins: evidence in patients with acute coronary syndromes. J Cardiovasc Pharmacol. 2009;53:440-5.
35. Reeder GS, Gersh BJ. Modern management of acute myocardial infarction. Curr Probl Cardiol. 1993;18:81-155.
36. Ambrosioni E, Borghi C, Magnani B. The effect of the angiotensin-converting-enzyme inhibitor zofenopril on mortality and morbidity after anterior myocardial infarction. The Survival of Myocardial Infarction Long-Term Evaluation [SMILE] Study Investigators). N Engl J Med. 1995;332:80-85.

CHAPTER 3

Echocardiography in the Critical Care Unit

Anthony S McLean

INTRODUCTION

The application of ultrasound in the emergency and intensive care departments within a hospital is considered essential in the 21st century. The development of smaller, mobile, and less expensive machines brings the modality within the grasp of the majority of health systems, even in the developing countries. Assessing cardiac function is paramount in patients in circulatory distress and any ultrasound machine that is purchased within the critical care environment should have echocardiographic capability.

Separation of competency levels for echocardiography into two levels has brought about a useful roadmap to guide the novice physician in applying the device, and for those with some experience on how to use it to further enhance diagnosis and patient treatment. International competency guidelines, established over many years, have been created for these purposes. A description of competency levels, the use of echocardiography in commonly encountered conditions in critically ill patients, and the central role of echocardiography in the management of the shocked patient are examined in the sections below.

COMPETENCY LEVELS

With the use of echocardiography in the critical care environment spreading throughout the world, there became a need to define what competency the operator should aspire to. International experts representing critical care societies in a number of European countries, North America, South America, and Asia held face-to-face meetings over a period of years, and ultimately identified two levels of competency in critical care ultrasound.[1] Although general ultrasound was also included in the international consensus, the focus of this chapter is on the application of echocardiography.

Basic Level

Every physician undergoing specialist critical care training should gain competency at this level. Initial training consists of a 2-day workshop, learning how to use an ultrasound machine and attain adequate images of the heart via the transthoracic approach [transthoracic echocardiography (TTE)]. This is followed by the performance of 30–50 supervised studies in the workplace. M-mode and two-dimensional (2D) echocardiography techniques only are utilized, but not the application of Doppler techniques which are required for the advanced level of competency. The echocardiographic examination on the patient seeks to answer four questions; left ventricular contractility, right heart function, presence of cardiac tamponade, and assessing intravascular volume. A popular example of such a course is RACE—"Rapid Assessment by Cardiac Echocardiography."[2]

Achieving basic level competency allows the attending doctor to rapidly assess the heart in a decompensating patient noninvasively and at any time day or night. The majority of cardiac pathologies requiring immediate attention can be identified with a basic study. Examples

Echocardiography in the Critical Care Unit

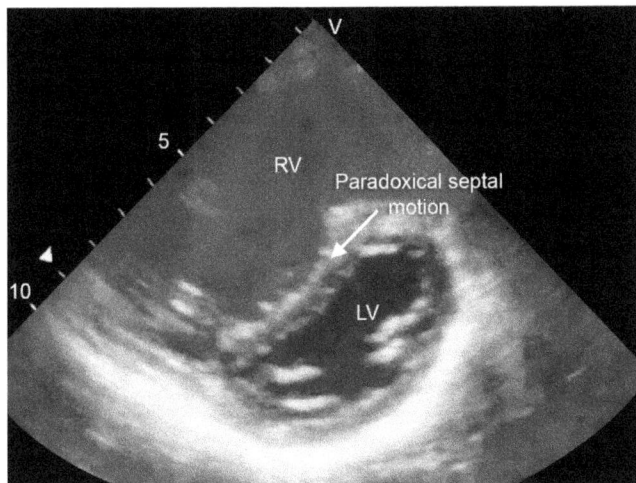

FIGURE 3.1: Paradoxical septal motion. The RV is enlarged and the LV is small with the ventricular septum bowing in the opposite direction to normal. This indicates marked elevation of right ventricular pressure/volume and in the acute situation is highly suggestive of an acute pulmonary embolus. (LV: left ventricle; RV: right ventricle)

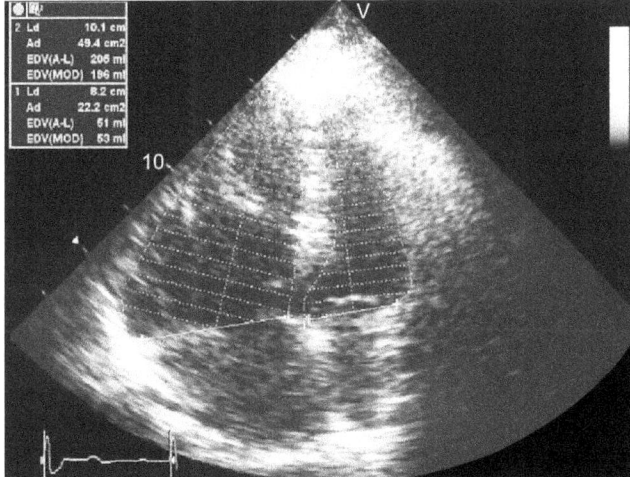

FIGURE 3.2: A comparison of the RV and LV sizes as seen from the apical four-chamber view. The RV is much bigger than the LV. (RV: right ventricular; LV: left ventricular)

of readily identified pathologies are demonstrated in Figures 3.1 and 3.2. Obviously, in some situations, further sophisticated echocardiographic examination will be necessary, usually in routine working hours when such expertise is more readily available.

Advanced Level

The addition of Doppler echocardiography requires extended training.[3] Components of the training are the attendance of 40 hours at quality advanced courses, performance of a required number of studies, competent supervision for all studies, taken over at least a 2-year period. Some current certification systems mandate the inclusion of transesophageal echocardiography (TEE), while others offer this component as a separate certificate. Examinations are considered necessary by most critical care societies.

By utilizing Doppler techniques, this more advanced level can provide a stunning array of clinically relevant information. Increased diagnostic ability is matched by the ability to perform hemodynamic assessment. It is noninvasive and using it displaces the need for pulmonary artery catheters and other invasive techniques, providing not only less pain to the patients but also bringing budgetary advantages as well. Obtaining pulmonary artery pressures, cardiac output (CO), left ventricular diastolic function, valvular stenosis, and regurgitation severity, in addition to more accurate assessment of right and left ventricular contraction, is possible in the majority of patients.

EVALUATION OF PATHOLOGIES COMMONLY ENCOUNTERED IN CRITICALLY ILL PATIENTS

Acute Pulmonary Embolus

Although Doppler is necessary to measure pulmonary artery pressure, the diagnosis of acute right heart failure resulting from an acute pulmonary embolus can often be inferred from 2D echocardiography alone (Fig. 3.1). Indeed, the decision whether to thrombolyze the patient is often made from a basic examination alone. The prognosis from pulmonary embolus depends upon right heart dysfunction with a dilated right ventricle, paradoxical septal motion, and small end-diastolic left ventricular volumes attesting to the presence of severe pulmonary hypertension. Contraction of the right ventricle can be variable with it being hyperdynamic in the early stages and hypodynamic later on. Estimating pulmonary artery pressures by measuring the tricuspid regurgitant pressure gradient or having a pulmonary acceleration time less than 90 ms adds more certainty to the diagnosis. Occasionally, an actual embolus is visible in the heart or pulmonary arteries, an important observation when considering the need for thrombolysis therapy (Fig. 3.3).

Heart Failure

Reduced CO secondary to right and/or left ventricular contractile impairment is a common finding patients presenting in the emergency department or intensive care unit. In some people, this may be on the background of a

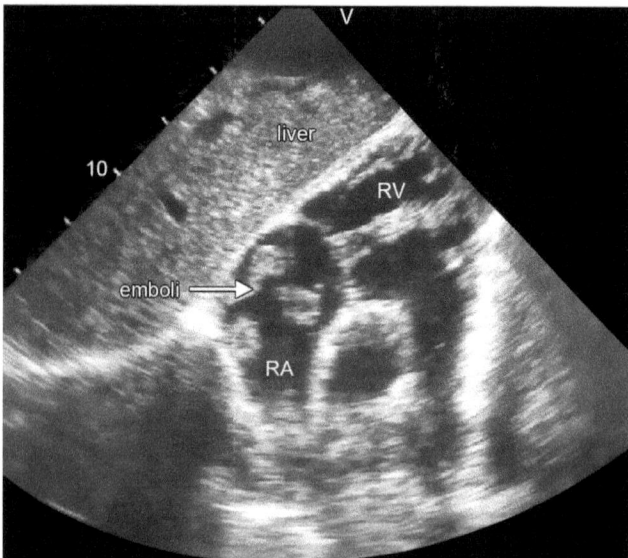

FIGURE 3.3: A subcostal of the heart in which multiple emboli are revealed within the RA. (RA: right atrium; RV: right ventricle)

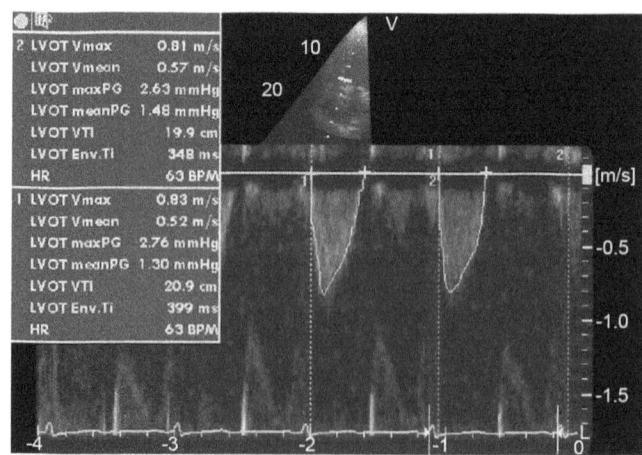

FIGURE 3.4: A pulsed-wave Doppler placed in the LVOT with the VTI measurement obtained as a surrogate for the cardiac output. (LVOT: left ventricular outflow tract; VTI: velocity time integral)

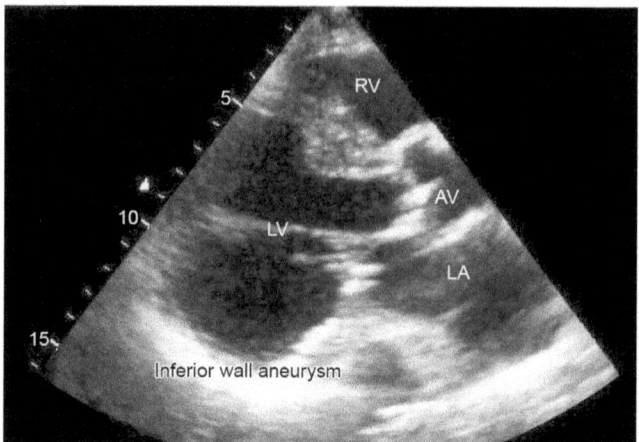

FIGURE 3.5: A PLAX view where the inferolateral wall of the left ventricle is markedly aneurysmal, indicating a segmental wall motion abnormality resulting from a right coronary artery occlusion. (AV: aortic valve; LA: left atrium; PLAX: parasternal long axis; RV: right ventricle)

chronic condition, recognized or otherwise, such as long-standing ischemic heart disease or cardiomyopathy, while in other situations, it reflects an acute condition, such as an acute myocardial infarction. Basic echocardiography allows for a relatively rapid assessment with the left ventricular ejection fraction (LVEF) being subjectively divided into normal, mild, or moderately reduced, and severe impairment. More experienced sonographers can attempt to be more objective by actually measuring LVEF or applying Doppler techniques to measure CO or its surrogate, such as the velocity time integral of the left ventricular outflow tract outflow (Fig. 3.4). Even more sophisticated techniques, such as speckle tracking and strain measurements, are becoming increasingly available in the critical care setting.[4] A very important component of the examination is that of identifying segmental wall motion abnormalities, especially when there are distinctive patterns indicating obstruction of a major epicardial artery (Fig. 3.5). As to whether acute obstruction of a coronary artery is present becomes an urgent determination as the need for rapid coronary angiography and subsequent maneuvers to recreate arterial patency is vital to survival and long-term morbidity.

Stress-induced cardiac syndromes are associated with a wide range of critical illnesses, best exemplified in severe sepsis with Takotsubo syndrome in its various forms. The spread of echocardiography in the management of septic patients has uncovered cardiac dysfunction which would have otherwise gone undiagnosed. Sometimes the pattern of left ventricular wall dysfunction resembles that of an acute myocardial infarction, resulting in the need for urgent coronary imaging. With the application of contrast echocardiography (in skilled hands), this can be performed at the bedside, negating the need for patient transfer to the catheter laboratory.

While the right ventricle is more difficult to assess because of its U shape and thin myocardium, it is important to obtain some measure of contraction. There may be segmental wall motion changes indicating underlying myocardial ischemia of stress-induced cardiomyopathy although global dysfunction of the right ventricle is more often observed. Fortunately the application of speckle-tracking and strain techniques is adding to our ability to evaluate right ventricular function as current techniques are imperfect (Fig. 3.6).

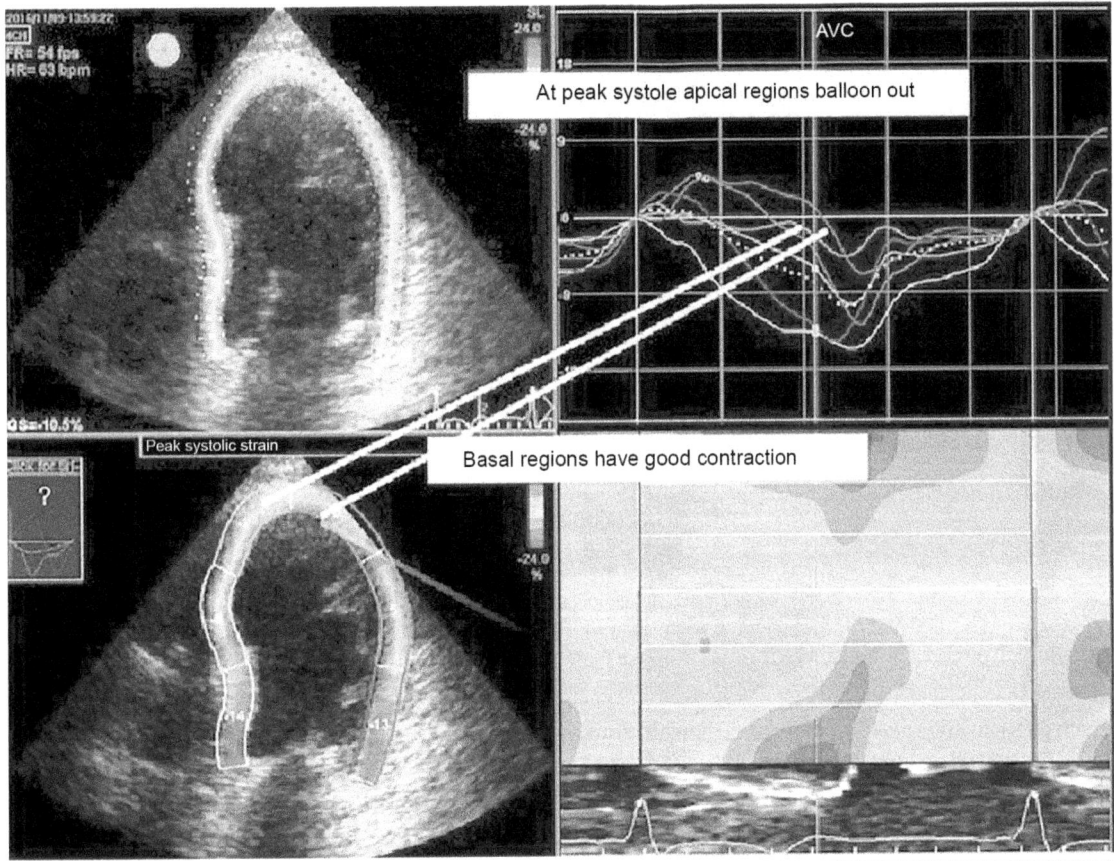

FIGURE 3.6: Speckle tracking and strain analysis demonstrating the LV apical wall segments contraction poorly compared to other wall segments, a typical finding in Takotsubo syndrome. (LV: left ventricular; AVC: artioventricular canal)

Abnormal Left Ventricular Diastolic Dysfunction

While a RACE may give indications of significant left ventricular diastolic dysfunction, such as when marked left ventricular wall hypertrophy is seen, Doppler techniques are necessary to assess it properly. Even in experienced hands, the diagnostic algorithms are challenging although the International Guidelines published in 2016 brought a lot more clarity to a complex subject.[5] Most importantly, these guidelines gave the clinician a workable roadmap. This is very important as half of the patients presenting with heart failure symptoms have normal left ventricular contraction, making diastolic dysfunction a management focus.

Severe Valvular Disease

Although accurate evaluation of valve dysfunction is more the purview of cardiologists, the presence of valve dysfunction should be considered with every critical care echocardiographic study. Both anatomical and functional evaluation, however limited, should be undertaken. During a RACE study, where right and ventricular function are assessed, the tricuspid, mitral, and aortic valves should be inspected. Although the absence of Doppler interrogation negates full functional evaluation, the appearance of the valve including thickening/calcification of leaflets or cusps, reduced opening, and/or irregular anatomy, such as flail leaflets or vegetations, will alert the sonographer to the need for a more advanced evaluation. The advanced evaluation requires the use of continuous-wave Doppler, pulsed-wave Doppler, color Doppler, and occasionally the performance of a TEE (Fig. 3.7). Often multiple techniques are used as a single method may not suffice, such as with severe aortic stenosis. Confounding factors, such as impaired left ventricular contraction, need to be factored into any calculation. The advice of colleagues, particularly experienced cardiologists, should be readily sought when uncertainty exists.

Acute Aortic Dissection

Although encountered rarely, acute thoracic dissection should be considered where symptoms and signs indicate the possibility. Aortic root dilatation, the possible presence

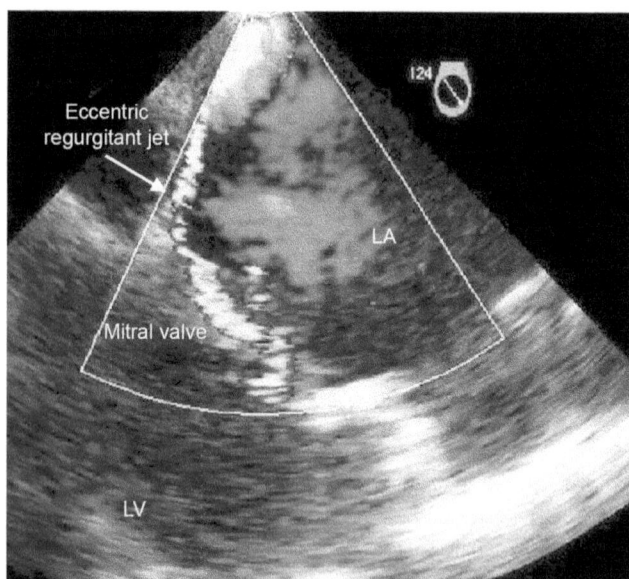

FIGURE 3.7: A TTE view of the mitral valve where color Doppler reveals a long, wall hugging, and eccentric jet of mitral regurgitation. (LV: left ventricle; LA: left atrium; TTE: transthoracic echocardiography)

of a dissection membrane, new onset aortic regurgitation, and pericardial effusion may be seen on a TTE, and occasionally the diagnosis can be made with certainty even though views are limited. Any changes are best seen in the parasternal long axis and parasternal short axis views. The absence of positive findings on TTE does not rule it out, and TEE is the preferred approach when the diagnosis is suspected. With TEE the root and ascending portion are well seen as well as the distal arch and descending aorta (Fig. 3.8).

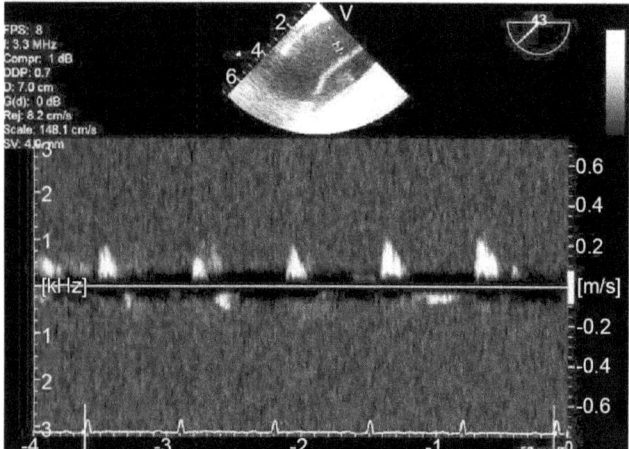

FIGURE 3.8: A TEE view of the descending thoracic aorta in a patient with Type A dissection, the pulsed-wave Doppler demonstrating minimal blood flow in the false lumen. (TEE: transesophageal echocardiography)

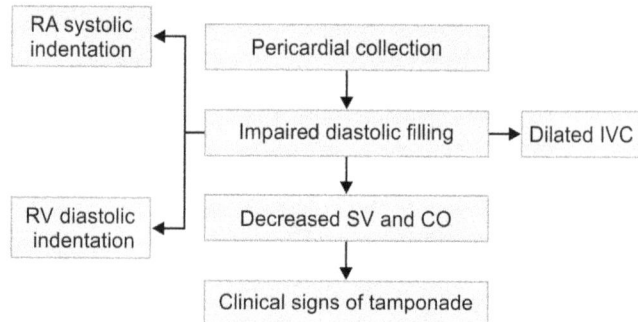

FLOWCHART 3.1: Tamponade—a basic echocardiography algorithm.

(RA: right atrium, RV: right ventricular; IVC: inferior vena cava; SV: stroke volume; CO: cardiac output)

Pericardial Effusion/Tamponade

The rapid identification of fluid in the pericardial space causing hemodynamic compromise exemplifies the use of echocardiography by the critical care physician. Confirming the presence of fluid is generally not difficult but determining the presence of tamponade needs to be a carefully made diagnosis as when present urgent pericardiocentesis, with attendant risks, is required. Fortunately for the basic operator, a simple algorithm, which does not require the use of Doppler, can usually make the diagnosis with certainty (Flowchart 3.1).

Elevated Left Atrial Pressure

The critical care physician frequently performs echocardiography to evaluate and monitor hemodynamic variables in an attempt to optimize the circulation. Left ventricular performance is central to this evaluation, and an idea of the left ventricular end diastolic pressure (LVEDP) can greatly assist. LVEDP is closely aligned with left atrial pressure, and this can often be estimated noninvasively by echocardiography. Similar measured parameters to those used in assessing left ventricular diastolic dysfunction are used, and once again the recently published International Guidelines are very helpful.[5] Advanced techniques including the application of spectral Doppler and tissue Doppler imaging are essential.

Endocarditis in the Critically Ill Patient

Echocardiography is an essential tool in the diagnosis and management of endocarditis. The lesion may be the primary source of systemic infection as is often found in intravenous drug users, or secondary to a source of sepsis originating in another part of the body, such as a vertebral staphylococcus infection. Being less invasive, a TTE is commonly used initially, but the absence of vegetations where endocarditis is suspected, necessitates the application of TEE which has diagnostic superiority. Often even where the presence of a vegetation is suspected the diagnosis is not easy as degenerative valvular abnormalities may cloud the picture, or the identified organism is one uncommonly associated with endocarditis. The modified Duke's criteria are a suitable roadmap to aid the clinician.[6] The two major criteria, necessary for a definite diagnosis, are the finding of two or more positive blood cultures for typical organisms consistent with infectious endocarditis and a positive echocardiogram. The positive echocardiographic features of a valvular lesion indicating that it is a vegetation are low reflectance, attachment to the upstream side of the valve, an irregular or amorphic shape, oscillating mobility, associated tissue changes, and associated valvular regurgitation. A possible diagnosis is indicated by the presence of one major criterion plus one minor criterion, or else three minor criteria. The minor criteria include classical peripheral stigmata, predisposition, fever >38.5°C, and microbiological criteria, such as an atypical organism or serological evidence, in the absence of positive cultures.

ECHOCARDIOGRAPHY IN THE MANAGEMENT OF THE SHOCK

Should a patient presenting with either differentiated or undifferentiated shock not be responding to initial fluid replacement and prescription of a vasopressor, hemodynamic assessment with echocardiography is recommended.[7] A RACE or basic echocardiographic examination will generally identify the type of shock within minutes, although the application of Doppler techniques can assist greatly in the challenge.[8] Not uncommonly the picture is mixed, such as when a person with underlying previous myocardial impairment from ischemic heart disease develops shock from urosepsis.

Cardiogenic shock reveals a poorly contracting left ventricle, often with the presence of segmental wall motion abnormalities indicating the presence of underlying coronary artery disease. Alternatively, severe valvular dysfunction may be inferred from structural changes. In advanced echocardiography the use of Doppler will clarify any significant valve dysfunction, in addition to measuring CO and determining left atrial pressure, allowing the contribution of diastolic dysfunction to the shock state to be also assessed. Hypovolemic shock is diagnosed where small left ventricular systolic volumes exist, and the classical sign of "kissing walls" of the left ventricle is seen. Static measurements such as the inferior vena cava and superior vena cava diameters and collapsibility, especially the latter, may be helpful but dynamic maneuvers are recommended. The advanced operator can then evaluate changes in CO (or surrogate measures) to either carefully titrated fluid boluses or passive leg raising.[9]

Obstructive shock is where echocardiographic examination is crucial to the diagnosis and prognosis, whether the underlying etiology be acute pulmonary embolism, pericardial tamponade, left ventricular outflow obstruction, or constrictive pericarditis.

Vasoplegic shock, one of the four most common types of shock, is where the contribution by echocardiography is less direct but is helpful in ruling out alternative types of shock and also providing clues as to the presence of reduced cardiac afterload. In a shocked patient, where echocardiographic examination does not identify cardiogenic, hypovolemic or obstructive shock, the possibility of vasoplegic shock is raised. An example is in a patient with high output septic shock where the left ventricle is hyperdynamic. The measured CO will be elevated, and there is usually an associated tachycardia. Unfortunately the ability to actually measure ventricular afterload remains elusive.

SUMMARY

The application of echocardiography is becoming standard practice in the daily management of the critically ill patient. Benefits range from more accurate and timely patient care, to negating the need for more invasive procedures and/or transfer of the patient outside the intensive care unit or emergency room for complex medical imaging. More precise and tailored management can be provided to the patient once the echocardiographic examination is performed.

REFERENCES

1. Cholley BP. International expert statement on training standards for critical care ultrasonography. Intensive Care Med. 2011;37:1077-83.
2. McLean A, Huang S (Eds). Critical care ultrasound manual. Australia: Elsevier; 2011.
3. Mayo PH, Vieillard-Baron A. International consensus statement on training standards for advanced critical care echocardiography. Intensive Care Med. 2014;40:654-66.
4. Huang SH, Orde S. From speckle tracking echocardiography to torsion: research tool today, clinical practice tomorrow. Curr Opin Crit Care. 2013;19(3):250-7.

5. Nagueh SF, Smiseth OA, Appleton CP, et al. Recommendations for the evaluation of left ventricular diastolic function by echocardiography: an update from the American Society of Echocardiography and the European Association of Cardiovascular Imaging. J. Am Soc Echocardiogr. 2016;29:277-314.
6. Baddour LM, Wilson WR, Bayer AS, et al. Infective endocarditis in adults: diagnosis, antimicrobial therapy, and management of complications: a scientific statement for healthcare professionals from the American Heart Association. Circulation. 2015;132:1435-86.
7. Cecconi M, De Backer D, Antionelli M, et al. Consensus on circulatory shock and hemodynamic monitoring. Task force of the European Society of Intensive Care. Intensive Care Med. 2014;40:1795-815.
8. McLean AS. Echocardiography in shock management. Crit Care. 2016;20(275):2-10.
9. Vignon P, Represse X, Begot E, et al. Comparison of echocardiographic indices used to predict fluid responsiveness in ventilated patients. Am J Respir Crit Care Med. 2017;195(8):1022-32.

CHAPTER 4

Assessment of Nutritional Status in Critically Ill

Andrew Li, Amartya Mukhopadhyay

BACKGROUND

After an acute event (such as sepsis, trauma, operation, or burns) that requires the patient to be placed in the intensive care unit (ICU), achieving hemodynamic stability, and maintenance of oxygenation and ventilation takes, precedence over starting nutrition. However, provision of adequate calorie and protein after the initial stabilization is equally important for patients' long-term outcomes should he/she survive the initial insult.

Deterioration of nutritional status in critically ill patients is rapid and related to the proinflammatory state, catabolism due to the increase in stress-related cytokines/hormones, and high sympathetic drive. Resulting malnutrition is common in ICU, even in patients with previous good nutritional status. Many patients admitted to ICU have a period of pre-ICU illness, either in hospital or at home when relatively low calorie and/or protein intake precedes their critical illnesses. Therefore, provision of adequate calorie and protein is essential for patients who are expected to stay in the ICU for more than 48 hours.[1]

PROVISION OF ENERGY IN CRITICALLY ILL

Current guidelines recommend starting nutrition preferably by an enteral route within 24–48 hours following the critical illness or ICU admission and slowly increased to achieve calorie and protein adequacy of ≥80% within 48–72 hours.[1] Adequate caloric and protein intake benefit those who are significantly malnourished as well as those are overweight prior to the ICU admission. However, there have been concerns that initiating feeds early would inhibit autophagy, an important physiologic process that takes place very early in critical illnesses. Autophagy is designed to remove damaged proteins, mitochondria, bacteria, and viruses with concurrent production of adenosine triphosphate for energy and protein synthesis. Insufficient autophagy can lead to inability to clear products of cellular damage and potentially prevent organs from recovering.[2]

PROVISION OF PROTEIN IN CRITICALLY ILL

Since amino acids (AAs) cannot be stored in the body, muscles are the only source. Under normal physiological state, AAs are absorbed in the blood after consumption of dietary protein, and the increased supply of essential AAs leads to muscle protein synthesis. In the post-absorptive state when there is no further absorption of AAs from the diet, obligatory oxidation of the essential AAs originating from muscle protein breakdown maintains the physiological functions. This periodic cycling of net protein synthesis and net protein breakdown maintains the overall muscle mass. In the state of critical illnesses, metabolic rates and the resting energy expenditure (EE) are increased. Although energy can be met with either enteral or parenteral calorie supplementation, protein breakdown always exceeds protein synthesis, and the negative nitrogen balance cannot be easily corrected. Increased availability of AAs due to the muscle breakdown stimulates protein synthesis to a certain extent but is insufficient to compensate for excessive breakdown.

After the initial insult, a period of relative "anabolic resistance" develops where increased supply of AA cannot simply stimulate adequate protein synthesis. This suggests that supplying higher amount of protein (therefore AAs) through diet or intravenously has limited impact on the protein synthesis. This is because intracellular availability of AA is of great importance for protein synthesis and in catabolic state, there is impaired transport of essential AAs in the cells. Anabolic resistance is also common in old age, leading to sarcopenia which in contrast to critical illness is slow in onset. Increased inflammation both in critical illness and old age may be responsible, and insulin resistance plays a role. Significant muscle wasting occurs early and rapidly during the critical illness, particularly among the patients who are sicker with more organ dysfunction and positively correlates with systemic inflammation.[3]

We aim to discuss how to assess of nutritional status and some of the controversies in ICU nutrition in this chapter.

NUTRITIONAL RISK ASSESSMENT

Due to the varied case mix, age, diagnosis, and different levels of illness, nutritional assessment in ICU poses significant challenges to the team. Body weight may change during resuscitation or dialysis due to rapid fluid infusion or withdrawal, respectively. Measurements, such as body mass index (BMI), therefore can be inaccurate. Traditional nutritional scoring systems that are useful in the general ward or community cannot be used in ICU due to inability of the patient to provide history, and the details of food intake are often not available.

Unlike in the general ward, nutritional risk assessments in critically ill patients are related to their severity of illness, and only two nutrition risk scores incorporating the disease severity are recommended.[1] The nutrition risk in the critically ill (NUTRIC) score[4] is most widely used (Table 4.1). As interleukin 6 is not routinely tested, modified NUTRIC score (without interleukin 6) has been validated in different ICU populations[5,6] (Tables 4.1 and 4.2). The other nutrition risk assessment score is the Nutrition Risk Screening 2002[7] (Table 4.2). However, it is important to highlight that these scores are not malnutrition screening; rather they suggest which groups of patients are at risk from nutrition point and will benefit from supplementation.

DETERMINING ENERGY REQUIREMENTS

Traditionally, the gold standard of assessing EE is with the indirect calorimetry (IC).[8] During the procedure of IC, measurements of the inspired and expired oxygen and carbon dioxide are taken to determine the VO_2, VCO_2, and EE. However, the use of IC has not been widely practiced because of the varied preconditions that must be met before the results can be interpreted accurately (Table 4.3). Many critically ill patients will require high ventilatory support and renal replacement therapy, thus becoming ineligible for IC measurements. IC is also expensive, resource intensive and requires specific training to operate the system.

Predictive equations are usually used as an alternative to facilitate EE calculation. Some of the commonly used equations are the Harris-Benedict and the Ireton-Jones equations, which are predominantly based on anthropometric measurements. However, these equations have been found to be inaccurate as they do not take into account the different metabolic states and body compositions of the patients.[9] At present, a weight-based equation of 25–30 kcal/kg/day is recommended in the absence of an IC.[1] The actual body weight should be used in the equation. In patients with BMI of 30–50 kg/m², 11–14 kcal/kg/day of actual body weight would be appropriate. However, in patients with BMI greater than 50 kg/m², 22–25 kcal/kg/day of ideal body weight should be used instead.

FEEDING STRATEGIES

Route and Timing of Feeding

Current guidelines recommend starting nutrition preferably by enteral route within the first 24–48 hours following critical illness or ICU admission.[1] However, enteral nutrition (EN) should be delayed in those critically ill patients with uncontrolled shock, hypoxemia and acidosis, upper gastrointestinal bleeding, bowel ischemia or obstruction, abdominal compartment syndrome, and high-output fistula.[10]

Vasopressors usage may disproportionately decrease blood flow to the gastrointestinal tract, and there had been concerns that EN among critically ill patients who are on vasopressors would lead to mesenteric ischemia. CALORIES and NUTRIREA-2 trials had included such patients but documented up to fourfold increase in vomiting and gastrointestinal side effects and associated increased ventilator-associated pneumonia; however, these side effects did not translate to prolonged mechanical ventilation or increased mortality.[11,12] Other studies have shown that EN within the first 24–48 hours help to reduce infection, hospital length of stay (LOS), and mortality without inducing any harm.[10] EN helps to maintain the structural and functional gut integrity, thus reducing bacterial translocation and intestinal permeability. Even among the patients for gastrointestinal surgeries, early postoperative feeding still helped to reduce complications without any adverse effects.[13]

Table 4.1: NUTRIC score.

Age	<50	0
	50–74	1
	≥75	2
APACHE II	<15	0
	15–19	1
	20–28	2
	≥29	3
SOFA	<6	0
	6–9	1
	≥10	2
Number of comorbidities	0–1	0
	≥2	1
Days from hospital to ICU admission	<1	0
	≥1	1
Scoring		
If IL-6 available	6–10	High risk
	0–5	Low risk
If IL-6 not available (Modified NUTRIC score)	5–9	High risk
	0–4	Low risk

(NUTRIC: nutrition risk in the critically ill; APACHE: Acute Physiology and Chronic Health Evaluation; SOFA: sequential organ failure assessment; IL: interleukin)

Table 4.2: Nutritional Risk Screening (NRS 2002).

Impaired nutritional status		Disease severity	
Normal nutrition status	0	Normal nutritional requirements	0
Weight loss >5 % in 3 months		Hip fracture	
Food intake below 50–75% of normal requirements in preceding week	1	Chronic patients, i.e. COPD, liver cirrhosis	1
Weight loss >5% in 2 months		Chronic hemodialysis, diabetes, oncology	
BMI 18.5–20.5 + impaired general condition	2	Major abdominal surgery, stroke	2
Food intake 25–50% of normal requirements in preceding week		Severe pneumonia, hematological malignancy	
Weight loss >5% in 1 month		Head injury	
BMI <18.5 + impaired general condition	3	Bone marrow transplantation	3
Food intake 0–25% of normal requirements in preceding week		Intensive care patients	
Scoring			

Determine score 0–3 for each section
Total up the score and add 1 to the total score if age ≥ 70 years old
if NRS ≥ 3, high risk
(BMI: body mass index; COPD: chronic obstructive pulmonary disease; NRS: nutrition risk screening)

Table 4.3: Conditions where indirect calorimetry measurements may not be valid.

Physical agitation or unstable sedation/analgesia	Unstable pH (± 0.1 change over the last hour)
Air leaks/pneumothorax	FiO_2 >60%
Unstable body temperature(>1°C change over the last hour)	Renal replacement therapy
ECMO	Liver dialysis

(ECMO: extracorporeal membrane oxygenation; FiO_2: fraction of inspired oxygen)

How Much Should We Feed?

Controversy has persisted with regards to the best feeding strategy. Current recommendations for enteral feeding are based on calories. Feeding is not well tolerated in ICU patients and stopped in many for surgeries, procedures, or transport for radiological investigations. Therefore, iatrogenic underfeeding remains common in the ICU.[14] Starting EN early, implementing a volume-based protocol, and empowering bedside nurse to increase feeding when it was stopped for several hours (PEP-uP strategy) can improve both calorie and protein adequacies.[15,16]

Recent observational studies utilizing IC data have shown that the optimal outcomes are achieved when 70% of resting EE is met.[17] It is important not to allow overfeeding, as it can lead to increased fat deposition in the liver and production of carbon dioxide, resulting in liver dysfunction and prolonged ventilator support.[18] Endogenous glucose production is maximum during the early phases of critical illness and may be further aggravated due to overfeeding.[17] Caloric requirements in the early phases of critical illness are much lower compared to the subsequent phases of critical illness. This has led to studies on early goal-directed nutrition (EGDN) by utilizing IC. Feeding to the EE measured by IC showed a trend toward improved hospital survival by per-protocol analysis in the Tight Calorie Control Study trial.[19] However, there was increased ICU LOS and prolonged mechanical ventilation with higher infection rates. Since EGDN does not appear to improve functional outcomes, it is yet to be endorsed by guidelines.

On the other hand, several recent trials have suggested that "permissive underfeeding" (defined as feeding up to 40-60% of caloric requirements) and "trophic feeding" (defined as 10–20 mL/kg/day or 500 kcal/day) may be possible.[20,21] However, many of these studies were restricted to patients with certain diseases, e.g. acute respiratory failure and may not be generalizable to all critically ill patients. Others believe that underfeeding can be detrimental. In the original NUTRIC score study[4] and multiple subsequent validation studies,[5,6] higher energy supplies have been associated with better outcomes including shorter LOS and even improved functional status at 3 months.[22]

PROTEIN INTAKE

Guidelines recommend daily protein intake of 1.2–2.0 g/kg actual body weight.[1] Adequate protein intake has been shown to improve mortality and potentially better functional outcomes upon discharge, particularly among those with high NUTRIC scores.[23] It may also reduce ICU LOS. Growing evidence now emphasizes the importance of adequate protein supply rather than full energy intake. However, since most EN formulas are calorie based, the protein requirements are not entirely met and the intake remains inadequate.[14] Therefore many ICUs practice additional protein supplementation. Protein delivery can also be improved by starting the feeding early and using EN with high protein content. Adequate delivery of protein can be assessed by reviewing daily intake and measurement of muscle loss by bedside ultrasound. Biochemical markers for adequate protein delivery are mainly used for research.

TOTAL PARENTERAL NUTRITION

Total parenteral nutrition (TPN) has always been viewed with some mistrust due to multiple associated complications (Table 4.4). In addition the timing of administering TPN has remained controversial. Early TPN in patients who were not able to take EN for a short period of time showed no difference in mortality and infection rates.[24] It even delayed recovery regardless of disease severity or type of macronutrient. This was further corroborated by the EPaNIC study,[25] where late TPN administration was associated with fewer ICU infections, shorter ICU LOS, and duration of mechanical ventilation. Importantly, it showed that early TPN could result in significant overfeeding. A negative dose–response relationship was also evident in the EPaNIC study. However the CALORIES trial did not demonstrate any mortality or infection rates difference when comparing early TPN and EN.[12] The subsequent supplemental parenteral nutrition study showed that it is possible to deliver early TPN to patients who have yet to receive at least 60% of their energy target from EN.[26] This highlights the potential advantage of TPN, where effective caloric delivery can be instituted when early EN is not able to achieve the energy requirements, provided no overfeeding occurs.

The current guidelines[1] has advocated TPN use in these three indications: (1) low-nutrition risk patients who have not been able to tolerate EN over a week following ICU admission; (2) high-nutrition risk or severely malnourish patients, when EN is not feasible; and (3) in patients who were not able to achieve at least 60% of energy and protein requirements via EN after 7–10 days.

CONCLUSION

While the broad principles of ICU nutrition have been laid out above, the studies were conducted in a mixed group of ICU patients with multiple comorbidities and different nutritional status. Not all critically ill patients are the same, and individualizing ICU nutrition to each patient would require intimate knowledge of the disease course, the patient's comorbidities, and the ability to deliver and meet both energy and protein requirements. Many nutrition-related questions in critically ill patients remain unanswered: how to best achieve the calorie and protein adequacy and if achievement of the recommended adequacy will translate to improved functional outcome, best time to apply higher protein supplementation, effect of increased volume with higher nutrition adequacies and outcome of patients, etc. Future research will answer some of them. Many modern ventilators incorporate IC measurements now and in the near future further data on diverse medical conditions using IC will be available.

Table 4.4: Complications of TPN.

Metabolic	Infection	Line-related problems
Hepatosteatosis, hepatocellualr injury	Fungal infection	Pneumothorax
Hyperglycemia	Line sepsis	Bleeding
Refeeding syndrome		Catheter occlusion
Thiamine deficiency		Air embolism
Metabolic bone disease		Venous thrombosis
Fluid overload		

(TPN: total parenteral nutrition)

REFERENCES

1. McClave SA, Taylor BE, Martindale RG, et al. Guidelines for the provision and assessment of nutrition support therapy in the adult critically ill patient: Society of Critical Care Medicine (SCCM) and American Society for Parenteral and Enteral Nutrition (A.S.P.E.N.). JPEN J Parenter Enteral Nutr. 2016;40(2):159-211.

2. Gunst J. Recovery from critical illness-induced organ failure: the role of autophagy. Crit Care. 2017;21(1):209.
3. Puthucheary ZA, Rawal J, McPhail M, et al. Acute skeletal muscle wasting in critical illness. JAMA. 2013;310(15):1591-600.
4. Heyland DK, Dhaliwal R, Jiang X, et al. Identifying critically ill patients who benefit the most from nutrition therapy: the development and initial validation of a novel risk assessment tool. Crit Care. 2011;15(6):R268.
5. Rahman A, Hasan RM, Agarwala R, et al. Identifying critically-ill patients who will benefit most from nutritional therapy: Further validation of the "modified NUTRIC" nutritional risk assessment tool. Clin Nutr. 2016;35(1):158-62.
6. Mukhopadhyay A, Henry J, Ong V, et al. Association of modified NUTRIC score with 28-day mortality in critically ill patients. Clin Nutr. 2017;36(4):1143-8.
7. Kondrup J, Rasmussen HH, Hamberg O, et al. Nutritional Risk Screening (NRS 2002): a new method based on an analysis of controlled clinical trials. Clin Nutr. 2003;22(3):321-36.
8. Oshima T, Berger MM, De Waele E, et al. Indirect calorimetry in nutritional therapy. A position paper by the ICALIC study group. Clin Nutr. 2017;36(3):651-62.
9. Wichansawakun S, Meddings L, Alberda C, et al. Energy requirements and the use of predictive equations versus indirect calorimetry in critically ill patients. Appl Physiol Nutr Metab. 2015;40(2):207-10.
10. Reintam Blaser A, Starkopf J, Alhazzani W, et al. Early enteral nutrition in critically ill patients: ESICM clinical practice guidelines. Intensive Care Med. 2017;43(3):380-98.
11. Reignier J, Boisrame-Helms J, Brisard L, et al. Enteral versus parenteral early nutrition in ventilated adults with shock: a randomised, controlled, multicentre, open-label, parallel-group study (NUTRIREA-2). Lancet. 2018;391(10116):133-43.
12. Harvey SE, Parrott F, Harrison DA, et al. Trial of the route of early nutritional support in critically ill adults. N Engl J Med. 2014;371(18):1673-84.
13. Zhuang CL, Ye XZ, Zhang CJ, et al. Early versus traditional postoperative oral feeding in patients undergoing elective colorectal surgery: a meta-analysis of randomized clinical trials. Dig Surg. 2013;30(3):225-32.
14. Heyland DK, Dhaliwal R, Wang M, et al. The prevalence of iatrogenic underfeeding in the nutritionally 'at-risk' critically ill patient: results of an international, multicenter, prospective study. Clin Nutr. 2015;34(4):659-66.
15. McClave SA, Saad MA, Esterle M, et al. Volume-based feeding in the critically ill patient. JPEN J Parenter Enteral Nutr. 2015;39(6):707-12.
16. Heyland DK, Cahill NE, Dhaliwal R, et al. Enhanced protein-energy provision via the enteral route in critically ill patients: a single center feasibility trial of the PEP uP protocol. Crit Care. 2010;14(2):R78.
17. Singer P, Berger MM, Weijs PJM. The lessons learned from the EAT ICU study. Intensive Care Med. 2018;44(1):133-4.
18. Reid C. Frequency of under- and overfeeding in mechanically ventilated ICU patients: causes and possible consequences. J Hum Nutr Diet. 2006;19(1):13-22.
19. Singer P, Anbar R, Cohen J, et al. The tight calorie control study (TICACOS): a prospective, randomized, controlled pilot study of nutritional support in critically ill patients. Intensive Care Med. 2011;37(4):601-9.
20. Arabi YM, Aldawood AS, Haddad SH, et al. Permissive underfeeding or standard enteral feeding in critically ill adults. N Engl J Med. 2015;372(25):2398-408.
21. Rice TW, Wheeler AP, Thompson BT, et al.; National Heart, Lung, and Blood Institute Acute Respiratory Distress Syndrome (ARDS) Clinical Trials Network. Initial trophic vs full enteral feeding in patients with acute lung injury: the EDEN randomized trial. JAMA. 2012;307(8):795-803.
22. Wei X, Day AG, Ouellette-Kuntz H, et al. The association between nutritional adequacy and long-term outcomes in critically ill patients requiring prolonged mechanical ventilation: a multicenter cohort study. Crit Care Med. 2015;43(8):1569-79.
23. Compher C, Chittams J, Sammarco T, et al. Greater protein and energy intake may be associated with improved mortality in higher risk critically ill patients: a multicenter, multinational observational study. Crit Care Med. 2017;45(2):156-63.
24. Doig GS, Simpson F, Sweetman EA, et al. Early parenteral nutrition in critically ill patients with short-term relative contraindications to early enteral nutrition: a randomized controlled trial. JAMA. 2013;309(20):2130-8.
25. Casaer MP, Mesotten D, Hermans G, et al. Early versus late parenteral nutrition in critically ill adults. N Engl J Med. 2011;365(6):506-17.
26. Heidegger CP, Berger MM, Graf S, et al. Optimisation of energy provision with supplemental parenteral nutrition in critically ill patients: a randomised controlled clinical trial. Lancet. 2013;381(9864):385-93.

CHAPTER 5

Prognosis and Risk Factors for Poor Outcome in Critically Ill Patients with Respiratory Illness

Amit Kansal, Dhanvijay Shekhar Yadavrao

INTRODUCTION

This chapter will discuss the prognosis and risk factors for poor outcome among the critically ill patients admitted with commonly encountered respiratory diseases.
- Pneumonia [community-acquired pneumonia (CAP) and hospital-acquired pneumonia (HAP)]
- Acute respiratory distress syndrome (ARDS)
- Chronic obstructive pulmonary disease (COPD) exacerbation.

PROGNOSIS AND RISK FACTORS FOR POOR OUTCOME IN COMMUNITY-ACQUIRED PNEUMONIA

SUMMARY
- CAP is associated with very high mortality among critically ill patients admitted to intensive care units (ICU) as well as high mortality among less sick hospitalized patients, especially in elderly population and patients with significant comorbidities
- Many risk factors and scores may predict poor outcome
- CAP is also associated with the risk of developing cardiovascular complications, both short- and long-term

Mortality: Mortality rates among patients hospitalized with CAP have been reported to be between 8% and 13% and higher (36.5%) among sicker patients who require admission to the intensive care units (ICU).[1,2] Patients usually die due to infective pathology (mostly pneumonia) and acute cardiovascular events.

Inhospital mortality: Various factors are associated with inhospital mortality, most of these indicate the severity of acute illness:[3]
- Bacteremia
- Respiratory rate (RR) >30 breaths/min
- PaO_2 <60 mm Hg or oxygen saturation <90%
- Mechanically ventilated
- Systolic blood pressure (BP) <90 mm Hg
- Arterial pH <7.35
- Blood urea nitrogen (BUN) >11 mmol/L
- Comorbidities

Several additional factors correlate with high inhospital mortality:
- Failure of initial therapy[2,4]
- Hyperglycemia on admission[5]

On the contrary, early ICU admission seems to confer survival benefit.[6]

Postdischarge mortality (short-term as well as long-term): A significant proportion of survivors die postdischarge from the hospital; 7% mortality at 1 year in one large prospective study.[7]

Mortality was higher among patients who were discharged alive after ICU admission; the 30-day mortality among survivors was 11%, increasing to 27% at 1 year.[8]

Following factors correlate with 1-year mortality:
- Dementia, COPD, diabetes mellitus (DM), cancer
- A 30-day readmission after discharge from the hospital
- Premorbidly long-term care resident

Long-term mortality significantly increased by more than 50% when a higher number of risk factors were present.

Several of these risk factors have been utilized to develop scores that predict mortality among hospitalized patients:[9]

CURB-65 score—[Confusion, age >65 years, BUN >20 mg/dL (7 mmol/L), systolic BP <90 mm Hg or diastolic BP ≤ 60 mm Hg, and RR >30/min]: The 30-day mortality seems to directly correlate with the number of risk factors present.

Pneumonia severity index (PSI): Gender, age, nursing home residence, comorbidities, physical examination, and laboratory and radiographic parameters.

Pneumonia severity index can predict 30-day mortality, facilitate triage CAP patients who are at low risk of dying (which in turn helps to recognize the need for ICU admission) and predict long-term mortality.

Predisposition, insult, response, and organ dysfunction (PIRO) score in ICU patients—[PIRO—comorbidities (COPD, immunocompromised status), elderly >70 years, shock, severe hypoxia, ARDS, multilobar involvement on chest X-ray, acute kidney injury, and bacteremia].[10]

The PIRO performed better than the Acute Physiology and Chronic Health Evaluation-II score, as well as the American Thoracic Society/Infectious Disease Society of America (ATS/IDSA) criteria in predicting mortality among the CAP patients admitted to the ICU.[10]

The Infectious Disease Society of America/ATS minor criteria: The 2007 IDSA/ATS identified the following criteria for direct admission to ICU:[2,9]
- One of the major criteria: Vasopressor-dependent septic shock and respiratory failure requiring mechanical ventilation or
- At least three minor criteria: Confusion, RR ≥ 30 breaths/min, PaO_2/FiO_2 ratio ≤250, multilobar involvement on chest X-ray, BUN ≥20 mg/dL (blood urea 7 mmol/L), leukopenia, thrombocytopenia, hypothermia, or hypotension requiring fluid resuscitation.

The minor criteria seem to predict 30-day mortality as good as PSI.

Biomarkers: Biomarkers, such as procalcitonin, may have prognostic value.[11] A meta-analysis, including 14 trials (4,211 patients with respiratory tract infection), reported that an initially elevated procalcitonin level was associated with a high likelihood of treatment failure and increased mortality in patients with CAP. On the contrary, initial procalcitonin levels did not show any correlation with the outcome among the sicker patients who required ICU admission, and the optimal threshold for predicting adverse events has not been determined. Serial procalcitonin levels may be more predictive than single values.

Etiology: Gram-negative organisms (*Pseudomonas aeruginosa*, *Klebsiella*, *Escherichia coli*) and *Staphylococcus aureus* are associated with very high mortality; 41 and 32%, respectively. In comparison the mortality rate with *Mycoplasma pneumoniae* is low (1.4%) and intermediate with *Streptococcus pneumoniae* and *Chlamydia pneumoniae* (12 to 15%) and influenza A (9%).[2,12]

The nonresponding patient: Studies suggest that up to 15% of immunocompetent patients do not respond to initial antibiotic therapy at 72 hours, and the mortality rates may be substantially high in these patients (up to 25 to 27%).[2,4] The failure rate may be even higher (up to 40%) among sicker patients who needed ICU admission initially.

Factors associated with the slower rate of resolution include:
- Comorbidities
- Age
- Severity of initial disease
- Infectious agent: *M. pneumoniae*, nonbacteremic *S. pneumoniae*, *Chlamydia* species, and *Moraxella catarrhalis* are associated with faster resolution compared to other pathogens

Vaccination: Prior pneumococcal and influenza vaccination appears to improve outcomes (including better survival) in patients with CAP, including the elderly patients.[4]

Cardiovascular complications among CAP patients: CAP patients seem to have an increased risk of new-onset cardiovascular disease (short- and long-term)—ischemic heart disease, heart failure, and cerebrovascular accident. These patients also have protracted clinical course and increased 30- and 90-day mortality.[13]

PROGNOSIS AND RISK FACTORS FOR POOR OUTCOME IN HOSPITAL-ACQUIRED PNEUMONIA AND VENTILATOR-ASSOCIATED PNEUMONIA

Hospital-acquired pneumonia and ventilator-associated pneumonia (VAP) are associated with significantly increased risk of death. However the attributable mortality remains uncertain. Various studies have reported the all-cause mortality associated with VAP from 20% to 50%; the attributable mortality has been estimated at 13%.[14]

Variables that are shown to correlate with higher mortality include:
- Elderly patients
- Severity of acute illness

- Bacteremia
- Comorbidities
- Multidrug-resistant infections
- Multilobar, cavitating, or rapidly progressive infiltrates on lung imaging
- Delayed antimicrobial therapy.

PROGNOSIS AND RISK FACTORS FOR POOR OUTCOME IN ACUTE RESPIRATORY DISTRESS SYNDROME

SUMMARY
- ARDS is associated with increased mortality and survivors demonstrate significant long-term morbidity
- Numerous factors seem to predict poor outcomes (in-hospital mortality and long-term morbidity)

Mortality: ARDS is associated with increased mortality, various studies suggesting from 26% to 58%.[15,16]

Interestingly, patients do not seem to die of respiratory failure commonly; instead, the patients usually die because of the underlying cause of the ARDS in the early part of their illness and sepsis and nosocomial pneumonia in later part of the clinical course.

Despite high mortality, the overall trend appears to be improving over time. Likely reasons behind improving mortality trend remain uncertain and may include a better understanding of the disease process over time, better critical care support, and improvements in specific management strategies, such as low-tidal-volume ventilation.[16]

Numerous factors seem to correlate with poor outcomes in terms of inhospital mortality and long-term morbidity. However, no single factor is superior to the others.[17-25]
- Age
- Obesity—conflicting evidence[18]
- Chronic alcohol abuse[19]
- Trauma-related ARDS appears to have better survival compared to the patients with other causes of ARDS[20]
- Disease severity (respiratory)
  - Driving pressure[21]
  - Gas exchange: Failure of oxygenation to improve, severe hypercarbia ($PaCO_2 \geq 50$ mm Hg)[22]
  - Pulmonary vascular dysfunction—as determined by mean pulmonary artery pressure and the pulmonary artery occlusion pressure
  - Extravascular lung water index and pulmonary vascular permeability indices
  - Increased dead space
  - Lung biopsy showing diffuse alveolar damage[23]
- Nonrespiratory disease severity *including*
  - Positive fluid balance and
  - Packed red blood cell transfusion[24]
- Delayed intubation:[25] Although it is not clear whether the use of noninvasive ventilation (NIV) or subsequent delay in intubation is the cause.

Morbidity among survivors: Survivors of ARDS commonly have significant cognitive, psychological, and physical morbidities; many of those present at long-term follow-ups. These manifestations resolve very slowly and may have a considerable impact upon the subsequent quality of life.

On a brighter note, one follow-up study reported that 50–70% of those who were working prior to the onset of acute illness were able to return to work; mostly within 2 years after discharge.
- *Cognitive*: Cognitive dysfunction incidence ranges from 30% to 55% in various studies; the rates were comparable to those reported among the survivors of critical illness in general.[26]
- *Psychiatric*: Depression (36% to 40% at 1 and 2 years, respectively) and anxiety/post-traumatic stress disorder (more than 60% at 1 year) are commonly reported in survivors of ARDS. One of the studies[28] identified younger patients, females, premorbidly unemployed, alcohol abusers, and greater opioid use while admitted in the ICU as high-risk factors, whereas the severity of disease and ICU length of stay had no association with the psychiatric symptoms.[27,28]
- *Physical*: Survivors of ARDS frequently have physical disabilities, persistent as well as progressively worse on long-term follow-up. Up to 38% of survivors may have muscle weakness at discharge, while impaired physical function has been demonstrated in more than 60% of survivors at 2-year follow-up. Prolonged ICU stay and premorbid depressive symptoms were significant risk factors for physical dysfunction.[29,30]

Studies have also demonstrated an association between muscle weakness at hospital discharge and increased 5-year mortality.[30]
- *Lung function and radiological recovery*: Lung function is commonly impaired following ARDS. However, the contribution of impaired lung function toward physical decline is uncertain. Only a small number of survivors have residual deficits, and very few require supplemental oxygen.[31] Similarly, a small percentage of patients have persistent radiological abnormalities and such patients tend to have worse pulmonary function and reduced quality of life; even though most patients show good radiologic recovery over a few months postdischarge.[32]

❑ *Complications of intubation*: Given the high incidence of prolonged mechanical ventilation (endotracheal intubation or tracheostomy) among ARDS patients, related complications are common—laryngotracheal stenosis, tracheomalacia, and speech or swallowing impairment.

Over last few years, extracorporeal membrane oxygenation (ECMO) is being increasingly used for management of sick ARDS patients, although inhospital mortality among this group of patients remains very high (ranging between 35% and 45%).[33]

Following factors seem to be correlated with poorer outcome among ARDS patients on ECMO:
❑ Age
❑ Immunosuppressed patients
❑ Poor respiratory system compliance
❑ Severity of extrapulmonary organ dysfunction
❑ Noninfluenzae pathogen.

PROGNOSIS AMONG CRITICALLY ILL PATIENTS WITH CHRONIC OBSTRUCTIVE PULMONARY DISEASE

SUMMARY
- The in-hospital mortality and morbidity among patients hospitalized with respiratory failure secondary to COPD are determined by the severity of current acute illness, rather than the premorbid chronic disease status alone
- On the contrary, the chronic health status and the severity of COPD are the factors primarily influencing the long-term survival of COPD patients

Prognosis in Patients Hospitalized with Acute Exacerbations

Patients with COPD require frequent hospital admissions for acute infective exacerbations, the outcome being determined by the severity of current acute illness, rather than the premorbid chronic disease status alone.[34]

Factors associated with inhospital mortality include:
❑ Advanced age
❑ Prolonged hospital length of stay prior to ICU admission
❑ Severity of respiratory dysfunction
❑ Severity of nonrespiratory organ dysfunction.

Hypercapnia: Hypercapnia induced by an acute exacerbation of COPD does not predict increased mortality compared to patients with eucapnia. In contrast, patients who develop chronic hypercapnia, have a decreased 5-year survival.[35]

Prognosis in Mechanically Ventilated Chronic Obstructive Pulmonary Disease Patients

Chronic obstructive pulmonary disease patients with acute respiratory failure, who require mechanical ventilation have significantly high ICU mortality (37 to 64%), stay ventilated longer and increased ICU length of stay in comparison with the patients without COPD.

Prognosis in ventilated COPD patients appears to be affected by both the severity of the premorbid COPD as well as the severity of the acute disease (e.g. multiorgan failure, high illness severity score, and ARDS). Other factors indicating poor prognosis include failure of NIV and infections caused by virulent pathogens, such as *Pseudomonas* and *Aspergillus*.[36]

Prognostic Factors Associated with Reduced Life Expectancy

Life expectancy of COPD patients is negatively influenced by many factors (which includes modifiable and nonmodifiable):[37-41]
❑ Genetic predisposition, male gender, advanced age
❑ Environmental exposure, cigarette smoking
❑ Chronic health status and comorbidities, human immunodeficiency virus infection
❑ Low body mass index (BMI ≤21)
❑ Diminished physical function—decreased exercise capacity
❑ Accelerated lung function decline
❑ The severity of disease—forced expiratory volume in 1 second (FEV_1), chronic hypercapnia,[35] histamine-induced airway hyperresponsiveness, peak oxygen consumption (VO_2) as calculated by cardiopulmonary exercise testing.

BODE index—is a multidimensional index [four factors determine the overall score—body mass index, dyspnea (Medical Research Council dyspnea score), exercise capacity as determined by six-minute walk distance, and airway obstruction (FEV_1)].

BODE index performed better compared to unidimensional assessment based only on the FEV_1 value. The index can also predict the risk of death and the risk of hospitalization.
❑ Chest computed tomography showing the presence of emphysema
❑ Increased airway bacterial load
❑ Frequent COPD exacerbations

Chronic Obstructive Pulmonary Disease and Risk of Developing Other Comorbid Conditions[42]

Chronic obstructive pulmonary disease has also been shown to be associated with the development of cardiovascular diseases (e.g. hypertension, coronary heart disease, and stroke), DM, renal failure, osteoporosis, psychiatric illness (e.g. depression and anxiety), and cognitive impairment.

To summarize, critically ill patients with respiratory illnesses have a significantly high burden of mortality and morbidity.

REFERENCES

1. Mandell LA, Wunderink RG, Anzueto A, et al. Infectious Diseases Society of America/American Thoracic Society consensus guidelines on the management of community-acquired pneumonia in adults. Clin Infect Dis. 2007;44(Suppl 2):S27-72.
2. Fine MJ, Smith MA, Carson CA, et al. Prognosis and outcomes of patients with community-acquired pneumonia. A meta-analysis. JAMA. 1996;275(2):134-41.
3. Metersky ML, Waterer G, Nsa W, et al. Predictors of in-hospital vs postdischarge mortality in pneumonia. Chest. 2012;142(2):476-81.
4. Garcia-Vidal C, Carratalà J. Early and late treatment failure in community-acquired pneumonia. Semin Respir Crit Care Med. 2009;30(2):154-60.
5. Lepper PM, Ott S, Nüesch E, et al. Serum glucose levels for predicting death in patients admitted to hospital for community acquired pneumonia: prospective cohort study. BMJ. 2012;344:e3397.
6. Restrepo MI, Mortensen EM, Rello J, et al. Late admission to the ICU in patients with community-acquired pneumonia is associated with higher mortality. Chest. 2010;137(3):552-7.
7. Adamuz J, Viasus D, Jiménez-Martínez E, et al. Incidence, timing and risk factors associated with 1-year mortality after hospitalization for community-acquired pneumonia. J Infect. 2014;68:534-41.
8. Sligl WI, Eurich DT, Marrie TJ, et al. Only severely limited, premorbid functional status is associated with short- and long-term mortality in patients with pneumonia who are critically ill: a prospective observational study. Chest. 2011;139(1):88-94.
9. Singanayagam A, Chalmers JD, Hill AT. Severity assessment in community-acquired pneumonia: a review. QJM. 2009;102(6):379-88.
10. Rello J, Rodriguez A, Lisboa T, et al. PIRO score for community-acquired pneumonia: a new prediction rule for assessment of severity in intensive care unit patients with community-acquired pneumonia. Crit Care Med. 2009;37(2):456-62.
11. Kutz A, Briel M, Christ-Crain M, et al. Prognostic value of procalcitonin in respiratory tract infections across clinical settings. Crit Care. 2015;19(1):74.
12. Kothe H, Bauer T, Marre R, et al. Outcome of community-acquired pneumonia: influence of age, residence status and antimicrobial treatment. Eur Respir J. 2008;32(1):139-46.
13. Corrales-Medina VF, Musher DM, Shachkina S, et al. Acute pneumonia and the cardiovascular system. Lancet. 2013;381(9865):496-505.
14. Kalil AC, Metersky ML, Klompas M, et al. Management of adults with hospital-acquired and ventilator-associated pneumonia: 2016 clinical practice guidelines by the Infectious Diseases Society of America and the American Thoracic Society. Clin Infect Dis. 2016;63(5):e61-111.
15. Bellani G, Laffey JG, Pham T, et al. Epidemiology, patterns of care, and mortality for patients with acute respiratory distress syndrome in intensive care units in 50 countries. JAMA. 2016;315(8):788-800.
16. Villar J, Blanco J, Añón JM, et al. The ALIEN study: incidence and outcome of acute respiratory distress syndrome in the era of lung protective ventilation. Intensive Care Med. 2011;37(12):1932-41.
17. Chen W, Ware LB. Prognostic factors in the acute respiratory distress syndrome. Clin Transl Med. 2015;4:23.
18. Memtsoudis SG, Bombardieri AM, Ma Y, et al. Mortality of patients with respiratory insufficiency and adult respiratory distress syndrome after surgery: the obesity paradox. J Intensive Care Med. 2012;27(5):306-11.
19. Clark BJ, Williams A, Feemster LM, et al. Alcohol screening scores and 90-day outcomes in patients with acute lung injury. Crit Care Med. 2013;41(6):1518-25.
20. Calfee CS, Eisner MD, Ware LB, et al. Trauma-associated lung injury differs clinically and biologically from acute lung injury due to other clinical disorders. Crit Care Med. 2007;35(10):2243-50.
21. Amato MB, Meade MO, Slutsky AS, et al. Driving pressure and survival in the acute respiratory distress syndrome. N Engl J Med. 2015;372(8):747-55.
22. Nin N, Muriel A, Peñuelas O, et al. Severe hypercapnia and outcome of mechanically ventilated patients with moderate or severe acute respiratory distress syndrome. Intensive Care Med. 2017;43(2):200-8.
23. Cardinal-Fernández P, Bajwa EK, Dominguez-Calvo A, et al. The presence of diffuse alveolar damage on open lung biopsy is associated with mortality in patients with acute respiratory distress syndrome: a systematic review and meta-analysis. Chest. 2016;149(5):1155-64.
24. Netzer G, Shah CV, Iwashyna TJ, et al. Association of RBC transfusion with mortality in patients with acute lung injury. Chest. 2007;132:1116.
25. Kangelaris KN, Ware LB, Wang CY, et al. Timing of intubation and clinical outcomes in adults with acute respiratory distress syndrome. Crit Care Med. 2016;44(1):120-9.
26. Mikkelsen ME, Christie JD, Lanken PN, et al. The adult respiratory distress syndrome cognitive outcomes study: long-term neuropsychological function in survivors of acute lung injury. Am J Respir Crit Care Med. 2012;185(12):1307-15.
27. Bienvenu OJ, Friedman LA, Colantuoni E. Psychiatric symptoms after acute respiratory distress syndrome: a 5-year longitudinal study. Intensive Care Med. 2018;44(1):38-47.
28. Huang M, Parker AM, Bienvenu OJ, et al. Psychiatric symptoms in acute respiratory distress syndrome survivors: a 1-year national multicenter study. Crit Care Med. 2016;44(5):954-65.

29. Mehta S, Povoa P. Long-term physical morbidity in ARDS survivors. Intensive Care Med. 2017;43(1):101-3.
30. Dinglas VD, Aronson Friedman L, Colantuoni E, et al. Muscle weakness and 5-year survival in acute respiratory distress syndrome survivors. Crit Care Med. 2017;45(3):446-53.
31. Neff TA, Stocker R, Frey HR, et al. Long-term assessment of lung function in survivors of severe ARDS. Chest. 2003;123(3):845-53.
32. Burnham EL, Hyzy RC, Paine R 3rd, et al. Chest CT features are associated with poorer quality of life in acute lung injury survivors. Crit Care Med. 2013;41(2):445-56.
33. Rozencwajg S, Pilcher D, Combes A, et al. Outcomes and survival prediction models for severe adult acute respiratory distress syndrome treated with extracorporeal membrane oxygenation. Crit Care. 2016;20:392-401.
34. Singanayagam A, Schembri S, Chalmers JD. Predictors of mortality in hospitalized adults with acute exacerbation of chronic obstructive pulmonary disease. Ann Am Thorac Soc. 2013;10(2):81-9.
35. Costello R, Deegan P, Fitzpatrick M, et al. Reversible hypercapnia in chronic obstructive pulmonary disease: a distinct pattern of respiratory failure with a favorable prognosis. Am J Med. 1997;102(3):239-44.
36. Domenech A, Puig C, Martí S, et al. Infectious etiology of acute exacerbations in severe COPD patients. J Infect. 2013;67:516-23.
37. Celli BR. Predictors of mortality in COPD. Respir Med. 2010;104(6):773-9.
38. Martinez FJ, Foster G, Curtis JL, et al. Predictors of mortality in patients with emphysema and severe airflow obstruction. Am J Respir Crit Care Med. 2006;173(12):1326-34.
39. Vestbo J, Prescott E, Almdal T, et al. Body mass, fat-free body mass, and prognosis in patients with chronic obstructive pulmonary disease from a random population sample: findings from the Copenhagen City Heart Study. Am J Respir Crit Care Med. 2006;173(1):79-83.
40. Haruna A, Muro S, Nakano Y, et al. CT scan findings of emphysema predict mortality in COPD. Chest. 2010;138(3):635-40.
41. Van Hirtum PV, Sprooten RTM, Van Noord JA, et al. Long term survival after admission for COPD exacerbation: a comparison with the general population. Respir Med. 2018;137:77-82.
42. Brown JP, Martinez CH. Chronic obstructive pulmonary disease comorbidities. Curr Opin Pulm Med. 2016;22(2):113-8.

CHAPTER 6

Blood Transfusion in Critically Ill Patients

Ruchira W Khasne, Pradnya Atul Kulkarni, Atul Prabhakar Kulkarni

INTRODUCTION

Blood transfusion (BT) is one of the most common procedures performed in hospitals all over the world. There are considerable variations in transfusion practices among geographic regions.[1] BT may be lifesaving in some situations, but many studies have shown an increased morbidity and mortality associated with BT.[2] It is an independent predictor of organ dysfunction, nosocomial infection, acute respiratory distress syndrome and mortality.[3] At present, there are no randomized controlled trials (RCTs) suggesting that BT would really improve oxygen delivery or clinical outcomes in critically ill patients.[4] The indications for BT in the critically ill remain poorly defined and have been the subject of considerable debate. However, routine use of red blood cell (RBC) transfusion to treat anemia in hemodynamically stable critically ill patients without evidence of active bleeding is not supported by published studies.[5] This adds to a dilemma for the clinician to determine the optimum transfusion "trigger" which poses an additional challenge.

This review is restricted to the determination of transfusion trigger in critically ill patients and restrictive transfusion strategy, BT in various clinical situations, storage lesions, other strategies to reduce transfusion requirements, and current place of artificial blood.

EPIDEMIOLOGY

More than one-fourth of critically ill patients receive BT during their intensive care unit (ICU) stay. There has been little change in this statistics over the past decade in spite of scrutiny of transfusion practices. As per a recent audit,[1] the present percentage of patients who receive RBC transfusion was lower (26%), compared to those reported in older studies European Anemia and Blood Transfusion in Critical Care (ABC) study (37%), North American CRIT study (44%),[6] and the European Sepsis Occurrence in Acutely Ill Patients (SOAP) study.[6-8]

TRANSFUSION TRIGGER

Due to variable transfusion practices, the exact transfusion trigger has not been defined. It varies according to evidence of ongoing bleeding, hemodynamic instability, comorbid conditions (ischemic heart disease), severity scores, patient wishes (Jehovah's witness), and geographic region. However as per a worldwide audit of transfusion practices published in 2018, transfusion trigger is slightly lower in patients admitted to the ICUs in Western Europe (8.1 g/dL) or North America (7.9 g/dL) than those reported in the older studies, such as ABC (8.4 g/dL) and CRIT (8.6 g/dL).[6] A transfusion trigger of 7 g/dL, with a target hemoglobin (Hb) range of 7–9 g/dL, should be the default for all critically ill patients, except in conditions where comorbidities or acute illness-related factors alter clinical decision-making. But definitely it should not exceed 9 g/dL in most critically ill patients.[7] Clinical Practice Guideline from the American Association of Blood Banks (AABB) strongly recommends transfusion at Hb of 8 g/dL or less or for symptoms, such as chest pain, orthostatic hypotension, or tachycardia unresponsive to fluid resuscitation.[8]

Following recommendations are made by an American Society of Anesthesiologist's Task Force:[9]
- Hemoglobin level is above 10 g/dL: Transfusion is rarely indicated.
- Hemoglobin level is below 6 g/dL: Transfusion is almost always indicated.
- The determination of transfusion in patients whose Hb level is 6–10 g/dL should be based on any ongoing indication of organ ischemia, the rate and magnitude of any potential or actual bleeding, the patient's intravascular volume status, and risk of complications due to inadequate oxygenation.

IMPACT OF BLOOD TRANSFUSION ON PATIENT OUTCOMES

Following is the summary of the current evidence of impact of BT on the outcome of critically ill patients.
- A recent worldwide audit on transfusion practices showed that in patients who received transfusion at any time during the ICU stay had higher severity scores [simplified acute physiology score II (39.7 ± 17.7 vs 45.7 ± 17.1, P <0.001) and sequential organ failure assessment scores (5.4 ± 3.7 vs 8.1 ± 4.3, P <0.001)]. Transfusion was associated with longer ICU length of stay (LOS) (ICU-LOS) [in all patients 3.0 (1.0–8.0), in no transfusion group 2.0 (1.0–6.0), and in transfusion group, it was high 7.0 (2.5–15.0) P <0.001]. It has been also observed that more the number of transfused RBC units, more was the ICU and hospital mortality (21.5% vs 14.3% and 30.0% vs 19.6%, both P <0.001). However in multivariable analysis the relative risk (RR) of inhospital mortality was slightly lower after transfusion [hazard ratio (HR), 0.98; confidence interval (CI), 0.96–1.00; P = 0.048]. On further subgroup analysis, they found that there was a stepwise decrease in HR for mortality associated with transfusion as the severity of illness increased.[1]
- CRIT study by Corwin et al. in 2004 involving 284 ICUs (n = 4,892) observed that the number of RBC transfusions is independently associated with morbidity and mortality, ICU admission, hospital LOS, and increased in the cost.[7]
- The ABC study[10] showed that ICU and overall mortality rates were significantly higher in patients who received BT compared to those who did not (ICU mortality 18.5% vs 10.1%, P <0.001; overall mortality rate 29.0% vs 14.9%, P <0.001; and 28-day mortality 22.7% vs 17.1%, P = 0.02). They compared patients with similar degrees of organ dysfunction and that those who received BT were found to have higher mortality rate.
- The ABC trial reported contradictory findings to SOAP trial. It was a multicenter trial including 3,147 patients. They observed that though transfused patients were sicker with higher ICU and hospital mortality, but on adjusting for confounding factors using a Cox regression model on multivariate analysis, they found that BT was not significantly associated with death. In fact, transfused patients have had a better survival.[11] ABC and SOAP studies had same protocols but the results were different. Authors opined that there is a possibility that changes in practice such as more awareness about BT, and more use of leukodepleted blood in SOAP study (46% in ABC vs 76% in SOAP) led to improved outcome.

As per the current literature, RBC transfusion can improve patient outcomes provided severity of illness is taken into account, and the need for transfusion is decided on an individual basis.[1]

ASSOCIATION OF ANEMIA IN INTENSIVE CARE UNIT AND BLOOD TRANSFUSION

Healthy individuals maintain oxygen consumption by increasing cardiac index and oxygen extraction, but for critically ill patients, this may not be possible. Anemia may be less well tolerated and is associated with worst outcome during critical illness, particularly in patients with cardiovascular diseases (CVDs).[7] Anemia is an independent predictor of major adverse cardiovascular events in these patients.[12] This thus produces a therapeutic dilemma for the clinician when deciding about BT. It is important to assess the patient clinically in terms of tolerance for anemia and then decide about transfusion. Patients with CVD may benefit from higher transfusion thresholds than those without. After transfusion, there is no difference in 30-day mortality; however, there is increase in the risk of acute coronary syndrome (ACS) in patients with pre-existing CVD with restrictive transfusion category. Thus higher threshold for BT (Hb of 8 g/dL) should be accepted in this group of patients.[13] There is an increase in the perioperative risk of death, with a low preoperative Hb, particularly in patients with CVD.[14] A restrictive strategy is usually appropriate but risk should be stratified according to physiological reserve considering age, cardiac comorbidity, and risk of bleeding to determine threshold for transfusion. Optimal management of the anemia of critical illness is an area of controversy, and further research is needed.

RESTRICTIVE TRANSFUSION STRATEGY

Restrictive transfusion strategy (transfusion at Hb concentration 7.0–9.0 g/dL) has many advantages over liberal strategy. However, there is little information about absolute Hb levels or a specific clinical condition; in which, transfusions are known to improve oxygen delivery. Following RCTs have suggested that restrictive transfusion thresholds result in better outcomes than higher thresholds:

- The AABB guidelines on RBC transfusion strongly recommend adherence to restrictive transfusion strategy (7–8 g/dL) in hospitalized, stable patients.[8] The same guidelines have reported that 11 out of 19 trials showed lower mortality with restrictive transfusion strategy (RR, 0.85; 95% CI, 0.7–1.03).[8]
- Restrictive transfusion strategy is supported by a Cochrane review, which included 19 trials (6,264 patients). This strategy was associated with a reduction in RBC transfusion by 39% (RR, 0.61; 95% CI, 0.52–0.72). The average units of RBCs transfused were reduced by 1.19 U (95% CI, 0.53–1.85 U). However, heterogeneity between trials was statistically significant (P <0.00001; I^2 93%) for these outcomes. They added that restrictive transfusion strategies that did not impact the rate of adverse events compared to liberal transfusion strategies; in terms of mortality, cardiac events, myocardial infarction, stroke, pneumonia, and thromboembolism. In fact, restrictive transfusion strategies were associated with a statistically significant reduction in hospital mortality (RR, 0.77; 95% CI, 0.62–0.95) but not 30-day mortality (RR, 0.85; 95% CI, 0.70–1.03). However, this review did not comment on transfusion strategies in patients with ACS.[15]
- In 1999, a Canadian trial [The Transfusion Requirements in Critical Care (TRICC) trial] introduced the concept of restrictive transfusion strategy. Results of this study have influenced the practice in ICUs by raising concerns related to BT and encouraged intensivists to limit the use of BT. They randomly assigned patients into liberal BT strategy (Hb concentration kept at 10–12 g/dL) with a restrictive transfusion practice (Hb concentration maintained at 7–9 g/dL) with possible exception of patients with acute myocardial infarction and unstable angina. Liberal group received more units of RBCs (5.6 vs 2.6, P <0.01) compared with restrictive group. They found nonsignificant trend toward lower 30-day mortality for the restrictive group (18.7% restrictive vs 23.3% liberal, P = 0.11). However, the mortality rate during hospitalization was significantly lower in the restrictive-strategy group (22.2% vs 28.1%, P = 0.05). They concluded that Hb concentrations should be maintained between 7.0 g/dL and 9.0 g/dL.[16]
- The results of the TRICC study have been validated by two recent studies, the Transfusion Requirements After Cardiac Surgery (TRACS) study[17] and FOCUS (Functional Outcomes in Cardiovascular Patients Undergoing Surgical Hip Fracture Repair).[18] TRACS trial (502 postcardiac surgical patients) compared liberal strategy (hematocrit ≥30%) to a restrictive strategy (hematocrit ≥24%). The 30-day mortality was similar between groups (10% liberal vs 11% restrictive; between-group difference, 1%; 95% CI, -6% to 4%; P = 0.85). However, the study also suggested that irrespective of transfusion strategy, the number of transfused RBC units was an independent risk factor for clinical complications or death at 30 days (HR for each additional unit transfused 1.2; 95% CI, 1.1–1.4; P = 0.002). FOCUS trial showed that even in elderly patients, it is acceptable to limit the transfusion except for those with either symptoms of anemia or an Hb of 8 g/dL. Average Hb level in liberal strategy was 1.3 g/dL higher as compared to restrictive-strategy (P <0.001). They observed that the mortality rate or an inability to walk without human assistance at 60-day follow-up was similar in liberal strategy and restrictive-strategy groups (35.2% vs 34.7%, P = 0.90).
- A meta-analysis of three trials (2,364 participants) showed that a restrictive transfusion strategy using an Hb transfusion trigger of <7 g/dL results in a significant reduction in ACS (RR, 0.44; CI, 0.22–0.89), pulmonary edema (RR, 0.48; CI, 0.33–0.72), rebleeding (RR, 0.64; CI, 0.45–0.90), bacterial infections (RR, 0.86; CI, 0.73–1.00), and inhospital mortality (RR, 0.74; CI, 0.60–0.92), and total mortality (RR, 0.80; CI, 0.65–0.98), compared with a more liberal strategy. Also there was a reduction in the number of units transfused by 40%, with an average of 2 U less per person.[4]
- Another study reported no significant differences in 90-day mortality, numbers of ischemic events, adverse reactions, and use of life support in patients with lower Hb threshold transfusion strategy versus higher Hb threshold. The patients with lower threshold group received 50% less units of blood compared to higher threshold group.[19]
- A systematic review of 31 randomized trials (9,813 patients) found that with restrictive transfusion, the incidence of myocardial infarction remained unaltered (RR, 1.28; 95% CI, 0.66–2.49; P = 0.46; 4,730 patients). Thus restrictive transfusion strategies were found to be safer, and liberal transfusion strategy did not offer any benefit.[20] This is also supported by Cochrane review of six trials (2,722 participants) of RBC transfusion for patients undergoing hip fracture surgery.[21]

In conclusion, current evidence suggests that critically ill patients can be successfully managed with restrictive RBC transfusion strategy (Hb concentrations: 7–9 g/dL), with the possible exception of patients with acute myocardial infarction and unstable angina.[22] In restrictive transfusion, there is reduction in RBC use and a lower mean Hb concentration.[8]

ASSOCIATION OF BLOOD TRANSFUSION WITH MORTALITY IN CARDIAC PATIENTS

Whether BT benefits patients with myocardial infarction is debatable. In a meta-analysis, liberal BT strategy was associated with higher risk for mortality independent of baseline Hb level, nadir Hb level, and change in Hb level during the hospital stay in a multivariate analysis. It showed an increase in all-cause mortality with a strategy of BT versus no BT (18.2% vs 10.2%) (RR, 2.91; 95% CI, 2.46–3.44; P <0.001), with a weighted absolute risk increase of 12%. In addition to that, BT was significantly associated with a higher risk for subsequent myocardial infarction (RR, 2.04; 95% CI, 1.06–3.93; P = 0.03).[23] Thus, practice of routine or liberal BT in cardiac patients should not be encouraged.

The AABB guidelines suggest adherence to a restrictive strategy in hemodynamically stable hospitalized patients with pre-existing CVD. Transfusion should be considered for patients associated with symptoms or Hb level of 8 g/dL or less because overall mortality has not been shown to be increased. Use of fewer RBC transfusions reduces cost and risks for adverse effects of transfusion.[10]

However, there is some uncertainty about the risk for perioperative myocardial infarction associated with a restrictive transfusion strategy. Evidence supporting this is not large enough to define the risks and benefits of BT in this setting.

As per British Committee for Standards in Haematology guidelines, in patients with ACS, consider transfusion to keep Hb at >8 g/dL, maintain Hb >7 g/dL if the patient is anemic and has stable angina.[7]

Blood Transfusion in Sepsis

The Surviving Sepsis Campaign guidelines 2016 have strongly recommended that RBC transfusion should occur only when Hb concentration decreases to <7.0 g/dL in adults in the absence of myocardial ischemia, severe hypoxemia, or acute hemorrhage.[24] The Transfusion Requirements In Septic Shock trial, a prospective randomized multicenter trial, included patients with septic shock. They compared a transfusion threshold of 7 versus 9 g/dL.[19] The lower threshold group received less number of transfusions (median of 1 U of blood vs median of 4 U). They found a similar 90-day mortality (43.0% vs 45.0% in lower vs higher threshold group; with RR, 0.94; 95% CI, 0.78–1.09; P = 0.44). The number of patients with ischemic events and use of life support were similar in both groups.

Blood Transfusion in Trauma

Trauma is one of the leading causes of mortality worldwide and massive bleeding leading to hypovolemia remains the primary cause of death in initial 24 hours after injury. Traditionally, resuscitation has been initiated with large volumes of crystalloid, accompanied by treatment with RBCs if hemodynamic instability persists.[25] Administration of large crystalloid volumes is independently associated with increased hemorrhage and decreased survival rates in trauma. Damage control resuscitation strategy, i.e. rapid control of bleeding along with early supplementation of blood components, has been recommended. Patients with severe hemorrhage should undergo the massive transfusion (MT) protocol to restore the blood volume and clotting factors.[26]

Following are the strategies for transfusion in actively bleeding patient:[25]

- *Fixed-ratio approach*: It involves transfusion of RBCs, fresh frozen plasma (FFP), and platelets in a fixed ratio, i.e. 1:1:1, in order to provide a composition similar to whole blood. The Pragmatic Randomized Optimal Platelet and Plasma Ratios (PROPPR) trial compared transfusion of FFP, platelets, and RBC in a 1:1:1 versus a 1:1:2 ratio in severely bleeding trauma patients. No significant differences in mortality at 24 hours or at 30 days were observed. However, in 1:1:1 group, more number of patients achieved greater hemostasis and lower mortality due to exsanguinations.[27]
- *Thromboelastometry-guided approach*: It is based on the current understanding of the pathophysiology of trauma, coagulopathy, and selective replacement of blood products. Currently available blood tests for coagulation, such as prothrombin time, international normalized ratio, activated partial thromboplastin time, fibrinogen level/activity, and platelet count, are not designed for the diagnosis of coagulopathy or to guide hemostatic therapy. These tests also require prolonged turnaround time. Thus goal-directed therapy for the replacement of coagulation factors is specifically required.

The use of viscoelastic testing, i.e. rotational thromboelastometry (ROTEM) or thromboelastography (TEG), has become accepted standard of care in such settings. TEG provides a more appropriate approach to monitor hemostasis, as it quickly provides information about the polymerization of fibrin in the presence of platelet activity, fibrinogen deficiency assessment, and factor XIII deficiency.[25]

Tapia et al. have shown that MT guided by TEG is superior in resuscitating patients with penetrating trauma when compared to standard MT practice.[28] Meyer et al. demonstrated that ROTEM clot firmness at 10 minutes is helpful in predicting who would require MT in a trauma population.[29]

STATA (Strategy of Transfusion in Trauma Patients): a randomized trial by Rodrigues et al. included patient with severe trauma and high injury severity score and compared fixed-ratio protocol (1:1:1) versus TEG-guided approach. The primary outcome was organ dysfunction at day 1, 5, 7, and 28, and secondary outcomes were number of transfusions within 48 hours, LOS in hospital, duration of ventilator free days, and cost of treatment.[25] The results of this trial are awaited.

Blood Transfusion in Neurocritical Care

Although anemia is consistently associated with worse outcomes among patients with traumatic brain injury (TBI), there is insufficient evidence to make strong recommendations regarding the relative benefit of a liberal over a restrictive transfusion strategy.

In patients with TBI the target Hb can be kept between 7 g/dL and 9 g/dL. Those with TBI associated with evidence of cerebral ischemia consider target Hb >9 g/dL and with subarachnoid hemorrhage (SAH) the target Hb should be between 8 g/dL and 10 g/dL. If patients are presenting with an acute ischemic stroke, the Hb should be maintained above 9 g/dL.[7] There is clear agreement in literature that critically ill patients with TBI and Hb less than 7 g/dL should be transfused. However, the exact threshold between 7 g/dL and 10 g/dL remains a debatable issue.

Although the overall quality of the evidence is low, recent data from a review article found no difference in neurological outcomes between the restrictive and liberal transfusion strategies.[30]

In a recent international survey conducted on RBC transfusion practices for patients with acute brain injury in five critical care medicine societies; 54% intensivists reported an Hb threshold of less than 8 g/dL. However, more than 50% of these physicians transfused blood at higher Hb values.[31]

Randomized trials evaluating the optimal transfusion threshold for TBI patients are currently ongoing, which may answer this question in near future.

Other Strategies to Reduce Transfusion Requirements in Trauma Patients

Several other strategies to reduce the BTs in ICU can be implemented because of the concerns of safety, storage lesions, limited availability, and costs associated with blood products.[7,9]

- Measures should be undertaken to stop ongoing bleeding.
- Correct the lethal triad of hypothermia, acidosis, and coagulopathy.
- Consider stopping unnecessary anticoagulation and antiplatelet agents.
- Use of antifibrinolytic agents {tranexamic acid or epsilon-aminocaproic acid especially in early trauma [Clinical Randomization of an Antifibrinolytic in Significant Hemorrhage 2 (CRASH II) trial]}.
- Techniques of cell salvage during surgery.
- Use blood conservation devices while sampling.
- Administration of recombinant erythropoietin and iron supplementation. For both these strategies the evidence for improvement in outcome is awaited.
- Artificial oxygen carriers are under investigation but these have their own problems.

STORAGE LESIONS

Blood storage lesions is also an interesting area of debate. These are adverse effects associated with the storage of blood which usually begins after about 2 weeks of storage and progresses with duration of storage (RBC age). Current regulations permit the storage of red cells for up to 42 days depending on manufacturing process, additive solution, and local policies. The "storage lesion" refers to the multiple complex biochemical and biomechanical alterations that occur during ex vivo storage. Prolonged storage has been associated with changes that may render red cells ineffective as oxygen carriers and lead to accumulation of substances that have untoward biologic effects.[32] Critically ill patients may be particularly vulnerable to the effects of storage lesions, and longer the storage duration of RBC units prior to transfusion, worst is the outcome. However, the evidence base is insufficient to support the routine administration of "fresher blood" to critically ill patients.[7] Following are the main components of storage lesions:[33]

- *Changes occurring in RBC*:
  - Metabolic changes: Decreased 2-3 diphosphoglycerate, thereby impaired oxygen delivery, decreased phosphate and adenine pool [adenosine monophosphate, adenosine diphosphate, and adenosine triphosphate (ATP)], decreased glutathione

levels, decreased S-nitroso-Hb and increased lactate levels.
- Oxidative stress: Protein oxidation including cytoskeleton, lipid peroxidation (generation of lysophospholipids may cause transfusion-related acute lung injury), generation of prostaglandins, and isoprostanes.
- Changes in shape and membrane: Shift from early reversible echinocytes to irreversible spheroechinocytes, generation of microvesicles with procoagulant properties, increased RBC rigidity and adherence to vascular endothelium, decreased cluster of differentiation 47 expression, and increased phosphatidylserine exposure.

❏ *Changes occurring in the supernatant:*
- Decreased power of hydrogen.
- Increased potassium concentrations (decreased Na–K–ATPase activity) with increased risks of hyperkalemia.
- Release of various molecules: Proinflammatory cytokines [interleukin (IL)-1beta, IL-6, IL-8, and tumor necrosis factor-alpha] and complement, biologically active lipids, such as platelet-activating factor, free Hb prone to scavenge nitric oxide of the recipient, heme and iron with potential redox injuries, cytotoxicity, and inflammation.

A systemic review by Lebure and Vincent, which included 55 studies, looked at the association between RBC storage and outcomes in adult patients. Morbidity outcomes included hospital and ICU-LOS, infections, multiple organ failure, microcirculatory alterations, cancer recurrence, thrombosis, bleeding, vasospasm, SAH, and cognitive dysfunction. Twenty-six studies (47%) suggested detrimental effects of RBC storage on any clinical endpoint, whereas the remainder (53%) did not show any significant difference. However this comparison is difficult to interpret due to high degree of heterogeneity in study population. First, the review included different patient populations, such as cardiac surgery, trauma, sepsis, cancer patients, with varying percentage of deleterious impact of older RBCs on any end point. In addition to that, the study population had different outcome end points and with variable criteria for organ dysfunction. In addition, there were variable ways of reporting the age of transfused RBCs (mean age of all RBCs transfused, maximum age of RBCs, mean of the two oldest units, and proportion of RBCs older than a given number of days). This systematic review has found no definitive argument to support the superiority of fresh over older RBCs for transfusion.[33]

Another systematic review of 18 observational studies (409,840 patients) and three RCTs (126 patients) suggested that the transfusion of older RBC compared with newer RBC was associated with a 16% increase in the risk of death.[34] Wang et al. (meta-analysis 21 studies, 410,000 patients) in predominantly cardiac surgery and trauma patients found that the use of older stored blood is associated with significantly increased mortality risk (odds ratio 1.16).[35] A prospective, multicenter observational study, including 47 ICUs studied for 5-week period involving 757 critically ill adult patients, observed that exposure to older RBCs (22.7 days) was independently associated with an increased risk of death (21.3% vs 13.2%) compared to fresh RBCs (7.7 days).[35] Many studies have shown no significant difference on impact of RBC storage duration on patient outcome (Table 6.1).

ROLE OF LEUKODEPLETED BLOOD

Leukoreduction (LR) aims to attenuate transfusion-associated reactions by filtering donor leukocytes from packed RBC units. However, it has its own drawbacks too. Up to 10% of RBCs may be inadvertently removed during the filtering process. RBCs have also been shown to get hemolyzed during processing which affects its oxygen-

Table 6.1: Association of RBC storage duration with mortality and morbidity.

Study	Population	Type of study	Sample size	Outcome
ABLE Trial[36]	Critically ill adults with a high risk of death	Double-blind, multicentre RCT	2430	No significant difference in 90 day mortality
INFORM Trial[37]	Hospitalized patient who required BT >18 years	Unblinded, randomized	10,578	No significant difference in 90 day mortality
TRANSFUSE Trial[32]	Critically ill adult patient	Multicenter, RCT	4,919	The age of transfused red cells has no affect 90-day mortality among critically ill
RECESS Trial[38]	12 years or more, undergoing complex cardiac surgery	Multicenter, RCT	1,098	The duration of red-cell storage is not associated with significant differences in the organ dysfunction

(ABLE: age of blood evaluation; BT: blood transfusion; INFORM: Informing Fresh versus Old Red Cell Management; RCT: randomized controlled trial; RECESS: Red Cell Storage Duration Study)

delivering capacity.[39] As per current evidence, LR is effective for the prevention of human leukocyte antigen and human platelet antigen immunization and platelet refractoriness, especially in high-risk patients. LR has shown decreasing trends of alloimmunization and graft rejection in the cases of multiple surgeries related to solid organ transplants.[40] There is also a role of cytomegalovirus (CMV)-seronegative and leukodepleted blood components in preventing the risk of CMV transfusion transmission. LR is effective in reducing the rate of febrile nonhemolytic transfusion reaction.[41] It also plays a key role in the prevention of transfusion-transmitted Epstein-Barr virus, human T-lymphotropic virus type infections. With prion reduction filters, it provides promising results for the prevention of transfusion of Creutzfeldt-Jakob disease. However, clinical benefits of LR are not large as per the current evidence. Further studies are required to elucidate the benefits of LR with an additional concern about the cost-effectiveness.[41]

CURRENT EVIDENCE FOR THE USE OF ARTIFICIAL BLOOD

Blood transfusion carries risks, is expensive, and often its supply is scarce. Newer development of artificial RBC substitutes or synthetic oxygen transporters products is under intensive focus due to current ongoing increase in demand for blood products. The products studied are of mainly two types: Perfluorocarbon and Hb-based oxygen carriers (HBOCs) (polymerized HBOCs, cross-linked HBOCs, and conjugated HBOCs).[42] The risk of spreading an infectious disease is eliminated with the use of these products. However these products have limitations due to short half-life (most of the Hb-based products last not more than 20–30 hours in the body). And they do not perform other functions of blood, such as coagulation. Thus the current status of artificial blood products is limited to only short-term blood replacement applications. In the future, it is anticipated that new materials to carry oxygen in the body will be found having longer half-life and less side effects.

CONCLUSION

Anemia is common in the ICU and is associated with adverse consequences. Paradox exists regarding transfusion trigger practices in critically ill patients. RBC transfusion can be associated with better outcomes provided that the severity of illness and need for transfusion is taken into account and individualized. An assessment of the risk-to-benefit ratio of transfusion to improve O_2-carrying capacity is a key consideration to optimize patient outcomes. General attempts to minimize the use of blood products and nontransfusion-based strategies (e.g. antifibrinolytic drugs, such as tranexamic acid) and other measures to control bleeding, use of blood conservation devices while sampling should be pursued. Restrictive strategy (7-9 g/dL) has almost replaced liberal strategy which would have a large effect on RBC use and related risks of complications. RBC transfusion should be encouraged when Hb drops to <7.0 g/dL in hemodynamically stable critical patients in the absence of circumstances, such as myocardial ischemia, severe hypoxemia, or acute hemorrhage. In later conditions, higher Hb threshold of 7-9 g/dL is generally accepted. New development of artificial RBC substitutes would open a new horizon in the field of transfusion.

REFERENCES

1. Vincent JL, Jaschinski U, Wittebole X, et al. Worldwide audit of blood transfusion practice in critically ill patients. Crit Care. 2018;22:102.
2. Lelubre C, Vincent JL. Red blood cell transfusion in the critically ill patient. Ann Intensive Care. 2011;1:43.
3. Marik PE, Corwin HL. Efficacy of red blood cell transfusion in the critically ill: a systematic review of the literature. Crit Care Med. 2008;36:2667-74.
4. Salpeter SR, Buckley JS, Chatterjee S. Impact of more restrictive blood transfusion strategies on clinical outcomes: a meta-analysis and systematic review. Am J Med. 2014;127:124-31.e3.
5. Hébert PC, Tinmouth A, Corwin HL. Controversies in RBC transfusion in the critically ill. Chest. 2007;131:1583-90.
6. Corwin HL, Gettinger A, Pearl RG, et al. The CRIT study: anemia and blood transfusion in the critically ill—current clinical practice in the United States. Crit Care Med. 2004;32:39-52.
7. Retter A, Wyncoll D, Pearse R, Fink MP, Levy MM, Abraham E, et al. Guidelines on the management of anaemia and red cell transfusion in adult critically ill patients. Br J Haematol. 2013;160:445-64.
8. Carson JL, Grossman BJ, Kleinman S, Tinmouth AT, Marques MB, Fung MK, et al. Annals of internal medicine clinical guideline red blood cell transfusion : a clinical practice guideline from the AABB. Ann Intern Med. 2012;157:49-58.
9. American Society of Anesthesiologists Task Force on Perioperative Blood Transfusion and Adjuvant Therapies. Practice guidelines for perioperative blood transfusion and adjuvant therapies: an updated report by the American Society of Anesthesiologists Task Force on Perioperative Blood Transfusion and Adjuvant Therapies. Anesthesiology. 2006;105:198-208.
10. Vincent JL, Baron JF, Reinhart K, Gattinoni L, Thijs L, Webb A, et al. Anemia and blood transfusion in critically ill patients. JAMA. 2002;288:1499-507.
11. Vincent JL, Sakr Y, Sprung C, Harboe S, Damas P, et al; Sepsis Occurrence in Acutely Ill Patients (SOAP) Investigators, et al. Are blood transfusions associated with greater mortality rates? Anesthesiology. 2008;108:31-9.

12. Sabatine MS, Morrow DA, Giugliano RP, Burton PB, Murphy SA, McCabe CH, et al. Association of hemoglobin levels with clinical outcomes in acute coronary syndromes. Circulation. 2005;111:2042-9.
13. Docherty AB, Walsh TS. Anemia and blood transfusion in the critically ill patient with cardiovascular disease. Crit Care. 2017;21(1):61.
14. Carson JL, Duff A, Poses RM, Berlin JA, Spence RK, Trout R, et al. Effect of anaemia and cardiovascular disease on surgical mortality and morbidity. Lancet. 1996;348:1055-60.
15. Carson JL, Stanworth SJ, Roubinian N, Fergusson DA, Triulzi D, Doree C, et al. Transfusion thresholds and other strategies for guiding allogeneic red blood cell transfusion. Cochrane Database Syst Rev. 2016;2016:1-69.
16. Hebert PC. TRICC trial—a multicenter, randomized, controlled clinical trial of transfusion requirements in critical care. N Engl J Med. 1999;340:409-17.
17. Hajjar LA, Vincent JL, Galas FR, Nakamura RE, Silva CM, Santos MH, et al. Transfusion requirements after cardiac surgery: the TRACS randomized controlled trial. JAMA. 2010; 304: 1559-67.
18. Carson JL, Terrin ML, Noveck H. Liberal or restrictive transfusion in high-risk patients after hip surgery. N Engl J Med. 2011;365:2453-62.
19. Holst LB, Haase N, Wetterslev J, Wernerman J, Guttormsen AB, Karlsson S, et al. Lower versus higher hemoglobin threshold for transfusion in septic shock. N Engl J Med. 2014;371:1381-91.
20. Holst LB, Petersen MW, Haase N, Perner A, Wetterslev J, et al. Restrictive versus liberal transfusion strategy for red blood cell transfusion: systematic review of randomised trials with meta-analysis and trial sequential analysis. BMJ. 2015;350:h1354.
21. Brunskill SJ, Millette SL, Shokoohi A, Pulford EC, Doree C, et al. Red blood cell transfusion for people undergoing hip fracture surgery. Cochrane Database Syst Rev. 2015:CD009699.
22. Hébert PC, Yetisir E, Martin C, Blajchman MA, Wells G, Marshall J, et al. Is a low transfusion threshold safe in critically ill patients with cardiovascular diseases?. Crit Care Med. 2001;29:227-34.
23. Chatterjee S, Wetterslev J, Sharma A, Lichstein E, Mukherjee D, et al. Association of blood transfusion with increased mortality in myocardial infarction: a meta-analysis and diversity-adjusted study sequential analysis. JAMA Intern Med. 2013;173:132-9.
24. Rhodes A, Evans LE, Alhazzani W, Lichstein E, Mukherjee D, et al. Surviving Sepsis Campaign: international guidelines for management of sepsis and septic shock: 2016. Intensive Care Med. 2017;43(3):304-77.
25. Rodrigues R, Oliveira R, Lucena L, Lucena L, Paiva H, Cordeiro V, et al. STATA—Strategy of Transfusion in Trauma Patients: a randomized trial. J Clin Trials. 2016;6:287.
26. Sihler KC, Napolitano LM. Massive transfusion: new insights. Chest. 2009;136:1654-67.
27. Holcomb JB, Tilley BC, Baraniuk S, Fox EE, Wade CE, Podbielski JM, et al. Transfusion of plasma, platelets, and red blood cells in a 1:1:1 vs a 1:1:2 ratio and mortality in patients with severe trauma: the PROPPR randomized clinical trial. JAMA. 2015;313:471-82.
28. Haas T, Fries D, Tanaka KA, Asmis L, Curry NS, Schöchl H. Usefulness of standard plasma coagulation tests in the management of perioperative coagulopathic bleeding: Is there any evidence?. Br J Anaesth. 2015;114:217-24.
29. Laursen TH, Meyer MAS, Meyer ASP, Gaarder T, Naess PA, Stensballe J, et al. Thrombelastography early amplitudes in bleeding and coagulopathic trauma patients: results from a multicenter study. J Trauma Acute Care Surg. 2018;84:334-41.
30. East JM, Viau-Lapointe J, McCredie VA. Transfusion practices in traumatic brain injury. Curr Opin Anaesthesiol. 2018;31:219-26.
31. Badenes R, Oddo M, Suarez JI, Antonelli M, Lipman J, Citerio G, et al. Hemoglobin concentrations and RBC transfusion thresholds in patients with acute brain injury: an international survey. Crit Care. 2017;21:1-10.
32. Cooper DJ, McQuilten ZK, Nichol A, Ady B, Aubron C, Bailey M, et al. Age of red cells for transfusion and outcomes in critically ill adults. N Engl J Med. 2017;377:1858-67.
33. Lelubre C, Vincent JL. Relationship between red cell storage duration and outcomes in adults receiving red cell transfusions: a systematic review. Crit Care. 2013;17:R66.
34. Lacroix J, Hébert PC, Fergusson DA, et al. Age of transfused blood in critically ill adults. N Engl J Med. 2015;372:1410-8.
35. Pettilä V, Westbrook AJ, Nichol AD, Tinmouth A, Cook DJ, Marshall JC, et al. Age of red blood cells and mortality in the critically ill. Crit Care. 2011;15:R116.
36. Lacroix J, Hébert P, Fergusson D, Tinmouth A, Blajchman MA, Callum J, et al. The Age of Blood Evaluation (ABLE) randomized controlled trial: study design. Transfus Med Rev. 2011;25:197-205.
37. Eikelboom JW, Cook RJ, Barty R, Liu Y, Arnold DM, Crowther MA, et al. Rationale and design of the Informing Fresh versus Old Red Cell Management (INFORM) trial: an international pragmatic randomized trial. Transfus Med Rev. 2016;30:25-9.
38. Steiner ME, Ness PM, Assmann SF, Triulzi DJ, Sloan SR, Delaney M, et al. Effects of red-cell storage duration on patients undergoing cardiac surgery. N Engl J Med. 2015;372:1419-29.
39. Kim Y, Xia BT, Chang AL, Pritts TA. et al. Role of leukoreduction of packed red blood cell units in trauma patients: a review young. Int J Hematol Res. 2017;2:124-9.
40. Sarkar RS, Philip J, Yadav P. Transfusion medicine and solid organ transplant—update and review of some current issues. Med J Armed Forces India. 2013;69:162-7.
41. Bianchi M, Vaglio S, Pupella S, Marano, G, Facco, G, Liumbruno, G. M, et al. Leucoreduction of blood components: an effective way to increase blood safety? Review. Blood Transfus. 2016;14:214-27.
42. Moradi S, Jahanian-Najafabadi A, Roudkenar MH. Artificial blood substitutes: first steps on the long route to clinical utility. Clin Med Insights Blood Disord. 2016;9:33-41.

CHAPTER 7

Antibiotics in Intensive Care Unit

Alexis Tabah, Jeffrey Lipman

INTRODUCTION

Infections in the intensive care unit (ICU) are present in more than half of the patients and represent a very wide range of different conditions. The backbone of their treatment is urgent appropriate antimicrobials[1] and effective source control.[2]

By the way of selection pressure, antibiotics are responsible for the emergence of multidrug-resistant (MDR) bacteria. Side effects include *Clostridium difficile*-associated diarrhea, allergic reactions, liver and kidney injury. Research has shown benefit to a conservative approach.[3] In the absence of a definite clinical infection or hemodynamic instability, we recommend this approach where antibiotics are withheld awaiting microbiology results.

Antibiotics are used to prevent and treat bacterial infections. Antimicrobials include treatments used to treat bacteria and other agents, such as virus, fungi, and parasites. They may either be bactericidal and kill or bacteriostatic and inhibit the growth of the pathogens. Antibiotic dosing complexity is increased in the ICU by pharmacokinetic and pharmacodynamic (pk/pd) specificities to this patient group.

Hospitals and ICU's should develop stewardship programs and have written guidelines to which antibiotic to use for each clinical circumstance.[4] International guidelines describe best practice in specific conditions and diseases.[5-7] This chapter describes the principles underlying the optimal antibiotic prescription and does not aim to replace these resources and the knowledge acquired from specific sections of this book.

RATIONAL ANTIBIOTIC USE

Early and Appropriate Antibiotics for Severe Infections

Delays and inadequate antimicrobial therapy are associated with increased mortality.[8,9] Empirical treatment is the initial antibiotic given when the infection is first suspected, before the diagnosis is confirmed. Appropriate empiric treatment should include molecules active against all the likely pathogens.[10]

Empiric treatment choice should take in account:
- Epidemiology of bacteria responsible for each condition.
- Penetration and activity of each antibiotic at the suspected source of infection.
- The setting: Community-, hospital-, or ICU-acquired infections.
- Local epidemiology of resistance within each setting (the antibiogram).
- The carriage of MDR organisms. Detective work to obtain previous culture results is a key to treatment appropriateness.

Common examples of probabilistic antimicrobials include:
- Community-acquired pneumonia (CAP): *Streptococcus pneumoniae*, *Haemophilus influenzae*, and intracellular pathogens (*Legionella*, *Chlamydia*, *Mycoplasma*). In

severe infections, we use a combination of ceftriaxone and azithromycin.
- Intra-abdominal infections and fecal soiling are often polymicrobial, including Gram-negative bacilli (GNB), anaerobes, and Gram-positive bacteria (GPB). A beta-lactams with antianaerobe activity, such as amoxicillin and clavulanic acid, is used in the absence of MDR.
- Urinary tract infections: Mostly caused by GNB and should be treated with a beta-lactam, such as cefotaxime, as it is excreted in the urine.

For other conditions, we refer the reader to specific sections of this textbook.

In critically ill patients at high risk of MDR colonization, it is commonly recommended to initially prescribe broad-spectrum empiric antimicrobial therapy. Most often a broad-spectrum beta-lactam, and sometimes combination therapy with a companion antibiotic (glycopeptide and/or aminoglycoside), to ensure all potential pathogens are covered. This will be followed by antibiotic de-escalation (ADE) when culture results are available by reducing the spectrum of the pivotal beta-lactam and/or stopping the companion antibiotic when they are not required.[11]

Emergence of Resistance

Antibiotics are grouped into classes by chemical structure, mechanisms of action, and spectrum of activity. Different antibiotic molecules are effective against different kind of pathogens. Bacteria will be intrinsically sensitive or resistant to each agent[5] and may acquire resistance to agents they are normally sensitive to.[12]

Within bacterial populations, random mutations happen and provide some colonies with resistance genes. Selection pressure will only enable a resistant isolate to survive and amplify within a more susceptible bacterial population. Resistance can also be transferred from the environment, from other patients by cross contamination or even between different bacterial species that may share genetic material.[12]

When the concentration of antibiotics is too low at the site of infection the probability that a resistant clone will survive is increased. This may happen with insufficient or inappropriate dosing, or deep-seated abscesses where the antibiotics will only reach the outer layer of the infection.

Further, by destroying the anaerobic intestinal barrier flora, antibiotics allow pathogenic microorganisms initially present in very small amounts to survive. This may include C. difficile, fungus, and resistant GNB.

Broader spectrum antibiotics and sometimes combination therapy are required to treat those resistant bacteria. In turn, exerting increased selection pressure.

Even brief exposure to imipenem has been shown to cause colonization with carbapenem-resistant organisms.[13]

In the recent years, we have witnessed the emergence of MDR extremely, and even pan drug-resistant bacterium that has become resistant to those broader spectrum antibiotics. For those, there are little treatment options left.[2,14]

Source Control

Source control is the process of physically removing the focus of the infection, including removal of foreign bodies or infected materials, drainage and debridement of infected fluids and tissues, and prevention of ongoing or further microbial contamination.[15]

Deep-seated infections cannot be treated with antibiotics alone.[2,16] As for antibiotics, delays in source control are associated with poor outcomes.[2]

Microbiology

Multiples specimens should be sent for culture prior to starting or modifying antibiotic therapy. The bare minimum is a set of aerobe–anaerobe blood cultures and specimens from the source of the infection. At least 10 mL of blood should be drawn in each bottle. Appropriate sterile technique, amount of fluid, handling, and urgent processing are important. Specimens should be sent for at the time of source control and at each intervention.[16] The results will allow to adjust or to streamline the empirical treatment.[11]

Specimens should not delay urgent antimicrobial therapy. Examples are meningitis and peritonitis where antibiotics should be given after a set of blood cultures but before a specimen is obtained from the source.

Communication with the microbiologist is the key. The laboratory may process some specimens more urgently or use specific techniques if they are informed of the clinical problem, including which antibiotics are ongoing. Novel and rapid molecular diagnostic techniques may be available to give urgent results on the causing pathogen and their likely resistance patterns.

In some ICUs, surveillance cultures are taken systematically and targeted to identify colonization with specific resistant pathogens, such as methicillin-resistant *Staphylococcus aureus* (MRSA), vancomycin-resistant *Enterococcus* (VRE) or extended spectrum beta-lactamase, and carbapenem-resistant GNB.

Adequacy and Streamlining Antimicrobial Therapy

Appropriate antimicrobial therapy is defined as the use of agents with in vitro activity against the etiologic pathogens. To be considered adequate, it should also be at the optimal dose, correct route of administration, and with an antibiotic that will penetrate and reach sufficient concentration at the site of infection.[10]

The initial microscopic examination and Gram staining will inform on the presence of GBP or GNB. Specific agents may be added if those are not covered.

Cultures will take 2–3 days to inform on the growth and the type of bacteria and an antibiogram will take another day.

Treatment should then be reassessed considering the following options:
1. An infection is clinically confirmed, and the bacteria are sensitive to the treatment: the antibiotic is appropriate. Dosing regimen and duration of treatment may require adjustment.
2. The bacteria are resistant to the ongoing treatment. Escalation is required to a regimen active on that pathogen.
3. The pathogen is sensitive, but the spectrum is too broad. ADE may be performed.[11]
4. Cultures remain negative. Two possibilities are as follows:
   - There was no infection and antibiotics should be stopped.
   - There was an infection, but it is undocumented. Causes may include antibiotics preceding cultures, poor specimen quality, or difficult to grow bacteria. Treatment should be continued for a set duration according to the clinical diagnosis.
5. There is some bacterial growth, but the infection is not clinically likely. Antibiotics should be stopped. This has been shown to decrease the emergence of bacterial resistance and superinfection without affecting mortality.[17]

Treatment duration should be kept to its minimum to ensure clinical cure.[18] All recent research comparing durations of antibiotics has shown safety of the shorter option.

In the Case of Treatment Failure

If the patient is not improving, develops a new fever, or clinically deteriorates, the answer is not to simply escalate to broader spectrum antibiotics.

Differentials to consider include:
- Complications of the initial infection or its management
- Superinfection with a resistant organism
- Drug reactions
- *Clostridium difficile*-associated diarrhea
- Intensive care unit-related complications
- Infectious, such as central line-related bloodstream infections, catheter-related urinary tract infections, and ventilator-associated pneumonia
- Noninfectious, such as myocardial infarction, mesenteric ischemia, or pulmonary embolism.

Complete clinical examination, new microbiological specimens, and investigations targeted to the clinical differential are necessary. If appropriate, broadening the spectrum of the antibiotics should be done considering previous results.

A Broad Differential and the Difference Between Colonization and Infection

Signs of infection are that of inflammation and infections mimickers are multiple. In a study of patients with suspected septic shock, when no clear diagnosis was available at 24 hours, 44% were finally diagnosed an alternate noninfections conditions.[19]

Colonization is the presence of bacteria without infection. It is extremely common, and virtually all patients receiving mechanical ventilation will have colonization of their respiratory tract. How to differentiate colonization from infection is difficult and one of our reasons for intensive care medicine to exist as a specialty.

A patient with distributive shock or with clinical signs indicative of infection should most often be treated with antibiotics. However, a broad differential, at admission and each daily reassessment, is necessary to avoid unnecessary antimicrobials and delays to the management of an alternate diagnosis.

OTHER IMPORTANT ASPECTS TO CONSIDER

Antibiotic Allergy

Penicillin allergy is reported in about 10% patient's files, of which 90–99% are not truly allergic. This has been associated with an increased rate of health care–associated infections, including 30, 14, and 23% increased odds of VRE, MRSA, and *C. difficile* respective rates of colonization or infection. Recent reports show increased rates of surgical site infection and increased mortality in hematological malignancy when patients have a reported penicillin allergy.[20]

Anaphylactic reactions and toxic epidermal necrolysis are life-threatening reactions that should be avoided at all cost; in-depth history taking should be triggered by any allergy reported in the patient's chart to determine the reality of the allergy.

Antibiotic Prophylaxis

Prophylactic antibiotics are indicated for some (not all) surgical and percutaneous procedures usually immediately prior to the procedure. They should not be continued after the procedure is completed, "just in case" there may be an infection. Guidelines from the relevant scientific societies should be followed.

Patients receiving immunosuppressants, such as organ transplant recipients or severe rheumatologic conditions, may require lifetime prophylaxis for opportunistic conditions. When such patients are admitted with an acute infection, infectious disease (ID) stewardship and primary specialty should be consulted to target investigations and probabilistic management.

PHARMACOKINETIC PRINCIPLES

Initial recommendations for antibiotic dosing considered pk/pd data from healthy volunteers. This information usually included guidance on dose reduction in the cases of renal impairment.

Intensive care unit patients with septic shock have an increased volume of distribution (Vd), decreased albumin levels, and a high cardiac output. This may lead to a phenomenon called augmented renal clearance.[21] Adding to the complexity, some patients may receive renal replacement therapy.

This may lead to the initial dose of antibiotics to achieve lower than expected maximum serum concentration during a dosing interval (C_{max}) and to be eliminated faster and reach lower than expected trough serum concentration (C_{min}).

Recent research describes the requirement for much higher dosing that initially recommended. While overdosing may increase toxicity, achieving proper concentrations is vital to avoid treatment failure and emergence of antibiotic resistance.

Continued dosing should be adjusted according to clinical progress and organ failures. Where available it is important to use therapeutic drug monitoring (TDM) and pk software to accurately define drug exposure and the need for altered dosing.

MAIN ANTIBIOTIC CLASSES

Four commonly used antibiotic classes have been chosen as examples to describe common pk/pd principles. See Figure 7.1 for targets in each case.

Beta-Lactams

Beta-lactam antibiotics are bactericidal by inhibiting the synthesis of the peptidoglycan layer of the bacterial cell wall.

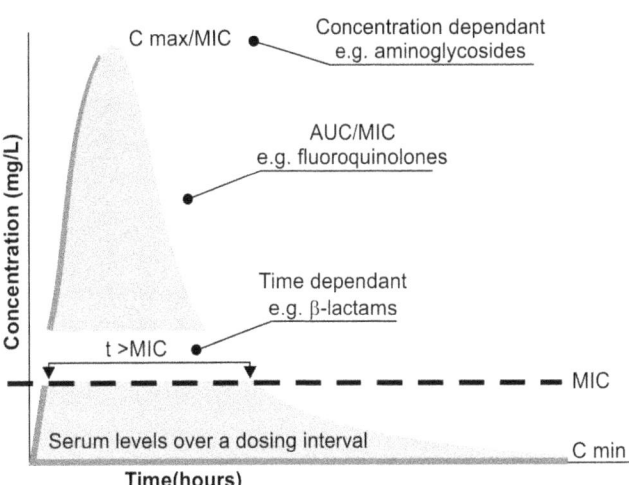

FIGURE 7.1: Pharmacodynamic targets of different classes of antibiotics.
(MIC: minimum inhibitory concentration; AUC: area under the inhibitor curve)

This class includes multiple agents and subclasses that have in common the beta-lactam ring. Spectrum ranges from narrow spectrum for penicillin, extended spectrum ureidopenicillins-carboxypenicillins active against *Pseudomonas* species, five generations of cephalosporins and carbapenems.

Carbapenems were long considered the antibiotic active against all problematic MDR. In the recent years, carbapenem resistance has been spreading to become endemic in many regions.

In general, the bactericidal activity of beta-lactams is slow, time dependent, and maximal at relatively low concentrations. It is related to the time that plasma and tissue levels exceed a certain threshold.[21] Increasing the time that concentration of the antibiotic is above the minimum inhibitory concentration (MIC) to 50 or 100% may be necessary to improve clinical outcomes.[22] Some beta-lactams may require the use of extended (more than 3 hours) or continuous infusions (CI) to reach adequate pk/pd targets. This is currently being investigated in a large multinational multicenter trial.

Fluoroquinolones

Broad-spectrum antibiotics are active against many GPB and GNB, including *Pseudomonas* species; they are lipophilic molecules with activity against intracellular pathogens, such as *Legionella*. Fluoroquinolones are bactericidal by targeting deoxyribonucleic acid (DNA) gyrase and topoisomerase, preventing DNA strand rejoining. The bactericidal activity is largely related to concentration-dependent kill characteristics, but also some concentration-dependent effects. Recommended target is to achieve high area under the inhibitor curve (AUC) with an AUC/MIC more than 125 being a commonly recognized target.[23]

Dosing is complicated in ICU patients, and TDM is not widely available. Problematic side effects include confusion and QT prolongation with a risk of torsade de pointe in the ICU population. Their potential to cause the emergence resistance has led some institutions to restrict their use as reserve antibiotics for difficult to treat GNB that have become resistant to beta-lactams.

Aminoglycosides

Aminoglycosides are most often used as a companion antibiotic, part of combination therapy for severe infections with GNB.[11] They have weak activity against GPB and none against anaerobic GNB. They are bactericidal by binding to the ribosomes and disrupting protein synthesis.[24]

Aminoglycosides kill characteristics are concentration dependent with a significant postantibiotic effect.[23] Current recommendation is to target a maximum serum concentration (C_{max}) of eight times the MIC. Their Vd is increased in critically ill patients, and higher doses than previously recommended are required to achieve these targets.[25] There is concern of significant nephrotoxicity and ototoxicity. This may be decreased by once daily dosing and short treatment duration.

Glycopeptides

Vancomycin is the most commonly used glycopeptide. It is slowly bactericidal on GPB by inhibition of peptidoglycan and bacterial cell wall synthesis. It has no activity on GNB.

It is renally excreted, and the best determinant of vancomycin efficacy is the AUC/MIC.[23]

A loading dose of 25 mg/kg should be administered at no more than 1,000 mg/h. Further dosing can be administered as an intermittent infusion (II) or a CI, with dosing based on renal function and subsequent adjustment on TDM. Targets are of 15–20 mg/L on II and 20–25 mg/L for CI.

PRACTICE PRESCRIPTION

Those are summarized in the following rules:
- Antibiotics should be given urgently to patients with severe infections. Probabilistic antibiotics should target the most probable pathogens.
- Cultures should be taken before the antibiotic is given but not delay its administration.
- Communication with the microbiology laboratory and IDs stewardship services is important.
- Microbiology results should be followed at least daily.
- The antibiotic regimen needs to be evaluated daily for continuation or modification.
- Antibiotic course should be as short as necessary, and they should be stopped as soon as possible:
  - If there is no infection.
  - When the infection is cured.
- In the case of failure to improve, worsening, or treatment failure, consider and investigate a wide differential before broadening the antibiotics.

REFERENCES

1. Levy MM, Evans LE, Rhodes A. The Surviving Sepsis Campaign Bundle: 2018 update. Intensive Care Med. 2018;44(6):925-8.
2. Tabah A, Koulenti D, Laupland K, et al. Characteristics and determinants of outcome of hospital-acquired bloodstream infections in intensive care units: the EUROBACT International Cohort Study. Intensive Care Med. 2012;38:1930-45.
3. Hranjec T, Rosenberger LH, Swenson B, et al. Aggressive versus conservative initiation of antimicrobial treatment in critically ill surgical patients with suspected intensive-care-unit-acquired infection: a quasi-experimental, before and after observational cohort study. Lancet Infect Dis. 2012;12:774-80.
4. Barlam TF, Cosgrove SE, Abbo LM, et al. Implementing an antibiotic stewardship program: guidelines by the Infectious Diseases Society of America and the Society for Healthcare Epidemiology of America. Clin Infect Dis. 2016;62:51-77.
5. Torres A, Niederman MS, Chastre J, et al. International ERS/ESICM/ESCMID/ALAT guidelines for the management of hospital-acquired pneumonia and ventilator-associated pneumonia: guidelines for the management of hospital-acquired pneumonia (HAP)/ventilator-associated pneumonia (VAP) of the European Respiratory Society (ERS), European Society of Intensive Care Medicine (ESICM), European Society of Clinical Microbiology and Infectious Diseases (ESCMID) and Asociación Latinoamericana del Tórax (ALAT). Eur Respir J. 2017;50(3).1-6.
6. Habib G, Lancellotti P, Antunes MJ, et al. 2015 ESC guidelines for the management of infective endocarditis: The Task Force for the Management of Infective Endocarditis of the European Society of Cardiology (ESC). Endorsed by: European Association for Cardio-Thoracic Surgery (EACTS), the European Association of Nuclear Medicine (EANM). Eur Heart J. 2015;36(44):3075-128.
7. Tunkel A, Hartman BJ, Kaplan SL, et al. Practice guidelines for the management of bacterial meningitis. Clin Infect Dis. 2004;39(9):1267-84.
8. Bloos F, Rüddel H, Thomas-Rüddel D, et al. Effect of a multifaceted educational intervention for anti-infectious measures on sepsis mortality: a cluster randomized trial. Intensive Care Med. 2017;43:1602-12.

9. Liu VX, Fielding-Singh V, Greene JD, et al. The timing of early antibiotics and hospital mortality in sepsis. Am J Respir Crit Care Med. 2017;196:856-63.
10. Siempos II, Ioannidou E, Falagas ME. The difference between adequate and appropriate antimicrobial treatment. Clin Infect Dis. 2008;46:642-4.
11. Tabah A, Cotta MO, Garnacho-Montero J, et al. A systematic review of the definitions, determinants, and clinical outcomes of antimicrobial de-escalation in the intensive care unit. Clin Infect Dis. 2016;62:1009-17.
12. Barbier F, Luyt CE. Understanding resistance. Intensive Care Med. 2016;42:2080-3.
13. Armand-Lefèvre L, Angebault C, Barbier F, et al. Emergence of imipenem-resistant gram-negative bacilli in intestinal flora of intensive care patients. Antimicrob Agents Chemother. 2013;57:1488-95.
14. Magiorakos A, Srinivasan A, Carey RB, et al. Multidrug-resistant, extensively drug-resistant and pandrug-resistant bacteria: an international expert proposal for interim standard definitions for acquired resistance. Clin Microbiol Infect. 2012;18(3):268-81.
15. Marshall JC, Maier RV, Jimenez M, et al. Source control in the management of severe sepsis and septic shock: an evidence-based review. Crit Care Med. 2004;32(Suppl. 11):S513-26.
16. Sartelli M, Catena F, Abu-Zidan FM, et al. Management of intra-abdominal infections: recommendations by the WSES 2016 consensus conference. World J Emerg Surg. 2017;12:22.
17. Singh N, Rogers P, Atwood CW, et al. Short-course empiric antibiotic therapy for patients with pulmonary infiltrates in the intensive care unit. A proposed solution for indiscriminate antibiotic prescription. Am J Respir Crit Care Med. 2000;162:505-11.
18. Garnacho-Montero J, Arenzana-Seisdedos A, De Waele J, et al. To which extent can we decrease antibiotic duration in critically ill patients?. Expert Rev Clin Pharmacol. 2017;10:1215-23.
19. Contou D, Roux D, Jochmans S, et al. Septic shock with no diagnosis at 24 hours: a pragmatic multicenter prospective cohort study. Crit Care. 2016;20(1):360.
20. Blumenthal KG, Ryan EE, Li Y, et al. The impact of a reported penicillin allergy on surgical site infection risk. Clin Infect Dis. 2018;66:329-36.
21. Udy AA, Roberts JA, Lipman J. Clinical implications of antibiotic pharmacokinetic principles in the critically ill. Intensive Care Med. 2013;39(12):2070-82.
22. Roberts JA, Paul SK, Akova M, et al. DALI: defining antibiotic levels in intensive care unit patients: are current ß-lactam antibiotic doses sufficient for critically ill patients?. Clin Infect Dis. 2014;58:1072-83.
23. Roberts JA, Lipman J. Pharmacokinetic issues for antibiotics in the critically ill patient. Crit Care Med. 2009;37:840-51.
24. Kohanski MA, Dwyer DJ, Collins JJ. How antibiotics kill bacteria: from targets to networks. Nat Rev Microbiol. 2010;8:423-35.
25. Tabah A, Lipman J, Roberts JA. Are new gentamicin dosing guidelines suitable for achieving target concentrations in patients with sepsis and septic shock?. Anaesth Crit Care Pain Med. 2016;35:311-2.

CHAPTER 8

Sedation in the Critically Ill

Andrew Li, Amartya Mukhopadhyay

INTRODUCTION

The art of sedation among the critically ill in the intensive care unit (ICU) is a difficult one. The zeal of controlling the ICU triad of pain, agitation, and delirium (PAD) underscores the oft-neglected intricate relationship of how the different classes of sedatives and analgesics in different combinations interact with one another. Advances have been made in recent years on sedative strategies and even nonpharmacological methods to help to improve sedation-related outcomes. This chapter summarizes the current evidence available aimed at improving the sedation practices in the critically ill.

Pain is an unpleasant sensory and emotional experience associated with tissue damage.[1] Pain is common among the critically ill who may undergo multiple ICU and surgical interventions, with more than 50% reporting pain.[2] Even routine nursing interventions, such as turning, dressing change, and tracheal suctioning, can inflict pain. In addition, these patients are relatively immobile, resulting in musculoskeletal stiffening and neuropathies, thus further contributing to pain. Inadequate pain control will eventually lead to increased energy expenditure, oxygen consumption, and endogenous catecholamine activity. Inadequate pain control can also inhibit effective cough reflex and deep breathing, contributing to respiratory complications. Pain is often assessed by directly asking the patient; however, if the patient is unable to respond, the Behavioral Pain Scale (BPS) or Critical Care Pain Observation Tool (CPOT) is recommended to ensure that analgesic dosage is carefully titrated.[3,4]

Critically ill patients need to be appropriately sedated to synchronize with mechanical ventilation, reduce anxiety, and allow nursing care. Ideally, they should be comfortable, calm, and able to cooperate and engage with caregivers and family. "Light" sedation is currently recommended and can be assessed either by Richmond Agitation–Sedation Scale or Sedation–Agitation Scale.[1]

COMMONLY USED SEDATIVES AND ANALGESICS IN THE INTENSIVE CARE UNIT

Table 8.1 summarizes the onset of action, half-lives, and side effects of common agents.[5]

Opioids

Opioids form the mainstay of analgesia in the ICU. The most frequently used opioids are morphine and fentanyl. Opioids act on the µ1 opioid receptor inhibiting pain response in the central nervous system. Due to the higher bioavailability and easier dose titration, intravenous route is preferred compared to enteral route or patches. Opioids are primarily metabolized in the liver followed by renal clearance of the metabolites. Some metabolites (e.g. morphine-3-glucuronide and morphine-6-glucuronide) have potent analgesic effects and may accumulate in

Table 8.1: Pharmacology of commonly used sedatives and opioids.

Drug	Onset	Half-life	Dose	Purpose	Side effects	Action
Sedative agents						
Midazolam	2–5 minutes	3–12 hours	0–15 mg/h	Sedation, hypnotic, anticonvulsant effects	Respiratory depression, metabolites accumulates in renal failure	Acts on GABA receptor
Lorazepam	5–20 minutes	10–20 hours	0.01–0.1 mg/kg/h	Sedative, analgesia, sympatholytic, anti-delirium effects	Hypotension, bradycardia	
Dexmedetomidine	5–10 minutes	2 hours	0.2–1.5 μg/kg/h			
Propofol	30–45 seconds	10 minutes	0.5–3 mg/kg/h	Sedative, hypnotic, anxiolytic, amnestic, anticonvulsant effects	Vasodilatory hypotension, propofol infusion syndrome	α2 agonist acting on locus coeruleus inhibiting norepinephrine release
Ketamine	30 seconds	10 minutes	0.05–0.1 mg/kg/h	Hypnotic, amnestic, analgesia	Increased catecholamine increased cerebral blood flow, bronchodilation	NMDA antagonist
Opioids						
Morphine	5 10 minutes	3–4 hours	0–25 mg/h	Analgesia	Metabolite accumulate in renal failure, histamine release	Act on μ1 opioid receptor, weak δ and κ receptor agonist
Fentanyl	1 minute	2–4 hours	25–250 μg/h	Analgesia	High dose leads to muscle rigidity. Can accumulate in renal failure	Act on μ1 opioid receptor
Remifentanil	1–3 minutes	3–10 minutes	0.02–0.2 μg/kg/min	Analgesia, sedative	Vomit, constipation	Act on μ1 opioid receptor

(GABA: gamma-aminobutyric acid; NMDA: N-methyl-D-aspartate)

renal failure. Fentanyl has no active metabolites and has a shorter duration of action; hence, many ICUs use fentanyl as their first-line analgesic.[6] Adverse effects include development of drug tolerance and dose-related respiratory depression. Fentanyl in high doses can paradoxically cause muscle rigidity. Morphine has an added effect of histamine release, thus contributing to hypotension and unstable hemodynamics. In patients with chronic opioid use, hyperalgesia may occur with worsening agitation. Remifenanil is a new very short-acting synthetic opioid and has the potential to reduce duration of mechanical ventilation and ICU length of stay (LOS).[7]

Benzodiazepines

Benzodiazepines (BZD) possess anxiolytic, sedative, and hypnotic effects. BZDs bind to the gamma-aminobutyric acid receptors in the brain and have opioid-sparing effect by modulating anticipatory pain response. Commonly used BZDs are midazolam and lorazepam (Table 8.1). Midazolam has faster onset of action by crossing the blood–brain–barrier more easily than lorazepam. Like opioids, BZD and their metabolites can accumulate with renal and liver failure.

Despite their popularity and lower cost, recent studies have shown that BZD are deliriogenic compared to other sedative agents.[8-10] BZDs worsen sleep architecture, delay emergence from sedation, prolong mechanical ventilation duration and ICU LOS. This could be due to the alteration of levels of potentially deliriogenic neurotransmitters, such as acetylcholine, dopamine, and serotonin.[5] BZD also potentiate post-traumatic stress disorder in a dose-related fashion, and with large doses of lorazepam, propylene glycol (solvent) toxicity may occur.[5] However, BZD are still indicated in refractory status epilepticus, intractable agitation, palliation, and alcohol withdrawal syndromes.

Propofol

Propofol has sedative, hypnotic, and amnestic properties. It is also an anticonvulsant and has added effect of reducing intracranial pressure. Importantly, propofol clearance is not altered by liver or renal failure. Its rapid onset and offset of action makes it an easily titratable sedative to use (Table 8.1) and is recommended as the first-line sedative agent by the PAD guideline.[1] Propofol is dissolved in fat and provides 1.1 kcal/mL of energy.

Main adverse side effects are hypotension due to systemic vasodilation, immunosuppressant effects, and the development of propofol infusion syndrome (PRIS).[11] PRIS is rare and usually occurs only at high propofol infusion doses. The risk exponentially increases if the infusion rate is more than 4 mg/kg/hour for at least 48 hours.[11] PRIS resembles mitochondrial disorders, where energy production is reduced through inhibition of the intracellular transport of long-chain fatty acids and the respiratory chain. This results in rhabdomyolysis, renal failure, hepatomegaly, hypertriglyceridemia, metabolic acidosis, and cardiovascular collapse. The production of phenols and uric acid gives rise to the green urine. Treatment is mainly supportive and cessation of the propofol infusion.[11]

Compared to BZD, propofol has lower delirium incidence, reduces duration of mechanical ventilation, and facilitates earlier ICU discharge.[9]

Dexmedetomidine

Dexmedetomidine belongs to the family of α2 agonists acting on the locus coeruleus to inhibit norepinephrine release. It has sedative, analgesic, anti-delirium, and sympatholytic properties. Importantly, it does not cause respiratory depression and can be used for short procedures even in nonintubated patients.[12] However, it can cause hypotension and bradycardia in a dose-related fashion.

Dexmedetomidine is effective as a sedative agent comparable to propofol and BZD.[13] It can attain sedation targets more easily with less delirium or coma incidence. Possible immunomodulatory effect and trend of mortality benefit among patients with sepsis were suggested in the MENDS study.[8] Recent studies have also emphasized on dexmedetomidine's anti-delirium effect. Adding dexmedetomidine nocturnally up to 0.7 µg/kg/min reduced the incidence of delirium by 30%.[14] Dexmedetomidine is safe even among non-intubated patients with hyperactive delirium and may facilitate extubation even when the patient is delirious. It reduces both delirium duration and incidence compared to BZD. Due to the analgesic effect, the concurrent sedatives and opioids doses can be minimized. Satisfactory sedation levels were still achieved, and there were cost savings due to the reduction in ICU LOS.

Volatile Anesthetic Agents

Examples include sevoflurane, desflurane, and isoflurane. They have a rapid onset of action, minimal adverse effects with little concerns of drug tolerance. Rapid offset is aided by pulmonary exhalation, without the need to perform dose adjustments in renal or liver failure.

However, they require specialized ventilators and miniature vaporizers. Studies have been limited to their usage in the short-term postoperative setting. Their impacts on hemodynamic, neurological state, and the kidneys are yet to be fully explored. Since they are eliminated via lungs, their use may not be suitable among patients who require lung-protective ventilation strategies.[15]

THE PAIN, AGITATION, AND DELIRIUM SYNDROME IN INTENSIVE CARE UNIT

Pain

More than 50% of ICU patients have suboptimal pain control.[2] Barriers to achieving adequate pain control include inability of patient to communicate, failure to assess and acknowledge the existence of pain, fear of precipitating opioid addiction, and personal bias and perception.[2] In order to overcome the barriers, the updated guidelines have proposed an evidence-based multimodal analgesic strategy, targeting different parts of the nociceptive pathways.[1] The analgesia can then be titrated to the objective pain assessment tools to achieve optimal control. During pain assessments, observing patient's vital signs (blood pressure, heart rate, and respiratory rate) are not accurate. Instead, self-reporting scales, such as the Numerical Rating Scale, are commonly used.[1] When self-reporting is not possible, the BPS and the CPOT have evidence for reliability and validity.[3,4] CPOT has been validated even among delirious patients.[16]

The first-line analgesic is an opioid. However, given the dose-related adverse effects, a multimodal strategy is now advocated to maximize opioid-sparing effects. Dexmedetomidine, low-dose ketamine infusion, and intravenous paracetamol are good adjuncts. For patients with neuropathic pain, adjunctive gabapentin or carbamazepine can be used. Nonsteroidal anti-inflammatory drugs, while effective, are not usually recommended in ICU due to the risk of stress ulcers and renal impairment.

Patient-controlled analgesia is another possible alternative to aid in minimizing opioid use. Thoracic epidural anesthesia is now the recommended postoperative analgesia in patients undergoing operation for abdominal aortic aneurysm and traumatic rib fractures.[1] Challenges include the technical difficulties in block placement, catheter insertion, bleeding, and infection risks associated with the catheters. Given the lack of evidence, no other recommendation for regional or neuraxial anesthesia has been made. Other possible opioid-sparing strategies are nonpharmacological. Concurrent music and relaxation therapy, massages, application of heat or cold packs, and early mobilization are some of the suggested measures. Early removal of drains and lines is helpful.

The timing of analgesia administration is also important. Preemptive analgesia and intermittent increases in analgesia for procedure-related pain are helpful. An example would be administering a fentanyl bolus to reduce the pain prior to turning the patient. In the present era, analgosedation is suggested as one of the main strategies, where pain management remains the top priority (see later).

Agitation

At present, deep sedation has only proposed for those with severe respiratory failure with patient-ventilator asynchrony, paralysis, prone position, status epilepticus, therapeutic hypothermia, and severe brain injury with raised intracranial pressure. Studies have shown that deeper sedation levels within the first 48 hours increased the risks of death up to 2 years, even in the emergency department setting.[17] Deep sedation can lead to respiratory depression, diaphragmatic dysfunction with increased risk of prolonged mechanical ventilation, weaning, and ICU LOS.[17] There are presently three proposed sedation minimization strategies, which are as follows:

1. *Analgosedation*: Less sedation is required with adequate pain control; therefore, is of paramount importance.[2] A 2010 study in Denmark[18] showed that a strategy of only morphine administration and without any sedation reduced days on the mechanical ventilator. However, this group of patients may have increased delirium and a higher staffing ratio was required.

2. *Light sedation*: This implies titrating sedation to objective scoring systems. Successful implementation requires a combination of the correct choice of sedative agent and close titration of the sedative intensity. The aim is to prevent sedation-related harm, rather than focusing on reactive interventions to reverse responsiveness. Given the impact of early deep sedation, some have advocated early goal-directed sedation, analogous to early goal-directed resuscitation.[19]

3. *Daily interruption of sedation*: Daily spontaneous awakening trial and spontaneous breathing trial have individually demonstrated their ability to reduce the duration of mechanical ventilation without impacting patients' comfort or safety.[20] When combined, they led to even longer mechanical ventilator-free days, shorter ICU stays, and coma duration[21] without any increased incidence of post-traumatic stress disorder. However, there was no difference in psychological or cognitive outcomes. With early mobilization, the synergistic effect helped further reduce the duration of mechanical ventilation, delirium, and improved functional outcomes.[22] This is likely due to the reduction in sedation use and sedation-induced immobility. By achieving independence more quickly, patients avoided pressure wounds, ventilator-associated events, and delirium. This has led to the promulgation of the Awakening and Breathing Coordination, Delirium Monitoring and Management, and Early Mobility (ABCDE) approach.[22] Despite the evidence, the ABCDE approach has yet to be fully implemented due to lack of nursing acceptance, concerns of device dislodgement, patient discomfort, and respiratory compromise.

Combination of strategies: One strategy may not be superior to the other, and various combinations of strategies have been attempted. A RCT had shown that addition of daily sedation interruption to a protocolized sedation does not reduce duration of ventilation or ICU stay.[23] However, in this study, BZD was the main sedative agent. The adherence to daily sedation interruption was poor and the amount of sedation used in the intervention group was higher. One proposal is the eCASH concept (early comfort using analgesia, minimal sedatives, and maximal humane care) combines the strategies of adequate analgesia with targeted light sedation to effect sequential process-of-care intervention and facilitate patient-centered care.[24]

Delirium

Delirium is defined as a syndrome characterized by the acute onset of cerebral dysfunction with a change or fluctuation in baseline mental status, inattention, and either disorganized thinking or an altered conscious level[25] and may affect up to 80% of mechanically ventilated patients.[10] During critical illness, it has been postulated that inflammation can lead to the degradation of the blood–brain barrier, endothelial dysfunction, alterations in the cerebral blood flow, and neurotransmitter levels (acetylcholine and monoamines).[10] Delirium can be hypoactive, hyperactive or mixed and may lead to increased nursing care burden, patient-ventilator asynchrony, and poor sleep quality. A delirious agitated patient may receive higher sedation rather than elucidating the primary cause of agitation.

The risk factors for delirium are many and found in Table 8.2. The prediction of delirium in ICU patients' equation was created to help predict the development of delirium within 24 hours of ICU admission.[26] Objectively, delirium can be difficult to evaluate, given its waxing and waning nature. The Confusion Assessment Method for the ICU (CAM-ICU) and Intensive Care Delirium Screening Checklist (ICDSC) has been validated to detect delirium.[10]

A multidisciplinary approach is required to both treat and prevent ICU delirium. Nonpharmacological interventions include reorientation by the nurses, use of hearing aids and clocks, allowing day–night orientation by exposure to sunlight, and ensuring better sleep. Maintenance of the circadian rhythm by dimming lights at night, earplugs, and reducing the alarm and environmental noise at night can be useful.[10] The ABCDE approach has been shown to effectively reduce delirium, particularly with early mobilization.[22]

Currently, the mainstay pharmacological options are dexmedetomidine and antipsychotics. The evidence with dexmedetomidine has already been mentioned. Haloperidol can be used to treat acute delirium, but prophylactic haloperidol has no benefit in preventing delirium or reducing ICU LOS. Intravenous haloperidol is preferred as this route has less extrapyramidal side effects. In addition, quetiapine is the preferred antipsychotic, helping to improve agitation and delirium more quickly with less haloperidol required. Sedation minimization strategies and avoiding BZD can help to minimize delirium.

USE OF SEDATIVES IN ELDERLY

Elderly patients are more sensitive to BZD and may also take longer to wake up from sedation. Fentanyl has minimal pharmacokinetic problem with age, but elderly patients are twice as sensitive to the pharmacodynamic effect of fentanyl compared to the younger patients. Propofol has classic three-compartment model of distribution: A central, rapidly equilibrating peripheral and slowly equilibrating peripheral compartments. With advanced age, the central compartment is smaller, leading to higher peak propofol levels after bolus doses. Patients with hypovolemia also have reduced volume of central compartment, making them further susceptible to the hypotensive effects of propofol. Interaction of commonly used analgesia and sedatives is also important in elderly patients with multiple comorbidities including renal and liver impairments.

CONCLUSION

Advances in sedation have provided new evidence to decide strategies, but there are many barriers to overcome. A multifaceted, multimodal evidence-based strategy is paramount to ensure good sedation practices, with the aim of adequate pain control and minimizing sedative use. This can lead to a reduction in delirium, shorter duration of mechanical ventilation, and ICU stay.

REFERENCES

1. Barr J, Fraser GL, Puntillo K, et al. Clinical practice guidelines for the management of pain, agitation, and delirium in adult patients in the intensive care unit. Crit Care Med. 2013;41(1):263-306.

Table 8.2: Risk factors of development of delirium.

Modifiable factors	Non-modifiable factors
Length of ICU stay	Age
No visible daylight	Dementia hypertension
Lack of hearing and visual aids	APACHE II score
Night time interruptions	Mechanical ventilation
Amount of sedation	Emergency surgery
Type of sedation (BZD)	Organ failure
Number of infusions	Metabolic acidosis
Use of restraints	Coma
Use of centrally acting medication	
Presence of urinary catheters, central catheters, gastric tubes	

(APACHE: Acute Physiologic Assessment and Chronic Health Evaluation; BDZ: benzodiazepine; ICU: intensive care unit)

2. Sigakis MJ, Bittner EA. Ten myths and misconceptions regarding pain management in the ICU. Crit Care Med. 2015;43(11):2468-78.
3. Gelinas C, Harel F, Fillion L, et al. Sensitivity and specificity of the critical-care pain observation tool for the detection of pain in intubated adults after cardiac surgery. J Pain Symptom Manage. 2009;37(1):58-67.
4. Aissaoui Y, Zeggwagh AA, Zekraoui A, et al. Validation of a behavioral pain scale in critically ill, sedated, and mechanically ventilated patients. Anesth Analg. 2005;101(5):1470-6.
5. Devlin JW, Roberts RJ. Pharmacology of commonly used analgesics and sedatives in the ICU: benzodiazepines, propofol, and opioids. Crit Care Clin. 2009;25(3):431-49, vii.
6. Patel SB, Kress JP. Sedation and analgesia in the mechanically ventilated patient. Am J Respir Crit Care Med. 2012;185(5):486-97.
7. Zhu Y, Wang Y, Du B, et al. Could remifentanil reduce duration of mechanical ventilation in comparison with other opioids for mechanically ventilated patients? A systematic review and meta-analysis. Crit Care. 2017;21(1):206.
8. Pandharipande PP, Pun BT, Herr DL, et al. Effect of sedation with dexmedetomidine vs lorazepam on acute brain dysfunction in mechanically ventilated patients: the MENDS randomized controlled trial. JAMA. 2007;298(22):2644-53.
9. Lonardo NW, Mone MC, Nirula R, et al. Propofol is associated with favorable outcomes compared with benzodiazepines in ventilated intensive care unit patients. Am J Respir Crit Care Med. 2014;189(11):1383-94.
10. Jackson P, Khan A. Delirium in critically ill patients. Crit Care Clin. 2015;31(3):589-603.
11. Diedrich DA, Brown DR. Analytic reviews: propofol infusion syndrome in the ICU. J Intensive Care Med. 2011;26(2):59-72.
12. Venn RM, Hell J, Grounds RM. Respiratory effects of dexmedetomidine in the surgical patient requiring intensive care. Crit Care. 2000;4(5):302-8.
13. Jakob SM, Ruokonen E, Grounds RM, et al. Dexmedetomidine vs midazolam or propofol for sedation during prolonged mechanical ventilation: two randomized controlled trials. JAMA. 2012;307(11):1151-60.
14. Skrobik Y, Duprey MS, Hill NS, et al. Low-dose nocturnal dexmedetomidine prevents ICU delirium. A randomized, placebo-controlled trial. Am J Respir Crit Care Med. 2018;197(9):1147-56.
15. Jerath A, Parotto M, Wasowicz M, et al. Volatile anesthetics. Is a new player emerging in critical care sedation?. Am J Respir Crit Care Med. 2016;193(11):1202-12.
16. Kanji S, MacPhee H, Singh A, et al. Validation of the critical care pain observation tool in critically ill patients with delirium: a prospective cohort study. Crit Care Med. 2016;44(5):943-7.
17. Stephens RJ, Dettmer MR, Roberts BW, et al. Practice patterns and outcomes associated with early sedation depth in mechanically ventilated patients: a systematic review and meta-analysis. Crit Care Med. 2018;46(3):471-9.
18. Strom T, Martinussen T, Toft P. A protocol of no sedation for critically ill patients receiving mechanical ventilation: a randomised trial. Lancet. 2010;375(9713):475-80.
19. Shehabi Y, Bellomo R, Reade MC, et al. Early goal-directed sedation versus standard sedation in mechanically ventilated critically ill patients: a pilot study. Crit Care Med. 2013;41(8):1983-91.
20. Kress JP, Pohlman AS, O'Connor MF, et al. Daily interruption of sedative infusions in critically ill patients undergoing mechanical ventilation. N Engl J Med. 2000;342(20):1471-7.
21. Girard TD, Kress JP, Fuchs BD, et al. Efficacy and safety of a paired sedation and ventilator weaning protocol for mechanically ventilated patients in intensive care (Awakening and Breathing Controlled trial): a randomised controlled trial. Lancet. 2008;371(9607):126-34.
22. Schweickert WD, Pohlman MC, Pohlman AS, et al. Early physical and occupational therapy in mechanically ventilated, critically ill patients: a randomised controlled trial. Lancet. 2009;373(9678):1874-82.
23. Mehta S, Burry L, Cook D, et al. Daily sedation interruption in mechanically ventilated critically ill patients cared for with a sedation protocol: a randomized controlled trial. JAMA. 2012;308(19):1985-92.
24. Vincent JL, Shehabi Y, Walsh TS, et al. Comfort and patient-centred care without excessive sedation: the eCASH concept. Intensive Care Med. 2016;42(6):962-71.
25. Reade MC, Finfer S. Sedation and delirium in the intensive care unit. N Engl J Med. 2014;370(5):444-54.
26. van den Boogaard M, Pickkers P, Slooter AJ, et al. Development and validation of PRE-DELIRIC (PREdiction of DELIRium in ICu patients) delirium prediction model for intensive care patients: observational multicentre study. BMJ. 2012;344:e420.

CHAPTER 9

Delirium: Prognosis and Outcome

Ruchira W Khasne, Atul Prabhakar Kulkarni

INTRODUCTION

Delirium is a neuropsychiatric syndrome, which is transient and usually reversible. It is defined as a disturbance in attention, awareness, and cognition that develops over a short period of time and fluctuates in severity.[1] It is a very common phenomenon in intensive care unit (ICU) yet an underdiagnosed form of organ dysfunction. High-risk populations include elderly and mechanically ventilated ICU patients.[2] It can be particularly challenging to diagnose delirium in patients with preexisting cognitive impairment, dementia, or psychiatric conditions. Delirium significantly affects the outcome of patients, which warrants us to implement definitive strategies toward early recognition of delirium, which is predictable, preventable, and treatable with appropriate monitoring.

EPIDEMIOLOGY

Incidence and prevalence of delirium is variable across studies depending on the patient population examined and the method of diagnosis. Incidence of delirium has been reported from 16% to 89% of hospitalized patients.[3] It is highest in mechanically ventilated patients (80%).[4] Elderly and postoperative patients are most vulnerable. Incidence of postoperative delirium varies from 10% to 70%.[5] A large international multicenter survey including 104 ICUs from 11 countries has shown the prevalence of delirium to be 32.3%. Patients who developed delirium had higher severity illness on admission, and this was associated with an increased ICU mortality (20% vs 5.7%; P = 0.002) and hospital mortality (24% vs 8.3%; P = 0.0017).[6] Implementation of ICU team practices to systematically evaluate patients for delirium improves the outcome of patients.

SUBTYPES OF DELIRIUM

Three subtypes of delirium are identified as hyperactive, hypoactive and mixed.[7] A prospective cohort study observed that delirium occurred in 43% of 325 patients. Out of these, 43% patients with delirium, 19 (15%) were hyperactive, 24 (19%) were hypoactive, 65 (52%) had a mixed picture, and 17 patients (14%) had no symptoms. Hypoactive delirium is the most common motor subtype. Elderly patients are more vulnerable to have hypoactive delirium and it is associated with worse prognosis. The 6-month mortality in hypoactive delirium compared with other types of delirium was higher (32% vs. 8.7%).[8]

PATHOPHYSIOLOGY

The pathophysiology of delirium is complex, multifactorial, and poorly understood. There is interaction of different pathways leading to disruption of neuronal networks causing imbalance in neurotransmitters that normally control cognitive function, behavior, and mood.[9]

Factors contributing to delirium as postulated are as follows:[9,10]

- Altered neurotransmitters: An excess of dopamine or depletion of acetylcholine (major contributor) and less

commonly γ-aminobutyric acid, serotonin, endorphins, and glutamate are supposedly involved.
- Systemic inflammation leading to systemic hypotension and hypoxia resulting in impaired cerebral perfusion pressure, oxidative metabolism, and ischemia.
- Availability of large neutral amino acids leading to elevated levels of dopamine and norepinephrine.
- Abnormal stress response, due to cortisol-related decline in cognition and aging.

CLINICAL FEATURES

The diagnosis of delirium is frequently missed or misdiagnosed in multiple clinical settings, such as dementia, depression, mania, psychotic disorders or a typical response of the aging of brain. It can occur at any age, but it occurs more commonly in elderly patients and with prior or present cognitive impairment. Signs and symptoms are described in Table 9.1.[4]

RISK FACTORS FOR DELIRIUM[4,11,12]

Delirium is usually multifactorial in origin, and it is potentially reversible. The presence of factors associated with increased risk of delirium warrants a closer clinical monitoring. Four baseline risk factors associated with the development of ICU delirium are pre-existing dementia, history of hypertension and/or alcoholism, and a high severity of illness at admission. In addition to that, coma is an independent risk factor for the development of delirium in ICU patients. Traditionally benzodiazepines (BZD) have been preferred sedative agents in ICU, but various studies have identified BZD as a risk factor for the development and worsening of delirium in adult ICU patients[13] (Table 9.2).

Table 9.1: Clinical features of delirium.

Signs/Symptoms as a hallmark of delirium	Acute onset, fluctuating course, poor attention, disorganized thinking, altered level of consciousness Other features: Disorientation, memory impairment, day–night reversal (increased agitation in late afternoon or early evening), psychomotor agitation and slowness, hallucination
Behavioral	Hyperactivity, hypoactivity, fear, irritability and combativeness, attempt to run or attack others or remove indwelling catheters, acute sensitivity to sound and light, vocal disturbance
Functional impairment	Incontinence, falls, dependence on others for care

Table 9.2: Risk factors for delirium.

Risk factors	Nonmodifiable	Modifiable
Baseline or predisposing risk factors	• Advanced age • History of cognitive impairment • Hypertension, other comorbidities, e.g. renal, liver disease, stroke	• Alcohol misuse • Use of psychoactive drugs (narcotics) • Benzodiazepine dependence • Cigarette smoking
Acute illness and illness-related factors	High severity of illness score Coma	• Hypotension • Hypoxia • Sepsis • Metabolic disturbances • POD
ICU environmental or treatment related		• Medication-induced coma, e.g. BZD use • Pain • Immobility • Physical restraints • Disorientation (e.g. no eyeglasses or hearing aid) • Sleep deprivation • Isolation • Indwelling catheters

(BZD: benzodiazepines; ICU: intensive care unit; POD: postoperative delirium)

DELIRIUM MONITORING TOOLS

Various delirium monitoring tools are available, such as Intensive Care Delirium Screening Checklist (ICDSC), Nursing Delirium Screening Scale, Cognitive Test for Delirium, Confusion Assessment Method (CAM), CAM-ICU, Delirium System Interview, and Delirium Detection Score.[14] The CAM-ICU and ICDSC are currently the two valid reliable instruments with high interrater reliability when tested by ICU nurses and intensivists as described in Table 9.3.[4] These tests facilitate identification of history or time course of any cognitive changes that may otherwise go undiagnosed. Delirium detected by these tests is associated with adverse clinical outcomes including increased duration of mechanical ventilation (MV), ICU and hospital length of stay (LOS), increased health-care costs, cognitive impairment, physical disability, and death.[14,15]

As per Tomasi et al, delirium patients diagnosed by CAM-ICU or ICDSC presented similar clinical profile; however, CAM-ICU is a better predictor of outcome.[16]

Table 9.3: Assessment of delirium tools.

Assessment tools	Component of assessment tools	Sensitivity (%)	Specificity (%)	Scoring
CAM-ICU	4 cardinal symptoms of delirium plus attention screening examination	95–100	89–93	• The CAM-ICU reports a dichotomous assessment at a single time point • Positive CAM if 1 and 2 components present
ICDSC	Total 8 components	99	64	• Observed over a period of time • Score ≥4 suggestive of delirium

(CAM-ICU: confusion assessment method for the intensive care unit; ICDSC: intensive care delirium screening checklist)

IMPACT OF DELIRIUM ON PATIENT'S OUTCOME

The dose–response effect is observed between association of delirium with various clinical outcomes after adjusting clinical covariates, such as preexisting comorbidities, severity of illness and age.[17] Delirium affects both the short-term and long-term outcomes of patients.

Association with Mortality

Delirium is an independent predictor of mortality (three times higher risk of 6-month mortality) even after adjusting for various covariates.[2,5,6,18]

E Wesley Ely in a study involving 275 patients found that patients with delirium had higher 6-month mortality rates (34% vs 15%, P = 0.03).[2]

Salluh et al. conducted a meta-analysis of 28 studies. The odd ratio for death in patients with delirium was 2.19 (95% CI, 1.78–2.70; P <0.001) and adjusted risk of mortality considering covariates remained high in the delirium group (OR 2.72, 95% CI, 1.75–3.69).[6]

An international survey undertaken by Salluh et al. in 104 ICUs from 11 countries reported that delirium was associated with increased ICU (20% vs 5.7%; P = 0.002) and hospital mortality (24% vs 8.3%; P = 0.0017) as compared to nondelirious patients. In the multivariate analysis, delirium was an independent predictor of ICU (OR = 3.14, 95% CI; 1.26–7.86); and hospital mortality (OR = 2.5, 95% CI; 1.1–5.7).[18]

Length of Stay

Delirium is an independent risk factor associated with prolonged ICU and hospital stay in those receiving MV even after adjusting for covariates.[2,4,5] The delirium patients have twice the risk of prolonged ICU stay as compared to nondelirious patients and have 60% more risk of prolonged hospital stay after ICU discharge [adjusted hazard ratio (HR), 2.0; 95% CI, 1.4–3.0; P <0.001]. A meta-analysis of 28 studies reported that length of stay is significantly longer in patients with delirium (standardized mean difference 1.38, 95% CI, 0.99–1.77; P < 0.001) compared with nondelirious patients.[6] An international multicenter survey reported similar findings.[18]

Duration of Mechanical Ventilation

Duration of MV is longer in patients with delirium than in those without it (1.79 days, ranges 0.31–3.27 days; P < 0.001).[6]

Duration of Delirium and Outcomes

It is not only the presence of delirium but also the number of days spent in a delirious state that determines the mortality, days of MV, and length of ICU stay. These deleterious effects are predominantly observed in early period of brain dysfunction that is within a period of 4 days.

There is a significant nonlinear relationship between number of days of delirium and mortality (P < 0.001 and = 0.02 for the nonlinear effect). Patients having delirium on only one day showed all-cause 30-day mortality of 14.5% (N = 8 of 55), whereas it increased to 39% (N = 52 of 132) for those with 3 days or more of delirium.[17] Association of delirium with increased mortality is estimated as a 10% increase in the relative risk of death for each day of delirium within 1 year of post ICU admission.[19] It also affects total number of days spent in hospital (20% increased risk) and in wards (10% risk).[2]

Postoperative delirium (POD): It is commonly observed in postoperative geriatric patients. A meta-analysis which included 34 studies (7,338 patients undergoing noncardiac surgery), tried to assess a causal relationship between new onset (incident) delirium and postoperative mortality. Among the included trials were studies with significant heterogeneity and high risk of bias. Postoperatively 10.8% of those who developed delirium died as compared to 8.7% of the nondelirious patients. The unadjusted OR for mortality in patients with incident delirium was 4.12 (95% CI, 3.29–5.17), seemingly higher than those without delirium. However, once the confounding factors were adjusted for, this difference reduced substantially. This seems to suggest that either the effect of incident delirium on postoperative mortality is lower than previously assumed or delirium simply reflects the severity of illness rather than being independent predictor of mortality.[20]

Accidental falls: Delirious patients often have risk of fall and causing self-injuries. Fall prevention programs should be implemented to recognize undiagnosed delirium, patient safety, functioning, and quality of life.[21]

Functional dependence: Delirium causes acute functional decline thus resolved delirium results in faster functional recovery compared to persistent delirium.[22]

Health-care cost: Delirium impacts the outcome, requiring prolonged institutionalization, and thus increases the cost incurred.[11]

Long-term consequences: Delirium is a predictor and is an independent risk factor of long-term cognitive impairment in ICU patients.[2,4,5,23,24] It was seen to cause mild (OR, 2.41; 95% CI, 1.57–3.69) to severe (3.10; 95% CI, 1.10–8.74) cognitive dysfunction, after multivariate analysis was carried out in a prospective study in 1,101 patients by Wolters.[25] However, same study showed that it was not associated with long-term mortality or worsening of self-reported health-related quality of life (HRQoL) after adjusting for confounding factors including severity of illness throughout ICU stay (HR, 1.26; 95% CI, 0.93–1.71) and HRQoL (regression coefficient: –0.04; 95% CI, –0.10 to 0.01).[25] Van Den Boogaard et al. also reported similar finding of long-term cognitive impact because of delirium.[26]

MANAGEMENT

Identification, screening, prevention, and treatment are the mainstays of the management of patients with delirium. The most important step in delirium management is early recognition. There are no diagnostic tests (laboratory, electrophysiological, or imaging tests) to diagnose delirium. Diagnosis of delirium remains clinical. A delirium management algorithm is described in Flowchart 9.1. Both prevention and treatment should focus on the minimization and/or elimination of predisposing and

FLOWCHART 9.1: Clinical approach and management algorithm for delirium.

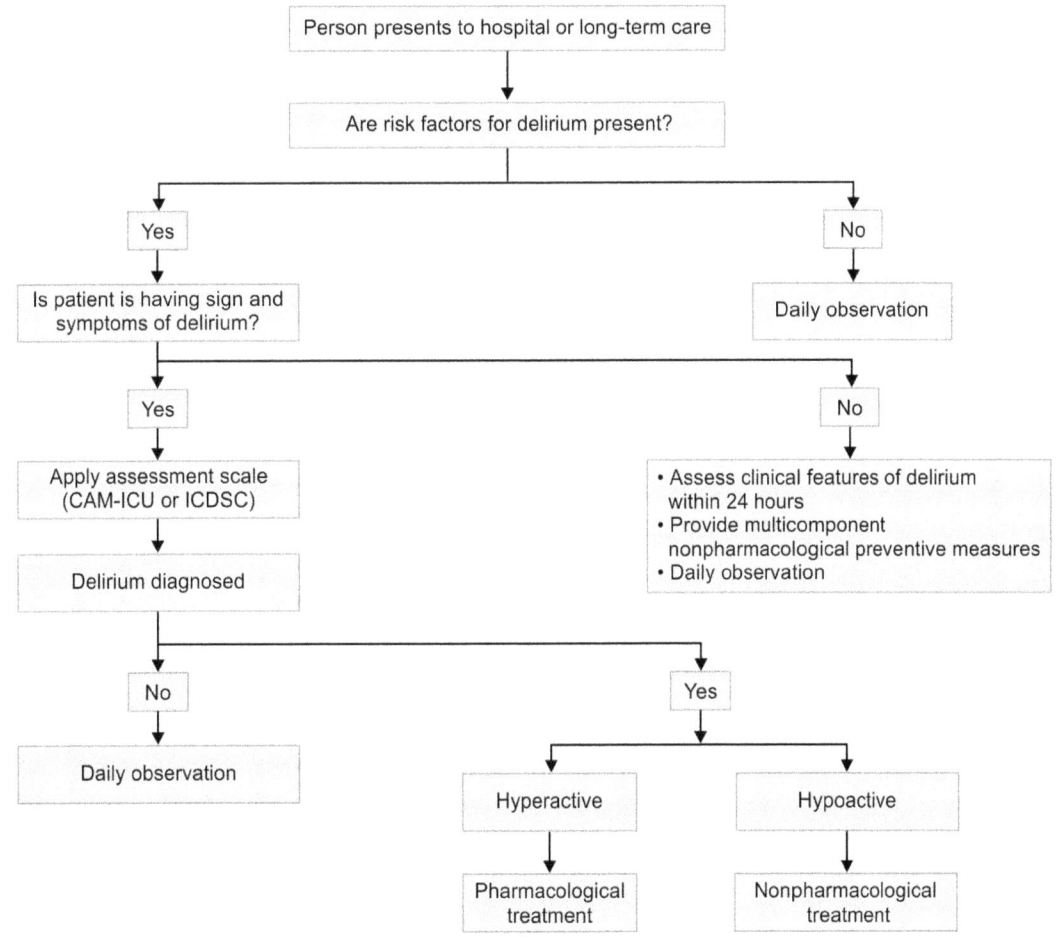

precipitating factors. Recognition of hypoactive delirium is particularly challenging, and usually there is an overlap between hypoactive delirium and reduced arousal states. It is often missed, or it may be confused with other central nervous system (CNS) conditions, such as Wernicke's encephalopathy, withdrawal (alcohol), hypertensive encephalopathy, hypoglycemia, metabolic/endocrine disorders, CNS infections, such as encephalitis, intracranial disease, e.g. traumatic brain injury, seizures, tumors, substance abuse, organ dysfunctions, such as renal failure, hepatic failure, cardiac insufficiency, and respiratory insufficiency.

Delirium prevention and treatment strategies can be categorized as nonpharmacologic, pharmacologic, and combined approaches.[6]

Nonpharmacological Therapies for Prevention and Treatment of Delirium

Prevention is a key factor in the management of delirium. Primary prevention with nonpharmacologic multi-component approach should be implemented not only to prevent delirium but also its persistence. The burden of delirium can be reduced with following nonpharmacologic measures.

Early and (frequent) Ambulation of Intensive Care Unit Patients

In ICU, patient mobilization at early stages of illness improves outcome,[27] shortens duration of delirium, and increases ventilator-free days compared with standard care.[28] Therapy can progress from passive range of motion to active range of motion, exercise in bed, sitting, standing, walking, and activity of daily living, the training depending on a patient's sedation level and physical abilities.

Sleep Hygiene

Intensive care unit is characterized by frequent interruptions of patient's normal sleep due to various factors, such as continuous alarms, lights, beepers, care-related interruptions, pain, anxiety, and ventilator dyssynchrony, as well as continuous medications.[29] Evidence suggests that promotion of normal sleep patterns through nonpharmacologic means can reduce the incidence of delirium. Noise-reduction strategies (such as earplugs), normalizing day–night illumination, minimizing care-related interventions during normal sleeping hours, and interventions promoting patient comfort and relaxation are low risk and inexpensive and should be implemented to prevent delirium.[30]

Remove Lines and Tubes

Invasive devices, such as vascular, urethral catheters, and endotracheal tubes (ETTs), can be a significant cause of discomfort to ICU patients leading to delirium. The presence of invasive lines and tubes can also prevent patients from participating in early mobilization efforts, which contributes to delirium. Daily review of these devices and use of criterion-based reminders to remove invasive devices, such as ICU daily rounding checklists, facilitates early discontinuation of invasive devices and also allows for early mobilization reducing delirium.[31]

Avoid Physical/Chemical Restraints

Use of physical restraints is a modifiable risk factor for development of delirium.[32] BZD are often administered as a chemical restraint. It precludes patients from participating in early mobilization efforts and also exerts a deliriogenic effect. Hence judicious and limited use of restraints helps in minimizing ICU delirium.

Reorient Intensive Care Unit Patient

Reorienting patients is an effective strategy for reducing and preventing ICU delirium. Reorientation techniques involve familiarization of the patient with surroundings, involving patient and family during ICU rounds, training the staff so that they introduce themselves, provision of visual and hearing aids, cognitive stimulation programs with avoidance of sensory deprivation.[29] Let patient know their schedule and keep them involved in their own care. Colombo et al. found that adding reorientation strategies, such as environmental, acoustic, and visual stimulation, to an ICU process of care reduced the incidence of delirium from 35% to 22% (P = 0.020).[33]

Eliminate Deliriogenic Medications

Assessment of polypharmacy is a high-yield procedure. Delirium risk appears to be increased with opioids (OR, 2.5, 95% CI, 1.2–5.2), benzodiazepines (OR 3.0, 95% CI 1.3–6.8), dihydropyridines (OR 2.4, 95% CI 1.0–5.8) and possibly antihistamines (OR 1.8, 95% CI 0.7–4.5). Drugs, such as H_2 antagonists, tricyclic antidepressants, antiparkinson medications, steroids, nonsteroidal anti-inflammatory drugs, and antimuscarinics, have uncertainty to cause delirium, whereas no increased risk is associated with neuroleptics (OR 0.9, 95% CI 0.6–1.3) or digoxin (OR 0.5, 95% CI 0.3–0.9).[13,34] Hence patient should be frequently assessed for the need of prescribed medications, and unnecessary agents should be discontinued as soon as possible.[31]

Nutrition Supplementation and Avoidance of Dehydration

Often these patients are not able to take care of themselves due to functional dependency. Hence supportive care, including nutrition and hydration, should be always provided.

Preventing Delirium through Pharmacologic Interventions

At present, no medications are approved by the US Food and Drug Administration (FDA) for the prevention of ICU delirium.[35]

Prophylactic administration of antipsychotics, cholinesterase inhibitors are intended to prevent delirium may be indicated in elderly postoperative patients, but the results to date suggest that their use is not warranted in critically ill patients. Haloperidol or atypical antipsychotics should not be used prophylactically to prevent delirium.[4] A recent randomized controlled trial, Haloperidol Effectiveness in Intensive Care Unit Delirium, has shown no difference in days alive and free of delirium or coma between patients prophylactically treated with intravenous Haloperidol (2.5 mg every 8 hours) compared to placebo. In addition to that, in Haloperidol group, oversedation was a common adverse effect.[36] Implementation of appropriate sedation protocol and optimum analgesics have definitive role in reducing delirium.

Use of Appropriate Sedative Agents

Multiple studies have found that BZD-based sedation practices are associated with higher incidence of delirium. BZD-sparing sedative agents should be incorporated in sedation protocol in ICU, along with daily assessment and interruption of sedative agents.[13] Addition of daily spontaneous breathing trials to a sedation protocol, as described in Awakening and Breathing Controlled Trial, further reduces the duration of acute brain dysfunction significantly.[30]

Non-BZD sedative agents, such as propofol[37] and dexmedetomidine,[38] are preferred sedative agents over BZD in mechanically ventilated patients. These studies have demonstrated faster awakening time and shorter duration of MV. In a randomized trial comparing dexmedetomidine with BZD, the SEDCOM (Safety and Efficacy or Dexmedetomidine COmpared with Midazolam) trial, patients sedated with midazolam had a 23% higher delirium prevalence than those receiving dexmedetomidine.[39] Patients requiring deep sedation, e.g. those with ALI should be more frequently assessed for delirium. With adherence to quality implement project, there was significant reduction of sedatives whereas increase in days awake without delirium.[40] Addition of physical, occupational therapy in early days of critical illness reduced the duration of delirium, compared to sedation interruption alone (median 2.0 vs 4.0 days, $P = 0.02$). In addition to that, there were more ventilator-free days and return to independent functional status at hospital discharge occurred more frequently in the intervention group (59% vs 35%, P = 0.02).[28]

Pain Management

Pain is a modifiable risk factor for delirium, and inadequate pain control is a frequent cause for agitation and delirium in the ICU. ICU patients are sedated many times and cannot report their pain, even if they experience pain during routine ICU procedures.

Inadequate pain assessment and/or pain control results in undue use of sedative medications particularly BZD[41] which have deliriogenic potential. Opioids, the most commonly preferred analgesics, have been associated with a reduced risk of delirium. Therefore, patients should undergo regular pain assessment and should have adequate pain control.

Nonpharmacologic pain management strategies include positioning and turning, heat/cold therapy, and injury stabilization should be done to manage pain whenever essential.

Pharmacologic treatment: Consider pharmacologic measures only if nonpharmacologic prevention strategies have failed. In addition to that, those at risk to harm self or others and if having severe distressing psychotic symptoms (hallucinations, delusions) need pharmacologic measures. There are no FDA-approved drugs for the treatment of delirium. Pharmacologic treatment often includes the use of typical (e.g. Haloperidol) and atypical (e.g. Olanzapine, Quetiapine, and Ziprasidone) antipsychotics (*see* Table 9.4). These medications may themselves cause delirium or increase sedation and have variable pharmacokinetics in ICU patients.[42] Cholinesterase inhibitors, such as Rivastigmine, Donepezil, and Galantamine, should not be used to reduce the duration of delirium. There are concerns regarding their efficacy, adverse effects, such as bradycardia, interactions with drugs, such as succinylcholine (increased levels of succinylmonocholine).[4,43]

Role of Dexmedetomidine in the Management of Delirium

Various studies have supported use of dexmedetomidine for ICU sedation instead of BZD, unless delirium is not due to BZD withdrawal or related to alcohol.[4] Dexmedetomidine group experienced more days alive without delirium

Table 9.4: Pharmacologic treatment for delirium.

Drugs	Comments	Evidence
Haloperidol	• Minimum risk of sedation, risk of QT prolongation and EPS • Cautious use with baseline prolonged QT or with concomitant medication which prolong QT interval, previous history of torsades de pointes	• Reserve for the short-term management of acute agitation[44] • No published evidence on prophylaxis and treatment[4] • Results are inconsistent for short-term use of haloperidol to reduce the incidence and/or severity of POD in high-risk older patients[45]
Ziprasidone	• Consider for hypoactive delirium • Less sedating, less risk of QT prolongation. Can cause EPS	• Comparative pilot study of 103 patients with haloperidol, ziprasidone, or placebo showed no significant differences in the number of days that patients survived without delirium or coma[46]
Quetiapine	• Atypical antipsychotics may reduce the duration of delirium[4] • Consider for hyperactive delirium or agitated mixed delirium • Risk of sedation and QT prolongation but minimum risk of EPS	• In a double-blind, randomized trial Quetiapine added to as-needed intravenous Haloperidol resulted in faster delirium resolution, less agitation, and a greater rate of transfer to home or rehabilitation. But no differences in mortality or ICU length • Adverse effects similar between both groups[47]
Olanzapine	• Should be considered in patients with hyperactive delirium • Safe, alternative to Haloperidol in delirious patients particularly in whom Haloperidol is contraindicated. But more risk of EPS compared to Quetiapine	• Study comparing haloperidol with olanzapine showed equivalent efficacy[48] • Its use for the prevention of POD is not recommended[45]

(EPS: extrapyramidal symptoms; POD: postoperative delirium)

or coma compared to lorazepam and lower prevalence of coma.[48] Compared to midazolam,[40] propofol,[49] and morphine, dexmedetomidine has lower incidence of delirium in various studies through the attainment of light sedation and the sparing effect on other sedatives. Thus, it improves outcome with lower rates of agitation. However, there is no definitive evidence supporting the role of dexmedetomidine for the treatment of delirium.[24] The most notable adverse effect of dexmedetomidine is bradycardia.

Quality Improvement Techniques

Delirium in the ICU is frequently multifactorial, so it is unlikely that a single intervention can prevent or reduce delirium. Therefore, a bundled approach including the "pain, agitation, and delirium" guidelines[4] and the "spontaneous awakening and breathing coordination, attention to the choice of sedation, delirium monitoring, and early mobility and exercise" (ABCDE) bundle[50] should be implemented to improve the outcome of delirium. This will shorten the duration of MV, length of stay in the ICU and hospital, improve functional outcomes, and improve survival. These guidelines emphasize on comprehensive approach in improving team communication, standardizing the ICU care, prioritizing the methods to lighten sedation and facilitate early mobilization and extubation. Implementation of this ABCDEF bundle has a dose-dependent response in patients so that even partial implementation and application of this bundle is beneficial to critically ill patients.

Multicomponent interventions (MIs) have been used in preventing delirium in the elderly. These interventions, such as physical therapy, cognitive stimulation programs, and nutritional supplementation, are included. There is a nearly 30% reduction in delirium rates while using MIs regardless of the setting and also in cognitive decline. It should be implemented as a standard of care,[51] and this approach is also supported by National Institute for Health and Care Excellence guideline.[11]

Hospital Elder Life Program,[52] an MI strategy with proven effectiveness and cost-effectiveness in the prevention of delirium and functional decline through targeting risk factors, is widely used approach in hospitals utilizing nonpharmacological measures.

Complications: Multiple clinical complications have been associated with delirium.
- Short-term complications
  - Inadvertent removal of indwelling catheters: Unintentional removal of ETT/Ryle's tube/central lines/urinary catheters
  - Reintubation
  - Malnutrition, fluid and electrolyte abnormalities
  - Aspiration pneumonia
  - Nosocomial pneumonia
  - Pressure ulcers
  - Weakness, decreased mobility, and decreased function
  - Falls and combative behavior leading to injuries and fractures

- Wandering and getting lost
- Extended/increased length of stay and cost of treatment
- Hospital-acquired infections
- Worsening of preexisting dementia and increase in the risk of development of de novo dementia.

❑ Long-term complications
- Prolonged immobility
- Mortality
- Long-term cognitive impairment
- Delayed recovery of cognitive dysfunction associated with long-term functional disability and poor quality of life
- Health-care costs
- Functional dependence.

CONCLUSION

Delirium is a multifactorial disorder, which is frequent in occurrence, often underestimated, and needs multidisciplinary approach for management. It is recognized as an independent predictor of negative clinical outcomes in ICU patients, including increased mortality, ICU LOS, hospital LOS, cost of care, and long-term cognitive impairment. ICU-acquired risk factors are potentially modifiable and are closely interconnected. Multicomponent strategies can effectively limit these risk factors, and integration of these strategies into daily ICU practice improves clinical outcomes. Validated screening tools (CAM-ICU or the ICDSC) are recommended for the early detection of delirium and should be incorporated into the daily work plan. Treatment is aimed at addressing underlying causes and managing symptoms principally by nonpharmacological measures. The efficacy of pharmacological prevention and treatment for delirium is still unclear. Although more pharmacological trials are awaited, the mainstay of treatment remains minimization and correction of risk factors along with regular screening of patients.

REFERENCES

1. American Psychiatric Association. Diagnostic and statistical manual of mental disorders. Arlington: American Psychiatric Association; 2013.
2. Ely EW, Speroff T, Gordon SM, Speroff T, Gordon SM, Harrell FE Jr, et al. Delirium as a predictor of mortality in mechanically ventilated patients in the intensive care unit. JAMA. 2004;291:1753-62.
3. Devlin JW, Fong JJ, Fraser GL, Riker RR. Delirium assessment in the critically ill. Intensive Care Med. 2007;33:929-40.
4. Barr J, Fraser GL, Puntillo K, Ely EW, Gélinas C, Dasta JF, et al. Clinical practice guidelines for the management of pain, agitation, and delirium in adult patients in the intensive care unit: executive summary. Am J Health Pharm. 2013;70:53-8.
5. Schenning KJ, Deiner SG. Postoperative delirium in the geriatric patient. Anesthesiol Clin. 2015;33:505-16.
6. Salluh JIF, Wang H, Schneider EB, Nagaraja N, Yenokyan G, Damluji A, et al. Outcome of delirium in critically ill patients: systematic review and meta-analysis. BMJ. 2015;350:h2538.
7. Liptzin B, Levkoff SE. An empirical study of delirium subtypes. Br J Psychiatry. 1992;161:843-5.
8. Robinson TN, Raeburn CD, Tran ZV, Brenner LA, Moss M. The motor subtypes of post-operative delirium in elderly. Arch Surg. 2011;146:295-300.
9. Girard TD, Pandharipande PP, Ely EW. Delirium in the intensive care unit. Crit Care. 2008;12(Suppl. 3):S3.
10. Slooter AJC, Van De Leur RR, Zaal IJ. Delirium in critically ill patients. In: Wijdicks EFM, Kramer AH (Eds). Handbook of clinical neurology, vol. 141, 1st edition. Elsevier BV; 2017. pp. 449-466.
11. O'Mahony R, Murthy L, Akunne A, Young J. Guideline Development Group. Synopsis of the National Institute for Health and Clinical Excellence guideline for prevention of delirium. Ann Intern Med. 2011;154:746-51.
12. Inouye SK, Westendorp RGJ, Saczynski JS, Pun BT, Wilkinson GR, Dittus RS. Delirium in elderly people. Lancet. 2014;383(9920):911-22.
13. Pandharipande PP, Shintani A, Peterson J, et al. Lorazepam is an independent risk factor for transitioning to delirium in intensive care unit patients. Anesthesiology. 2006;104:21-6.
14. Brummel NE, Vasilevskis EE, Han JH, Pun BT, Ely EW. Implementing delirium screening in the ICU: Secrets to success. Crit Care Med. 2013;41:2196-208.
15. Hayhurst CJ, Pandharipande PP, Hughes CG. Intensive care unit delirium. Anesthesiology. 2016;125:1229-41.
16. Tomasi CD, Grandi C, Salluh J, Soares M, Giombelli VR, Cascaes S, et al. Comparison of CAM-ICU and ICDSC for the detection of delirium in critically ill patients focusing on relevant clinical outcomes. J Crit Care. 2012;27:212-7.
17. Shehabi Y, Riker RR, Bokesch PM. Delirium duration and mortality in lightly sedated, mechanically ventilated intensive care patients. Crit Care Med. 2010;38:2311-8.
18. Salluh JI, Soares M, Teles JM, Ceraso D, Raimondi N, Nava VS, et al. Delirium epidemiology in critical care (DECCA): an international study. Crit Care. 2010;14:R210.
19. Pisani MA, Kong SYJ, Kasl SV. Days of delirium are associated with 1-year mortality in an older intensive care unit population. Am J Respir Crit Care Med. 2009;180:1092-7.
20. Hamilton GM, Wheeler K, Di Michele J, Lalu MM, McIsaac DI. A systematic review and meta-analysis examining the impact of incident postoperative delirium on mortality. Anesthesiology. 2017;127:78-88.
21. Lakatos BE, Capasso V, Mitchell MT, Kilroy SM, Lussier-Cushing M, Sumner L, et al. Falls in the general hospital: association with delirium, advanced age, and specific surgical procedures. Psychosomatics. 2009;50:218-26.
22. Boettger S, Breitbart W, Jenewein J, Boettger S. Delirium and functionality: the impact of delirium on the level of functioning. Eur J Psychiatry. 2014;28:86-95.

23. Girard T, Pun BT, Thompson JL, Pun BT, Thompson JL, Shintani AK, et al. Delirium as a predictor of long-term cognitive impairment in survivors of critical illness. Crit Care Med. 2010;38:1513-20.
24. Reade MC, Finfer S. Sedation and delirium in the intensive care unit. N Engl J Med. 2014;370:444-54.
25. Wolters AE, van Dijk D, Pasma W, Cremer OL, Looije MF, de Lange DW, et al. Long-term outcome of delirium during intensive care unit stay in survivors of critical illness: a prospective cohort study. Crit Care. 2014;18:1-7.
26. Van Den Boogaard M, Schoonhoven L, Evers AWM, van der Hoeven JG, van Achterberg T, Pickkers P. Delirium in critically ill Patients: Impact on long-term health-related quality of life and cognitive functioning. Crit Care Med. 2012;40:112-8.
27. Morris PE, Griffin L, Berry M, Thompson C, Hite RD, Winkelman C, et al. Receiving early mobility during an ICU admission is a predictor of improved outcomes in acute respiratory failure. Am J Med Sci. 2012;341:373-7.
28. Schweickert WD, Pohlman MC, Pohlman AS, Nigos C, Pawlik AJ, Esbrook CL, et al. Early physical and occupational therapy in mechanically ventilated, critically ill patients: a randomised controlled trial. Lancet. 2009;373:1874-82.
29. Cooper AB, Thornley KS, Young GB, Slutsky AS, Stewart TE, Hanly PJ. et al. Sleep in critically ill patients requiring mechanical ventilation. (Chest. 2000;117:809-18.
30. Brummel NE, Girard TD. Preventing delirium in the intensive care unit. Crit Care Clin. 2013;29:51-65.
31. Blair GJ, Mehmood T, Rudnick M, Kuschner WG, Barr J. Nonpharmacologic and medication minimization strategies for the prevention and treatment of ICU delirium: a narrative review. J Intensive Care Med. 2018:885066618771528.
32. McPherson JA, Wagner CE, Boehm LM, Hall JD, Johnson DC, Miller LR, et al. Delirium in the cardiovascular ICU: exploring modifiable risk factors. Crit Care Med. 2013;41:405-13.
33. Colombo R, Corona A, Praga F, Minari C, Giannotti C, Castelli A, et al. A reorientation strategy for reducing delirium in the critically ill. Results of an interventional study. Minerva Anestesiol. 2012;78:1026-33.
34. Clegg A, Young JB. Which medications to avoid in people at risk of delirium: a systematic review. Age Ageing. 2011;40:23-9.
35. Nelson S, Muzyk AJ, Bucklin MH, Brudney S, Gagliardi JP. Defining the role of dexmedetomidine in the prevention of delirium in the intensive care unit. Biomed Res Int. 2015;2015:635737.
36. Page VJ, Ely EW, Gates S, Zhao XB, Alce T, Shintani A, et al. Efficacy of intravenous haloperidol on the duration of delirium and coma in critically ill patients (Hope-ICU): a randomised, placebo-controlled trial. Lancet Respir Med. 2013;1:515-23.
37. Pradelli L, Povero M, Bürkle H, Kampmeier TG, Della-Rocca G, Feuersenger A, et al. Propofol or benzodiazepines for short- and long-term sedation in intensive care units? An economic evaluation based on meta-analytic results. Clin Outcomes Res. 2017;9:685-98.
38. Jakob SM. Dexmedetomidine vs midazolam or propofol for sedation during prolonged mechanical ventilation. JAMA. 2012;307:1151-60.
39. Riker RR, Shehabi Y, Bokesch PM, Ceraso D, Wisemandle W, Koura F, et al, for SEDCOM Study Group. Dexmedetomidine vs midazolam for sedation of critically ill patients: a randomised trial. JAMA. 2009;301:489-99.
40. Hager DN, Dinglas VD, Subhas S, Rowden AM, Neufeld KJ, Bienvenu OJ, et al. Reducing deep sedation and delirium in acute lung injury patients: a quality improvement project. Crit Care Med. 2013;41:1435-42.
41. Payen JF, Bosson JL, Chanques G, Mantz J, Labarere J; DOLOREA Investigators. Pain assessment is associated with decreased duration of mechanical ventilation in the intensive care unit. Anesthesiology. 2009;111:1308-16.
42. King J, Gratrix A. Delirium in intensive care. Contin Educ Anaesth Crit Care Pain. 2009;9:144-7.
43. Gage L, Hogan DB. (2014). 2014 CCSMH Guideline Update: The Assessment and Treatment of Delirium. Toronto: Canadian Coalition for Seniors' Mental Health (CCSMH). [online] Available from www.ccsmh.ca. [Accessed September 24, 2018].
44. Girard TD, Kress JP, Fuchs BD, Thomason JW, Schweickert WD, Pun BT, et al. Efficacy and safety of a paired sedation and ventilator weaning protocol for mechanically ventilated patients in intensive care (Awakening and Breathing Controlled trial): a randomised controlled trial. Lancet. 2008;371(9607):126-34.
45. Girard TD, Pandharipande PP, Carson SS, Schmidt GA, Wright PE, Canonico AE, et al. Feasibility, efficacy, and safety of antipsychotics for ICU delirium: the MIND randomized, placebo-controlled trial. Crit Care Med. 2010;38:428-37.
46. Devlin JW, Roberts RJ, Fong JJ, Skrobik Y, Riker RR, Hill NS, et al. Efficacy and safety of quetiapine in critically ill patients with delirium: a prospective, multicenter, randomized, double-blind, placebo-controlled pilot study. Crit Care Med. 2010;38:419-27.
47. Skrobik YK, Bergeron N, Dumont M, Gottfried SB. Olanzapine vs haloperidol: treating delirium in a critical care setting. Intensive Care Med. 2004;30:444-9.
48. Pandharipande PP, Pun BT, Herr DL, Maze M, Girard TD, Miller RR, et al. Effect of sedation with dexmedetomidine vs lorazepam on acute brain dysfunction in mechanically ventilated patients: the MENDS randomized controlled trial. JAMA. 2007;298:2644-53.
49. Xia ZQ, Chen SQ, Yao X, Xie CB, Wen SH, Liu KX. Clinical benefits of dexmedetomidine versus propofol in adult intensive care unit patients: a meta-analysis of randomized clinical trials. J Surg Res. 2013;185:833-43.
50. Marra A, Frimpong K, Ely EW. The ABCDEF implementation bundle. Korean J Crit Care Med. 2016;31:181-93.
51. Martinez F, Tobar C, Hill N. Preventing delirium: should non-pharmacological, multicomponent interventions be used? A systematic review and meta-analysis of the literature. Age Ageing. 2015;44:196-204.
52. Singler K, Thomas C. HELP—Hospital Elder Life Program—ein multimodales Interventionsprogramm zur Delirprävention bei älteren Patienten. Internist. 2017;58:125-31.

CHAPTER 10

Brain Death

Elizabeth Louise Trent, Timothy Martin Wilkinson

INTRODUCTION

It is 50 years since the Harvard Ad Hoc Committee provided the blueprint by which a person could be determined dead by neurological rather than circulatory criteria.[1,2] Their primary incentive was to provide certainty to the grieving family that their loved one was dead and to avoid ongoing treatment of "the hopelessly unconscious patient." The facilitation of transplantation was a secondary consideration, and it is vital that death determination remains a distinct and separate entity in health policy and research although there is a close intersection.

Death by neurological criteria specifies a clinical point beyond which capacity for consciousness and brainstem function is permanently lost. That these criteria do indeed entail death is clinically and legally accepted in many countries. Whether it is socially accepted is another question. Comparatively few people give much thought to brain death but, at least in many societies, brain death is not widely disagreed with.

Variations in guidelines and practice inconsistencies in the determination of brain death are reported between countries and jurisdictions;[3,4] however, there are also fundamentals of clinical practice that are consistent globally. These could effectively be said to constitute a minimum international standard with the current absence of international consensus.[5]

The history of humanity's efforts to understand the concept of death is essential to understanding the current meaning of death today and what paradigms may evolve in the future.[6] Bernat said "Over the last 50 years brain death has matured from its origin as an instrumental concept to its present state as a philosophical concept."[7] It is therefore important to understand the biophilosophical arguments as these are still being deliberated.

BIOPHILOSOPHICAL ARGUMENTS EXPLAINED

When considering death, including brain death, it helps to bear in mind that the following questions are separate from each other:

1. What is death? A plausible answer here is the total and permanent irreversible cessation of life, although the question then arises, what is life?
2. What is it that makes someone dead? That is, what conditions are essential to carrying on living such that their loss would entail death? The answers here would in some way have to follow from the answers to the first question. Examples might include the loss of some or all brain function, the loss of integrated function, and the loss of spontaneous respiration.
3. How do we know whether someone is dead? Again, the answer would depend in part on the answer to the previous questions. Examples might include the clinical examination for determining neurological death and imaging to confirm no cerebral blood flow (CBF), if brain function is essential for life, or testing

for respiration and circulation if these are essential for life.
4. What is the ethical and legal significance of death? In many societies, death entails dissolving marriages, reading wills and reallocating property, and, of course, allowing the retrieval of organs otherwise required for life. The ethical and legal implications of death do not follow in any obvious way from the answers to questions 1-3.

This section focuses on the first two questions, and the remainder of the chapter deals with the third. The ethical and legal significance of death is a large separate topic.[8]

Why is brain death supposed to be death? Two main reasons have been given. The first is that brain death implies the total and permanent loss of mental states. The second is that brain death implies the biological organism ceases to exist. Obviously these reasons are very different from each other. We first show how they relate to fundamentally different conceptions of what entities we are. Then we ask whether it is a good reason to conclude that brain death is death.

The concept of death presupposes the concept of life, and life is often thought to presuppose existence. To know what death is for entities like us, we need to know what our existence conditions are or, put another way, what is essential for our survival. For that, we need to know what sort of entities we are.

Western philosophy is split. Many philosophers have thought that we are essentially persons, and being a person requires the capacity for mental states. But others think that we are animals that "each of us is identical with, is one and the same thing as, an animal."[9] To continue to exist as an animal need not require mental states. It may require only persisting as an integrated biological organism. Neither view can be easily dismissed.

To return to death the total and permanent loss of mental states would be death if mental states are fundamental to our existence, while ceasing to exist as a biological organism would be death if we are animals. It may then seem with either view, brain death would be death.

Unfortunately, this convenient conclusion is not sustainable. On the one hand, if death is the total and permanent loss of mental states, then brain death is more than necessary for death. On the other hand, brain death is not enough to make the organism cease to have integrated functioning. The brain dead organism would not function without critical care organ support; but, with support, brain dead organisms can continue to function in an integrated way and to some degree independently of support. An example would be a brain dead pregnant woman having a fetus brought to term. How could that be possible if the organism were dead?[10]

Brain death has sometimes been described as a conservative criterion, and it may indeed be better to be conservative and err on the side of caution. But brain death is a conservative criterion if death is the loss of mental states; it is not conservative if death is ceasing to exist as a biological organism, because some entities could be brain dead but still alive as biological organisms.

A different approach would be to consider what is valuable in life. Perhaps only mental states confer value on our lives and, without mental states, life would not be worth living. If so, critical care for the brain dead would be valueless and may be ethically withdrawn. While this conclusion may be correct, it is quite different from saying that without mental states we would not be alive.

PHYSIOLOGICAL AND BIOLOGICAL PLAUSIBILITY OF BRAIN DEATH

Dying is a biological and physiological process during which cellular activities and organ function progressively cease. Death is the moment in time during the dying process when an individual passes from the state of being alive to that of being dead.[11]

Death occurs after the brain has lost ability to use oxygen. This may be because of the absence of systemic blood flow or less commonly from raised intracranial pressure (ICP) causing cessation of CBF.[12] When the brain sustains a severe insult, edema results. Edema increases intracranial tissue volume, and as the skull is rigid and fluid is incompressible, the ICP rises. Elevated ICP reduces cerebral perfusion pressure and CBF creating a vicious cycle of increasing ICP and reducing CBF producing further edema until the ICP exceeds the systemic arterial blood pressure. Transtentorial herniation of the cerebral cortex into the brainstem causes progressive loss of brainstem function and "coning" occurs at the foramen magnum with total occlusion of intracranial blood flow permanent loss of brain function results. The occlusion is external, and the arteries are not immediately thrombosed.[13] Absent CBF can be determined by neuroimaging when neurological death cannot be confirmed by clinical tests.

Understanding death in terms of function rather than anatomy places emphasis on the permanently non-functioning brain. Shemie defines being dead as "absent brain function with no biological potential in the brain to reinstate sufficient cell function required to achieve emergence to consciousness and self-awareness."[5] In the discussion of pathophysiology of brain death, almost all of the brain's complex work falls into three central functions, being cognitive function, hormonal function, and integrative function.[14] Loss of cortical function is a component of current practical brain death testing guidelines, but "higher brain death" alone is not accepted worldwide as death. Hormonal function may be lost in whole brain death; but in some patients, the hypothalamic function is preserved.[15] It is the loss of integrative function between the brain and body in response to stimuli (brainstem integrative function) that is the basis of the clinical examination that determines neurological death.[14] Permanent loss of *all* intracranial neurological functioning is not and is not required to be confirmed during clinical examination to determine brain death. Truog said recently brain injury occurs on a spectrum of severity where "brain death" is near the very bottom of that spectrum, representing the loss of most—but not necessarily all the functions of the brain.[16] This point on the spectrum is permanent apneic areflexic coma, those functioning above that line are legally alive and those below that line are legally dead.[16] The United Kingdom, India, Taiwan, Hong Kong, Singapore, and some other commonwealth countries refer to death by neurological criteria as brainstem death rather than brain death or total brain death.[17] Brainstem death has a lower burden of proof than whole brain death.[18]

At a cellular level, brain ischemia and then subsequent reperfusion trigger a complex process involving reactive oxygen species, calcium-mediated vasospasm, and inflammatory cascades that lead to brain swelling and that can eventually cause physical destruction of brain cells. There is not a discrete cellular event that can be called death.[19] Neuropathologic examination is not diagnostic of brain death.[20] There is no specific biological marker to precisely identify brain death, but it has been theorized that biomarkers related to the mitochondrial integrity of crucial brain cells may provide one option in the future.[12]

The physiologic and anatomic correlates of the minimum required functional brain loss that results in cessation of brain function will no doubt continue to evolve with scientific advancements; however, there may never be a discrete biological transition to a state called death.[12,19]

Guidelines show a trend toward describing phenomena observed in the determination of brain death rather than assumed mechanisms. For example, "apnea" rather than loss of respiratory center and "diabetes insipidus" rather than loss of function of the hypothalamus.

CLINICAL PRACTICE

Different countries produce comprehensive practical documents for the neurological determination of death, and each describe the detailed systematic process and tests needed to confirm death. Individuals should obviously adhere to their own jurisdictions legal and protocol requirements. Despite much attention to the differences in codes of practice for determining brain death around the world, it is in fact the similarities that bind them. Neurological determination of death guidelines generally have fundamental clinical components; evidence of sufficient intracranial pathology to cause permanent coma, absence of reversible or confounding factors, absence of cortical or brainstem-mediated motor responses, absent brainstem reflexes, and loss of capacity to breath.[5]

The concept of brain death is broadly accepted around the world; however, the implementation and practice is variable. A survey of 91 countries in 2015 showed 70% had legal provision and 77% had institutional protocols for brain death.[3] This varied between income levels with 22% of low income versus 97% of high-income countries having an institutional protocol. The reasons for no institutional protocol were mostly lack of expertise and technology. Within 16 countries surveyed in the World Health Organization (WHO) Southeast Asian and Western Pacific regions, 10 had a law and 9 had an institutional protocol for brain death determination. The major areas of variability occur in technical procedures used to arrive at the clinical diagnosis, the process of the apnea test, and the need for ancillary tests. There are minor variations in the number of physicians required to certify and qualifications, time to brain death declaration and pediatric criteria.[3] Pediatric criteria for brain death are not covered in this review.

The Australian and New Zealand Intensive Care Society (ANZICS) statement on death and organ donation is based on review of the law, medical literature, and committee consensus and is the practice standard for Australia and New Zealand.[21]

Some of ANZICS recommendations are included below and discussed in relation to variations within the Asia-Pacific region.

Caring for the dying patient and their family is of utmost importance. It is an uncertain and immensely distressing time for families of patients in intensive care with catastrophic neurological injury. The intensive care doctor and their team should meet early with all families and have regular subsequent meetings to detail the treatment, communicate prognosis, and involve them in consensus decision-making. If it becomes clear that the patient is dying, this should be communicated with sensitivity, cultural humility, and compassion.[21,22] Family and patient-centered care with clear communication, mutual trust, rapport with and respect for the family over the period leading up to the confirmation of death helps in the delivery of this devastating news. Brain death should be determined when it has occurred, and it is the clinical team's responsibility to ensure the family understands that this is death. Families may have minimal understanding of death by neurological criteria, and it may be difficult for them to accept this conceptually so careful choice of language, and explanation is crucial to understanding and acceptance.[21] Families may benefit from observing the clinical examination with a trained chaperone as it helps them understand the irreversibility of neurological death and is reported not to have an adverse effect on psychological well-being.[23]

ANZICS recommendation 1:

Neurological determination of death is carried out by two doctors, who must each independently determine death according to this statement, and meet the requirements of jurisdictional legislation.

The number of doctors needed to perform the clinical brain death testing differs between countries. Most Asian-Pacific countries require two doctors with India requiring four and South Korea four to six staff with at least two doctors.[17,24] The qualification of the doctors stipulated also varies, with intensivists, neurosurgeons, and neurologists being involved most often.[3,17,24] The necessity of repeating the whole clinical examination sequence lacks evidence;[25] however, within the Asia/Pacific area, all countries except Singapore require repeat clinical testing. The time interval between repeat testing can be variable, from nonspecified to generally less than 6 hours in adults. In children the interval between testing may be up to 48 hours.[3,17]

ANZICS recommendation 2:

For neurological determination of death to take place, there must be definite clinical or neuroimaging evidence of acute brain pathology consistent with deterioration to permanent loss of all neurological function. In the cases of hypoxic ischemic brain injury, clinical history alone may provide sufficient evidence.

ANZICS recommendation 3:

There is a minimum 4-hour observation period prior to neurological determination of death using clinical examination alone. Throughout this observation period, all preconditions are met, the patient has a Glasgow Coma Scale of 3, with pupils nonreactive to light, absent cough/tracheal reflex, and apparent apnea on a ventilator. Following an acute hypoxic–ischemic brain injury or hypothermia (<35°C) of duration greater than 6 hours, there should be a waiting period of 24 hours before determination of death using clinical examination alone.

Preconditions are very similar throughout Asia-Pacific and the world and must be met prior to and during clinical examination.[24] There must be an established etiology of the severe brain injury that is capable of causing brain death. Other preconditions include normothermia, normotension, exclusion of effects of sedative drugs, absence of severe metabolic or endocrine disturbances, absence of acute liver failure or decompensated chronic liver disease, intact neuromuscular function, ability to examine the cranial nerve (CN) reflexes in at least one ear and eye, and the ability to perform apnea testing.[21,25]

CLINICAL EXAMINATION

The fundamental three criteria of clinical examination needed to determine brain death are profound unresponsive coma, absence of brainstem reflexes, and no spontaneous breathing effort.[21,25] There is general agreement amongst different institutional protocols that responsiveness and testable brainstem reflexes should be absent.

Application of noxious stimuli to all four limbs, the trunk, and the CN distribution tests responsiveness. "There must be absent motor response in the CN distribution to noxious stimulation of the face, trunk, and four limbs *and* absent response in the trunk or limbs to noxious stimulation within the CN distribution."[21]

To confirm the absence of brainstem reflexes the following should be tested sequentially: the pupils must be nonreactive to light (CN II, III). There must be no corneal reflexes (CN V, VII). There must be no facial movement to noxious stimuli (CN V, VII). The eyes must be immobile with absent oculocephalic and/or oculovestibular reflexes (CN III, IV, VI, VIII). The gag reflex (CN IX, X) and the cough reflex (CN X) must be absent. The oculocephalic reflex test is a submaximal stimulus and often not included in many guidelines including ANZICS.

Testing for apnea should be performed last. There are exacting procedures associated with confirming apnea, which should be strictly adhered to.[21,25] The code of conduct for the apnea tests has the most variation between countries.[3] For example, there are different blood gas requirements for confirming apnea although the majority in the Asia-Pacific region requires a $PaCO_2 > 60$ mm Hg with a rise in $PaCO_2$ of greater than 20 mm Hg above baseline.[17] For patients receiving extracorporeal membrane oxygenation an adapted apnea test involving adjusting settings until adequate hypercarbia has occurred can be used.[26]

The presence of spinal reflexes is consistent with brain death. Many complex spinal reflex forms are described.

Ancillary tests assess brain function or blood flow. Any ancillary test has pitfalls, and they should not be used to supplant bedside clinical examination or relied on when at odds with a clinical neurological examination.[4,27] Evaluation for CBF are now preferred in most jurisdictions as these are less affected by confounding factors.[28]

ANZICS recommendation 5:

When imaging to demonstrate the absence of brain perfusion is required, it must be preceded by those parts of the clinical examination that are possible and responsiveness, all testable brainstem reflexes and breathing effort must be absent.

Imaging is used to demonstrate the absence of brain perfusion when parts of the clinical examination are not possible or reliable. This may be inability to examine all the CN reflexes, inability to conduct the apnea test, or when confounding factors are present. All parts of the clinical examination that are possible must be performed and have absent findings before imaging is undertaken. Imaging tests must have a 100% specificity to avoid wrongly declaring absent CBF in a patient who does not meet brain death criteria, as well as a high sensitivity.[21]

ANZICS recommendation 6:

If assessment of brain perfusion is required, three- or four-vessel angiography or radionuclide imaging is preferred. Computed tomography angiography is acceptable if recommended radiological guidelines are followed. Magnetic resonance imaging or angiography and transcranial Doppler should not be used.

The ANZICS 2018 recommendation lists and explains three acceptable techniques for assessing cerebral perfusion. Intra-arterial catheter angiography with digital subtraction is considered the gold standard, followed by radionuclide imaging using technetium 99m radiolabeled hexamethylprophylene amine oxime radionuclide. Computed tomography angiography can be used if the other two are unavailable and certain strict technical criteria are adhered to.[21]

Other ancillary tests that measure brain electrophysiology, such as the electroencephalogram (EEG), somatosensory evoked potentials are used around the world. The EEG is frequently used and is considered an important validated confirmatory test with sensitivity and specificity of 90%. EEG can be prone to artifact in the intensive care unit.[25,28]

Further research and standardization is required in this area to improve ancillary test reliability. In some countries, e.g. China, Japan, South Korea, ancillary testing is routinely required before brain death can be certified.[17]

This clinical process lends itself well to a checklist to ensure completeness and should be done in every death certification.

ANZICS recommendation 11:
Documentation of neurological determination of death should be made using a specific form to demonstrate explicitly that all criteria set out in this statement are met, whether or not donation occurs. The same criteria should be listed in local hospital forms.

Efforts to ensure best practice in the determination of brain death are essential for public confidence and the acceptance of brain death as death. Brain death is a relatively rare occurrence for an individual clinician. Specific training in the determination of death is therefore important for physicians working in the intensive care and should decrease variation in practice within countries. A simulation-based training program showed markedly improved adherence to the American Academy of Neurology criteria.[29] Courses, an education module and work-based assessments, are a mandatory educational requirement for Australia and New Zealand trainees in Intensive Care Medicine.[21] Intensivists can access this education and can readily obtain telephone advice and support when clinically needed from on-call specialists in both countries. More broadly formal end-of-life communication training is an essential component of best practice for all staff caring regularly for dying patients.[22]

International guideline development for the determination of death has been underway since 2012. This group proposes a single operational unified determination of death based on cessation of brain function which occurs over two pathways, either permanent absence of circulation or subsequent to catastrophic brain injury.[11] A harmonized international clinical practice guideline would reduce variation of practice between countries and improve public and professional confidence in the process. It seems unclear currently whether worldwide consensus for either the definition or the criteria is achievable given complex challenges identified by the World Health Organization (WHO).[5]

SUMMARY

The primary purpose of certifying brain death is to bring closure to families. In order to do this, it is an important feature of the certification of brain death that it is reliable. If done thoroughly and precisely, the stepwise clinical examination for neurological determination of death is accurate, reproducible and can be reliably performed by doctors properly trained in the process; ancillary testing is only infrequently required. However, certifying brain death is only one aspect of bringing closure. Another aspect is the acceptance that brain death is final. A large question is whether brain death is really death. While brain death has become clinically and legally accepted as death in many countries, the nature of death is ultimately a philosophical rather than clinical or legal matter and it is one without a consensus. Nonetheless, it can be argued that it is reasonable to regard brain dead people as being dead either because they are dead or because no harm could be done since whatever life remains is of no value to the person.

REFERENCES

1. Wijdicks M. Deliberating death in the Summer of 1968. N Engl J Med. 2018;379(5):412-5.
2. [No authors listed]. A definition of irreversible coma. Report of the Ad Hoc Committee of the Harvard Medical School to Examine the Definition of Brain Death. JAMA. 1968;205:337-40.
3. Wahlster S, Eelco F, Pratik VP, et al. Brain death declaration: practices and perceptions worldwide. Neurology. 2015;84:1870-9.
4. Ghoshal S, Greer D. Why is diagnosing brain death so confusing?. Curr Opin Crit Care. 2015;21:107-12.
5. Shemie S, Baker A. Uniformity in brain death criteria. Semin Neurol. 2015;25:162-8.
6. De Georgia M. History of brain death as death: 1968 to the present. J Crit Care. 2014;29:673-8.
7. Bernat J. Death by neurologic criteria 1968-2014: changing interpretations. Forward. J Crit Care. 2014;29:671-2.
8. Wilkinson TM. Ethics and acquisition of organs. Oxford: Oxford University Press; 2011.
9. Snowdon PF. Persons, animals, ourselves. Oxford: Oxford University Press; 2014.
10. Singer P. Rethinking life and death: the collapse of traditional ethics. Macmillian Publishing; 1996.
11. Shemie S, Hornby L, Baker A, et al. International guideline development for the determination of death. Intensive Care Med. 2014;40:788-97.
12. Baker A, Shemie S. Biophilosophical basis for identifying the death of a person. J Crit Care. 2014;29(4):687-9.
13. Langfitt TW, Kassell NF. Non-filling of cerebral vessels during angiography: correlation with intracranial pressure. Acta Neurochir (Wien). 1966;14(1):96-104.
14. Shutter L. Pathophysiology of brain death: what does the brain do and what is lost in brain death. J Crit Care. 2014;29:683-6.
15. Nair-Collins M, Northrup J, Olcese J. Hypothalamic-pituitary function in brain death: a review. J Intensive Care Med. 2016;31:41-50.
16. Truog R. Defining death—making sense of the case of Jahi McMath. JAMA. 2018;319(18):1859-60.
17. Chua HC, Kuek TK, Morihari H. Brain death: the Asian perspective. Semin Neurol. 2015;35:152-61.
18. Smith M. Brain death: time for an international consensus. Br J Anaesth. 2012;108(108):6-9.
19. Wowk B. The future of death. J Crit Care. 2014;29:1111-3.
20. Wijdicks EF, Pfeifer EA. Neuropathology of brain death in the modern transplant era. Neurology. 2008;70:1234-7.
21. Australian and New Zealand Intensive Care Society. (2018). The ANZICS statement on death and organ donation. Draft after consultation. Melbourne: ANZICS. [online] Available from http://www.anzics.com.au/.
22. Australian and New Zealand Intensive Care Society. The ANZICS statement on death and organ donation. Draft after consultation. ANZICS. Melbourne. July 2018. Online. Available via: http://www.anzics.com.au/. [Accessed August 22, 2018].
23. Tawil I, Brown LH, Comfort D, et al. Family presence during brain death evaluation: a randomized controlled trial. Crit Care Med. 2014;42(4):934-43.
24. Ganapathy K. Brain death revisited. Neurol India. 2018;66:308-15.
25. Wijdicks E. Brain death Guidelines explained. Semin Neurol. 2015;35:105-15.
26. Goswami S, Evans A, Das B, et al. Determination of brain death by apnoea test adapted to extracorporeal cardiopulmonary resuscitation. J Cardiothorac Vasc Anesth. 2013;27(2):312-4.
27. Wijdicks EF. The case against confirmatory tests for determining brain death in adults. Neurology. 2010;75(1):77-83.
28. Kramer A. Ancillary testing in brain death. Semin Neurol. 2015;35:125-38.
29. MacDougall B, Robinson J, Kappus L, et al. Simulation-based training in brain death determination. Neurocrit Care. 2014;21:383-91.

CHAPTER 11

Organ Donation

Michael J O'Leary

INTRODUCTION

Organ transplantation is the preferred treatment for many patients with end-stage organ failure. In Australia, over 25% of heart recipients and 40% of adult liver recipients are alive 25 years following transplant. Over 80% of kidney recipients are well and off of dialysis 5 years after transplant. While living donor programs for organ transplantation have been well developed in some parts of the world, in general the majority of organs for transplant have to be sourced from deceased donors. Transplantation is expensive, however, in countries that have a well-developed deceased donor kidney transplant program the cost savings associated with removing patients from dialysis can significantly subsidize the costs of transplantation of other organs. Internationally, there is a large gap between the need for deceased donor organs for transplant and supply, and it is estimated that current transplant procedures represent less than 10% of the global need. Many countries have implemented "reform programs" in an effort to increase diseased donor organ supply, and generally these are similar in approach.[1]

In order to successfully transplant an organ from a deceased donor, it is vital that organ warm ischemia is avoided or minimized. Consequently, only patients that die with brain death or have life-sustaining treatment withdrawn and develop circulatory standstill shortly thereafter are suitable to donate. This means that all potential deceased organ donors will be cared for in an intensive care unit (ICU) (or possibly an emergency department) immediately prior to death. Given the disparity between the need for transplants and the availability of organs a guiding principle is that in every end-of-life care situation where donation of organs is apparently possible, the chance to donate should be offered, through discussion with family. The identification of potential donors, the family approach, and the subsequent donor management prior to organ retrieval surgery are clearly the remit of an intensive care specialist. The pathway to deceased organ donation comprises a number of steps (Fig. 11.1), the careful conduct of each of which is vital to success.

POTENTIAL DONOR IDENTIFICATION

The majority of deceased organ donors have suffered a devastating brain injury that has progressed to the development of brain death [donation after brain death (DBD)]. In recent years, in many countries, there has been increasing donation from patients with other reasons for receiving life support in the ICU, such as an isolated organ failure or circulatory failure [donation after circulatory death, (DCD)]. Identification of potential donors in patients with brain death is often straightforward; however, in patients with brain injury not causing brain death, or other reasons for receiving life support, the potential for donation may not be so readily recognized. A vital step to optimize organ donation opportunities is to put in place processes to ensure that potential donors are recognized early and are referred to key donation personnel within the hospital,

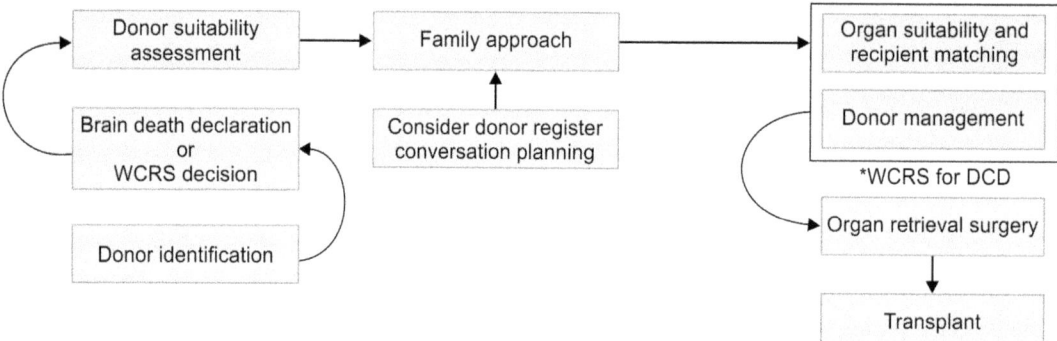

FIGURE 11.1: Steps in the pathway to deceased organ donation.
(WCRS: withdrawal of cardiorespiratory support)

or to an organ donation agency.[2] Early identification can be facilitated by the development of "clinical triggers" such as Glasgow Coma Scale ≤5, intubated, ventilated, and end-of-life care (Fig. 11.2) or simple mantras such as "I.E.: intubated, end-of-life → refer." Early identification and referral allows an early assessment of potential donor suitability to be made—this should rarely be decided by the local treating specialist as potential recipient requirements can change on a day-by-day basis.

While the possibility of organ donation as an outcome is usually readily apparent in patients with brain death, this may not be the case if a determination of brain death has not been made. Many specialists may only consider the determination of brain death when organ donation has already been considered as an option. This is a poor practice. Brain death should always be diagnosed when it is suspected as this permits accurate diagnosis and prognostication—death is death. It also potentially normalizes brain death as a standard method of death determination irrespective of whether organ donation is a possibility. Strategies that ensure that all patients with brain death are identified lead to an increase in the number of actual organ donors.[3,4] In adults the extra donors will generally be older with more comorbidities than standard brain dead organ donors.

Immediate Contraindications to Cadaveric Organ Donation

Contraindications are constantly changing, and intensive care specialists are always advised to check with their local donation agency or transplant teams for clarification. Metastatic cancer, hematological malignancies, human immunodeficiency virus (HIV) infection and Prion diseases would currently be considered absolute contraindications (Table 11.1). In addition, there are donor age cutoffs; however, these may vary between countries. For example, in Australia, the upper age limit for DCD is 70 years for kidneys and 75 years for lungs—consequently in the patients above these ages if brain death is not likely to occur donation can be considered contraindicated.

For donation to be possible following circulatory death (DCD), circulatory standstill has to occur soon after the withdrawal of cardiorespiratory support (WCRS) to limit damaging organ warm ischemia. The acceptable time to circulatory standstill is uncertain as it differs for individual organs and is not agreed across different transplant units and jurisdictions. Furthermore, there is no agreement regarding when warm ischemia starts. Some commence timing from the moment of WCRS, whereas others use a specific blood pressure step as a commencement target (such as systolic <90 mm Hg or mean <50 mm Hg). Clearly, if it is not anticipated that circulatory standstill will occur within the locally agreed timeframe for DCD then donation cannot proceed. Unfortunately, there is no reliable method to predict time to circulatory standstill in these situations. The opinion of the treating intensive care specialist is

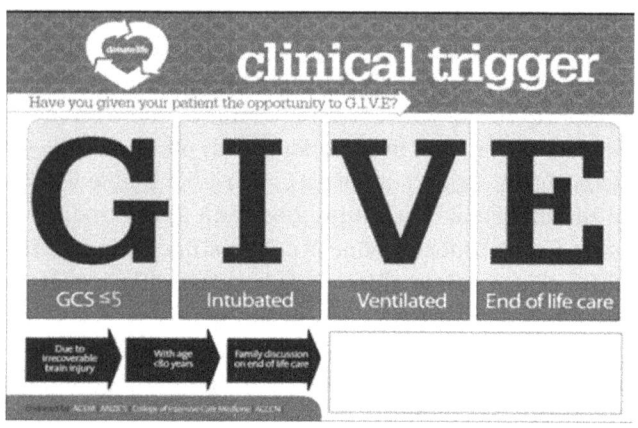

FIGURE 11.2: The "GIVE" clinical trigger—an example of a process measure to promote early potential donor identification in hospitals.

Table 11.1: Main contraindications (absolute and relative) to deceased organ donation.

Malignancy	• Current malignant neoplasms except nonmelanoma skin cancers and primary CNS tumors without metastases • Metastatic malignancy • Melanoma at any time • Hematologic malignancies
Premalignant conditions	Aplastic anemia, agranulocytosis, myelofibrosis
Premature neonates	<500 g or <32-week gestational age
Infection	• Active untreated infection (relative) • Tuberculosis • Intra-abdominal sepsis • HIV • Rabies • Prion diseases
Age (relative contraindications, may vary locally)	• Kidney DBD <80 years, DCD <70 years • Liver DBD <90 years, DCD <55 years • Heart <60 years • Lung <75 years

(CNS: central nervous system; DBD: donation after brain death; DCD: donation after circulatory death; HIV: human immunodeficiency virus)

probably the most reliable predictor.[5] Depending on the likely organs to be suitable to donate and the availability of a retrieval team a decision may need to be made as to whether it is appropriate to proceed with an attempt at DCD if it is uncertain that circulatory standstill will occur in a suitable time, and it may be decided that it is inappropriate to proceed with donation work-up.

ASSESSMENT OF POTENTIAL DONOR SUITABILITY

Medical suitability assessments should always be made by experts in organ donation and transplantation. Potential donor suitability is a dynamic entity as it can vary depending on the characteristics of available potential recipients. For example, a liver transplant team may consider a very marginal graft for a patient imminently coning with fulminant hepatic failure today that on any other day would be rejected. Active infection is never an absolute contraindication to donation, as it depends on the site of infection, the organism(s) involved, their susceptibility to treatment, and recipient factors. The changing prognosis of hepatitis C with the availability of effective antiviral treatment means that active donor infection is no longer a contraindication to donation. It may be that a similar view will apply to HIV infection in the near future. Assessment of individual organ suitability for transplantation will also involve blood group and human leukocyte antigen matching (where appropriate) and size/age matching for lung and liver transplantation.

FAMILY APPROACH FOR DONATION

Organ donation conversations occur at a traumatic time for the family of a patient who has died or will shortly die, so are often difficult and potentially emotional. Evidence shows that when clinicians have undergone specific training in the conduct of these conversations that they are more likely to obtain consent to donation. Of course, consent is not for everyone, and getting a refusal should not be considered a failure as the principle is to ensure that when the conversation is over one is confident that the family has made an enduring decision—that is one that they will be comfortable with into the future. It has been shown, however, that families are much less likely to regret a decision to proceed with donation than to refuse,[6] and furthermore from a societal viewpoint it is our duty as health professionals to optimize donation opportunities.

Australian data show that in addition to training, using specialists in organ donation (medical or nursing) is additive in increasing the likelihood of family consent. This is probably related to the experience these specialists gain from conducting regular conversations as even in busy ICUs, any individual intensive care specialist will only conduct a few conversations each year.

A number of key principles are important in the best practice conduct of donation conversations.[7] First is that the family should understand and have accepted the patient's prognosis—either that death has occurred, in the case of DBD, or that treatment is to be withdrawn in the case of potential DCD. Organ donation should not be discussed until these matters are certain. "Decoupling" is the term used to describe the process of conducting the breaking bad news conversation on death or withdrawal separately from the donation conversation. Best conversation outcomes are seen when the donation conversation is conducted by a different specialist from he/she who conducted the breaking bad news conversation.[7] A "planning meeting" or "huddle" should be held prior to the donation conversation. At this meeting the family dynamic is reviewed, what has already been said is discussed, and a plan for the donation conversation outlined. Conducting an effective donation conversation can take time. Occasionally, it may be appropriate to take a break or to offer the family some time for refreshment, so it is important that the specialist conducting the conversation is not subject to distraction from other work.

During the conversation the specialist should present the option of donation in a positive manner—using a neutral approach is not appropriate. In jurisdictions where potential donor registers are used, and it is known that the potential donor is registered, then it is appropriate to style the conversation along the lines of a discussion to outline how the person's wishes can be fulfilled rather than to gain consent. After each donation conversation a team review should be held to provide an opportunity to reflect and improve upon practice.

DONOR MANAGEMENT

Once donation has been agreed the focus of management of the patient changes from treatment and support in the expectation of survival to the support of organ function to make best outcomes from transplantation possible. In the case of the brain dead potential donor, there are no conflicts as in most countries the patient is now legally dead and there is no ethical issue with focusing completely on organ function. In potential DCD cases, however, there may be an issue with treatments, investigations, or interventions that have the potential to cause harm or discomfort to the patient, who is not yet dead, but will likely soon be so (note that in not all cases described have potential DCD donors died following WCRS). The ethics of such so-called premortem interventions are complex; however, many would consider that if the patients themselves had given consent to donation at any time during his/her life, then as part of this they would have the expectation that interventions might be done to ensure good organ function as they would wish any transplant to be as successful as possible. However, in some jurisdictions, such as NSW in Australia, families (surrogates) do not have the legal authority to consent for treatments that are not to improve a patient's own health and wellbeing.

During the development of brain death, herniation of the brainstem triggers autonomic, endocrine, and inflammatory changes. Hypotension (>80% of donors), diabetes insipidus (DI, >60% of donors), hypothermia, and hypernatremia are common, with disseminated intravascular coagulation, cardiac arrhythmias, pulmonary edema, and metabolic acidosis less frequently encountered. Several donor management guidelines and reviews have been published,[8] but there is still a paucity of evidence to guide clinical practice. The recommendations are largely based on physiological rationale, consensus statements, and limited clinical research. The following practice points are important:

- ❑ The time from brain death to organ retrieval surgery should be kept as short as possible.
- ❑ The goal of donor management is to optimize organ function in order to maximize the number of organs transplanted and maximize the transplantation outcome for the recipient.
- ❑ The key to optimal donor management is frequent clinical assessment of organ function and the response to interventions.

Cardiovascular System

Initially, brainstem ischemia leads to intense sympathetic activation with hypertension and possible pulmonary edema; however, this is usually transient and followed by hypotension which is frequently more prolonged. Early hypertension is best treated with short-acting agents such as esmolol or sodium nitroprusside. Hypotension if untreated can lead to end-organ ischemia. Initial management involves ensuring euvolemia (concomitant DI may result in rapid fluid shifts) and the administration of a vasoconstrictor catecholamine such as noradrenaline. Addition of vasopressin is useful if noradrenaline requirements are escalating and should be considered early if DI is present. Invasive hemodynamic monitoring can be a useful guide to therapy; central venous pressure and cardiac output monitoring being of most value. Poor cardiac function or ongoing instability despite volume, noradrenaline, and vasopressin should lead to the consideration of administration of hormonal replacement. Methylprednisolone, 15 mg/kg intravenous (IV) bolus and triiodothyronine by infusion 4 μg/hr are suggested.

Respiratory System

Many potential lung donors fail to eventuate due to potentially preventable causes such as atelectasis, pulmonary edema (neurogenic and fluid overload), and pneumonia. After brain death, ventilation management should change to a lung protective focus. The main target is to minimize lung trauma by using low tidal volumes (6-8 mL/kg), low mean airway pressures, and optimal positive end-expiratory pressure with recruitment maneuvers. The head of the bed should be elevated to 30°, and regular tracheal toilet using closed suction systems and chest physiotherapy performed. Bronchoscopy is often requested as part of donor assessment and may be used to obtain bronchoalveolar lavage samples for culture and to clear stagnant secretions. There should be a low threshold for the commencement of respiratory pathogen antimicrobials.

Diabetes Insipidus

Marked polyuria usually signifies DI and should be treated early with desmopressin or vasopressin as it can rapidly lead to hypovolemia, hemodynamic instability, and organ hypoperfusion, or the development of hypernatremia which negatively impacts on liver graft function. Desmopressin 1-4 μg 4-8 hourly is usually effective. Hypernatremia can be treated with nasogastric water or IV 5% glucose. (There is now no concern regarding any potential adverse cerebral effect of this).

General Care

The brain dead potential organ donor should otherwise be treated as any other intensive care patient with good nursing care concentrating on the dignity of the body and maintenance of normothermia and normoglycemia (using IV insulin in necessary). If enteric feeding is in progress, this should be continued.

Management of the Potential Donor after Circulatory Death

As these patients are not dead, but it has been determined that death is inevitable, the primary focus of management is on the person's comfort and dignity. Appropriate analgesic and sedative medications should be commenced or continued and titrated to comfort. Management that is solely related to the underlying condition can be ceased (as long as this will not hasten death, as the patient needs to be supported until organ retrieval is possible). Otherwise the strategy should be to maintain as normal as possible physiology and biochemistry until the time of WCRS. Nutrition should be continued, and other supportive treatments such as dialysis and inotropes are continued up to the time of WCRS.

Once circulatory standstill has occurred, it is necessary to rapidly access the patient's organs that are destined for transplant and infuse the cold preservative solutions. In order to limit the time for this to occur, it is recommended that WCRS occurs in the operating theater suite for potential DCD patients. This has logistic challenges but has been successfully implemented in many hospitals across Australia. The treating intensive care team is responsible for the conduct of WCRS and the administration of any palliative medications to the patient between the time of WCRS and the time of the patient's death. This should not be undertaken by the members of the organ donation team in order to prevent any impression of conflict of interest.

ORGAN DONATION AND THE COMMUNITY

There are marked differences in family donation consent rates internationally. The reasons for this are likely multifactorial. Often religious or cultural reasons are given as explanation; however, organ donation is permitted by all major religions, and cultures that have low acceptance of donation have little objection to receiving a transplant. Undoubtedly hospital processes involved in donor identification, assessment, consenting, and management play a vital role in determining the success of an organ donation program as has been clearly illustrated in Spain.[2] The effect of legislative approaches is unclear. Although most of the countries leading a league table of donors per million population have an "opt-out" system for donation, there are a number of "opt-out" countries at the bottom of the table as well. There is little evidence to support the value of organ donation registers in increasing donation; however, in Australia the family consent rate when a potential donor is registered is around 90%, compared with only 40% when there is no registration or family knowledge of wishes. Unfortunately, only about 30% of the population are registered, and this has been difficult to shift despite considerable government effort.

In almost all countries, whether "opt-out" or "opt-in," the family are always approached for their assent to donation before proceeding. Having community buy-in to the process is thus vital. Using the media to promote good news stories about the successes of transplantation is probably quite effective, and "high profile" donors always result in a transient increase in donation consents. High levels of trust in the healthcare system and that the donation and transplantation system is fair and equitable is most important. If any doubts are raised, this can have a serious adverse effect on donor numbers.[9]

REFERENCES

1. White SL, Hirth R, Mahíllo B, et al. The global diffusion of organ transplantation: trends, drivers and policy implications. Bull World Health Organ. 2014;92:826-35.
2. Matesanz R, Domínguez-Gil B, Coll E, et al. How Spain reached 40 deceased organ donors per million population. Am J Transplant. 2017;17:1447-54.
3. Zier JL, Spaulding AB, Finch M, et al. Improved time to notification of impending brain death and increased organ donation using an electronic clinical decision support system. Am J Transplant. 2017;17:2186-91.
4. Bendorf A, Kerridge IH, Stewart C. Intimacy or utility? Organ donation and the choice between palliation and ventilation. Crit Care. 2013;17:316.
5. Brieva J, Coleman N, Lacey J, et al. Prediction of death in less than 60 minutes after withdrawal of cardiorespiratory support in potential organ donors after circulatory death. Transplantation. 2014;98:1112-8.
6. Rodrigue JR, Cornell DL, Howard RJ. The instability of the organ donation decisions by next of kin and factors that predict it. Am J Transplant. 2008;8:2661-7.
7. Lewis VJ, White VM, Bell A, et al. Towards a national model for organ donation requests in Australia: evaluation of a pilot model. Crit Care Resusc. 2015;17:233-8.
8. Kotloff RM, Blosser S, Fulda GJ, et al. Management of the potential organ donor in the ICU. Crit Care Med. 2015;43:1291-325.
9. Schwettmann L. Decision solution, data manipulation and trust: the (un-)willingness to donate organs in Germany in critical times. Health Policy. 2015;119:980-9.

CHAPTER 12

Do-Not-Attempt Cardiopulmonary Resuscitation Decision-Making

Michael AJ Park, Kate Barnett, Ross C Freebairn

INTRODUCTION

Cardiac arrest is inevitable in the process of dying. Depending on the circumstances, cardiopulmonary resuscitation (CPR) can be an effective means of saving lives or an unwelcome and unnecessary intrusion in the natural dying process. It is now accepted that CPR is an inappropriate intervention for certain patients, and this has led to the development of CPR status decisions within health-care environments. For CPR to be indicated there needs to be an acceptable balance of benefit over harm. Therefore, it is important to identify beforehand those patients who either do not wish to undergo CPR in the event of a cardiac arrest or who suffer from pre-existing medical conditions that make CPR ineffective.

DEFINITION

Cardiopulmonary resuscitation is an emergency procedure that includes chest compressions often combined with artificial ventilation. Its role is to preserve brain function until further measures are taken to restore spontaneous circulation and breathing in a person whose heart has stopped.

A *do-not-attempt* CPR (DNACPR) decision is intended to prevent inappropriate CPR attempts where it clearly will not work or would not be wanted by a patient. Such attempts can cause significant harm and distress to a patient and their family, as it can be an undignified and highly traumatic process. However, a DNACPR decision relates only to the act of CPR and must not in itself place any limitations on other aspects of a patient's future medical treatment.[1,2]

PRINCIPLES

Indication for Cardiopulmonary Resuscitation

Cardiopulmonary resuscitation is indicated where there is a reasonable chance of a success in terms of restoring the pulse, reasonable neurologic outcome, and no unacceptable (by the patient) decrease in subsequent quality of life.

Cardiopulmonary Resuscitation is a Therapy

Cardiopulmonary resuscitation is like any other therapy and therefore must have indications and a therapeutic goal. Clinicians need to assess whether it is an appropriate treatment for the individual patient. Consideration of the likelihood of restoration of a pulse and respiration should be made initially along with the benefit for the patient.

What makes Cardiopulmonary Resuscitation Different from other Therapies?

Cardiopulmonary resuscitation differs from other therapies in that it cannot wait until the patient requires CPR before seeking consent.[3] To facilitate autonomy, we need to ask the patient in advance. The whole question that needs to be asked is "If CPR is deemed as an appropriate therapy for you, would you want it?"

Why do we need a Cardiopulmonary Resuscitation Status Decision?

The legislation regulating CPR differs in different countries and is often either not well articulated, or in many countries, law clearly requires that a patient be resuscitated where the procedure would be beneficial to him or her. All patients shall be presumed as having consented to CPR unless there is documentation in the medical record indicating the contrary.[4]

Cardiopulmonary resuscitation should be initiated in the event of cardiac or respiratory arrest unless a CPR status decision has been clearly documented. If in doubt, resuscitate.

If a decision is not documented for a hospitalized patient, this will effectively result in a for CPR order by default. Alternatively, it leaves the decision to be made at short notice by medical staff who may not be acquainted with the patient and at a time when it may be difficult to ascertain the patient's wishes. This is not ideal, and steps must be taken to avoid this default.[5] In some countries, DNACPR orders are not recognized, and physicians are required to provide CPR to patients irrespective of the patient's wishes or potential efficacy.[6,7]

DISCUSSION ABOUT CARDIOPULMONARY RESUSCITATION

A discussion with the patient about his/her wishes for CPR does not need to take place if the likelihood of such an event is low, i.e. a reasonable person in the patient's circumstances would not expect it to be discussed. This applies to patients admitted for minor surgery, childbirth, investigation of non-life-threatening disease, and any other patient where the chance of a cardiorespiratory arrest is remote.

Patients in whom there is an intermediate or high risk of cardiac or respiratory arrest should have a conversation to allow shared decision-making regarding CPR. This is to be undertaken by a senior clinician or delegated junior clinician involved with their care, at or as soon as is it is practical following hospital admission. However, a diagnosis is often necessary in order to give a realistic prognosis. Therefore discussion may need to be delayed until either or both diagnosis and prognosis can be determined. If CPR is deemed appropriate then CPR is the default until a conversation has taken place. It is a good idea to consider a support person from the family to be present during this conversation, and ideally the discussion should take place in an environment that provides privacy.

The following points should be covered in the discussion:
- The patient's diagnosis and prognosis
- The overall aims of treatment and realistic outcomes
- The nature of CPR response
- The reasons that will make CPR ineffective
- The likelihood of hospital survival and the possibility of permanent brain damage
- The effect and of a CPR status decision on the patient's current and future management.

A more limited discussion may be appropriate in urgent clinical circumstances. If the decision not to commence CPR is based on its ineffectiveness then:
- A discussion with the patient is not necessary before making this decision.
- A discussion with the patient and, if appropriate, those close to the patient should be conducted focusing on informing them of the nature of and reasons for the decision reached.

In some countries, notification of the CPR decision to the patient and family is mandatory by law, and in other countries, patient consent is required to withhold CPR. These laws and policies were made with the intention to encourage communication, but they can confuse the issues and may actually increase harm to patients because clinicians may choose to avoid discussion altogether.[4,8] However, it could also be argued that a clinician may not only breach the law by not informing the patients and their family of any DNACPR decision order but also breach the law if the clinicians have not discussed resuscitation with any patient who is at risk of having a cardiac arrest, irrespective of DNACPR decision-making.[9]

The clinician may feel that discussion with the patient/key person(s) regarding CPR status is inappropriate given an individual patient's circumstances, such as informing the patient will likely cause "physical or psychological harm," although this has not been defined.[10] However, it is essential that the patient and/or key person(s) must be aware that death due to illness/disease is certain and cannot be prevented. This allows for key person(s) to ask questions. If the patient lacks capacity to do this then advice from relatives should be sought on what they believe would be the patient's views. Principles of confidentiality should be maintained when involving those "close to the patient."

Role of the Surrogate Decision Maker

A surrogate decision maker may be appointed by a patient. Usually, any surrogate decision maker will only take effect if the patient loses capacity to make informed decisions. The law regarding surrogate decision-making can vary from country to country, and any clinician should familiar with local laws and regulations.[11,12]

A verbal discussion in a quiet and private environment is important. Staff must speak in clear lay language, avoiding the use of medical jargon. There is an ethical and moral obligation to discuss CPR in a manner that respects religious beliefs and cultural needs. It may be necessary to involve an interpreter or cultural or religious support people, especially if there is no family support.

Effectiveness of Cardiopulmonary Resuscitation

Cardiopulmonary resuscitation has a low success rate in terms of survival to hospital discharge. Success rates vary depending on the clinical state moments prior to the cardiopulmonary arrest. Those most likely to benefit from CPR are those with sudden, unexpected circulatory collapse or abrupt respiratory insufficiency in the setting of acute cardiovascular illness. All other patients have a lesser chance of a good outcome. The best results are achieved with rapid and effective CPR.

The effectiveness of CPR can be dynamic during a patient's hospital stay. This means that during the patient's course of their illness, there may be a period that CPR will have no effect, but CPR may become more effective as the patient recovers from their illness. Therefore DNACPR decisions should be regularly reviewed based on the patient's clinical state.

When to use DNACPR Decisions?

When the Patient Declines Cardiopulmonary Resuscitation?

According to some laws a competent patient has the legal right to refuse CPR, just like any other therapy.

Clinicians must ensure the patient is fully informed and understands the consequences of declining CPR.

Patients may have already considered the choice to decline CPR despite clinicians believing that it is an appropriate therapy. This may be expressed verbally or nonverbally or in accordance with a valid and applicable advance decision (advanced directive). Advance directives may be presented and must be applied unless there is reason to suppose that they are no longer valid.

A patient derived CPR decision (whether they accept or decline the provision of CPR) shall remain until revoked by the patient.

Assessment of capacity: Capacity is the ability to make an informed decision. Competence is the ability to understand the question and the consequences of the decision.
A person is unable to make an informed decision if they:
- Lack the insight and judgment
- Are unable to make a decision about a matter relating to his or her personal care and welfare
- Are unable to understand the nature of decisions about matters relating to his or her personal care and welfare
- Are unable to foresee the consequences of decisions about matters relating to his or her personal care and welfare or of any failure to make such decisions
- Are unable to communicate (verbally on nonverbally) about matters relating to his or her personal care and welfare.

Competence is always presumed present unless proven otherwise.

Where Attempting Cardiopulmonary Resuscitation will not be Effective?

This is a clinical decision and is based on a clinical assessment of the patient and whether CPR is appropriate. The role of the clinical team is to decide whether CPR would realistically have a successful outcome. If the therapy will not work then it is logical not to provide it. However, such decisions cannot involve quality of life judgments made only by the clinical team and must comply with accepted medical standards.

Where the Burdens of Attempting Cardiopulmonary Resuscitation Outweighs the Benefits?

If CPR is effective, the benefits of prolonging life must be weighed against the potential risks to the patient. These include:
- Prolonging of suffering
- Poor postarrest quality of life
- Potential for injury during the attempt
- The potential for a subsequent unsuccessful resuscitation.

It may be helpful to consider whether the patient would benefit from intensive care as this is the likely scenario following a "successful" prolonged CPR attempt. There are more outcomes from CPR than simply "life" and "death." Many people who survive need to cope with fractures, collapsed lungs, severe pain, and even internal hemorrhages. There is also a spectrum of disability, including coma, brain damage, and organ failure. Thought must be given to situations in which the expected benefit is outweighed by the potential risk. When an individual patient's condition is such that CPR will not alter the patient's expected death, the clinician does not have a duty to avert that death at all costs. Do you want everything done? is not a valid question in this circumstance. In discussing CPR, consideration should be given to things the patient values and what outcomes the patient would find acceptable or unacceptable. The conversation should focus on the patient rather than the decision and ideally should be linked with goals of care.[13,14]

It is essential that those patients who have capacity and have declined CPR, or those where such efforts are inappropriate, are identified and a natural death is allowed. Every case needs to be considered on an individual basis, especially the need for discussion with the patient and family. At all times, patients should be kept informed of their current medical state and appropriate treatment options. The appropriateness of performing or not performing CPR can change depending on the patient's clinical situation. A DNACPR decision relates only to the act of CPR and does not in itself place any limitations on other aspects of a patient's future medical treatment. It is not be confused with goals of care or palliative care.[15]

LIMITED RESUSCITATION

A limited cardiac arrest response, where the extent of resuscitation to be undertaken is documented, is a valid intervention when the limits are clearly stated in advance and agreed with the patient and the clinicians involved. Documenting limits on resuscitation, such as "for three shocks only," is not useful and can confuse clinical teams. The preference would be to limit cycles of CPR dependent on response. "Slow codes" or token attempts at resuscitation where ineffective resuscitation is knowingly provided in order to appear to be taking action are ethically unacceptable.

DOCUMENTATION

Any discussion must be fully documented in the patient's health record by the clinician involved even if an order is not made. In this way the discussion is recorded and communicated to all clinicians involved in the care of the patient. Documentation of the discussion must include:
- The date and time of discussion;
- The individuals present;
- The result of discussion;
- Whether the decision is at the request of the patient or medically initiated;
- The date and time of the decision being made;
- The decision DNACPR—allows a natural death;
- The indication for the decision;
- The name and signature of the person completing the order;
- The name of the consultant with whom the order has been discussed;
- The individuals with whom the decision has been discussed;
- A time for review if required.

IS A DNACPR STATUS PERMANENT?

In addition to readily reversible causes, it may be appropriate to temporarily suspend a DNACPR status during some procedures if the procedure itself could precipitate a respiratory or cardiac arrest. CPR would be appropriate while the reversible cause was treated unless the patient has specifically refused interventions in such circumstances.

If the patient's clinical condition improves but the patient lacks decision-making capacity, the DNACPR status should be reviewed by the clinical team. If the patient has decision-making capacity, the medical decision should be reviewed and discussed with the patient. Any previous request for a DNACPR status made by a patient can be cancelled at the subsequent request of the patient while they remain mentally competent. If the patient loses decision-making capacity, the decision they made regarding CPR while mentally competent should be respected.

CONFLICT RESOLUTION

- *If the patient and clinician differ in their opinions regarding CPR provision*: The patient is entitled to a second opinion.
- *If the family and clinician differ in their opinions regarding CPR status decisions*: The decision is ultimately the clinician's, but a second opinion should be sought and every effort made to explain to the family the rationale for the decision.

Ethical principles behind CPR status decisions:[16]
- *Patient autonomy*: A patient has the right to be informed of any proposed treatment or procedure and to consent to or refuse that treatment/procedure.
- *Principle of beneficence*: Clinicians and other health professionals are not obliged to provide treatments they do not regard as beneficial.
- *Principle of nonmaleficence*: Clinicians and other health professionals have a positive duty to refrain from providing treatment/procedures that have the potential only for harm.

There are numerous scenarios where DNACPR orders can cause both clinical and ethical dilemmas and practices may vary from country to country.[17] An example of a clinical dilemma is a patient who has a patient-initiated DNACPR order who undergoes surgery and develops an anaphylaxis from a medicine or dysrhythmia from central line insertion. An example of an ethical dilemma is where a patient has initiated a DNACPR order then a medical error leads to a cardiac arrest.

In both the above cases the cause is potentially reversible, and therefore the principle of beneficence can take precedence over the principle of autonomy. In some institutions, patients who are undergoing surgical procedures have their DNACPR order annulled because situations that may require CPR during surgery are likely to be more reversible.[18]

REFERENCES

1. Resuscitation Council. Decisions relating to CPR statement RC UK (2016). [online] Available from https://www.resus.org.uk/dnacpr/decisions-relating-to-cpr/. [Accessed December, 2018].
2. Resuscitation Council. Do not attempt CPR. [online] Available from https://www.resus.org.uk/dnacpr/do-not-attempt-cpr-model-forms/. [Accessed December, 2018].
3. Freebairn R. CPR for all? Ethical and medicolegal considerations. N Z Med J. 2011;124(1328):7-9.
4. Indian Health Service. Guide guidelines for withholding cardiopulmonary resuscitation. [online] Available from https://www.ihs.gov/ihm/pc/part-3/p3c25/ [Accessed December, 2018].
5. Medical Council of New Zealand. End of life issues. In: Cole's medical practice in New Zealand, 12th edition. Wellington: Medical Council of New Zealand.
6. Gibbs AJO, Malyon AC, Fritz ZBM. Themes and variations: an exploratory international investigation into resuscitation decision-making. Resuscitation. 2016;103:75-81.
7. Saifan AR, Alrimawi I, AbuAlruz ME, et al. The perspective of Palestinian physicians and nurses about the do-not-resuscitate order for terminally ill patients. Health Sci J. 2016;10(3):6.
8. Downar J, Warner M, Sibbald R. Mandate to obtain consent for withholding nonbeneficial cardiopulmonary resuscitation is misguided. CMAJ. 2016;188(4):245-6.
9. Etheridge Z, Gatland E. When and how to discuss "do not resuscitate" decisions with patients. Br Med J. 2015;350:h2640.
10. Macfarlane M, Shayler S, Nelms L, et al. Tracey judgement and hospice DNACPR orders: steady as she goes or seismic change? BMJ Support Palliat Care. 2018.
11. Freebairn R, Hicks P, McHugh GJ. Informed consent and the incompetent adult patient in intensive care—a New Zealand perspective. Crit Care Resusc. 2002;3:202-5.
12. Young R, King A. Consent for the critically ill patient. Crit Care Resusc. 2002;4:12-3.
13. Fritz Z, Slowter A, Perkins G. Resuscitation policy should focus on the patient, not the decision. Br Med J. 2017;356:j813.
14. Perkins GD, Griffiths F, Slowther A, et al. Do-not-attempt-cardiopulmonary-resuscitation decisions: an evidence synthesis. In: Health Services and Delivery Research, No. 4.11. Southampton, UK: NIHR Journals Library; 2016.
15. Srithan G, Mills AC, Levinson MR, et al. Doctors' attitudes regarding not for resuscitation orders. Aust Heath Rev. 2017;41:680-7.
16. Bossaert LL, Perkins GD, Askitopoulou H, et al. European Resuscitation Council guidelines for resuscitation 2015. Section 11. The ethics of resuscitation and end-of-life decisions. Resuscitation. 2015;95:302-11.
17. Mentzelopoulos SD, Bossaert L, Raffay V, et al. A survey of key opinion leaders on ethical resuscitation practices in 31 European Countries. Resuscitation. 2016;100:11-7.
18. Dawson SR, McBrien ME. Management of 'Do Not Attempt Cardiopulmonary Resuscitation' (DNACPR) decisions in the perioperative period. J Perioper Pract. 2015;25(7-8):126-8.

SECTION 2

Organ Dysfunction

Outlines

13. Atrial Fibrillation in Intensive Care Unit
14. Cardiogenic Shock (with Intra-aortic Balloon pump)
15. Asthma and Chronic Obstructive Pulmonary Disease
16. Acute Pulmonary Embolism
17. Chest Trauma
18. Traumatic Brain Injury
19. Encephalitis
20. Acute Liver Failure
21. Diarrhea in Intensive Care Unit
22. Gastric Stasis in Intensive Care Unit
23. Mesenteric Ischemia
24. Necrotizing Pancreatitis
25. Critical Care in Burns
26. Necrotizing Soft Tissue Infections
27. Metabolic Acidosis
28. Anaphylaxis
29. Organophosphate Poisoning
30. Snake Envenomation
31. Toxidromes

CHAPTER 13

Atrial Fibrillation in Intensive Care Unit

Muhammad Habibullah Rana, Monika Gulati Kansal, Hao Zheng Wong

INTRODUCTION

Atrial fibrillation (AF) is defined as a supraventricular tachyarrhythmia with uncoordinated atrial activation and consequently ineffective atrial contraction.[1] Although AF is the most common arrhythmia encountered in critically ill patients affecting about 10–46% of the studied cohort,[2-4] there is a limited evidence regarding its management. As a result, significant variation in clinical practice is noticeable among different intensive care unit (ICU) populations. AF is an indicator of the severity of the underlying disease and it also has a significant impact on the clinical outcome.[4,5] Multiple studies have reported its association with increased morbidity and mortality in different intensive care settings.[5-7]

ETIOPATHOLOGY

Multiple risk factors (Box 13.1) have been described in literature that are known to trigger AF.[8] Meierhenrich et al. reported in a prospective observational study that an increased level of C-reactive protein was associated with an increased incidence of AF in a patient with septic shock[9] indicating the role of inflammation to trigger AF. Certain interventions in ICU increase the risk of AF. In a prospective observational study, Seguin et al. found that insertion of the pulmonary artery catheter was an independent risk factor for AF.[10] The incidence of AF correlates with severity of illness described by different scoring systems, for example, Acute Physiology and Chronic Health Evaluation II and Simplified Acute Physiology Score II.[11] Hence, AF has been described as a marker of severity of underlying illness.

BOX 13.1: Risk factors for atrial fibrillation.

Patient's factors
- Advanced age
- Male sex
- Obesity
- Fluid overload
- Hypoxemia
- Hypotension
- Anemia
- Acid–base abnormalities
- Electrolyte abnormalities
- Disease severity (APACHE II > 20)

Comorbidities
- Ischemic heart disease
- Pre-existing calcium-channel blocker/beta-blocker use

Presenting diagnosis
- Shock
- Sepsis
- Heart failure
- Myocardial infarction
- Blunt thoracic trauma
- Thoracic surgery
- Trauma

Intensive care intervention
- Vasopressor use
- Withdrawal of beta-blocker
- Pulmonary artery catheter

(AF: atrial fibrillation; APACHE: Acute Physiology and Chronic Health Evaluation)

DIAGNOSIS OF ATRIAL FIBRILLATION

The diagnosis of atrial fibrillation is based on Electrocardiography criteria mentioned in Box 13.2 and Figures 13.1 and 13.2.

CLASSIFICATION (TABLE 13.1)

Terminology to Describe Atrial Fibrillation in Critically Ill Patient

- *New-onset atrial fibrillation*: It refers to AF occurring in response to different pathophysiological triggers in critically ill patients.
- *Pre-existing AF*: AF in critically ill patient known to have paroxysmal/persistent/permanent/long-standing AF.

BOX 13.2: Electrocardiography criteria.

- Irregular R-R interval
- Replacement of P wave with a fibrillatory wave that marks irregular, bizarre atrial activation
- Ventricular activation varies widely with usual ventricular rate of 100–180 beats/min
- The QRS complex is usually narrow but wide QRS complex (>20 ms) is possible with concurrent conduction abnormality (e.g. bundle branch block) or pre-excitation via an accessory pathway
- An additional feature of underlying pathology including myocardial ischemia, left ventricular hypertrophy, or conduction abnormalities

IMPACT OF ATRIAL FIBRILLATION

Atrial fibrillation leads to an adverse impact on cardiac dynamics. Ineffective atrial contraction impairs diastolic filling causing decreased left ventricular preload. The rapid ventricular rate driven by AF causes impaired cardiac contractility, leading to a decreased cardiac output and potentially resulting in worsening hemodynamic and pulmonary congestion.[12] Patients with underlying heart failure [heart failure with preserved ejection fraction (HFpEF) or heart failure with reduced ejection fraction (HFrEF)] tolerate tachyarrhythmia poorly.[13] Sometimes, asymptomatic diastolic failure is unmasked by fast AF.[14]

Atrial fibrillation may adversely affect duration of ventilator dependence, length of ICU stays, rates of thromboembolic events, and overall hospital mortality. In a retrospective observational study, Tseng et al. showed AF independently increased the risk of weaning failure and was associated with prolonged ventilator dependence.[15] In a prospective study, Moss et al. reported AF was associated with increased length of ICU stay and increased in-hospital mortality.[5] In a large retrospective study, Carrera et al. showed that new-onset AF (NOAF) was associated with greater disease severity and poorer short-term ICU outcome, but it was not independently associated with in hospital mortality.[16] In a retrospective analysis, Walkey et al.

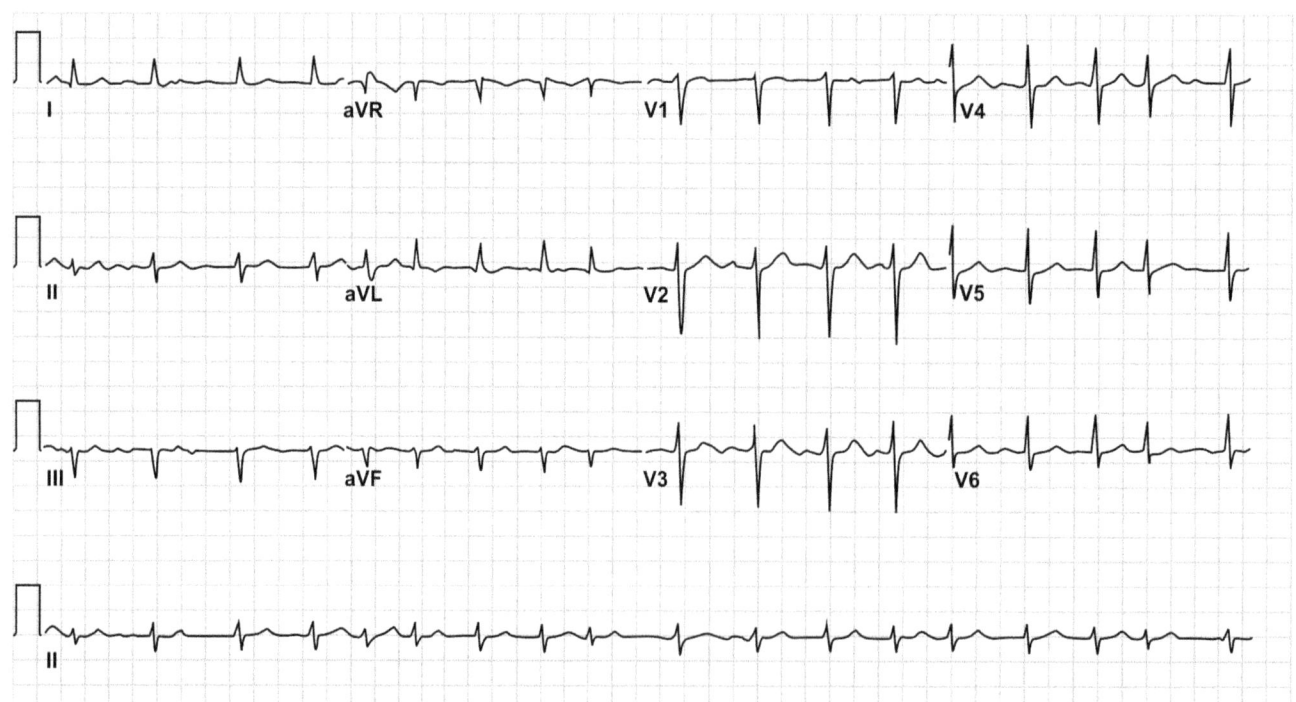

FIGURE 13.1: ECG showing AF with rapid ventricular rate. (AF: atrial fibrillation; ECG: electrocardiography)

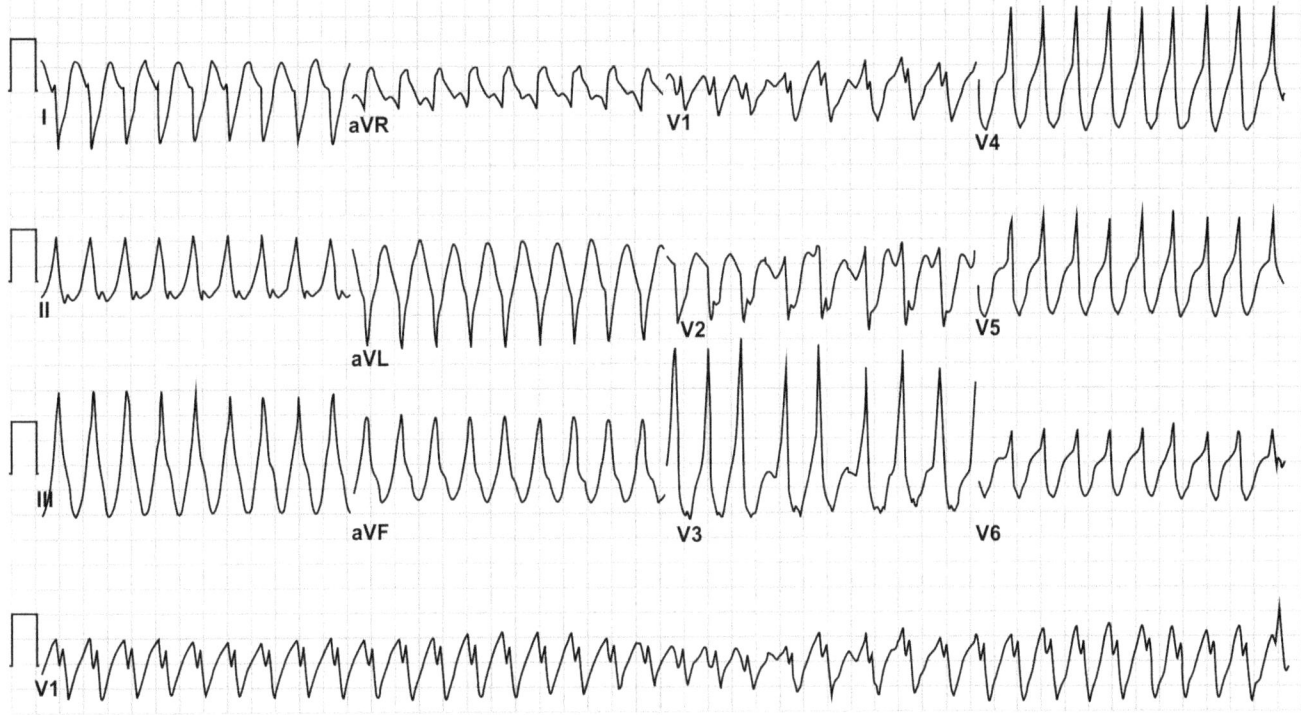

FIGURE 13.2: ECG showing AF with wide QRS complex.
(AF: atrial fibrillation; ECG: electrocardiography)

Table 13.1: Classification of atrial fibrillation.	
Paroxysmal AF	Terminates spontaneously or with intervention within 7 days
Persistent AF	Continuous AF that is sustained >7 day
Permanent AF	Continuous AF > 12 months in duration
Long-standing persistent AF	When the patient and the clinician make a joint decision to stop further attempts to restore and/or maintain sinus rhythm
Nonvalvular AF	AF in the absence of rheumatic mitral stenosis, a mechanical or bioprosthetic heart valve, or mitral valve repair

(AF: atrial fibrillation)

found a NOAF in a patient with sepsis was associated with an increase in post-discharge incidence of heart failure, ischemic stroke, and increased mortality when compared to a septic patient with pre-existing or no AF.[17]

EVIDENCE

Although, AF has a significant impact on the outcome, very limited evidence exists for the management of AF in ICU. Acknowledging this knowledge gap, Kanji et al. concluded no recommendation can be made on standard treatment for AF in a noncardiac critically ill adult patient.[18] Hence the evidence for management of AF in a critically ill patient is based on observational studies, expert opinion and is largely extrapolated from non-ICU settings.

MANAGEMENT

The principle of management of AF includes treatment of underlying pathological triggers, optimization of hemodynamic status, restoration of normal rhythm or controlling rate, and prevention of complications, such as stroke, systemic thromboembolism, and heart failure. The chosen treatment modality depends on underlying pathophysiology and the impact of AF on hemodynamic status.

Treatment of Modifiable Triggers

Identification and treatment of underlying pathophysiological conditions should be sought as most of the patients with AF will have one or more risk factors. Aggressive treatment of sepsis, ischemia, correction of electrolytes, hypoxia, treatment of concurrent volume overload or dehydration, and controlling temperature might reverse AF.

Rate versus Rhythm Control

At present, there is no evidence to compare rate versus rhythm-control strategy in intensive care patients. Evidence is mostly extrapolated from non-ICU settings for the long-term management of AF. Caldeira et al. in a meta-analysis comparing rate-control and rhythm-control strategy in medical patients, found no significant difference in outcome with either strategy.[19] Moreover, Sethi et al. in another meta-analysis found that rhythm-control strategy is associated with more serious adverse effect without any outcome benefit when compared with rate-control strategy.[20] However, the National Institute for Health and Care Excellence (NICE) guideline recommends a rate-control strategy in general except for the following patient group:[21]
- Atrial fibrillation with a reversible cause.
- Heart failure thought to be primarily caused by AF.
- New-onset AF.
- Atrial fibrillation is considered suitable for an ablation strategy to restore sinus rhythm.
- For whom a rhythm-control strategy would be more suitable based on clinical judgment.

It is not clear which strategy is more favorable for the critically ill patient. Kanji et al. showed that a pharmacological rhythm-control strategy was attempted for 76% of patient with NOAF which successfully restored sinus rhythm in 87% of treated patient, although 42% of patient had a recurrence. Interestingly, only 18% of this group of patients left ICU with AF.[18]

At present, evidence-based recommendation cannot be made to favor of any specific strategy. But probably rate control is more pragmatic for a patient with pre-existing AF, elderly age, or structural cardiac pathology. On the other hand, rhythm control might be a more favorable option for the young patient, NOAF, HFpEF, tachycardia-induced cardiomyopathy, or hemodynamic instability.

Rate-Control

A rate-control strategy tolerates AF but controls ventricular rate facilitating diastolic filling, to improve left ventricular preload and cardiac output. This approach improves morbidity, reduces tachycardia-induced cardiomyopathy and incidence of HFpEF. The optimum heart rate target for the critically ill patient is unknown. The American Heart Association (AHA) recommends a heart rate of 80 beats/min, but up to 110 beats/min might be reasonable if the patient is asymptomatic and does not have heart failure.[22] Pharmacological rate control can be achieved by beta-blockers, digoxin, the calcium-channel blockers, or combination therapy. Antiarrhythmic agents, such as amiodarone, dronedarone, sotalol, and to some extent, propafenone also, have rate-controlling properties.

The choice of agent depends on the presence or absence of symptoms, hemodynamic status, cardiac function, and underlying trigger. International guidelines recommend beta-blocker and calcium-channel blockers for acute rate control.[22-24] In a meta-analysis, Segal et al. showed that the efficacy of digoxin is inferior to beta-blockers and calcium-channel blockers in the presence of high sympathetic tone.[25] Similar findings were observed when Schreck et al. compared the effectiveness of diltiazem with digoxin in the emergency department for acute onset AF in a randomized controlled trial (RCT); diltiazem was found to be superior for controlling heart rate.[26] Despite this, selected patients with isolated cardiac pathology, especially those with a poor left ventricular function, may still benefit from digoxin.

Beta-Blockers

Beta-blockers reduce heart rate, cardiac excitability, delay conduction, optimize ventricular filling, and reduce cardiac workload and oxygen consumption. The negative inotropic effects of beta-blockers warrant cautious use in critically ill patients, especially for those with poor left ventricular ejection fraction. However, recent evidence assures the safety of beta-blocker even in the context of HFrEF. The European guideline recommends continuing beta-blocker if the patient was previously on it and to start beta-blocker at a small dose in acute heart failure patient.[23]

The efficacy and safety of multiple agents, including esmolol, metoprolol, bisoprolol, carvedilol, and nebivolol, has been established. Esmolol is a short-acting agent which is available in intravenous formulation and can be used for acute heart rate control, especially for patients with left ventricular dysfunction.

Calcium-Channel Blocker

Nondihydropyridine calcium-channel antagonists, such as verapamil or diltiazem, can be used for rate-control strategy. Verapamil is a more cardioselective drug that blocks both T- and L-type calcium channel, resulting in reduced excitability and conductivity. Diltiazem acts on the heart as well as blood vessels causing reduced excitability, conductivity, and vasodilation. Both drugs have negative inotropic action. Nondihydropyridine calcium-channel blockers should be used cautiously with beta-blockers and digoxin. Combination therapy can potentially lead to heart block or severe heart failure, especially in elderly patients.

Glycosides

The cardiac glycoside digoxin primarily inhibits Na–K adenosine triphosphatase (ATPase) pump leading to an increase in intracellular calcium ion. It has an inotropic action, but it increases vagal tone, hence reduces conductivity. The positive inotropic effect with simultaneous rate control effect makes digoxin a preferable agent for patients with HFrEF. Its action is of slow onset, and most often it fails to achieve rate control in a critically ill patient in the presence of high sympathetic tone. However, it can be effective for the selected patient groups either solely or in combination with another rate-limiting agent. Digoxin is primarily excreted by the kidney, so patients with renal failure should be monitored for toxicity while on digoxin therapy. Digoxin completes with potassium for its binding site of Na–K ATPase pump, hence hypokalemia should be avoided as it may potentiate toxicity.

Rhythm-Control

A rhythm-control strategy comprises restoring sinus rhythm by means of a pharmacological agent or by electrical cardioversion. AHA and NICE guideline recommend cardioversion for treatment of the hemodynamically unstable patient, but this recommendation might not be appropriately applied to the critically ill patient. In a critically ill patient, cause of shock is frequently multifactorial, and AF is commonly a manifestation of underlying pathology rather being the cause of shock. However, restoring normal sinus rhythm may improve hemodynamic status for patients with isolated cardiogenic shock or complex shock. Rhythm-control strategy may prevent arrhythmia-induced cardiomyopathy and improve synchronization with an intra-arterial balloon pump. Another consideration is that any intervention to restore sinus rhythm is frequently unsuccessful or nonsustained and lacks evidence of outcome benefit.

The choice of intervention to restore rhythm depends on the clinical context, for example, presence of the symptoms (such as chest pain, shortness of breath) or hemodynamic instability. Kanji et al. showed pharmacological cardioversion is a more commonly used strategy for the critically ill patient likely due to the complex nature of shock state.[18] Electrical cardioversion should be considered for a patient with acute symptomatic AF with or without hemodynamic instability when the shock is believed to be primarily caused by arrhythmia or when the reversal of arrhythmia is likely to improve a refractory shock state.

Electrical Cardioversion

Electrical cardioversion renders the highest success rate in restoring normal sinus rhythm in elective settings, but the response can be poor for critically ill patients; even when sinus rhythm is restored, the effect is usually transient, leading to recurrence of AF for most of the patients.[27] Concurrent treatment with a pharmacological agent might help to restore and retain sinus rhythm.

Electrical cardioversion is conducted for two groups of patients in ICU. Elective or semielective cardioversion is instituted for stable patients when restoring normal sinus rhythm is believed to improve long-term outcome. On the other hand, urgent cardioversion is conducted for patients with hemodynamic instability that are frequently in complex refractory shock state for further optimization of hemodynamic status by rhythm control. Unfortunately, cardioversion is often unsuccessful for the second group of patients and has failed to show any outcome benefit.

Cardioversion is performed by delivering a synchronized shock using electrode over the chest of the patient after necessary preparation. Kirchhof et al. in an RCT, showed the anterior–posterior placement of electrodes and biphasic waveform is associated with an increased success rate.[28] The initial energy level for the first cardioversion is controversial; shock is repeated with an increasing energy level if the initial attempts are unsuccessful. Glover et al. in an RCT, found a biphasic waveform with a higher initial energy level (200 J compared with 100 J) was associated with more successful cardioversion.[29] Obese patient with increased chest wall impedance frequently needs higher energy level.

Pharmacological Cardioversion

Commonly used pharmacological agent for rhythm-control strategy includes amiodarone, flecainide, propafenone, and ibutilide. A recent survey in the United Kingdom found that amiodarone was the most commonly used antiarrhythmic in ICU.[30] Amiodarone prolongs phase III of the action potential, slows conduction, and increases the refractory period of cardiac tissue. Amiodarone has less negative inotropic effect compared to other agents, and it is a comparatively safer agent for patients with structural heart disease. Amiodarone is a lipophilic agent with a high volume of distribution. Asymptomatic elevation of liver enzyme is common while the patient is on amiodarone; rarely life-threatening hepatotoxicity has been reported. Dronedarone is a multichannel blocker similar to amiodarone with better pharmacokinetic properties but was associated with increased incidence of heart failure, stroke, and death from cardiovascular event,[31] hence, the use of dronedarone is not recommended. Flecainide and propafenone are group Ic agent, effective in achieving rapid rhythm control but associated with an increased mortality in a patient with structural heart disease.[32] Intravenous magnesium a commonly used agent for NOAF in ICU and was found efficacious for control of rate and rhythm by Onalan et al. in a meta-analysis.[33] Ho et al., in another meta-analysis, showed adding magnesium to digoxin reduces ventricular response in NOAF. The effect of intravenous magnesium on the ventricular rate and its cardiovascular side effects are less significant than other calcium antagonists or amiodarone.[34]

Anticoagulation Strategy

The risk of embolic stroke and conversely the safety of anticoagulation are not established in the context of AF in the critically ill patient. Multiple scoring systems, e.g. $CHADS_2$, CHA_2DS_2-VASc are recommended for long-term risk stratification for ischemic stroke in a patient with nonvalvular AF,[21,22] but none of the scoring systems have been validated in the settings of intensive care. Although critical illness might predispose the patient to the prothrombotic state, disease-related coagulopathy, organ dysfunction, and impaired drug metabolism may increase the risk of anticoagulant-related complications. Darwish et al. in a retrospective observational study, found no septic patients with NOAF with high $CHADS_2$ score had a stroke during hospitalization despite not receiving anticoagulant treatment; rather, the risk of anticoagulant-related complication was increased.[35] In absence of clear evidence the use of anticoagulation should be justified on a case-to-case basis weighing risk and benefit.

PRACTICE PRESCRIPTIONS

- Critically ill patients underlying pathophysiological condition commonly lead to complex shock state; same pathological condition triggers fast AF. Hence, treatment of underlying pathophysiological state remains in the focus of management.
- When AF is cause of shock, immediate cardioversion is indicated.
- Rate-control strategy is indicated in general for hemodynamically stable patient. Beta-blockers are preferable agents for rate-control strategy, calcium-channel blockers should be considered in condition where beta-blocker is contraindicated (asthma). Digoxin should be considered for patients with HFrEF.
- Rhythm-control strategy should be considered for young patient, patient with HFpEF, tachyarrhythmia-induced cardiomyopathy, or when hemodynamic goal is not achieved by other strategy.
- Intravenous magnesium is effective for NOAF for both rate- and rhythm-control strategy.
- Use of anticoagulation should be justified on a case-to-case basis weighing risk and benefit.
- We propose a management algorithm for management of rapid AF in critically ill patient as shown in Flowcharts 13.1 and 13.2.

FLOWCHART 13.1: Algorithm to guide anticoagulation for patient with fast AF in ICU.

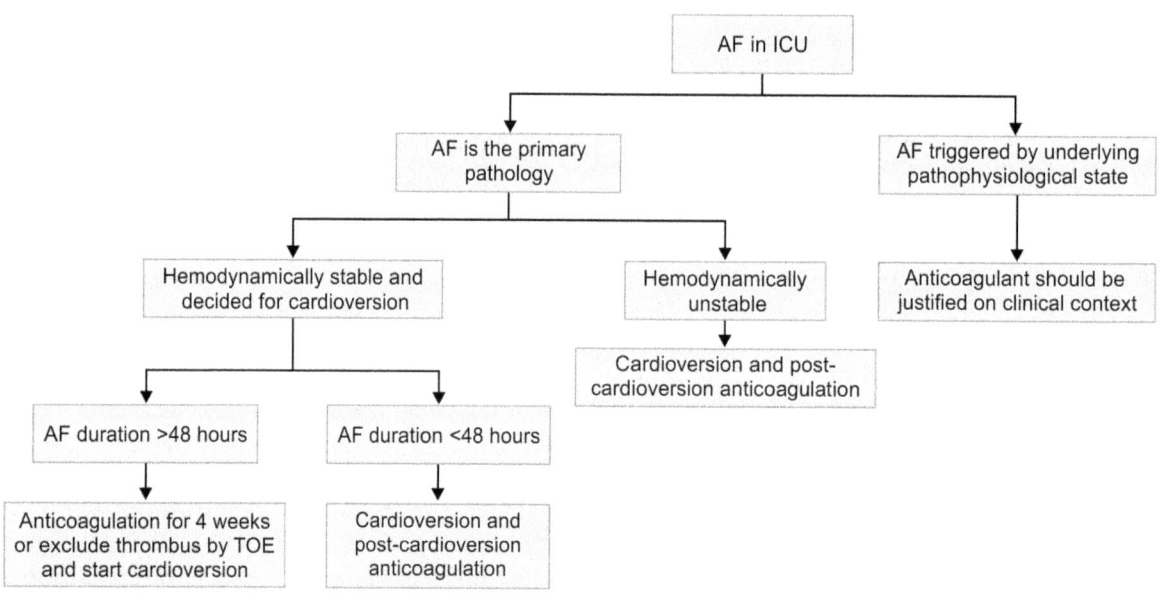

(AF: atrial fibrillation; ICU: intensive care unit; TOE: transoesophageal echocardiography)

FLOWCHART 13.2: Algorithm for management of fast atrial fibrillation in ICU.

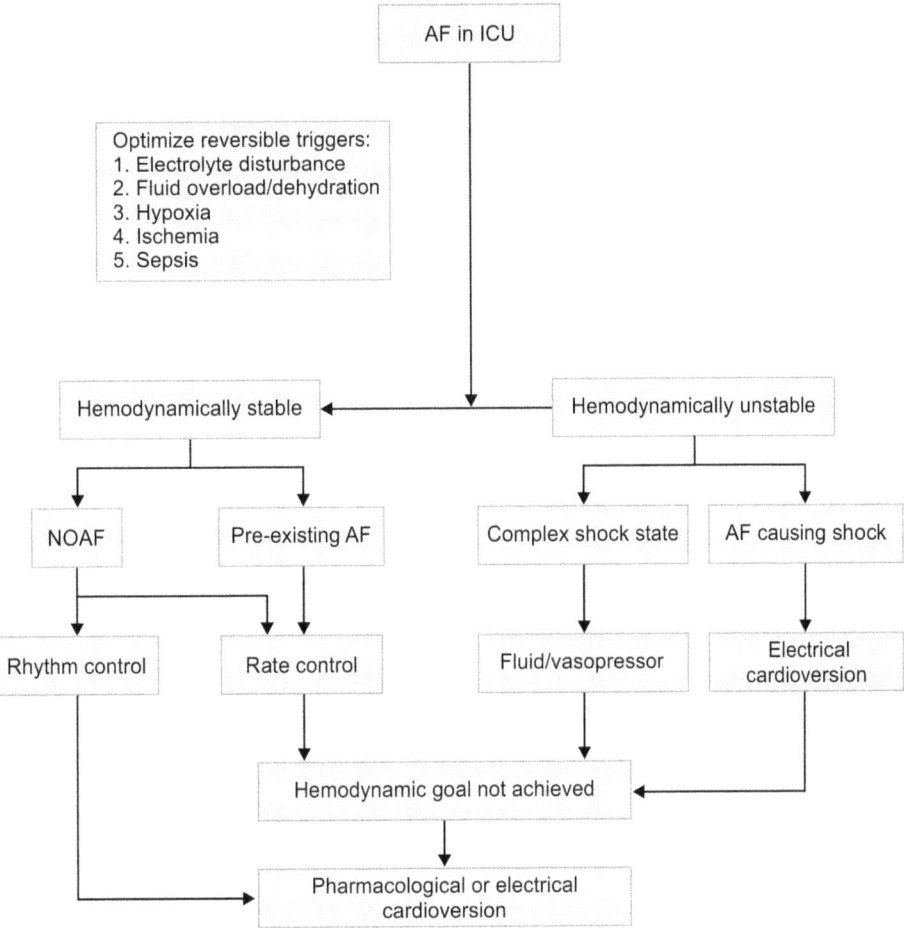

(NOAF: new-onset atrial fibrillation; AF: atrial fibrillation; ICU: intensive care unit)

REFERENCES

1. Fuster V, Rydén LE, Asinger RW, et al. ACC/AHA/ESC guidelines for the management of patients with atrial fibrillation: executive summary a report of the American College of Cardiology/American Heart Association task force on practice guidelines and the European Society of Cardiology committee for practice guidelines and policy conferences (committee to develop guidelines for the management of patients with atrial fibrillation) developed in collaboration with the North American Society of Pacing and Electrophysiology. Circulation. 2001;104(17):2118-50.
2. Klein Klouwenberg PM, Frencken JF, Kuipers S, et al. Incidence, predictors, and outcomes of new-onset atrial fibrillation in critically ill patients with sepsis. A cohort study. Am J Respir Crit Care Med. 2017;195(2):205-11.
3. Yoshida T, Uchino S, Yokota T, et al. The impact of sustained new-onset atrial fibrillation on mortality and stroke incidence in critically ill patients: a retrospective cohort study. J Crit Care. 2018;44:267-72.
4. Seguin P, Launey Y. Atrial fibrillation is not just an artefact in the ICU. Crit Care. 2010;14(4):182.
5. Moss TJ, Calland JF, Enfield KB, et al. New-onset atrial fibrillation in the critically ill. Crit Care Med. 2017;45(5):790.
6. Pangrazzi M, Lat I, Kress J. 753: Characterizing the impact of atrial fibrillation in the medical intensive care unit. Crit Care Med. 2012;40(12):1-328.
7. Preslaski C, Lat I, Mieure K, et al. 610: The impact of new-onset atrial fibrillation on clinical outcomes in the medical intensive care unit. Crit Care Med. 2011;39(12):168.
8. Sibley S, Muscedere J. New-onset atrial fibrillation in critically ill patients. Can Respir J. 2015;22(3):179-82.
9. Meierhenrich R, Steinhilber E, Eggermann C, et al. Incidence and prognostic impact of new-onset atrial fibrillation in patients with septic shock: a prospective observational study. Crit Care. 2010;14(3):R108.
10. Seguin P, Signouret T, Brangier B, et al. Incidence and risk factors of atrial fibrillation in a surgical intensive care unit. Crit Care. 2004;8(1):P92.
11. Yoshida T, Fujii T, Uchino S, et al. Epidemiology, prevention, and treatment of new-onset atrial fibrillation in critically ill: a systematic review. J Intensive Care. 2015;3(1):19.

12. Raymond RJ, Lee AJ, Messineo FC, et al. Cardiac performance early after cardioversion from atrial fibrillation. Am Heart J. 1998;136(3):435-42.
13. Dimarco JP. Atrial fibrillation and acute decompensated heart failure. Circ Heart Fail. 2009;2(1):72-3.
14. Nagarakanti R, Ezekowitz M. Diastolic dysfunction and atrial fibrillation. J Intervent Card Electrophysiol. 2008;22(2):111-8.
15. Tseng YH, Ko HK, Tseng YC, et al. Atrial fibrillation on intensive care unit admission independently increases the risk of weaning failure in nonheart failure mechanically ventilated patients in a medical intensive care unit: a retrospective case–control study. Medicine. 2016;95(20):e3744.
16. Carrera P, Thongprayoon C, Cheungpasitporn W, et al. Epidemiology and outcome of new-onset atrial fibrillation in the medical intensive care unit. J Crit Care. 2016;36:102-6.
17. Walkey AJ, Hammill BG, Curtis LH, et al. Long-term outcomes following development of new-onset atrial fibrillation during sepsis. Chest. 2014;146(5):1187-95.
18. Kanji S, Williamson DR, Yaghchi BM, et al. Epidemiology and management of atrial fibrillation in medical and noncardiac surgical adult intensive care unit patients. J Crit Care. 2012;27(3):326.e1-8.
19. Caldeira D, David C, Sampaio C. Rate versus rhythm control in atrial fibrillation and clinical outcomes: updated systematic review and meta-analysis of randomized controlled trials. Arch Cardiovasc Dis. 2012;105(4):226-38.
20. Sethi NJ, Feinberg J, Nielsen EE, et al. The effects of rhythm control strategies versus rate control strategies for atrial fibrillation and atrial flutter: a systematic review with meta-analysis and trial sequential analysis. PLoS One. 2017;12(10):e0186856.
21. NICE. Atrial fibrillation: management. Guidance and guidelines (2018). Nice.org.uk. [online] Available from https://www.nice.org.uk/guidance/cg180/resources [Accessed December, 2018].
22. January CT, Wann LS, Alpert JS, et al. 2014 AHA/ACC/HRS guideline for the management of patients with atrial fibrillation: a report of the American College of Cardiology/American Heart Association Task Force on practice guidelines and the Heart Rhythm Society. J Am Coll Cardiol. 2014;64(21):e1-76.
23. McMurray JJ, Adamopoulos S, Anker SD, et al. ESC guidelines for the diagnosis and treatment of acute and chronic heart failure 2012: the Task Force for the Diagnosis and Treatment of Acute and Chronic Heart Failure 2012 of the European Society of Cardiology. Developed in collaboration with the Heart Failure Association (HFA) of the ESC. Eur Heart J. 2012;33(14):1787-847.
24. Piepoli MF, Hoes AW, Agewall S, et al. 2016 European Guidelines on cardiovascular disease prevention in clinical practice: The Sixth Joint Task Force of the European Society of Cardiology and Other Societies on Cardiovascular Disease Prevention in Clinical Practice (constituted by representatives of 10 societies and by invited experts) Developed with the special contribution of the European Association for Cardiovascular Prevention & Rehabilitation (EACPR). Atherosclerosis. 2016;252:207-74.
25. Segal JB, McNamara RL, Miller MR, et al. The evidence regarding the drugs used for ventricular rate control. J Family Pract. 2000;49(1):47-59.
26. Schreck DM, Rivera AR, Tricarico VJ. Emergency management of atrial fibrillation and flutter: intravenous diltiazem versus intravenous digoxin. Ann Emerg Med. 1997;29(1):135-40.
27. Mayr A, Ritsch N, Knotzer H, et al. Effectiveness of direct-current cardioversion for treatment of supraventricular tachyarrhythmias, atrial fibrillation, in surgical intensive care patients. Crit Care Med. 2003;31(2):401-5.
28. Kirchhof P, Eckardt L, Loh P, et al. Anterior–posterior versus anterior-lateral electrode positions for external cardioversion of atrial fibrillation: a randomised trial. Lancet. 2002;360(9342):1275-9.
29. Glover BM, Walsh SJ, Mc Cann CJ, et al. Biphasic energy selection for transthoracic cardioversion of atrial fibrillation. The BEST AF Trial. Heart. 2008;94(7):884-7.
30. Chean CS, McAuley D, Gordon A, et al. Current practice in the management of new-onset atrial fibrillation in critically ill patients: a UK-wide survey. PeerJ. 2017;5:e3716.
31. Connolly SJ, Camm AJ, Halperin JL, et al. Dronedarone in high-risk permanent atrial fibrillation. N Engl J Med. 2011;365(24):2268-76.
32. Echt DS, Liebson PR, Mitchell LB, et al. Mortality and morbidity in patients receiving encainide, flecainide, or placebo: the Cardiac Arrhythmia Suppression Trial. N Engl J Med. 1991;324(12):781-8.
33. Onalan O, Crystal E, Daoulah A, et al. Meta-analysis of magnesium therapy for the acute management of rapid atrial fibrillation. Am J Cardiol. 2007;99(12):1726-32.
34. Ho KM, Sheridan DJ, Paterson T. Use of intravenous magnesium to treat acute onset atrial fibrillation: a meta-analysis. Heart. 2007;93(11):1433-40.
35. Darwish OS, Strube S, Nguyen HM, et al. Challenges of anticoagulation for atrial fibrillation in patients with severe sepsis. Ann Pharmacother. 2013;47(10):1266-71.

CHAPTER 14

Cardiogenic Shock (with Intra-aortic Balloon Pump)

Yatin Mehta, Ajmer Singh

INTRODUCTION

Cardiogenic shock (CS) is the most catastrophic manifestation of acute decompensated heart failure (HF), with clinical features of decreased cardiac output (CO) and tissue hypoxia despite adequate intravascular volume. Acute myocardial infarction (AMI) leading to CS is seen in 5–15% of patients, which means approximately 40,000–50,000 patients per year in the United States, and 60,000–70,000 in Europe.[1] Recent advancements in therapeutic management of CS, mainly by early revascularization, have reduced the mortality rates from 80% to 40–50% in patients with AMI.[2]

DIAGNOSIS

The earlier interpretation of CS included following parameters: persistent hypotension [systolic blood pressure 80–90 mm Hg or mean arterial pressure (MAP) 30 mm Hg below baseline] with severe reduction in cardiac index (1.8 L/min/m^2 without support or 2.0–2.2 L/min/m^2 with support) and adequate or elevated filling pressure [e.g. left ventricular (LV) end-diastolic pressure >18 mm Hg or right ventricular (RV) end-diastolic pressure >10–15 mm Hg].[3] At present, CS can be diagnosed on the basis of clinical criteria alone, without including advanced hemodynamic parameters. The accepted criteria for the diagnosis of CS include (1) systolic blood pressure <90 mm Hg for >30 minutes or vasopressors requirement to achieve a blood pressure >90 mm Hg; (2) pulmonary congestion or elevated LV filling pressure; and (3) signs of impaired organ perfusion with at least one of the following criteria: (a) altered mental status, (b) cold, clammy skin, (c) oliguria, and (d) increased serum lactate.[2]

ETIOLOGY

Left/right ventricular dysfunction resulting from AMI is the most common cause of CS, seen in about 80% of patients. Less common causes of CS include ventricular septal rupture, rupture of free wall of LV, acute mitral regurgitation, acute myocarditis, and arrhythmias. The detailed etiology of CS is shown in Box 14.1. Predisposing factors for CS in the setting of AMI include old age, hypertension, diabetes

BOX 14.1: Causes of cardiogenic shock.

1. Acute myocardial infarction (AMI)
2. Mechanical complications of AMI
   – Ventricular septal rupture, free wall rupture, papillary muscle rupture
3. Left/right ventricular dysfunction caused by acute myocarditis, pericarditis, stress-induced cardiomyopathy, hypertrophic cardiomyopathy, postpartum cardiomyopathy
4. Postcardiotomy, cardiac tamponade, postcardiac arrest
5. Refractory tachyarrhythmias
6. Aortic dissection, acute coronary dissection
7. Acute valvular regurgitation caused by endocarditis, chordal rupture, trauma
8. Acute stress in the setting of aortic or mitral stenosis
9. Massive pulmonary embolism
10. Others: Hemorrhage, infection, bowel ischemia, hypothyroidism, hyperthyroidism

mellitus, coronary artery disease involving multiple vessels, anterior wall MI, prior MI or angina, ST elevation MI (STEMI), history of HF, and left bundle branch block.[4]

PATHOPHYSIOLOGY

Severe LV dysfunction, RV dysfunction, and alteration in peripheral vasculature play a vital role in the pathogenesis of CS. The degree of LV dysfunction associated with CS is often severe enough to cause hypotension and compromised coronary blood flow. Impaired coronary perfusion decreases CO causing further decrease in the perfusion of vital organs including that of heart. Furthermore, there is release of catecholamines following hypoperfusion, which causes an increase in myocardial oxygen demand in addition to arrhythmogenic and cardiotoxic effects. Vasopressors and inotropes transiently improve peripheral perfusion and CO but do not adjourn this causal nexus. Intra-aortic balloon pump (IABP) support may relieve ischemia and support the circulation for a short period of time, but it is not a definitive therapy. Revascularization therapy in the form of percutaneous coronary intervention (PCI) or coronary artery bypass graft (CABG) surgery, by causing relief of coronary obstruction, interrupts the negative feedback loop and improves outcome.[5]

Right ventricular dysfunction contributes to about 5% of cases of CS, and it impairs LV filling by causing a reduction in CO, or change in geometry of interventricular septum, or both. In patients with CS resulting from RV dysfunction, RV-end diastolic pressure is often >20 mm Hg, which may cause shift of interventricular septum to the left. This can cause an elevation in left atrial pressure, impaired LV filling, and impaired LV systolic function.[6] Therefore, inotropic therapy, instead of aggressive fluid therapy, may be more helpful in patients with CS due to RV dysfunction. Perfusion of vital organs is maintained by constriction of peripheral arterioles resulting from catecholamines release, triggered by low CO. Furthermore, there is release of vasopressin and angiotensin II, which leads to improved coronary and systemic perfusion. An imbalance between angiopoietin-1 and angiopoietin-2 causes an impairment of microcirculation and vascular leakage. In addition, MI can also cause systemic inflammatory response syndrome, release of interleukin-6, and tumor necrosis factor-α, which in turn can lead to inappropriate vasodilatation, impaired gut perfusion, and myocardial depression.[7]

LABORATORY EVALUATION

In clinical practice, recommended laboratory investigations include complete blood count, arterial blood gas, serum electrolytes/lactate, serum creatinine, liver function tests, cardiac troponin, and natriuretic peptides. Chest X-ray and ultrasound provide details on the size of the heart and pulmonary vasculature and may establish diagnosis in many pathological conditions. A 12-lead electrocardiography is invaluable for the diagnosis of conditions, such as STEMI, non-STEMI, pulmonary embolism, and drug toxicity. A comprehensive transthoracic echocardiogram provides information on the etiology of CS, extent of myocardium in jeopardy, presence of mechanical complications, valvular insufficiency, cardiac tamponade, volume status, pulmonary artery (PA) pressure, and it can guide vasoactive therapy. Additional imaging with transesophageal echocardiography or computed tomography may be used whenever indicated.

MANAGEMENT

The management section will be discussed under the following headings: (1) revascularization, (2) hemodynamic management, (3) pharmacological treatment, and (4) mechanical circulatory support (MCS).

Revascularization

Antithrombotic therapy in the form of aspirin and heparin is recommended for the treatment of AMI. On the basis of results of coronary angiography, clopidogrel is indicated in patients undergoing PCI. The first innovation in the treatment of CS was achieved by the randomized SHOCK (SHould we emergently revascularize Occluded coronaries for Cardiogenic shocK) trial.[8] Although SHOCK trial did not show superiority of revascularization over medical therapy on 30-day mortality, but it did show an increase (13%) in 1-year survival in patients subjected to early revascularization in CS. Many other studies, including Swiss Multicenter Study of Angioplasty for Shock trial, have shown survival benefit of early revascularization across all age-groups.[9] American College of Cardiology/American Heart Association guideline for CS has recommended early revascularization for those <75 years of age (class I) and for suitable candidates ≥75 years of age (class IIa).[10] In the current European Society of Cardiology (ESC) guidelines, early revascularization (by either PCI or CABG) is a class 1B recommendation.[11] If a delay has occurred in transfer to PCI facility, or if PCI is impossible, thrombolysis is indicated. Mortality rates were lowest in CS patients undergoing primary PCI, when door-to-angioplasty times were <90 minutes.[8] Despite comparable mortality rates with CABG and PCI, CABG is rarely indicated in CS, and PCI of the culprit lesion is the usual practice. Furthermore, PCI of multiple critically stenosed vessels or unstable lesions in addition to the culprit lesion is class IIa B recommendation.[11] During PCI, use of ancillary anticoagulation including heparin, or direct thrombin inhibitors, is recommended along with antiplatelets.

Hemodynamic Management

Pulmonary artery catheter (PAC) is helpful to establish the diagnosis of CS, to measure the filling pressures/vascular resistances/CO, and to guide vasoactive medications. Cardiac power output (calculated as MAP × CO/451) strongly correlated with mortality in CS in SHOCK trial registry.[12] Routine usage of PAC, however, is on the wane, and its use is recommended only in severely hypotensive patients. Echocardiography, a noninvasive modality, can provide information about LV ejection fraction, PA systolic pressure, and PA wedge pressure.

Pharmacological Treatment

The basic therapy for CS includes use of fluids to maintain euvolemia and inotropes/vasopressors to maintain MAP above 65 mm Hg. β-Blockers and renin–angiotensin–aldosterone system antagonists should be avoided. Early use of statins is recommended in CS associated with MI. Inotropic agents and vasopressors are required to maintain coronary and systemic perfusion till a definitive therapy resolves the CS. Most inotropic agents cause an increase in myocardial oxygen consumption; hence, they should be used in lowest possible doses for a short duration. Norepinephrine (class IIb B), because of its high potency and less incidence of arrhythmia compared to dopamine (class IIa C) and dobutamine, is recommended for severely hypotensive patients.[10] Dobutamine, however, can be used along with norepinephrine in order to increase contractility. Levosimendan, a calcium ion sensitizer or phosphodiesterase inhibitors, cause an increase in myocardial contractility without increasing oxygen consumption and risk of vasodilation; however, their role in CS is very limited. Since they do not increase CO through β-receptor stimulation, they may be effective when downregulation of β-receptors has occurred due to chronic HF. Close monitoring of urine output should be done, and renal replacement therapy should be initiated whenever indicated. If noninvasive ventilation is ineffective, invasive ventilation with lung-protective approach should be used to avoid parenchymal injury. Positive end-expiratory pressure (PEEP) has favorable effect on gas exchange, lung recruitment, and airway patency. Moreover, it reduces LV afterload, preload, improves work of breathing, and optimizes delivery of oxygen to the myocardium. In patients with RV dysfunction, PEEP attenuates hypoxic pulmonary vasoconstriction and thereby reduces pulmonary vascular resistance and increases cardiac index, by attenuating pulmonary edema. Adjuvant therapy includes nutritional supplementation, glycemic control, thromboembolism and stress ulcer prophylaxis, and restrictive blood transfusion regimen. For unwitnessed cardiac arrest patients, therapeutic hypothermia is recommended to prevent brain injury.

Mechanical Circulatory Support

Mechanical circulatory support, in the form of IABP or LV assist device (LVAD), or extracorporeal life support (ECLS) system, is used to improve hemodynamics in patients unresponsive to standard therapy or to overcome the limitations of inotropes/vasopressors.

- *Intra-aortic balloon pump:* Intra-aortic balloon counter pulsation has long been the cornerstone therapy for CS, with an insertion rate of approximately 50,000 per year in the United States, and about 200,000 annually worldwide. First clinical use of IABP was described by Kantrowitz et al. in 1968.[13] IABP catheter is comprised of a polyurethane membrane, installed on a vascular 7–8-F catheter, and is placed in the descending thoracic aorta just distal to the left subclavian artery. The inflation and deflation events are timed with the cardiac cycle, and the electronics of the IABP console produce the counterpulsations. IABP improves coronary perfusion by augmentation of diastolic pressure with balloon inflation. In addition, it improves systemic perfusion with afterload reduction via systolic balloon deflation. Balloon inflation timing should coincide with aortic valve closure; otherwise, aortic insufficiency and LV strain may occur. Similarly, late inflation will result in impaired coronary perfusion. Early deflation will cause inappropriate loss of afterload reduction, and late deflation will increase LV work by causing an increase in afterload.

  The common indications for the use of IABP are CS following MI or CS with mechanical complications (25%), hemodynamic support during high-risk PCI (21%), weaning from cardiopulmonary bypass (16%), preoperatively in high-risk CABG (13%), and unstable angina refractory to medical therapy (12%). The presence of aortic dissection and severe aortic regurgitation are considered contraindications for the use of IABP. Use of IABP in CS was considered class I recommendation by American and European guidelines before 2012–2013. IABP indications have been downgraded to IIb B in the

2012 ESC guidelines and to IIa B in the 2013 American guidelines, based on the recent meta-analysis.[14,15] IABP-SHOCK II trial ($n = 600$) did not show significant difference in terms of 30-day mortality between the IABP group and conventional treatment group in CS patients.[16] There was no difference in the secondary end point (serum lactate, renal function, and inotrope requirement) and 12-month mortality in the two groups (52% IABP group vs 51% control group). IABP-SHOCK II trial's results have influenced recent ESC revascularization guidelines with a further downgrading of the IABP with a new class III A recommendation for the routine use in CS.[11] At present, the use of IABP is only indicated in mechanical complications of AMI (class IIa C recommendation).[12] The negative results of IABP-SHOCK II trial, however, should not be considered the demise of this therapy; it may inspire the future cardiovascular researchers to perform more randomized trials.

- *Left ventricular assist devices:* Temporary MCS with LVADs breaks off the vicious cycle of ischemia, hypotension, and myocardial dysfunction and allows for recovery of stunned and hibernating myocardium. The mechanism involves circulation of oxygenated blood through a device that drains blood from the left side of the heart and returns blood via pulsatile or continuous flow to the systemic arteries. Both percutaneous and surgically implanted LVADs, including TandemHeart, Impella (2.5, 3.5, 5.0), CP systems, paracorporeal pulsatile device iVAC 2L, HeartWare, and HeartMate Percutaneous Heart pump, are available. The TandemHeart drains blood from the left atrium via transseptal puncture using a cannula inserted through the femoral vein. Blood is then pumped to a systemic artery, usually the femoral, with retrograde perfusion of the abdominal and thoracic aorta. In randomized trials consisting of the TandemHeart versus IABP, better hemodynamics were seen in LVAD group, although the mortality rates were the same, in CS complicating MI.[17,18] Another percutaneous device, the Impella, is positioned across the aortic valve and has shown better survival at discharge.[19] In patients with refractory CS, use of percutaneous LVADs for circulatory support is recommended (class IIa C), without any predilection for device selection.

- *Extracorporeal life support* system consists of circulation of blood through extracorporeal membrane oxygenator by the blood pump. ECLS followed by LVAD have been used as bridge to heart transplant, with a survival rate of 74% to transplantation and 87% to hospital discharge. The disadvantages of the ECLS system include large cannula size causing limb ischemia, bleeding complications, lack of LV unloading, and limited time period for its use. The low cost of the system compared to LVAD is a distinct advantage.

CONCLUSION

Cardiogenic shock is multifactorial in origin and is frequently associated with multiorgan failure and high mortality. Patient management should focus on providing effective and timely hemodynamic support, and promptly referring the patient for definitive therapy. It often requires multidisciplinary care in a tertiary care center that has the facilities for medical, surgical, and mechanical therapies. The pathophysiology and therapeutic options for CS are poorly understood. Large population-based trials and registries are required to fill this knowledge gap, with the aim to reduce the morbidity and mortality associated with this condition.

REFERENCES

1. Goldberg RJ, Spencer FA, Gore JM, et al. Thirty-year trends (1975 to 2005) in the magnitude of, management of, and hospital death rates associated with cardiogenic shock in patients with acute myocardial infarction: a population-based perspective. Circulation. 2009;119:1211-9.
2. Thiele H, Ohman EM, Desch S, et al. Management of cardiogenic shock. Eur Heart J. 2015;36:1223-30.
3. Reynolds HR, Hickman JS. Cardiogenic shock. Current concepts and improving outcomes. Circulation. 2008;117:686-97.
4. Lindholm MG, Kober L, Boesgaard S, et al. Cardiogenic shock complicating acute myocardial infarction: prognostic impact of early and late shock development. Eur Heart J. 2003;24:258-65.
5. Beyersdorf F, Buckberg GD, Acar C, et al. Cardiogenic shock after acute coronary occlusion: pathogenesis, early diagnosis, and treatment. Thorac Cardiovasc Surg. 1989;37:28-36.
6. Jacobs AK, Leopold JA, Bates E, et al. Cardiogenic shock caused by right ventricular infarction: a report from the SHOCK registry. J Am Coll Cardiol. 2003;41:1273-9.
7. Kohsaka S, Menon V, Lowe AM, et al. Systemic inflammatory response syndrome after acute myocardial infarction complicated by cardiogenic shock. Arch Intern Med. 2005;165:1643-50.
8. Hochman JS, Sleeper LA, Webb JG, et al. Early revascularization in acute myocardial infarction complicated by cardiogenic shock: SHOCK Investigators: Should we emergently revascularize Occluded coronaries for Cardiogenic shocK. N Engl J Med. 1999;341:625-34.
9. Urban P, Stauffer JC, Bleed D, et al. A randomized evaluation of early revascularization to treat shock complicating acute myocardial infarction: the (Swiss) Multicenter trial of Angioplasty for Shock: (S)MASH. Eur Heart J. 1999;20:1030-8.

10. Antman EM, Anbe DT, Armstrong PW, et al. ACC/AHA guidelines for the management of patients with ST-elevation myocardial infarction—executive summary: a report of the American College of Cardiology/American Heart Association Task Force on Practice Guidelines (Writing Committee to Revise the 1999 Guidelines for the management of patients with acute myocardial Infarction). Circulation. 2004;110: 588-636.
11. Windecker S, Kolh P, Alfonso F, et al. 2014 ESC/EACTS guidelines on myocardial revascularization: the Task Force on Myocardial Revascularization of the European Society of Cardiology (ESC) and the European Association for Cardio-Thoracic Surgery (EACTS) Developed with the special contribution of the European Association of Percutaneous Cardiovascular Interventions (EAPCI). Eur Heart J. 2014;35:2541-619.
12. Fincke R, Hochman JS, Lowe AM, et al. Cardiac power is the strongest hemodynamic correlate of mortality in cardiogenic shock: a report from the SHOCK trial registry. J Am Coll Cardiol. 2004;44:340-48.
13. Kantrowitz A, Tjonneland S, Freed PS, et al. Initial clinical experience with intra-aortic balloon pumping in cardiogenic shock. JAMA. 1968;203:113-8.
14. Steg PG, James SK, Atar D, et al. ESC guidelines for the management of acute myocardial infarction in patients presenting with ST-segment elevation. Eur Heart J. 2012;33:2569-619.
15. O'Gara PT, Kushner FG, Ascheim DD, et al. 2013 ACCF/AHA guideline for the management of ST-elevation myocardial infarction: a report of the American College of Cardiology Foundation/American Heart Association Task Force on Practice Guidelines. Circulation. 2013;127:e362-425.
16. Thiele H, Zeymer U, Neumann FJ, et al. Intraaortic balloon support for myocardial infarction with cardiogenic shock. N Engl J Med. 2012;367:1287-96.
17. Burkhoff D, Cohen H, Brunckhorst C, et al. A randomized multicenter clinical study to evaluate the safety and efficacy of the TandemHeart percutaneous ventricular assist device versus conventional therapy with intraaortic balloon pumping for treatment of cardiogenic shock. Am Heart J. 2006;152:469.e1-8.
18. Thiele H, Sick P, Boudriot E, et al. Randomized comparison of intra-aortic balloon support with a percutaneous left ventricular assist device in patients with revascularized acute myocardial infarction complicated by cardiogenic shock. Eur Heart J. 2005;26:1276-83.
19. O'Neill WW, Theodore Schreiber T, Wohns DH, et al. The current use of Impella 2.5 in acute myocardial infarction complicated by cardiogenic shock: results from the USpella Registry. J Interv Cardiol. 2014;27:1-11.

CHAPTER 15

Asthma and Chronic Obstructive Pulmonary Disease

Sing Chee Tan, Amit Kansal

EPIDEMIOLOGY

Accurate estimates on the prevalence of asthma in Asia remain elusive, due to regional variations in data quality and diagnostic criteria applied. Available data suggest that the general prevalence of asthma in Asia remains lower than in Western nations; however, there is an upward trend paralleled by increasing levels of urbanization.[1]

In contrast the burden of chronic obstructive pulmonary disease (COPD) in Asia remains higher than in Western nations and is projected to rise in the coming decades. This is attributed largely to the widespread use of tobacco products as well as ongoing issues with air pollution.[2]

The growing prevalence of both diseases, combined with increasing population density and environmental challenges, suggests that acute exacerbations due to infectious and environmental triggers will continue to present a clinical challenge to critical care physicians.

PATHOPHYSIOLOGY

Although asthma and COPD have distinct underlying pathophysiology, similar changes occur in exacerbations of both the conditions—namely bronchial wall thickening, mucus plugging, and smooth muscle hyperreactivity, resulting in expiratory flow limitation with dynamic hyperinflation and gas trapping.

Respiratory tract infections and environmental pollution are the common triggers of acute exacerbations of both asthma and COPD, with a significant proportion of exacerbations having no identifiable trigger.[3]

PHARMACOTHERAPY

Inhaled Bronchodilator Therapies

Beta Agonists and Anticholinergics

Short-acting beta agonists remain the mainstay of treatment for acute exacerbations of asthma and COPD, with evidence that combination with anticholinergics enhance bronchodilator response. This synergistic effect is most consistent in asthmatics[4] but is less consistently found in the COPD population.[5]

The use of nonselective beta agonists, such as epinephrine, is not recommended due to limited efficacy with increased side effects.[6]

Delivery Routes

Pressurized metered-dose inhalers (pMDI) with spacers and nebulizers have been shown to be equipotent at producing bronchodilation. However, the proper use of a pMDI with spacer may be limited in the acutely unwell patient, and nebulizer therapy may be preferred for logistical reasons.[7] Various nebulizer techniques have been described (jet, ultrasonic, and mesh) with varying drug delivery characteristics, but there is no evidence of clinical superiority of any particular technique.[8] In severe exacerbations not responding to intermittent bronchodilator therapy, the use of continuous nebulized bronchodilator therapy may be beneficial.[9]

In intubated patients, both pMDIs and nebulizers may be effectively used, but the former requires coordination with the inspiratory phase of the ventilator to ensure appropriate delivery.[7] As such, where clinical effect is not observed with pMDI administration, nebulized therapy should be trialed.

Significantly higher doses are required due to deposition in the ventilator circuit; this is further exacerbated by the use of active humification systems or the presence of a heat-moisture exchanger. The exact dose adjustment varies based on technique, patient disease severity, and equipment variables and should be titrated to clinical effect.[10]

Intravenous Bronchodilator Therapies

Magnesium

In asthmatics with severe exacerbations the use of intravenous magnesium is safe and beneficial and should be routinely administered. There is considerable less evidence of efficacy in patients with exacerbations of COPD,[11] but it may nonetheless be considered in light of its low cost and relative safety. Serum magnesium levels do not correlate with clinical effects due to its predominant intracellular distribution, and targeting specific levels is unlikely to be useful.

Ketamine

Ketamine is known to have a bronchodilating effect, likely mediated by indirect catecholamine release and a vagolytic effect. Evidence for its use in asthma remains large restricted to case reports or small studies, with a lack of quality evidence to recommend routine use in addition to standard bronchodilator therapy. The evidence for ketamine in exacerbations of COPD is even more limited, and its use cannot be recommended in this population.

Beta Agonists and Adrenaline

Despite a theoretical basis for the use of parenteral beta agonists in severe asthma or COPD due to reduced ventilation and inhaled drug delivery, there is a lack of benefit over inhaled bronchodilators. Furthermore, there are significant increases in side effects, including paradoxical respiratory decompensation due to metabolic effects.[12] Although their routine use is not recommended, they may have a role as rescue therapy in moribund patients who have failed all other therapies.

Methylxanthines

Methylxanthines (e.g. aminophylline) are no longer recommended for routine use in asthma or COPD exacerbations due to their narrow therapeutic window, significant side effects, and lack of efficacy in patients already on beta agonists (Table 15.1).[13,14]

Table 15.1: Suggested doses of intravenous therapies.

Drug	Suggested dose
Salbutamol	200 µg over 1 minute Followed by infusion of 5 µg/min up to 10–20 µg/min
Magnesium	10 mmol over 20 minutes
Adrenaline	5 µg/kg as a slow push Followed by infusion of 1–20 µg/min
Ketamine	2 mg/kg
Aminophylline	5 mg/kg loading dose Followed by infusion of 0.5 mg/kg/hour

Steroids

Systemic steroids improve resolution of symptoms and reduce length of stay in exacerbations of both asthma and COPD, although its clinical effects do not become apparent for a number of hours postadministration. The rapid absorption and high bioavailability of enteral steroids lead to equipotency for both oral and intravenous routes; however, the latter may be necessary for critically unwell patients in whom the oral route is unavailable.

The optimal dose and duration of steroid therapy remains a matter of expert opinion. There is a growing body of evidence suggesting moderate doses (40-60 mg prednisolone daily equivalent) would be adequate for most exacerbations, with higher doses reserved for more severe cases.[15,16] The recommended duration of steroid therapy is 5-7 days, bearing in mind that prolonged courses of steroids increase the risk of intensive care unit (ICU)-acquired weakness (ICUAW), particularly if heavy sedation and neuromuscular blockade are used to facilitate ventilation.

Inhaled corticosteroids may be added to systemic steroids, but their role in acute exacerbations of asthma or COPD is unclear.[17]

Antibiotics

Antibiotics have been shown to improve outcomes in acute exacerbations of COPD, particularly in severe exacerbations requiring admission to the ICU, and should be routinely administered. Therapy should be targeted toward respiratory infections as guided by local antibiograms if available.[15]

There is no evidence for routine antibiotic treatment in asthmatic exacerbations, unless there is evidence of pulmonary infection (e.g. fever or radiological changes).[18]

MECHANICAL VENTILATION AND OXYGEN THERAPY

Oxygen Therapy

In exacerbations of COPD, oxygen therapy per se is not deleterious and should be can be safely administered for correction of significant hypoxemia without precipitating hypercarbic respiratory failure. In particular, titrating oxygen to achieve SpO_2 goals of 88–92% leads to improved outcomes as compared to higher SpO_2 targets.[19]

Amongst asthmatics, marked hypoxemia is uncommon and should alert the clinician to a life-threatening exacerbation or coexisting pathology, such as pneumonia. There is no evidence to support any particular oxygenation target, and oxygen therapy can be safely used to maintain SpO_2 above 92%.[18]

High-Flow Nasal Cannulae

High-flow nasal cannulae oxygen therapy, which is capable of delivering oxygen at flows of up to 60 L/min, has emerged as an alternative therapy for the management of hypoxic respiratory failure. Its role in hypercapnic respiratory failure, which often occurs in COPD and asthma, is less well established, although there is limited evidence of efficacy.[19] Its observed benefit in hypercapnic respiratory failure may be attributed to enhanced dead-space washout of CO_2 and providing (limited) positive end-expiratory pressure (PEEP), thereby reducing the work of breathing and improving respiratory mechanics. It may thus be trialed in selected patients [e.g. unable to use noninvasive ventilation (NIV), not for intubation, or patients demonstrating clinical improvement].

Noninvasive Ventilation

The use of NIV has a well-established role for acute exacerbations of COPD and reduces ICU length of stay and mortality compared to early intubation.[20]

Its role in asthma is less well established, with limited evidence suggesting a reduction in the rate of intubation,[21] potentially by reducing the work of breathing, preventing respiratory fatigue, and providing time for bronchodilator treatment effect. It is reasonable to perform a trial of NIV with frequent reassessment for signs of failure, bearing in mind that NIV is a temporizing measure that does not treat the underlying disease process.

Patients with acute exacerbations of COPD and asthma who fail NIV and require intubation have significantly worse outcomes. Although this may reflect the severity of the underlying disease, a failure to recognize signs of NIV failure and a delay to intubation may play a contributing role, necessitating meticulous attention to the progress of these patients once NIV has been commenced.[21,22]

Invasive Ventilation

In both conditions the ventilation strategy should be directed toward avoiding dynamic hyperinflation and excessively high intrinsic PEEP (iPEEP). This would necessitate low inspiratory:expiratory ratios, frequent assessments of plateau and end-expiratory pressures, and watchfulness for hemodynamic sequalae of gas trapping with elevated intrathoracic pressures (Fig. 15.1). Although

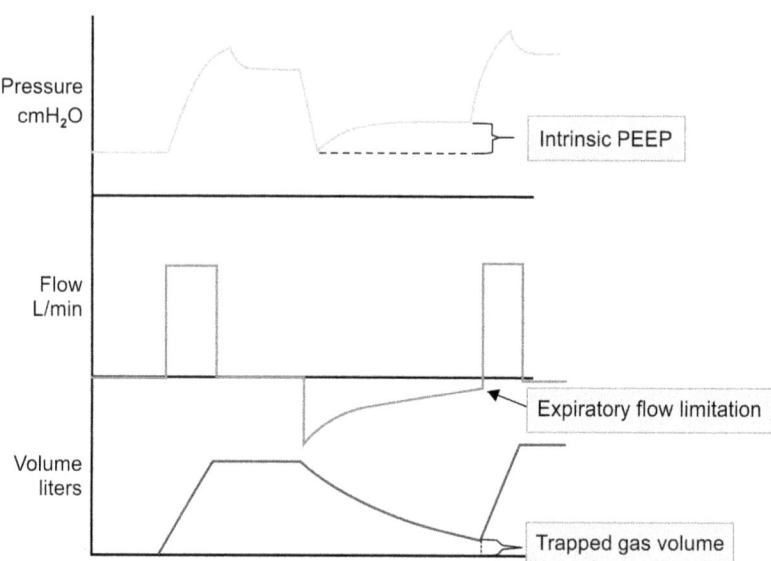

FIGURE 15.1: Ventilator waveform demonstrating intrinsic PEEP, expiratory flow limitation with incomplete exhalation, and gas trapping. (PEEP: positive end-expiratory pressure)

many modern ventilators provide the option of measuring iPEEP, this value should be interpreted with caution due to potential complete obstruction of small airways (with retained gas in the alveoli), leading to a falsely low iPEEP reading by the ventilator. Controversy still exists regarding the application of PEEP with the aim of counteracting iPEEP, and this should always be done in incremental steps with great caution.

In the weaning phase of ventilation the presence of residual iPEEP may significantly add to the spontaneous respiratory work of breathing, and this may be further compounded by breath stacking due to withdrawal of sedation.

Manual Chest Decompression

Following the institution of positive-pressure ventilation, dynamic hyperinflation may lead to difficulty in ventilation or hemodynamic instability. Active decompression occasionally suggested but should be done with caution; the presence of expiratory flow limitation may lead to a precipitous rise in intrathoracic pressures, loss of cardiac output with resultant hemodynamic collapse.

INTENSIVE CARE UNIT POLYNEUROMYOPATHY

Patients with exacerbations of COPD and asthma are at high risk of ICUAW due to the frequent use of neuromuscular blockade, high-dose steroids, deep sedation, and prolonged mechanical ventilation. This issue is particularly pronounced in the COPD population, who frequently has poor baseline nutrition and a chronic catabolic state. ICUAW develops in a more than third of these patients,[23,24] and attention should be paid to risk factor minimization, good nutritional support, and early mobilization.

NUTRITIONAL SUPPORT

Although there is no conclusive evidence on the optimal feeding strategy in the general ICU population, it is reasonable to ensure that enteral feeds are started as soon as possible, with a protein daily protein intake of 1.2–1.5 g/kg/day. Malnourished COPD patients may require higher protein intake of 1.5–2 g/kg/day, and consideration of reduced carbohydrate to fat ratios to minimize CO_2 production. Reassessment of the patient's respiratory status is required after the commencement of feeding, to avoid overfeeding which may confound ventilatory weaning.

PROGNOSIS

Despite frequent concerns regarding the prognosis of patients with COPD requiring mechanical ventilation, these patients actually have reasonable outcomes compared to patients with respiratory failure of other etiologies.[25,26] In the absence of poor prognostic markers, such as multi-organ dysfunction, it is reasonable to provide a trial of invasive ventilation, with a reassessment of treatment goals if there is a lack of clinical improvement.

Patients with acute exacerbations of asthma generally have good inhospital outcomes, which is potentially attributable to their younger age and smaller burden of comorbidities.[27]

SUMMARY

- Asthma and COPD patients should receive inhaled bronchodilators in the form of beta agonists and antimuscarinic agents, as well as systemic steroids.
- Patients with exacerbations of COPD should receive antibiotics; there is no role for routine antibiotics in asthmatics with acute exacerbations.
- Inhaled bronchodilators may be effectively given via spacer or nebulizer, with dose adjustment for intubated patients.
- Intravenous beta agonists, adrenaline, and methyl-xanthines should not be routinely used.
- Noninvasive ventilation should be used for COPD exacerbations; in asthma, a trial of NIV is reasonable. Intubation should occur early at the first signs of NIV failure.
- High-flow nasal cannulae may be of benefit in select patients and should be trialed if the patient is not in imminent need of intubation and is not tolerating NIV.
- Mechanical ventilation strategies should be aimed at minimizing dynamic hyperinflation and avoiding worsening of iPEEP.
- ICU-acquired weakness is potentially a major source of morbidity, and attention to strategies to minimize this should be adopted.
- Patients with COPD who require intubation have a reasonable chance of meaningful recovery and should be considered for a trial of invasive ventilation.

REFERENCES

1. Song WJ, Kang MG, Chang YS, et al. Epidemiology of adult asthma in Asia: toward a better understanding. Asia Pac Allergy. 2014;4:75-85.
2. Tan WC, Ng TP. COPD in Asia: where East meets West. Chest. 2008;133(2):517-27.
3. Pauwels RA. Similarities and differences in asthma and chronic obstructive pulmonary disease exacerbations. Proc Am Thorac Soc. 2004;1(2):73-6.
4. Kirkland SW, Vandenberghe C, Voaklander B, et al. Combined inhaled beta-agonist and anticholinergic agents for emergency

management in adults with asthma. Cochrane Database Syst Rev. 2017;11(1):CD001284.
5. McCrory DC, Brown CD. Anti-cholinergic bronchodilators versus beta2-sympathomimetic agents for acute exacerbations of chronic obstructive pulmonary disease. Cochrane Database Syst Rev. 2002;(4):CD003900.
6. Mondal P, Kandala B, Ahrens R, et al. Nonprescription racemic epinephrine for asthma. J Allergy Clin Immunol Pract. 2014;2(5):575-8.
7. Holland A, Smith F, Penny K, et al. Metered dose inhalers versus nebulizers for aerosol bronchodilator delivery for adult patients receiving mechanical ventilation in critical care units. Cochrane Database Syst Rev. 2013;(6):CD008863.
8. Hess DR. Aerosol delivery devices in the treatment of asthma. Respir Care. 2008;53(6):699-725.
9. Camargo CA, Spooner CH, Rowe BH. Continuous versus intermittent beta-agonists in the treatment of acute asthma. Cochrane Database Syst Rev. 2003;(4):CD001115.
10. Dhand R. Inhalation therapy with metered-dose inhalers and dry powder inhalers in mechanically ventilated patients. Respir Care. 2005;50(10):15.
11. Shivanthan MC, Rajapakse S. Magnesium for acute exacerbation of chronic obstructive pulmonary disease: a systematic review of randomised trials. Ann Thorac Med. 2014;9(2):77-80.
12. Travers AH, Milan SJ, Jones AP, et al. Addition of intravenous beta(2)-agonists to inhaled beta(2)-agonists for acute asthma. Cochrane Database Syst Rev. 2012;12:CD010179.
13. Barr RG, Rowe BH, Camargo CA. Methylxanthines for exacerbations of chronic obstructive pulmonary disease. Cochrane Database Syst Rev. 2003;(2):CD002168.
14. Addition of intravenous aminophylline to inhaled beta(2)-agonists in adults with acute asthma. Cochrane Database Syst Rev. 2012 Dec 12;12:CD002742.
15. GOLD. (2017). GOLD 2017 Global Strategy for the Diagnosis, Management and Prevention of COPD. Global Initiative for Chronic Obstructive Lung Disease—GOLD. [online] Available from http://goldcopd.org/gold-2017-global-strategy-diagnosis-management-prevention-copd/. [Accessed December, 2018].
16. National Heart, Lung, and Blood Institute. National Asthma Education and Prevention Program, third expert panel on the diagnosis and management of asthma. In: Expert panel report 3: guidelines for the diagnosis and management of asthma. Bethesda, MD: National Heart, Lung, and Blood Institute; 2007.
17. Edmonds ML, Milan SJ, Camargo CA, et al. Early use of inhaled corticosteroids in the emergency department treatment of acute asthma. Cochrane Database Syst Rev. 2012;12:CD002308.
18. GINA. (2018). 2018 GINA report: global strategy for asthma management and prevention. Global Initiative for Asthma—GINA. [online] Available from http://ginasthma.org/2018-gina-report-global-strategy-for-asthma-management-and-prevention/. [Accessed December, 2018].
19. Austin MA, Wills KE, Blizzard L, et al. Effect of high flow oxygen on mortality in chronic obstructive pulmonary disease patients in prehospital setting: randomised controlled trial. BMJ. 2010;341:c5462.
20. Osadnik CR, Tee VS, Carson-Chahhoud KV, et al. Non-invasive ventilation for the management of acute hypercapnic respiratory failure due to exacerbation of chronic obstructive pulmonary disease. Cochrane Database Syst Rev. 2017;13(7):CD004104.
21. Stefan MS, Nathanson BH, Lagu T, et al. Outcomes of noninvasive and invasive ventilation in patients hospitalized with asthma exacerbation. Ann Am Thorac Soc. 2016;13(7):1096-104.
22. Brochard L, Mancebo J, Wysocki M, et al. Noninvasive ventilation for acute exacerbations of chronic obstructive pulmonary disease. N Engl J Med. 1995;333(13):817-22.
23. Amaya-Villar R, Garnacho-Montero J, García-Garmendía JL, et al. Steroid-induced myopathy in patients intubated due to exacerbation of chronic obstructive pulmonary disease. Intensive Care Med. 2005;31(1):157-61.
24. Douglass JA, Tuxen DV, Horne M, et al. Myopathy in severe asthma. Am Rev Respir Dis. 1992;146(2):517-9.
25. Gadre SK, Duggal A, Mireles-Cabodevila E, et al. Acute respiratory failure requiring mechanical ventilation in severe chronic obstructive pulmonary disease (COPD). Medicine (Baltimore). 2018;97(17):e0487.
26. Esteban A, Anzueto A, Frutos F, et al. Characteristics and outcomes in adult patients receiving mechanical ventilation: a 28-day international study. JAMA. 2002;287(3):345-55.
27. Peters JI, Stupka JE, Singh H, et al. Status asthmaticus in the medical intensive care unit: a 30-year experience. Respir Med. 2012;106(3):344-8.

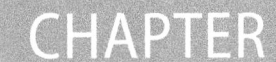

16

Acute Pulmonary Embolism

Dhanvijay Shekhar Yadavrao, Monika Gulati Kansal, Amit Kansal

INTRODUCTION

The term venous thromboembolism (VTE) comprises pulmonary embolism (PE) and deep venous thrombosis (DVT). It has an overall annual incidence of 100–200 per 100,000 inhabitants making it the third most frequent cardiovascular cause of death.[1] An acute pulmonary embolism (APE) is the most ominous presentation of VTE.

CLASSIFICATION OF PULMONARY EMBOLISM[2,3]

The classification details of pulmonary embolism are described in Table 16.1.

Mr Morris is a 54-year-old man. Day 5 post-internal fixation of a traumatic fracture of neck of the femur. The patient is referred to ICU for tachycardia and tachypnea.

The patient is awake. Heart rate: 108/min. Blood pressure: 106/54 mm Hg, Respiratory rate: 28/min, SpO_2: 97% on 2 L/min O_2

ECG: Sinus tachycardia. T inversion in V1-V3. CXR: Normal

Arterial blood gas (ABG) results: pH: 7.40, pCO_2: 30, paO_2: 88, HCO_3: 22

Troponin: Raised

Could Mr Morris have PE?

Table 16.1: Classification of pulmonary embolism (PE).

Hemodynamics	Category		Characteristics
Unstable	Massive PE (High risk PE)		• Systolic blood pressure <90 for 15 min or • Poor tissue perfusion or • Multiorgan failure along with • Extensive thrombosis such as Saddle PE or left or right main bronchus thrombus
Stable	Submassive PE (intermediate risk PE)	High risk (intermediate high risk PE)	Hemodynamically stable but moderate or severe right ventricular (RV) dysfunction or enlargement, coupled with biomarker elevation indicative of RV microinfarction and/or RV pressure overload
		Low risk (intermediate low risk PE)	Hemodynamically stable with RV dysfunction or biomarker elevation, but not both
	Small or moderate PE (Low risk PE)		Normal hemodynamics and normal RV size and function

Section 2: Organ Dysfunction

CLINICAL FEATURES

Dyspnea is the most common symptom, and tachypnea is the most common sign of PE. Table 16.2 lists the signs and symptoms of PE along with their frequencies.[4,5]

Hypotension and raised jugular venous pressure in the absence of alternate diagnosis (tension pneumothorax, acute myocardial infarction, pericardial tamponade or a new arrhythmia) strongly suggests a diagnosis of PE.[6]

INVESTIGATIONS

- *Chest radiograph*: Chest radiograph rules out alternative causes of the patient's symptoms. A normal chest radiograph in the presence of severe respiratory compromise is highly suggestive of PE.
  Hampton's hump and Westermark's sign are rare radiographic abnormalities but when present strongly suggest the diagnosis of PE (Figs. 16.1 and 16.2).
- *Electrocardiography*: ECG can exclude other differential diagnoses such as acute myocardial infarction or detect signs of right ventricular strain such as S1Q3T3 (though a rare abnormality), new right bundle branch block (RBBB), and inverted T waves in leads V1 to V4.
  More often though ECG is either normal, shows tachycardia or nonspecific ST-T changes in patients with PE.[4]
- *Arterial blood gas (ABG)*: Hypoxemia with a normal chest radiograph should raise the clinical suspicion for PE. However, 20% of patients with acute PE have a normal partial pressure of oxygen (paO_2). Most patients are also hypocapnic. But the discriminatory value of ABG in excluding PE is poor.[7]
- *Echocardiography*: Echocardiography can diagnose PE by detecting right ventricular clot if present. More

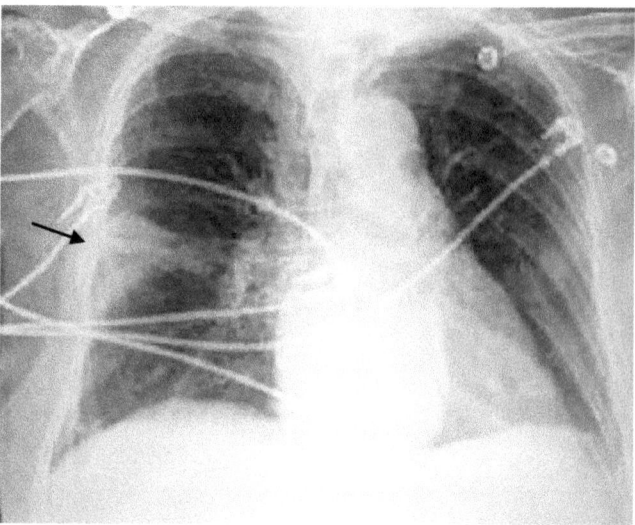

FIGURE 16.1: Hampton's hump.

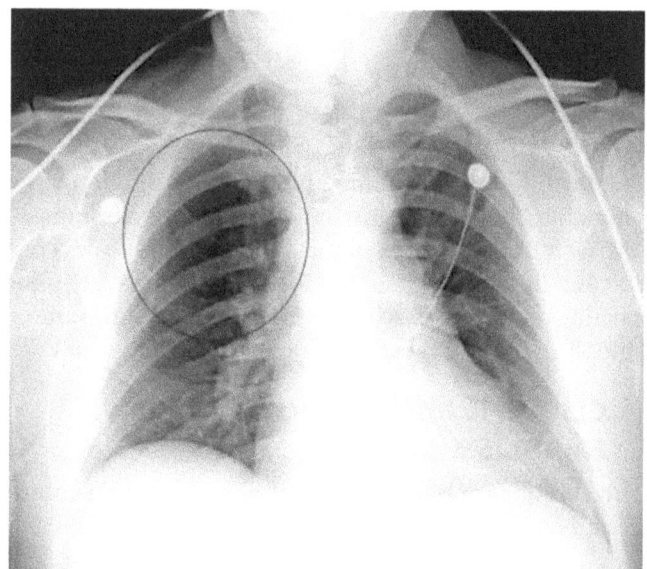

FIGURE 16.2: Westermark's sign.

often echocardiography is useful for detection of right ventricular strain among patients with established PE. Some of the signs of right ventricular (RV) strain on echocardiography are as follows:[8]

- *Right ventricular(RV)*: Left ventricular (LV) ratio more than 1 (Normal ratio: <0.6)
- Systolic dysfunction right ventricular
- Mid RV wall hypokinesis with apical sparing (McConnell's signs)
- Moderate to severe tricuspid regurgitation
- Paradoxical septal wall motion towards the left ventricle
- Atrial dilatation
- Right atrial or right ventricular thrombus

Table 16. 2: Signs and symptoms of pulmonary embolism.

Symptoms	Frequency
Dyspnea	73%
Pleuritic chest pain	66%
Cough	37%
Hemoptysis	13%
Signs	Frequency
Tachypnea	70%
Rales	51%
Tachycardia	30%
Fourth heart sound	24%
Accentuated pulmonic component of second heart sound	23%
Circulatory collapse	8%

- Absence of respiratory variation of inferior vena cava. In hemodynamically unstable patients with a high probability of PE in whom CT pulmonary angiogram (CTPA) is impractical, echocardiography (by diagnosing right heart stain) may help with the decision to start appropriate treatment (Flowchart 16.1).
- *Troponin*: Troponin levels while not having diagnostic value have a role in the assessment of RV dysfunction. They have significant prognostic implications as those patients with acute pulmonary embolism who also have raised troponin levels have increased risk of clinical worsening and death.[9]
- *B-type natriusetic peptide (BNP)*: Similar to troponin, elevated BNP has limited diagnostic value, but has significant prognostic implications.[10]
- *D-dimer*: Serum levels of D-dimer are raised in patients having any acute systemic illness. Hence elevated D-dimers levels are of not much use in the diagnosis of PE. However, when D-dimer levels are normal, PE could be practically ruled out.[11,12]
- *CT pulmonary angiogram*: A multidetector (≥16 detector rows) CTPA acquiring less than or equal to 2.5 mm section volumetric images of the chest after intravenous contrast is the imaging modality of choice for the diagnosis of PE with high sensitivity and specificity. The scan is timed precisely to yield maximal enhancement of the pulmonary arteries. CT scan can detect signs of right ventricular strain such as—(1) increased LV diameter ratio; (2) increased RV: LV volume ratio; (3) bowing or flattening of interventricular septum, and (4) reflux of contrast agent into the inferior vena cava.
- *Ventilation-perfusion scan (V/Q scan)*:[13] The radiation dose from a V/Q scan is significantly lower than that of a CTPA. It should be considered for patients in whom CTPA is contraindicated because of pregnancy, renal failure or contrast allergy. Results could be stratified into risk categories.
- Normal scan or a low probability scan (only 0–6% risk of having PE)
- High probability scan (56–96% risk of having PE)
- Non-diagnostic scan.[14]

Back to Mr Morris:

It is clear that for confirming the diagnosis and definitive treatment, he will need CTPA. However, the combination of clinical findings allows classification of patients with suspected PE into distinct categories of pre-test probability. This categorization increases the diagnostic yield of CTPA. One of the most commonly used and validated pre-test probability scores is the Wells Score (Table 16.3).[15]

This score categorizes patient into three categories (Table 16.4).

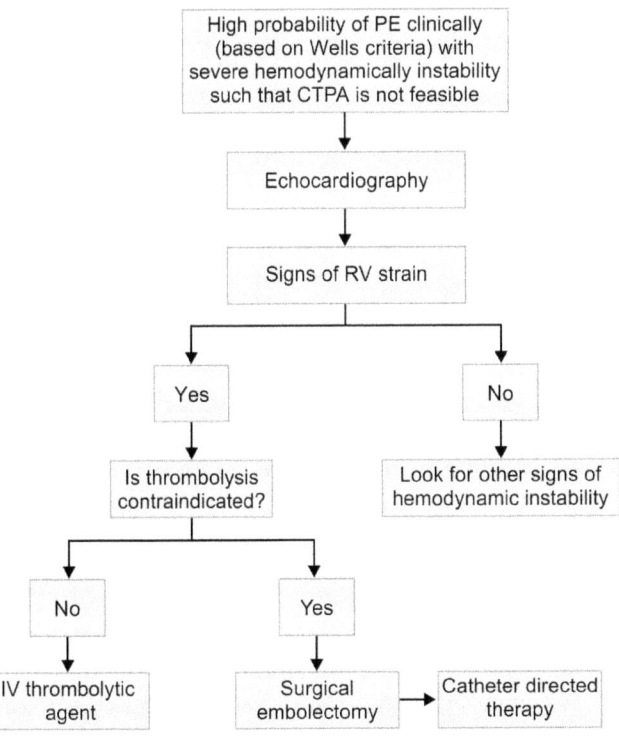

FLOWCHART 16.1: Management approach for a patient with suscpicion of acute pulmonary embolism but due severe hemodynamic instability CTPA is not feasible, e.g. a typical scenario will be cardiac arrest or peri arrest on wards.

(RV: right ventricular; IV: intravenous)

Table 16.3: Wells score.[15]

Items	Clinical score
Deep vein thrombosis (DVT) symptoms or signs	3
An alternative diagnosis is less likely than pulmonary embolism (PE)	3
Heart rate >100 beats/min	1.5
Immobilization or surgery within 4 weeks	1.5
Previous DVT or PE	1.5
Hemoptysis	1
Malignancy	1

Table 16.4: Categories based on Wells score.

Category	Scores
Low probability of pulmonary embolism (PE)	Score <2
Intermediate probability of PE	Score 2 to 6
High probability of PE	Score >6

Wells' Score for Mr Morris is 6, and hence he has an intermediate probability of having PE.

Appropriately CTPA is done, and it shows a large right pulmonary artery thrombus.

CTPA also shows that RV/LV ratio >1.5. There is reflux of contrast in IVC. The echocardiography also confirms the RV/LV ratio of >1.5. How do we treat Mr Morris?

PE could be ruled out if Wells' Score is less than 2 and the D-dimer is negative.

TREATMENT

- Supportive treatment
- Anticoagulation
- Primary reperfusion/advanced therapy

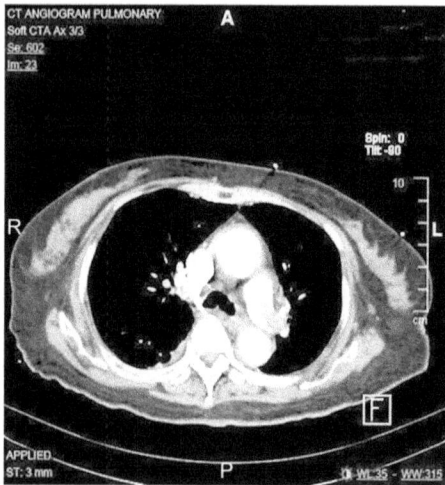

FIGURE 16.3: CT pulmonary angiogram showing large thrombus in right main pulmonary artery.

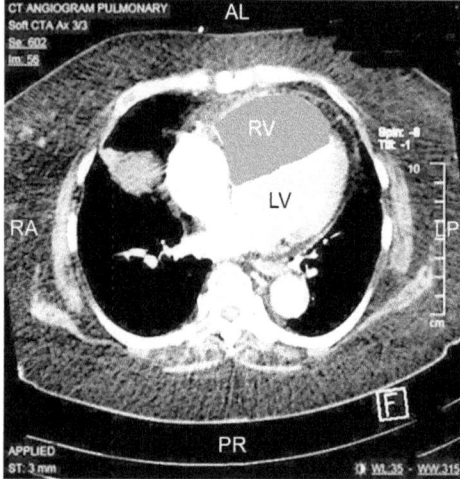

FIGURE 16.4: CT pulmonary angiogram with right ventricular to left ventricular ratio more than 1.5.

Supportive Treatment

Supportive treatment is often required in acute pulmonary embolism to stabilize the patient while definitive treatment is underway.

- *Hemodynamic support*
- *Fluid resuscitation*: Judicious fluid resuscitation can improve low cardiac output state,[3] but excessive fluid administration causes overstretching of right ventricle causing worsening of RV systolic dysfunction. RV overload can also shift interventricular septum to the left and cause reduced LV preload and hence reduced LV output.
- *Vasopressors/inotropes*: Vasopressors/inotropes can be supplemented when moderate fluid resuscitation is not able to achieve adequate organ perfusion. Noradrenaline and adrenaline may improve hemodynamics by improving RV contractility, LV contractility, and systemic blood pressure. Excessive rises in cardiac index, however, may worsen VQ mismatch.[3]
- *Vasodilators*: Vasodilators can improve RV dysfunction by reducing pulmonary vascular resistance. In this regard inhaled nitric oxide can improve hemodynamics and V/Q mismatch due to its local action on pulmonary vasculature without systemic side effects.[16]
- *Respiratory support*: Hypoxia in acute pulmonary embolism is usually responsive to oxygen therapy, and hence oxygen should be given to all patients with acute pulmonary embolism to achieve an oxygen saturation of more than or equal to 90%. In patients with severe hypoxia and or hemodynamic instability, mechanical ventilation might be necessary.

Anticoagulation

Anticoagulation is essential to the management of acute pulmonary embolism. Anticoagulation reduces the risk of death and the likelihood of recurrent embolism in patients with an acute pulmonary embolism.[17]

Low molecular weight heparin (LMWH) is preferred over unfractionated heparin (UFH) in patients with pulmonary embolism as it carries a lower risk of causing major bleeding and heparin-induced thrombocytopenia.[18-20] However, because of its short half-life and ease of reversal of its anticoagulation effects with protamine, UFH is recommended for patients who are considered for primary reperfusion therapy as well as for those with severe renal impairment due to its short half-life, the ease of monitoring and its rapid reversal by protamine.

Parenteral anticoagulation is to be continued for at least 5–10 days. Therapeutic anticoagulation should have been achieved for at least 2 consecutive days before transitioning to an oral anticoagulation regimen.

Duration of long-term anticoagulation required for patients with PE ranges from at least 3 months to the whole duration of life depending on the reversibility of risk factors.

Primary Reperfusion

Primary reperfusion in the context of pulmonary embolism is a term used to describe advanced therapies such as:
- Systemic thrombolysis
- Surgical embolectomy
- Catheter embolectomy

Mr. Morris is continued on oxygen therapy and started on anticoagulation with enoxaparin at therapeutic dose 1 mg /kg Q 12 hourly.

From echocardiography and CTPA and raised troponin results it is clear that Mr Morris has a right ventricular strain and signs of myocardial injury, i.e. submassive high-risk PE. So should Mr Morris be treated with primary reperfusion therapy?

Systemic Thrombolysis

Therapeutic thrombolysis restores pulmonary artery perfusion and reduces pulmonary artery pressure more rapidly than therapeutic anticoagulation alone. However, thrombolysis is associated with substantial risk of bleeding. The decision to thrombolyse needs to be tailored to the individual patient with careful consideration of risk-benefit ratio.

Following is a list of thrombolytic agents approved by Food and Drug Administration (FDA):[3]
Recombinant tissue plasminogen activator (rtPA) 100 mg given over 2 hours.
- 0.6 mg/kg given over 15 minutes (maximum dose 50 mg) (IU: international units; rtPA: recombinant tissue plasminogen activator).

Urokinase:
- Initial bolus dose: 4,400 IU/kg over 10 minutes
- Maintenance: 4,400 IU/kg per hour given over 12–24 hours
- Accelerated regimen: 3 million IU over 2 hours.

Streptokinase:
- Initial bolus dose: 250,000 IU over 30 minutes
- Maintenance dose: 100,000 IU/h given over 12–24 hours
- Accelerated regimen: 1.5 million IU given over 2 hours
    A meta-analysis that included 15 trials and involved a total of 2,057 patients showed that combination of thrombolytic therapy with heparin vs. heparin alone was associated with a significant reduction of overall mortality (OR; 0.59, 95% CI: 0.36–0.96). This reduction, however, was not significant statistically after exclusion of studies that included patients with high-risk PE. The combined endpoint of death or treatment escalation, PE-related mortality, and PE recurrence was significantly reduced with thrombolytic therapy. Major hemorrhage and fatal or intracranial bleeding were significantly more frequent among patients receiving thrombolysis.[21]

- *Primary perfusion in massive PE or high-risk PE:* Thrombolysis has shown to reduce mortality and recurrent PE in massive PE.[21,22] As a result, most guidelines accept thrombolysis as the treatment for massive PE.[23]
- *Primary perfusion in hemodynamically stable patients with PE:*
  - *Submassive high-risk PE (intermediate high-risk PE):* There exists a contentious issue of a possible clinical benefit of thrombolytic therapy in apparently stable patients with intermediate high-risk or submassive high-risk PE.

The PEITHO trial compared a single intravenous bolus of tenecteplase plus heparin with placebo plus heparin in 1,006 patients with submassive PE (intermediate high-risk PE) with signs of right ventricular dysfunction and a positive troponin. The primary composite outcome of all-cause death or hemodynamic decompensation/collapse within 7 days occurred less frequently in thrombolysis group than in the group receiving heparin alone. However, there was no significant reduction in mortality; there was a 10-fold rise in the rate of hemorrhagic strokes and 3-fold rise in major non-intracranial bleeds in patients allocated to tenecteplase.[24]

A meta-analysis of 16 randomized controlled trials (RCTs) in patients with PE showed that use of thrombolytics was associated with lower all-cause mortality but greater risks of major bleeding. However major bleeding was not significantly increased in the subgroup of patients who were 65 years and younger.[25]

So though these studies have shown improved outcome in terms of mortality, the bleeding risk is substantial.

This makes us wonder if halving the dose of thrombolytics might tilt this balance in favor of thrombolysis.

An RCT comparing effects of receiving half dose thrombolysis plus heparin vs. heparin alone on the incidence of pulmonary hypertension in patients with submassive PE showed that half dose thrombolysis group had a lower incidence of pulmonary hypertension at 28 days and that there was no difference in bleeding episodes between the two groups.[26]

This makes half dose thrombolysis a reasonable option. However, this study defined "submassive" PE using anatomical rather than functional criteria. Only 21% of patients had RV enlargement and 6% had RV hypokinesia.[26]

- *Submassive low-risk PE (intermediate low-risk PE) and nonmassive PE:* Include patients who are hemodynamically stable with either sign of RV failure or biomarker rise but not both. These patients should be treated with anticoagulation only. Thrombolysis should be considered in case of clinical worsening to massive or submassive high-risk PE.

Surgical Embolectomy

First introduced in 1924, emergency surgical embolectomy has re-emerged as a management option for patients having either massive PE or submassive PE with severe right ventricular dysfunction who have a contraindication for thrombolysis or have failed systemic thrombolysis. Surgically clots can be extracted from both pulmonary arteries down to the segmental level under direct vision after sternotomy and cardiopulmonary bypass. In the largest single-center case series, 115 patients underwent surgical pulmonary embolectomy. The overall 30-day mortality rate was 6.6%. In the subgroup of 56 patients with submassive PE, the operative mortality rate was 3.6%.[27]

Preoperative thrombolysis is not an absolute contraindication to surgical embolectomy though it does increase the risk of bleeding.

Catheter-directed therapy for pulmonary embolism:[28] The catheter-directed therapy typically uses one-fourth the dose of thrombolysis than that used for systemic thrombolysis. Moreover, interventional mechanical techniques could be performed either in conjunction with low-dose thrombolysis or by itself (in patients with absolute contraindications to thrombolysis). These techniques include mechanical fragmentation and aspiration of thrombus through a standard pulmonary artery catheter, clot pulverization with a rotating basket catheter, rheolytic thrombectomy, and pigtail rotational catheter embolectomy. Further balloon dilation or stenting of pulmonary artery could be undertaken to treat the residual stenosis.

In a review of interventional treatment that included 35 non-randomized studies covering 594 patients, clinical success, defined as stabilization of hemodynamic parameters, resolution of hypoxia and survival to discharge was 87%.

Low-intensity ultrasound-facilitated fibrinolysis is a novel approach. Ultrasound disaggregates fibrin strands, increases clot permeability, and disperses infused fibrinolytic drug into the clot through acoustic microstreaming effects. The SEATTLE II Trial studied 150 patients with massive or submassive PE to evaluate the safety and efficacy of ultrasound-facilitated, catheter-directed fibrinolysis using 24 mg of tissue plasminogen activator. No patient suffered intracranial hemorrhage. This procedure decreased right ventricular dilation, reduced pulmonary hypertension, and decreased the anatomic thrombus burden.[29]

So considering that Mr Morris has submassive high-risk PE and is younger than 65 years, following options could be considered in addition to anticoagulation:[8]

1. Anticoagulation only: Likely the most practical option. There will be a bleeding risk in view of patient's post surgery status.
2. *Half dose thrombolysis:* However, Mr. Morris is postoperative day 5 and risk of bleeding could be substantial.
3. *Catheter-directed mechanical +/- very low dose thrombolysis.*
4. *Surgical embolectomy.*

Options 3 and 4 could be considered only if the institution has expertise available or if he can be safely transferred to a facility whether such expertise is available.

If Mr. Morris becomes hemodynamically unstable, full dose thrombolysis will be the treatment.

However, if the risk of bleeding is considered unacceptable, surgical embolectomy or catheter-directed therapy would be reasonable options if such facilities are available.

REFERENCES

1. Heit JA. The epidemiology of venous thromboembolism in the community. Arterioscler Thromb Vasc Biol. 2008;28(3):370-2.
2. Jaff MR, McMurtry MS, Archer SL, et al. Management of massive and submassive pulmonary embolism, iliofemoral deep vein thrombosis, and chronic thromboembolic pulmonary hypertension: a scientific statement from the American Heart Association. Circulation. 2011;123(16):1788-830.
3. Konstantinides SV, Torbicki A, Agnelli G, et al. 2014 ESC guidelines on the diagnosis and management of acute pulmonary embolism. Eur Heart J. 2014;35(43):3033-69.
4. Stein PD, Saltzman HA, Weg JG. Clinical characteristics of patients with acute pulmonary embolism. Am J Cardiol. 1991;68(17):1723-4.
5. Stein PD, Terrin ML, Hales CA, et al. Clinical, laboratory, roentgenographic, and electrocardiographic findings in patients with acute pulmonary embolism and no pre-existing cardiac or pulmonary disease. Chest. 1991;100(3):598-603.
6. Guidelines on diagnosis and management of acute pulmonary embolism. Task Force on Pulmonary Embolism, European Society of Cardiology. Eur Heart J. 2000;21(16):1301-36.

7. Stein PD, Goldhaber SZ, Henry JW, et al. Arterial blood gas analysis in the assessment of suspected acute pulmonary embolism. Chest. 1996;109(1):78-81.
8. Rudoni RR, Jackson RE, Godfrey GW, et al. Use of two-dimensional echocardiography for the diagnosis of pulmonary embolism. J Emerg Med. 1998;16(1):5-8.
9. Meyer T, Binder L, Hruska N, et al. Cardiac troponin I elevation in acute pulmonary embolism is associated with right ventricular dysfunction. J Am Coll Cardiol. 2000;36(5):1632-6.
10. Kiely DG, Kennedy NS, Pirzada O, et al. Elevated levels of natriuretic peptides in patients with pulmonary thromboembolism. Respir Med. 2005;99(10):1286-91.
11. Bass AR, Fields KG, Goto R, et al. Clinical decision rules for pulmonary embolism in hospitalized patients: a systematic literature review and meta-analysis. Thromb Haemost. 2017;117(11):2176-85.
12. Le Gal G, Righini M, Roy PM, et al. Value of D-dimer testing for the exclusion of pulmonary embolism in patients with previous venous thromboembolism. Arch Intern Med. 2006;166(2):176-80.
13. PIOPED Investigators. Value of the ventilation/perfusion scan in acute pulmonary. Results of the prospective investigation of pulmonary embolism diagnosis (PIOPED). 1990;263(20):2753-9.
14. Anderson DR, Kahn SR, Rodger MA, et al. Computed tomographic pulmonary angiography vs ventilation-perfusion lung scanning in patients with suspected pulmonary embolism: a randomized controlled trial. JAMA. 2007;298(23):2743-53.
15. van Belle A, Bu¨ller HR, Huisman MV, et al. Effectiveness of managing suspected pulmonary embolism using an algorithm combining clinical probability, D-dimer testing, and computed tomography. JAMA. 2006;295(2):172-9.
16. Capellier G, Jacques T, Balvay P, et al. Inhaled nitric oxide in patients with pulmonary embolism. Intensive Care Med. 1997;23(10):1089-92.
17. Barritt DW, Jordan SC. Anticoagulant drugs in the treatment of pulmonary embolism: a controlled trial. Lancet. 1960;1(7138):1309-12.
18. Cossette B, Pelletier MÈ, Carrier N, et al. Evaluation of bleeding risk in patients exposed to therapeutic unfractionated or low-molecular weight heparin: a cohort study in the context of a quality improvement initiative. Ann Pharmacother. 2010;44(6):994-1002.
19. van Dongen CJ, Van den Belt AG, Prins MH, et al. Fixed dose subcutaneous low molecular weight heparins versus adjusted dose unfractionated heparin for venous thromboembolism. Cochrane Database Syst Rev. 2004;(4):CD001100.
20. Stein PD, Hull RD, Matta F, et al. Incidence of thrombocytopenia in hospitalized patients with venous thromboembolism. Am J Med. 2009;122(10):919-30.
21. Marti C, John G, Konstantinides S, et al. Systemic thrombolytic therapy for acute pulmonary embolism: a systematic review and meta-analysis. Eur Heart J. 2015;36(10):605-14.
22. Wan S, Quinlan DJ, Agnelli G, et al. Thrombolysis compared with heparin for the initial treatment of pulmonary embolism: meta-analysis of the randomized controlled trials. Circulation. 2004;110(6):744-9.
23. Kearon C, Akl EA, Ornelas J, et al. Antithrombotic therapy for VTE disease: CHEST Guideline and Expert Panel Report. Chest. 2016;149(2):315-52.
24. Meyer G, Vicaut E, Danays T, et al. Fibrinolysis for patients with intermediate-risk pulmonary embolism. N Engl J Med. 2014;371(6):581-2.
25. Chatterjee S, Chakraborty A, Weinberg I, et al. Thrombolysis for pulmonary embolism and risk of all-cause mortality, major bleeding, and intracranial hemorrhage: a meta-analysis. JAMA. 2014;311:2414-21.
26. Sharifi M, Bay C, Skrocki L, et al. Moderate pulmonary embolism treated with thrombolysis (from the "MOPETT" Trial). Am J Cardiol. 2013;111(2):273-7.
27. Neely RC, Byrne JG, Gosev I, et al. Surgical embolectomy for acute massive and submassive pulmonary embolism in a series of 115 patients. Ann Thorac Surg. 2015;100(4):1245-51.
28. Kuo WT, Gould MK, Louie JD, et al. Catheter-directed therapy for the treatment of massive pulmonary embolism: systematic review and meta-analysis of modern techniques. J Vasc Interv Radiol. 2009;20(11):1431-40.
29. Piazza G, Hohlfelder B, Jaff MR, et al. A prospective, single-arm, multicenter trial of ultrasound-facilitated, catheter-directed, low-dose fibrinolysis for acute massive and submassive pulmonary embolism: the SEATTLE II study. JACC Cardiovasc Interv. 2015;8(10):1382-92.

CHAPTER 17

Chest Trauma

Anthony David Holley, Alexis Kate Ford

INTRODUCTION

Thoracic trauma is one of the leading causes of trauma-related deaths. In the United States, chest trauma is responsible for up to 25% of traumatic deaths with 20% being the result of penetrating injuries, including stabbings or gunshot wounds.[1] Gunshot wounds are characterized as either low or high velocity injuries, with this differentiation having significant implications for management. Blunt thoracic injury is most frequently encountered secondary to motor vehicle accidents, falls, and sporting injuries. In Australasia and the United Kingdom, 90–95% of chest trauma results from blunt injury.[2] Injury following blunt trauma usually results from a combination of shear forces, direct compression, and acceleration/deceleration forces. Chest trauma is often managed nonoperatively with less than 20% of penetrating chest trauma requiring operative intervention.[3]

Thoracic injuries are diverse, and an anatomical approach combined with an evaluation of clinical features provides an effective approach, recognizing multiple structures are often involved in the injury complex. The critical care physician needs to consider whether the trauma patient has fractures of the ribs and sternum, disruption of the pleura, pulmonary laceration/contusion, bronchial tree disruption, injury of vascular intrathoracic structures, diaphragmatic injury, and finally cardiac injury (Table 17.1).

The initial priority in the patient with thoracic trauma is the primary survey, which includes urgent airway assessment, evaluation of the quality of respiration, and an assessment of hemodynamic stability. Urgent intervention is required, as remediable problems are identified. The life-threatening potential and time critical nature of chest trauma mandates a methodical approach. Every trauma patient should subsequently undergo a thorough secondary survey screening for all injuries, as well as more subtle evidence of thoracic injury not immediately apparent on the primary survey.

While clinical examination is useful in the detection of thoracic injuries, radiological investigation is mandatory to detect potentially occult life-threatening pathologies. Modern imaging algorithms utilize ultrasound, chest radiographs, and computed tomography (CT) with intravenous contrast to accurately diagnose and effectively treat patients with acute thoracic trauma. A portable chest radiograph is required as a bedside adjunct to the primary

Table 17.1: The six life-threatening injuries detected on the primary survey.

Injury	Intervention
Tension pneumothorax	Intercostal catheter
Flail chest	Mechanical ventilatory support
Massive hemothorax	Intercostal catheter and/or thoracotomy
Airway obstruction	Intubation or provision of surgical airway
Cardiac tamponade	Pericardiocentesis and/or thoracotomy
Open pneumothorax	Three-sided occlusive dressing

Table 17.2: Pathophysiology of thoracic trauma.	
Injury	Consequence
Cardiac injury	Decreased cardiac output/hypoperfusion
Vascular injury	Hypovolemia
Pulmonary parenchymal injury	Hypoxia
Pulmonary/Airway disruption	Hypoxia/Pneumothorax
Sternal/Rib fractures	Mechanical respiratory failure/Hypoxia

survey and often assists to identify chest wall injuries, hemopneumothoraxes, mediastinal trauma, and pulmonary contusion.[4] Ultrasound is also readily accessible at the bedside as part of an e-FAST (extended focused abdominal sonogram for trauma) which provides reliable information with respect to pneumothoraces, cardiac injury, and may potentially assist in identifying aortic injury.[5]

The complexity in managing chest trauma is explained by the potential for catastrophic hemorrhage, mechanical respiratory failure, direct cardiac injury, or a combination of these processes. Hypoperfusion, hypoxemia, and inflammatory response may subsequently further complicate management. The critical care physician must recognize that even apparently more minor chest trauma may harbor occult serious injury or lead to complications related to pain, immobilization, and respiratory failure (Table 17.2).

CHEST WALL

Chest wall injury is a frequent manifestation of trauma, with 70% of patients admitted to hospital following a motor vehicle accident having fractured ribs. Most commonly, ribs are fractured resulting in significant pain, immobility, and potential for respiratory compromise. When an entire segment of chest wall becomes discontinuous with the rest of the boney thorax because two or more ribs are fractured, in two or more places, it may represent a flail segment. In a flail chest, there are paradoxical chest wall movements such that the flail segment is drawn in, rather than expanded on inspiration. This is often associated with mechanical respiratory failure, significant pain, atelectasis, and subsequent pneumonia. Importantly it often signals the potential for severe underlying pulmonary contusion.

The mainstay of rib fracture management is an effective analgesia, which is often provided systemically, but introduces the risk of delirium and decreased mobility. Epidural catheters or paravertebral blocks are increasingly being recommended for pain control.[6]

In recent years, there has been renewed interest in the surgical management of rib fractures and flail segments. Slobogean et al.[7] performed a meta-analysis of nine observational studies and two randomized control trials which included 753 patients, comparing operative fixation to conservative therapy in the management of flail chest. Operative intervention was associated with a lower mortality, fewer ventilator days, a lower incidence of pneumonia, sepsis or need for tracheostomy. These findings were confirmed in 2017 by the same group.[8]

Severe chest trauma often mandates intubation and ventilation, but the decision to commence invasive mechanical ventilation is usually based on the degree of respiratory embarrassment and hypoxia. In the presence of significant thoracic cage injury, the associated pulmonary contusion may develop progressively over hours to days. Aside from pulmonary contusions with hypoxia or hypercapnia, the need for mechanical ventilation may be secondary to impedance to ventilation, resulting from a flail segment. The prevention of hypercapnia becomes critical in the setting of multitrauma patients with concurrent head injury.

The utility of noninvasive ventilation is controversial. Noninvasive ventilation can decrease the work of breathing and recruit regions of atelectasis, thereby improving oxygenation. Noninvasive ventilation may be a reasonable strategy in a select trauma patient population that is cooperative, hemodynamically stable, with no other indication for general anesthesia and neurologically intact, if employed early before the onset of fulminant respiratory failure.[9,10]

PULMONARY/PLEURAL INJURY

Pulmonary contusions occur in 30–70% of blunt chest trauma patients (Flowchart 17.1 and Fig. 17.1). They result from damage to the interstitial or alveolar tissue with subsequent edema and hemorrhage. Bleeding into adjacent lung segments results in bronchospasm and compromised alveolar function. There is often increased mucus production, impaired clearance of mucus by damaged airways, and finally decreased generation of surfactant by injured alveolar tissues. These processes contribute to pulmonary dysfunction and ultimately respiratory failure.[11] Computerized tomography is very sensitive in detecting contusions, where plain radiography may often fail to demonstrate the lesions until well advanced (Figs. 17.1 and 17.2). Similarly challenging is the diagnosis of small traumatic pneumothoraces. Computerized tomography has demonstrated that pneumothoraces following chest trauma are extremely common with nontension pneumothoraces

Section 2: Organ Dysfunction

FLOWCHART 17.1: Chest injury mechanisms and injury patterns.

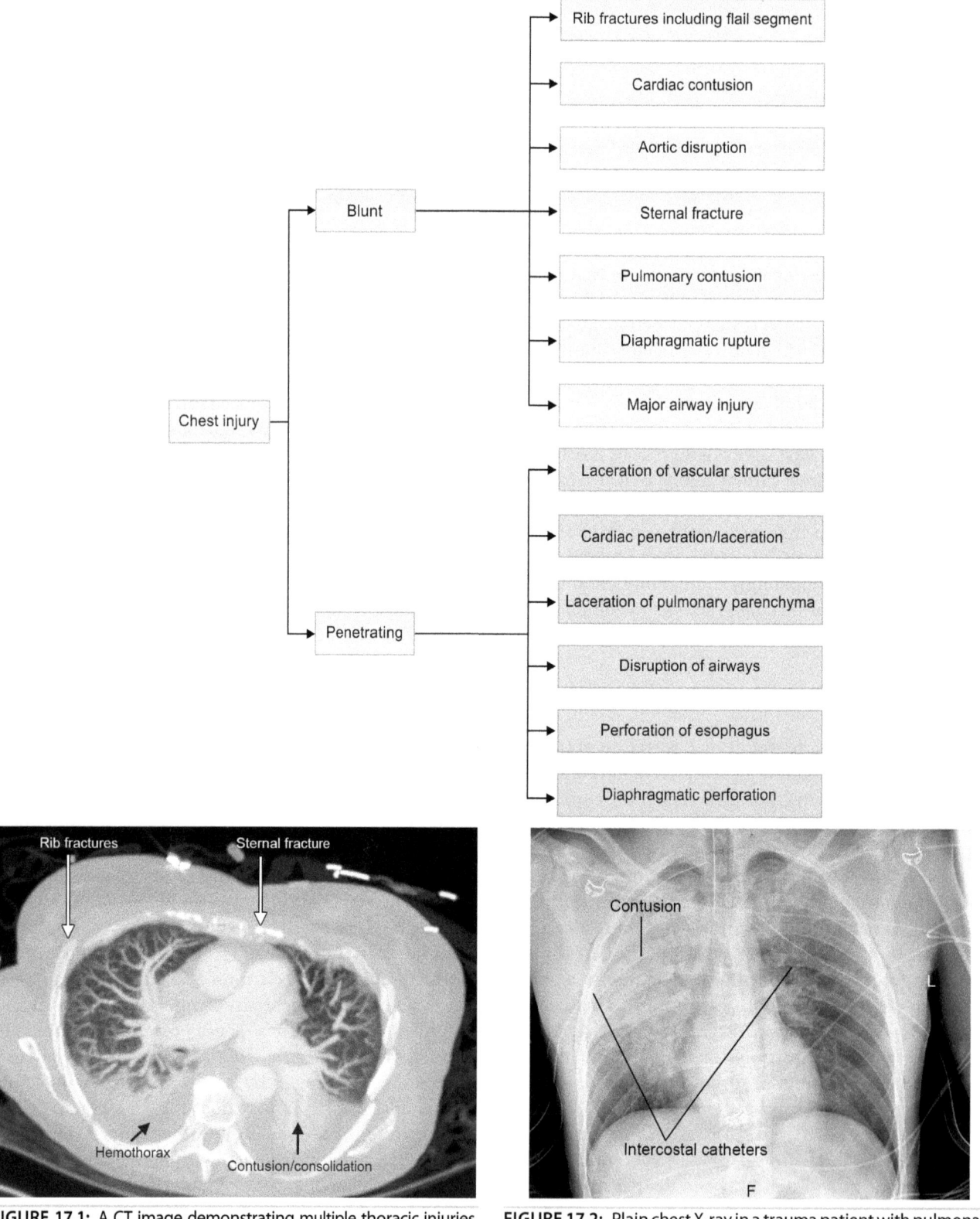

FIGURE 17.1: A CT image demonstrating multiple thoracic injuries. (CT: Computed tomography).

FIGURE 17.2: Plain chest X-ray in a trauma patient with pulmonary contusions.

estimated to have an incidence as high as 20%. There is a 20–35% false-negative rate of supine chest X-ray in detecting small pneumothoraces. If the patient is symptomatic, tube thoracostomy is indicated.

Penetrating trauma may result in an open pneumothorax. This usually occurs because of a penetrating wound that creates a direct connection between the pleural space and the ambient environment. This equilibrates the intrathoracic pressure with atmospheric pressure and disrupts the physiologic pressure gradient that drives respiration. If the defect is sufficiently large, the negative intrathoracic pressure generated during inspiration aspirates air into the thoracic cavity via the wound. This may then become a "sucking chest wound." The management includes an initial three-sided dressing that minimizes aspiration of air through the chest wall defect but facilitates expulsion of air on expiration. This should then be followed by a formal thoracostomy tube.

Placing of a thoracostomy tube (Fig. 17.3) requires monitoring of the patient, appropriate positioning, and identifying the anatomical landmarks, namely the fifth intercostal and the midaxillary line. A skin incision is made between the fourth and fifth intercostal space, between the midaxillary and anterior axillary lines. Followed by blunt dissection down to the parietal pleura allowing a finger to be passed into the pleural space and then guide the thoracostomy tube into the thoracic cavity. The thoracostomy tube is attached to an underwater seal and is then secured at the skin.

The challenge of managing small/occult pneumothoraces in the setting of positive-pressure ventilation and/or aeromedical transfer is more controversial. The evidence suggests that observation is at least as safe and effective as tube thoracostomy for the management of occult pneumothorax. If the critical care physician elects to manage these small pneumothoraces conservatively, there is a strict requirement for vigilance and serial chest radiographs.[12] Management of patients with pulmonary contusion is purely supportive and requires judicious fluid administration, with particular emphasis on avoiding fluid overload states.[13] The ventilation strategy should employ positive end-expiratory pressure (PEEP) to minimize the fraction inspired oxygen, minimize plateau pressures, and utilize tidal volumes of 6 mL/kg predicted body weight.[10,14]

TRACHEOBRONCHIAL INJURIES

Tracheobronchial injuries may result from either blunt or penetrating trauma. The incidence of tracheobronchial injury is probably underestimated as these injuries are both under-recognized and under-reported. Clinical findings are nonspecific and diverse and often result from a persistent air leak, including subcutaneous emphysema, pneumomediastinum, voice hoarseness, and pneumothorax. Pneumoperitoneum occurs when air escaping from the defect, particularly with positive-pressure ventilation, dissects the fascial plains into the abdomen. Pneumopericardium/Pneumomediastinum is frequent findings occasionally resulting in obstructive shock. Plain chest radiographs will demonstrate pneumomediastinum, subcutaneous emphysema, and/or pneumothoraces, while CT imaging may also be useful in delineating a greater detail on the underlying pathology.

Bronchoscopy provides the gold standard for the diagnosis, identifying the exact location and extent of tracheal or bronchial injury, and may also be utilized in therapeutic strategies.

An infrequent but severe complication of thoracic trauma is a bronchopleural fistula characterized by a persistent air leak secondary to a disruption of the visceral pleura or bronchus that communicates with the pleural space. If the leak is significant (>100 mL/breath), a large proportion of the tidal volume will not be involved in gas exchange, but rather directly flow into the pleural space. PEEP will also be dissipated, with further loss of alveolar ventilation. This will result in hypoxemia and respiratory acidosis. The initial treatment of these air leaks is decompression of the pleural cavity with a thoracostomy tube; this will avert the development of a tension pneumothorax.

The subsequent ventilation strategy should incorporate the following principles:
- Minimize mean airway pressures to decrease the pressure gradient across the fistula.

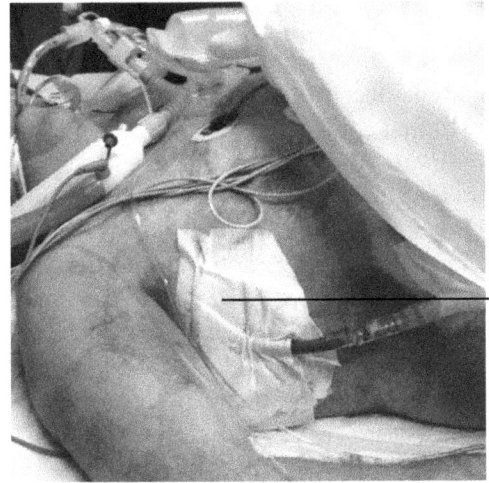

FIGURE 17.3: Trauma patient with an intercostal catheter. (4th/5th intercostal space between the mid and anterior axillary lines)

Section 2: Organ Dysfunction

- Maintain an optimal fraction inspired oxygen to avoid hypoxia.
- Avoid excessive extrinsic PEEP.
- Pressure support ventilation should be avoided as flow decrement will result in premature termination of inspiratory cycle.
- Positive-pressure ventilation should be expeditiously weaned.

Conservative treatment with appropriate respiratory support is often sufficient for resolution to occur. A surgical approach is required at times for complex, large, and persistent defects or those complicated by infection or injury to adjacent structures.[15]

Aortic Injury

Traumatic aortic injury frequently results in immediate death after major blunt trauma. Those patients with an incomplete laceration near the ligamentum arteriosum of the aorta have reasonable chance of survival if the pathology is identified and treated expeditiously. Survival occurs in the context of a contained hematoma preventing immediate exsanguination and death. Penetrating injury or free rupture of a transected aorta into the left hemithorax will usually result in death in a matter of minutes.

In order to avoid missing the diagnosis of an aortic injury a high index of suspicion is mandatory. While lacking sensitivity, there are some well-described findings suggestive of aortic injury on plain chest radiography which may be useful (Box 17.1).

Despite the presence of an aortic injury, the initial X-ray may be negative in as many as 10% of cases. Helical contrast-enhanced CT of the thorax is a reliable modality for evaluating patients with a suspected blunt aortic injury. The sensitivity and specificity of a properly performed helical contrast-enhanced CT is reported as close to 100%. Any uncertainty generated from the CT interpretation should prompt the gold standard investigation, namely aortography. Transesophageal echocardiography is also a useful investigation and has the advantage of being able to be performed at the bedside.

Once an aortic dissection is diagnosed, the treatment approach will be determined and may include open repair with resection and graft replacement of the torn segment or occasionally primary repair of the vessel may be performed. Endovascular repair is now the most common option for managing aortic injury with excellent results.

Once an aortic injury is diagnosed, it is important to fastidiously manage and prevent any hypertension. If no contraindications exist, the heart rate should be controlled with a short-acting beta blocker, targeting a heart rate of 60–80 beats/min. Once the tachycardia is controlled then a vasodilating agent can be safely introduced to ensure a systolic pressure of less than 120 mm Hg.[16]

Cardiac Injury

Significant chest wall trauma, including multiple rib or sternal fractures, lung contusion, pneumothorax or intrathoracic vascular injury, may predict an incidence of blunt cardiac injury as high as 15%. The clinical variability of cardiac injury presentation varies widely from cardiac arrest to the patient being asymptomatic. The standard 12-lead electrocardiography (ECG) is extremely useful in the initial evaluation and performed serially has demonstrated an 89% sensitivity for detecting cardiac injury. The most common abnormality reported on the ECG following blunt chest trauma is a right bundle branch block.[17] Combined with serial troponin assays the critical care physician is reliably able to select patients for echocardiography (Flowchart 17.2).

Penetrating thorax injury either secondary to projectiles or stabbing may result in myocardial laceration. The most frequently injured chamber of the heart is the right ventricle. Survival in penetrating chest injury is reported as high as 40% in centers experienced in the management of these injuries. Penetrating chest injury mandates an immediate bedside echocardiogram to demonstrate pericardial collections or myocardial laceration. All patients with chest injury with hemodynamically significant pericardial effusions identified on an e-FAST examination in the resuscitation room should urgently undergo transfer for a subxiphoid pericardial window. A pericardial window is preferentially performed over pericardiocentesis which is often complicated by clotting, technical difficulties, and an 80% false negative rate.

BOX 17.1: Chest X-ray findings suspicious for aortic injury.

- Widened mediastinum
- Tracheal deviation to the right
- Depression of left main stem bronchus
- Obliteration of the aortic knuckle
- Fractures of the first or second rib
- Loss of the aortopulmonary window
- Apical pleural cap
- Widened paratracheal stripe
- Left hemothorax
- Deviation of the esophagus (nasogastric tube) to the right

FLOWCHART 17.2: Approach to suspected blunt cardiac injury.

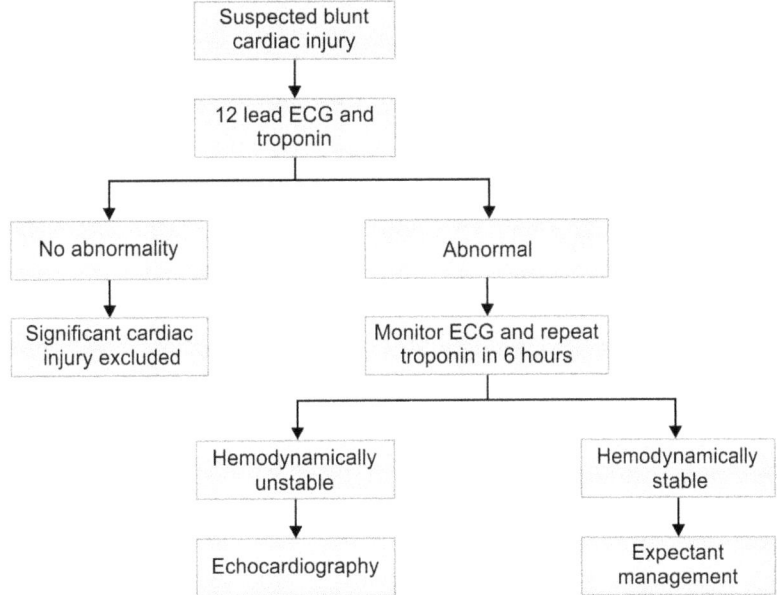

Resuscitative Thoracotomy

Emergency department resuscitative thoracotomy is frequently performed in the setting of thoracoabdominal penetrating or blunt chest trauma where the patient arrives in cardiac arrest. The indications for the procedure remain controversial. However, the goal of this procedure is clear (Box 17.2) and is to immediately restore cardiac output and to control major hemorrhage within the thorax and abdominal cavity.[18]

The broadly accepted indications for performing a resuscitative thoracotomy (Box 17.3) includes penetrating injuries, followed by cardiac arrest during transport and trauma patients with blunt or penetrating injuries suffering cardiac arrest which is witnessed by the resuscitation team.[19]

In patients with penetrating cardiac injuries, resuscitative thoracotomy has generated very encouraging results with survival reported as high as 15–50% in stab victims and about half that in gunshot victims. Outcomes in blunt trauma are much more variable, with a reported 1.5–25% survival,[20,21] it is critical that patients are carefully selected and the contraindications are acknowledged. For good outcomes to be achieved, patients must have vital signs on admission and/or receive an emergency thoracotomy within 15 minutes of cardiac arrest (Box 17.4).[22]

BOX 17.3: Accepted indications for resuscitative thoracotomy.

- Penetrating trauma with prehospital cardiac arrest
- Blunt and penetrating trauma with cardiac arrest on arrival to the hospital or in the emergency department
- Patients with blunt and penetrating trauma with cardiac arrest while in the operating theater undergoing surgical procedures
- Blunt trauma with witnessed cardiac arrest prior to hospital arrival

BOX 17.2: Aims of resuscitative thoracotomy.

- Relief of cardiac tamponade
- Immediate repair of cardiac injuries
- Control of hemorrhage
- Open cardiac massage and internal defibrillation
- Cross-clamping of the descending thoracic aorta to control abdominal hemorrhage
- Control of major thoracic vascular or pulmonary hilar injuries
- Treatment of air embolus

BOX 17.4: Contraindications for resuscitative thoracotomy.

- Blunt injury without witnessed cardiac activity (prehospital)
- Penetrating abdominal trauma without cardiac activity (prehospital)
- Severe multisystem injury
- Severe head injury
- Inadequate equipment
- Inadequate training

Diaphragmatic Injury

Blunt or penetrating chest trauma may result in diaphragmatic injuries. The incidence of diaphragmatic injury is reported as 10–15% with a penetrating mechanism of injury, and from 1% to 7% in patients with significant blunt trauma.[23] Importantly diaphragmatic injury is almost always associated with significant intra-abdominal injuries, thoracic injuries, fractures of the ribs, pelvis and long bones, head injuries, and occasionally aortic injuries.

Diaphragmatic injuries are potentially difficult to diagnose with the pathogenomic clinical findings being auscultation of bowel sounds in the chest, diminished breath sounds on the affected side, and respiratory failure. However, in many cases, there are minimal signs and symptoms, and the diagnosis may be delayed for months or even years.[24] Chest radiography is useful, but the classical findings of the nasogastric tube and/or abdominal viscera visualized in the hemithorax or a markedly raised diaphragm on the affected side are only seen in 50% of cases (Fig. 17.4). The sensitivity of plain chest radiography for right-sided diaphragmatic injury is even lower at approximately 17%,[25] diagnosis has been improved by the liberal use of CT scanning in the emergency department.

Magnetic resonance imaging (MRI) allows the diaphragm to be visualized as a discrete structure and hence a rupture of the diaphragm in the absence of a diaphragmatic hernia can often be diagnosed by this modality. There are, however, significant challenges in performing an MRI on an acutely injured patient.[26]

Thoracoscopy as a diagnostic tool for detecting diaphragmatic injury has a sensitivity of 98–100% and has been effectively utilized for more than a decade.[24]

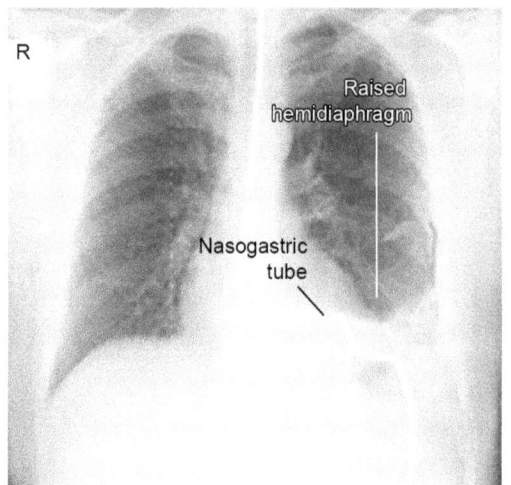

FIGURE 17.4: Plain radiography of a diaphragmatic injury.

Mortality in patients with acute traumatic diaphragmatic injury is entirely dependent on associated injuries and only rarely on the diaphragmatic injury itself. Repair of the diaphragm is achieved via laparotomy, thoracotomy, or a combination of these approaches. Endoscopic repair techniques are becoming more popular.

CONCLUSION

Chest injury is common in both blunt and penetrating trauma and is associated with significant morbidity and mortality. A systematic approach is required to prioritize the interventions involving airway, breathing and circulation that are urgently required, prior to a detailed secondary survey that will assist the critical care physician to identify all injuries. A sound understanding of mechanisms, structures, and injury patterns will allow for the appropriate investigations to be performed in a timely fashion. Finally advances in therapeutic strategies have allowed for a progressive reduction in associated mortality.

REFERENCES

1. Khandhar SJ, Johnson SB, Calhoon JH. Overview of thoracic trauma in the United States. Thorac Surg Clin. 2007;17(1):1-9.
2. Ludwig C, Koryllos A. Management of chest trauma. J Thorac Dis. 2017;9(Suppl 3):S172-7.
3. Alihodzic-Pasalic A, Grbic K, Pilav A, et al. Initial treatment of isolated thoracic injuries. Med Arch (Sarajevo, Bosnia and Herzegovina). 2013;67(2):107-10.
4. Tataroglu O, Erdogan ST, Erdogan MO, et al. Diagnostic accuracy of initial chest X-rays in thorax trauma. J Coll Physicians Surg Pak. 2018;28(7):546-8.
5. Trovato FM, Catalano D, Trovato GM. Thoracic ultrasound: an adjunctive and valuable imaging tool in emergency, resource-limited settings and for a sustainable monitoring of patients. World J Radiol. 2016;8(9):775-84.
6. O'Connell KM, Quistberg DA, Tessler R, et al. Decreased risk of delirium with use of regional analgesia in geriatric trauma patients with multiple rib fractures. Ann Surg. 2018;268(3):534-40.
7. Slobogean GP, MacPherson CA, Sun T, et al. Surgical fixation vs nonoperative management of flail chest: a meta-analysis. J Am Coll Surg. 2013;216(2):302-11.e1.
8. Swart E, Laratta J, Slobogean G, et al. Operative treatment of rib fractures in flail chest injuries: a meta-analysis and cost-effectiveness analysis. J Orthop Trauma. 2017;31(2):64-70.
9. Chiumello D, Coppola S, Froio S, et al. Noninvasive ventilation in chest trauma: systematic review and meta-analysis. Intensive Care Med. 2013;39(7):1171-80.
10. Simon B, Ebert J, Bokhari F, et al. Management of pulmonary contusion and flail chest: an Eastern Association for the Surgery of Trauma practice management guideline. J Trauma Acute Care Surg. 2012;73(5 Suppl 4):S351-61.
11. Cohn SM, Dubose JJ. Pulmonary contusion: an update on recent advances in clinical management. World J Surg. 2010;34(8):1959-70.

12. Zhang M, Teo LT, Goh MH, et al. Occult pneumothorax in blunt trauma: is there a need for tube thoracostomy? Eur J Trauma Emerg Surg. 2016;42(6):785-90.
13. Wiedemann HP, Wheeler AP, Bernard GR, et al. Comparison of two fluid-management strategies in acute lung injury. N Engl J Med. 2006;354(24):2564-75.
14. Brower RG, Matthay MA, Morris A, et al. Ventilation with lower tidal volumes as compared with traditional tidal volumes for acute lung injury and the acute respiratory distress syndrome. N Engl J Med. 2000;342(18):1301-8.
15. Dominguez E, De La Torre C, Sanchez AV, et al. Severe tracheobronchial injuries: our experience. Eur J Pediatr Surg. 2015;25(1):71-6.
16. Trust MD, Teixeira PGR. Blunt trauma of the aorta, current guidelines. Cardiol Clin. 2017;35(3):441-51.
17. Bellister SA, Dennis BM, Guillamondegui OD. Blunt and penetrating cardiac trauma. Surg Clin North Am. 2017;97(5):1065-76.
18. Pust GD, Namias N. Resuscitative thoracotomy. Int J Surg (London, England). 2016;33(Pt B):202-8.
19. Morse BC, Mina MJ, Carr JS, et al. Penetrating cardiac injuries: a 36-year perspective at an urban, Level I trauma center. J Trauma Acute Care Surg. 2016;81(4):623-31.
20. Narvestad JK, Meskinfamfard M, Soreide K. Emergency resuscitative thoracotomy performed in European civilian trauma patients with blunt or penetrating injuries: a systematic review. Eur J Trauma Emerg Surg. 2016;42(6):677-85.
21. Slessor D, Hunter S. To be blunt: are we wasting our time? Emergency department thoracotomy following blunt trauma: a systematic review and meta-analysis. Ann Emerg Med. 2015;65(3):297-307.e16.
22. Seamon MJ, Haut ER, Van Arendonk K, et al. An evidence-based approach to patient selection for emergency department thoracotomy: a practice management guideline from the Eastern Association for the Surgery of Trauma. J Trauma Acute Care Surg. 2015;79(1):159-73.
23. Scharff JR, Naunheim KS. Traumatic diaphragmatic injuries. Thorac Surg Clin. 2007;17(1):81-5.
24. Bosanquet D, Farboud A, Luckraz H. A review diaphragmatic injury. Respir Med CME. 2009;2(1):1-6.
25. Mihos P, Potaris K, Gakidis J, et al. Traumatic rupture of the diaphragm: experience with 65 patients. Injury. 2003;34(3):169-72.
26. Bonatti M, Lombardo F, Vezzali N, et al. Blunt diaphragmatic lesions: imaging findings and pitfalls. World J Radiol. 2016;8(10):819-28.

CHAPTER 18

Traumatic Brain Injury

Amit Madhukar Narkhede, Kapil Zirpe, Atul Prabhakar Kulkarni

INTRODUCTION

Traumatic brain injury (TBI) is one of the leading causes of disability and death worldwide and tremendously adds to the economic burden of health-care systems. Worldwide incidence of TBI has been rising, largely due to the increase in road traffic accident (RTA)–related and violence-related TBI in low- and middle-income countries.[1] These countries contribute nearly 90% of the global TBI-related mortality. The precise global incidence of TBI and associated mortality is difficult to estimate, predominantly due to underdeveloped reporting systems, prehospital deaths, and lack of epidemiological studies. In the United States alone, the incidence of TBI was estimated to be 2.8 million in the year 2013, including 2.5 million TBI-related emergency department visits, 264,000 hospitalizations, and 56,000 deaths.[2] RTAs are the leading cause of TBI in the developing countries, whereas falls are the leading cause of TBI in the developed countries.[1]

In India, RTAs were the leading cause of TBI, followed by falls and violence contributing 60, 25, and 10% of the disease burden, respectively.[3] However, a recent trial has shown that falls from a height (56%) have become the leading cause of TBI, followed by RTA (36%) (Figs. 18.1 and 18.2).[4]

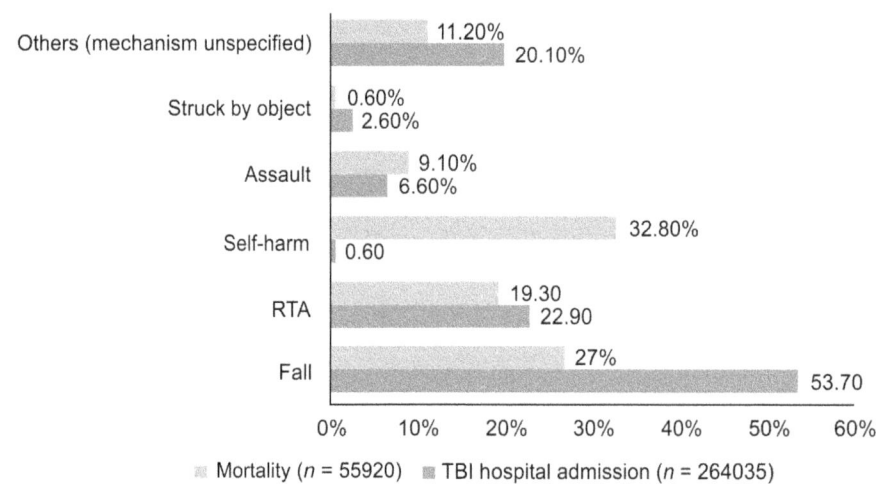

FIGURE 18.1: Causes of traumatic brain injury (TBI) and mortality in USA (2013).[2]

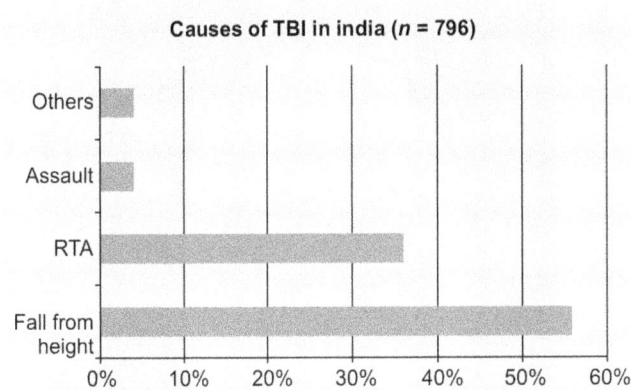

FIGURE 18.2: Causes of traumatic brain injury (TBI) in India.

PATHOPHYSIOLOGY OF TRAUMATIC BRAIN INJURY

The pathophysiology of TBI is studied under two distinct but interdependent categories:
1. Primary brain injury
2. Secondary brain injury

Primary Brain Injury

Primary brain injury is the injury to the brain tissue due to the external mechanical forces transferred to intracranial contents at the time of trauma. Mechanisms commonly implicated in primary brain injury include rapid deceleration–acceleration, shearing forces, direct impact, penetrating injuries, and blast waves. These various mechanisms lead to different morphological types of primary brain injuries, such as skull fractures with underlying neurovascular damage, hemorrhages (epidural, subdural, intraparenchymal, and intraventricular), contusion, and diffuse axonal injury (DAI). The primary brain injury leads to a cascade of processes which leads to loss of cerebrovascular autoregulation and disruption of blood brain barrier, leading to worsening of cerebral edema, intracranial hypertension, and decreased cerebral perfusion pressure (CPP).

Skull Fractures

Skull fractures result from a considerable contact force directly applied to the skull. Either the vault of the skull or base of the skull is involved. The fracture may have linear or stellate defect. Also, the skull bone may be depressed or nondepressed. Generally, the skull fractures by themselves are not detrimental to the patients. It is the damage caused to the underlying neurovascular tissues which leads to several consequences. Basilar fractures may disrupt the cribriform plate damaging olfactory nerves or involve internal auditory canal to damage facial or auditory nerves. They may also lead to cerebrospinal fluid (CSF) rhinorrhea and otorrhea which may act as portal of entry for bacterial infections causing meningitis. Fractures involving the squamous temporal bone may injure the middle meningeal artery, leading to an epidural hematoma (EDH).

Intracranial hemorrhages are present in around 46% patients presenting with TBI and are associated with increased mortality.[5]

Epidural hematoma: It is an extraaxial hematoma between the inner table of the skull bone and the dura mater and is lenticular in shape. It commonly results from rupture of middle meningeal artery or its branches and is associated with skull fractures. It does not cross suture lines where dura mater is tightly adherent to the bones. It is present in 22.5% patients with TBI and is associated with 27.7% mortality (Fig. 18.3).[5]

Subdural hematoma (SDH): They develop between the inner surface of the dura mater and the surface of the brain and are crescent shaped. It spreads beyond suture lines but is limited by the falx cerebri. It results from disruption of bridging veins on the surface of cerebral cortex or the dural venous sinuses. It occurs in 30.1% patients with TBI and is associated with 32.8% mortality (Fig. 18.4).[5]

Intracerebral hemorrhage (ICH): It is hemorrhage into the substance of the brain. It is associated with significant mass effect and surrounding edema. It occurs in 21.8% patients with TBI and is associated with 31.8% mortality.[5]

Subarachnoid hemorrhage (SAH): It results from the disruption of corticomeningeal vessels and does not produce mass effect. However, it may be associated with

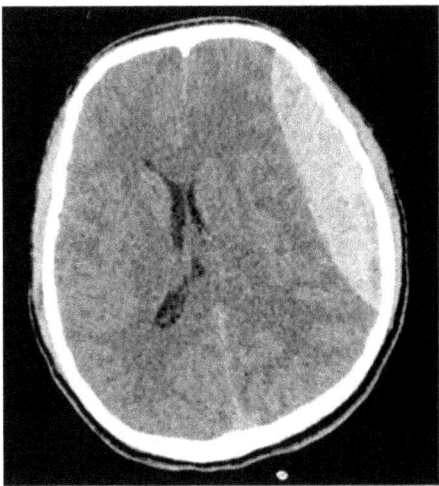

FIGURE 18.3: Epidural hematoma.

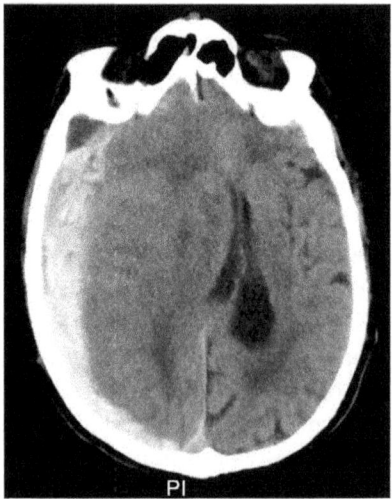

FIGURE 18.4: Subdural hematoma for TBI. (TBI: traumatic brain injury).

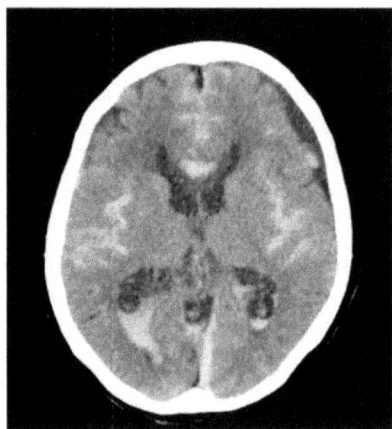

FIGURE 18.5: Subarachnoid hemorrhage.

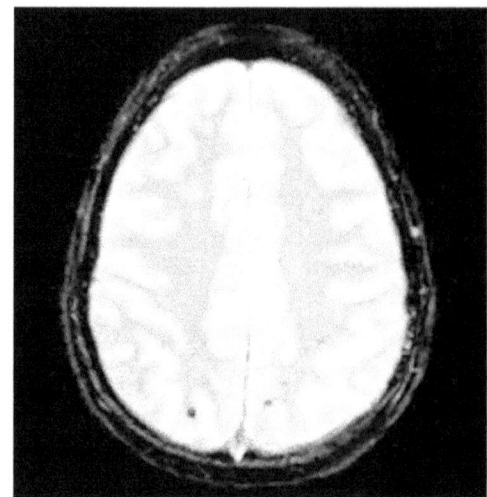

FIGURE 18.6: Diffuse axonal injury.

increased risk of cerebral vasospasm and lead to worse outcomes. It is present in 21.7% patients with TBI and associated with a mortality of 40.4% (Fig. 18.5).[5]

Intraventricular hemorrhage (IVH): It results from the disruption of subependymal vessels or extension of subarachnoid or intraparenchymal hemorrhage. Acute hydrocephalus is a common complication.

Contusions: Focal cerebral contusions consist of heterogenous lesions with punctate hemorrhages, edema, and necrosis. They are common after TBI and commonly found in inferior frontal and anterior temporal lobes. Acceleration–deceleration injuries are the most common mechanism. They can be subdivided into coup and counter-coup contusions.

Diffuse axonal injury: They result from the shearing forces between the gray and white matter caused by rotational or translational acceleration. They constitute punctate lesions with edema at interface between gray and white matter. The DAI was initially thought to be a purely mechanical injury; however, recent research has shown various biochemical and histological changes which show gradual evolution of the DAI.[6] Thus, DAI may at times be a secondary brain injury (Fig. 18.6).

Secondary Brain Injury

The TBI which occurs hours to days after the initial traumatic incident is called secondary brain injury. The initial trauma triggers a cascade of molecular mechanisms within hours and continuing for days together causing further neuronal damage. The secondary brain injury is further exacerbated by neurotransmitter excitotoxicity (such as glutamate), free radical injury, raised intracranial pressure (ICP), mitochondrial dysfunction, dyselectrolytemias (such as hyponatremia), cerebral vasospasm, ischemia, neuronal apoptosis, systemic inflammatory response, and lipid degeneration. Stress response to TBI may lead to catecholamine surge and organ dysfunction as also lead to hyperglycemia and worsen neurological outcomes. Neurocritical care primarily aims at reducing and preventing secondary brain injury and associated systemic effects.[7] A clearer understanding of the molecular mechanisms leading to secondary brain injury would guide the evolution of targeted therapies toward prevention and management of secondary brain injury.

Patients with TBI are likely to develop coagulopathy, or they may be on antiplatelet, anticoagulant medications. Coagulopathy is associated with increased size of hemorrhage, poor neurological outcomes, and death.

Monro-Kellie doctrine: It describes the cranium as a rigid structure containing the brain, CSF, and blood.

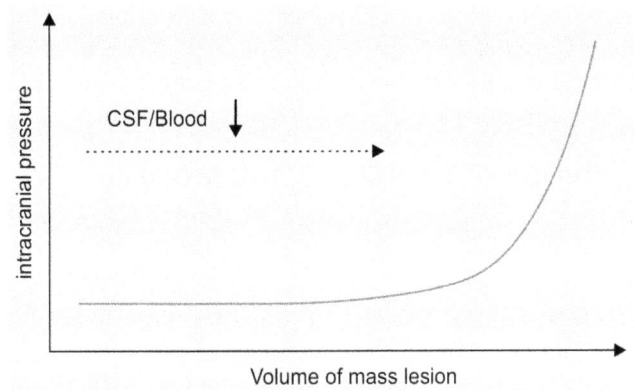

FIGURE 18.7: Monro-Kellie doctrine.

When there is any mass lesion or edema of the brain, the blood and CSF volumes decrease in an effort to prevent an increase in ICP. However, this capacity for compensation is limited, and as the compensation fails, an exponential rise in ICP occurs with increase in volume of mass lesion or edema. Ultimately, this rise in ICP leads to herniation (transtentorial, subfalcine, tonsillar, and reverse/upward herniation) of brain tissue, followed by terminal brainstem compression (Fig. 18.7).

Severity of Traumatic Brain Injury

Severity of TBI has traditionally been assessed based on the Glasgow Coma Scale (GCS). It is a universally accepted, simple, practical, easy to use, and reproducible clinical tool to assess severity of TBI with a good prognostic value. It consists of three components—motor responsiveness, eye opening, and verbal performance. It is scored as illustrated in Table 18.1.[8] TBI is classified as severe (GCS <8), moderate (GCS 9–12), and mild (GCS 13–15) based on the GCS (Table 18.2). However, certain factors, such as intoxication, sedation, paralysis, and endotracheal intubation, may limit its accuracy and practical application. It also does not test brainstem reflexes.

Table 18.1: Intracranial lesions associated with traumatic brain injury and mortality (n = 13,962).[5]

Lesion	Incidence (%)	Mortality (%)
EDH	22.5	27.7
SDH	30.1	32.8
ICH	21.8	31.8
SAH	21.7	40.4
No bleed	53.8	14.6

(EDH: epidural hematoma; ICH: intracerebral hemorrhage; SAH: subarachnoid hemorrhage; SDH: subdural hematoma)

Table 18.2: Glasgow Coma Scale.

Best motor responsiveness (M)	Verbal response (V)	Eye opening (E)	Score
Obeys commands	–	–	6
Localizing	Oriented	–	5
Normal flexion	Confused	Spontaneous	4
Abnormal flexion	Words	To sound	3
Extension	Sounds	To pressure	2
None	None	None	1

Maximum score: 15, minimum score: 3
TBI: mild <8, moderate 9–12, and severe 13–15
(TBI: traumatic brain injury)

The Full Outline of UnResponsiveness (FOUR) score: The FOUR score is a novel, simple, and more comprehensive tool for assessing the level of consciousness in patients with TBI. It has four components—eye responses, motor responses, brainstem reflexes, and respiration. Each component has a maximum score of 4 and a minimum score of 0. It is a 17-point scale ranging from minimum score of 0 to a maximum score of 16. It does not have a verbal response score and hence not affected by endotracheal intubation unlike the GCS (Table 18.3).[9]

Table 18.3: Full outline of unresponsiveness score.[9]

Score	Eye response	Motor response	Brainstem reflexes	Respiration
4	Eyelids open or opened, tracking, or blinking to command	Thumbs-up, fist, or peace sign	Pupil and corneal reflexes present	Not intubated, regular breathing pattern
3	Eyelids open but not tracking	Localizing to pain	One pupil wide and fixed	Not intubated, Cheyne-Stokes breathing pattern
2	Eyelids closed but open to loud voice	Flexion response to pain	Pupil or corneal reflexes absent	Not intubated, irregular breathing
1	Eyelids closed but open to pain	Extension response to pain	Pupil and corneal reflexes absent	Breathes above ventilator rate
0	Eyelids remain closed with pain	No response to pain or generalized myoclonus status	Absent pupil, corneal, and cough reflex	Breathes at ventilator rate or apnea

The Marshall computed tomography (CT) classification is the most commonly used CT classification system. It was first described in 1991 by Marshall et al. It classifies TBI based on three main variables—presence of mass lesion, appearance of perimesencephalic cisterns, and the extent of midline shift on CT scans.[10] It has six categories as described in Table 18.2. It was initially used as a descriptive tool; however, it has commonly been used as a prognostic tool also (Table 18.4).

The Rotterdam CT score: The Rotterdam CT score was developed by Maas et al. in 2005 using data from 2,269 TBI patients from Europe and North America. While the Marshall classification was a descriptive tool, Rotterdam CT score is a prognostic tool. It can reliably predict 6-month mortality outcome in TBI patients. It uses individual CT characteristic, such as status of basal cisterns, midline shift, traumatic SAH and/or IVH, and presence/absence of epidural mass lesions.[11] It is illustrated in Table 18.5.

PROGNOSTIC PREDICTION MODELS

The International Mission for Prognosis and Analysis of Clinical Trials Prognostic Model

The International Mission for Prognosis and Analysis of Clinical Trials (IMPACT) study database has pooled data of 9,205 TBI patients from eight randomized controlled trials and three observational studies. The IMPACT prognostic model uses patient admission characteristics to predict 6-month outcomes as assessed by the Glasgow Outcome Scale (GOS) which is an ordered outcome measure with five categories: (1) dead, (2) vegetative state, (3) severe disability, (4) moderate disability, and (5) good recovery.[12] The IMPACT prognostic model has three models depending on the number and complexity of variables. The core model consists of age, motor score, and papillary reaction to light. The extended model has hypoxia, hypotension, and CT characteristics in addition to the core model. The laboratory model has hemoglobin and blood glucose levels in addition to the extended model. The performance of the model improves with increasing numbers of variables.[13]

The Corticosteroid Randomization After Significant Head Injury Prognostic Model

The Corticosteroid Randomization after Significant Head Injury (CRASH) prognostic model is the result of the Medical Research Council-CRASH trial investigating the role of corticosteroids in 10,008 patients with TBI enrolled from 1994 to 2004. The CRASH prognostic model predicts

Table 18.4: Marshall CT classification of traumatic brain injury.[10]

Marshall CT class	CT findings
Diffuse injury I	No visible intracranial pathology seen on CT scan
Diffuse injury II	Cisterns are present with midline shift 0–5 mm and/or lesion densities present
	No high or mixed density lesion >25 cm³, may include bone fragments and foreign bodies
Diffuse injury III	Cisterns compressed or absent with midline shift of 0–5 mm
	No high or mixed density lesions >25 cm³
Diffuse injury IV	Midline shift >5 mm
	No high or mixed density lesions >25 cm³
Evacuated mass lesion	Any surgically evacuated lesion
Nonevacuated mass lesion	High or mixed density lesion >25 cm³ Not surgically evacuated

(CT: computed tomography)

Table 18.5: Rotterdam score.[11]

Score	CT characteristic			
	Basal cisterns	Midline shift	Epidural mass lesion	IVH or tSAH
0	Normal	None or ≤5 mm	Present	Absent
1	Compressed	>5 mm	Absent	Present
2	Absent	–	–	–

Add plus 1 to the above score to get the Rotterdam CT score which is used to predict 6-month mortality as stated below. The score range of 1–6 also makes it consistent with Marshall CT classification and motor component of GCS

Rotterdam score	1	2	3	4	5	6
Predicted 6-month mortality	0	6.8	16	26	53	61

(CT: computed tomography; GCS: Glasgow coma scale; IVH: intraventricular hemorrhage; tSAH: traumatic subarachnoid hemorrhage)

14-day mortality and 6-month neurological outcome on the GOS based on certain admission characteristics. It also has two models—the basic model incorporating age, GCS, pupillary reaction to light, and presence of major extracranial injury. The extended model contains CT scan characteristics in addition to the basic model. It has separate models for low-income and high-income countries.[14]

MANAGEMENT

The management of a TBI patient involves early identification, initial stabilization, followed by continued care to prevent further deterioration and maximize recovery. The impact of primary brain injury may be reduced only through effective preventive strategies, such as education, safety measures, and regulatory legislation. The main goals of neurocritical care management are to prevent and manage secondary brain injuries. In recent years, advances in management of TBI are related to systematic, protocol-guided management following international guidelines, such as the Brain Trauma Foundation Guidelines for the management of Severe Traumatic brain Injury, based on recent evidence and updated in a timely manner.[15]

Prehospital and Emergency Department Management

Sustained hypoxia (PaO_2 <60 mm Hg) and hypotension [systolic blood pressure (SBP) <90 mm Hg)] in the prehospital setting are known to be strongly associated with worse outcomes in patients with TBI.[16] Management of a TBI patient should always begin with assessment of the airway and securing the airway with stabilization of the cervical spine. The decision to intubate a patient may be based on factors, such as (1) GCS <9, (2) SpO_2 <92% despite oxygen supplementation, (3) signs of cerebral herniation, (4) signs of aspiration, or (5) compromised airway. Rapid sequence intubation with manual in-line stabilization is the recommended technique for securing the airway as it reduces sympathetic response, agitation, and transient increases in ICP and cervical spine injury.

Mechanical ventilation should be initiated to attain normocarbia (PCO_2 ~ 35-40 mm Hg) as hypercapnia will cause increase in ICP, and hypocapnia would lead to decreased cerebral perfusion through cerebral vasoconstriction. Maintain an SpO_2 >90% or PaO_2 >60 mm Hg to achieve adequate oxygenation of cerebral tissues. Therapeutic hyperventilation (PCO_2 ~ 30 mm Hg) should be only reserved for short periods in the case of (1) acute neurological deterioration due to cerebral herniation or (2) an acute rise in ICP refractory to medical management.

Hypotension (SBP <100 mm Hg) should be promptly corrected with isotonic fluids and blood products as required. Vasopressors may be used if hypotension is not responding to fluids and blood products. Maintaining SBP at >100 mm Hg for patients 50-69 years of age or at >110 mm Hg for patients 15-49 or >70 years old may be considered to decrease mortality and improve outcomes.[15] Any systemic injuries (hemothorax, hemoperitoneum, cardiac tamponade, and tension pneumothorax) should be promptly managed to improve circulation. Trials of permissive hypotension/hypotensive resuscitation and restricted/controlled resuscitation have excluded TBI patients and should be avoided in patients with TBI.[17] The rationale for this exclusion is the fact that permissive hypotension will cause or exacerbate secondary brain injury. A brief neurologic examination should be performed including GCS, papillary signs, and symmetry of limb movements. Neurologic status should be frequently assessed. Any signs of increased ICP and impending herniation, such as significant pupillary asymmetry, fixed and dilated pupils, decorticate or decerebrate posturing, and the "Cushing triad" of irregular respiration, bradycardia, and hypertension, should prompt immediate institution of measures to control ICP. Blood glucose, serum electrolytes, complete blood count, coagulation profile, blood alcohol level, and urine toxin screen should be measured in patients with TBI. The patient should be transferred to a center with neurosurgical facilities soon after stabilization.

All patients with TBI and GCS less than 15 should undergo a noncontrast-enhanced CT scan of the brain. Other indications for CT brain include the presence of vomiting, seizures, suspicion of skull fracture, age >65 or <2 years, and presence of intoxication. Follow-up CT scan may be required in the case of neurological deterioration. CT findings along with GCS and other neurological signs may prompt a neurosurgical intervention. CT scan may also be useful for detecting secondary brain injuries, such as cerebral edema, infarcts, and herniation.

Neurosurgical Management

The decision for an emergency neurosurgical intervention is guided by the GCS and findings on CT scan, such as location and volume of hematoma, midline shift, and mass effect. An EDH more 30 mL in volume and SDH >10 mm in thickness or midline shift >5 mm and ICH more than 50 mL in volume should be evacuated regardless of the GCS. Patients with GCS of 6-8 with frontal or temporal contusions greater than 20 cm^3 in volume with midline shift of at least 5 mm and/or cisternal compression on CT scan should undergo surgical intervention. Patients with EDH with GCS <9 with anisocoria should undergo neurosurgical intervention.[18,19] Decompressive craniectomy for medically refractory raised ICP has been shown to reduce mortality without reduction in poor neurological outcome. Two large recent trials–Decompressive Craniectomy (DECRA) trial and Randomised Evaluation of Surgery with Craniectomy for Uncontrollable Elevation of Intracranial Pressure (RESCUEicp) trial showed that decompressive craniectomy in refractory intracranial hypertension although appeared to decrease mortality but increased persistent vegetative state at 6 months.[20,21]

Management in the Intensive Care Unit

Intensive care management in moderate-to-severe TBI primarily aims at reducing secondary brain injury. The various aspects of intensive care management include ICP management, hemodynamic management, temperature management, glucose management, nutrition, and rehabilitation.

Intracranial Pressure Monitoring

Indications for ICP monitoring in TBI include (1) GCS≤8 with CT showing mass effect due to IC bleed; (2) GCS ≤8 with a normal CT scan if any two of the following—age >40 years, motor posturing and SBP <90 mm Hg.[15] An ICP target of <22 mm Hg is generally recommended. An external ventricular drain (EVD) is accurate, common, practical, and cost-effective technique of ICP monitoring. It also has a therapeutic advantage of CSF drainage to treat increased ICP. The primary disadvantage is its invasive nature and risk of infection. Also, insertion of EVD may be difficult in patients with cerebral edema with compression of ventricles. Intraparenchymal pressure monitoring consists of a fiber optic transducer inserted into the brain parenchyma. Advantages include ease of placement and lower risk of infection, and the disadvantage is the inability to drain CSF and loss of accuracy over time due to drift of baseline. Subarachnoid bolts and epidural optical transducers are less invasive with lower risk of infection or hemorrhage but are inaccurate. ICP waveforms include A, B, and C waves. The A waves are pathological, and they are seen when there is profound and sustained elevation in ICP. The A waves indicate loss of autoregulatory and compensatory mechanisms warranting urgent intervention to reduce ICP. B waves are due to respiratory variation in ICP, and C waves represent ICP variations due to arterial blood pressure variations. Transcranial Doppler velocity waveforms and optic nerve sheath diameter are noninvasive ways to monitor ICP but are less accurate and unable to quantify ICP measurements.

Intracranial hypertension is defined as sustained ICP elevations more than 20 mm Hg. CPP is the pressure gradient between systemic arterial pressures to the ICP and is a surrogate of the cerebral blood flow. CPP = mean arterial pressure (mm Hg) - ICP (mm Hg). A CPP target of 60-70 mm Hg has been recommended.[15] Maintaining higher CPP may not be beneficial and increases risk of hypoxemic respiratory failure.[22]

Intracranial Pressure Management

Head end of bed should be elevated by 30-45° to allow adequate venous drainage as well maintain cerebral perfusion. Venous drainage can further be optimized by maintaining neutral position of the neck, loosening of any endotracheal/tracheostomy tube ties, and cervical braces if too tight.

Provision of adequate analgesia and sedation helps ameliorate sympathetic response, decrease both cerebral metabolic rate, and patient-ventilator dyssynchrony. Short-acting agents, such as propofol, dexmedetomidine, and fentanyl, are commonly used and allow frequent neurological assessment. Neuromuscular blocking agents are generally discouraged but may be used in selected patients to avoid patient-ventilator dyssynchrony.

Maintain normocapnia as both hypercapnia and hypocapnia can be deleterious. Ventilation should be managed as described in the section on mechanical ventilation.

Cerebrospinal fluid drainage using an EVD is an easy way to reduce ICP in patients with EVD and ICP monitoring. An EVD system zeroed at the level of the midbrain/external auditory meatus with continuous drainage more effectively normalizes ICP than intermittent drainage.[15]

Osmotic Therapy

It involves use of osmotic agents, such as mannitol and hypertonic saline, to create an osmotic gradient across the blood brain barrier. This removes water from the brain parenchyma leading to a decrease in ICP. Effect of treatment diminishes over time; hence, prolonged use is not recommended. Also, osmotic agents should not be abruptly stopped due to the risk of rebound cerebral edema. Mannitol is used in a dose of 0.25-1 g/kg, four to six times a day. Hypertonic saline has been used in various concentrations 3-23.5%. Three-percent saline is commonly used as an infusion to target serum sodium levels of 145-155 mEq/L, whereas 23.4% saline is used as intermittent boluses. It has a theoretical advantage over mannitol in patients with hypovolemia, ongoing bleeding with less likelihood of leakage into brain tissue and renal failure. However, there is no convincing clinical evidence of superiority of hypertonic saline over mannitol in severe TBI.[23]

Therapeutic hypothermia has been proposed to manage raised ICP after severe TBI on account of its potential to reduce ICP, cerebral metabolic rate, and secondary brain injury. A recently conducted large randomized control trial, however, failed to show any benefit in improving outcomes.[24] Hyperthermia is harmful and should be avoided and promptly treated.

Induced barbiturate coma has been used in severe TBI to reduce ICP and cerebral metabolic rate to reduce secondary brain injury. Pentobarbital infusion with electroencephalography monitoring to achieve burst suppression is used. Barbiturate coma reduces ICP but causes hypotension and does not improve outcomes.[25] Prophylactic use of barbiturates is discouraged; however, they may be used in refractory intracranial hypertension with stable hemodynamics.[15]

Decompressive craniectomy, in refractory intracranial hypertension following TBI, may reduce the ICP and improve mortality, but it has not been shown to improve neurological outcomes in the long term (GOS at 6 months).[20,21]

Hemodynamic management involves maintaining CPP 60-70 mm Hg. It can be achieved using fluids and vasopressors as indicated. Isotonic crystalloids are generally recommended. Normal saline is the preferred fluid as balanced salt solutions may be relatively hypotonic. Glucose-containing fluids should be avoided. Colloids including albumin should be avoided.[26]

General Intensive Care Unit Management

Blood sugar levels should be maintained in a range of 140-180. Both hypoglycemia and hyperglycemia can be detrimental.

Prophylaxis against early post-traumatic epilepsy is recommended for up to 7 days. Phenytoin is commonly used, and levetiracetam is an equally effective alternative drug with better long-term neurological outcomes. Prolonged prophylaxis for post-traumatic epilepsy is not recommended.[15,27]

Venous Thromboembolism Prophylaxis

Patients with severe TBI are at increased risk of venous thromboembolism. All patients with moderate-to-severe TBI should receive venous thromboembolism prophylaxis with sequential compression devices. The risk of hematoma expansion is greatest in the first 24-48 hours.

Pharmacological prophylaxis may be initiated at 24-48 hours after admission in patients with low hemorrhagic risk TBI, once expansion of clot is ruled out by CT scan.[28]

Nutrition

Early enteral nutrition has been shown to improve mortality and should be considered in all hemodynamically stable patients with TBI as has been recommended in recent guidelines with weak level of evidence.[15,29,30] Postpyloric feeding may be considered to decrease incidence of ventilator-associated pneumonia in these patients.[15,31] Addition of nutritional supplements, such as docosahexaenoic acid and eicosapentaenoic acid, may be considered in patients with TBI.[29]

Rehabilitation and physical therapy should begin early during intensive care unit stay. Passive range of motion exercises and early mobilization may help reduce deep vein thrombosis and hasten recovery.

POTENTIAL USE OF BIOMARKERS IN TRAUMATIC BRAIN INJURY

Various biomarkers are under evaluation for potential role for prognostication in patients with TBI. CSF levels of tau protein, neurofilament light polypeptide, neuron-specific enolase, and S100β have been evaluated for the prognostication of TBI.[32]

CONCLUSION

Traumatic brain injury is a major cause of morbidity and mortality worldwide. Education and implementation of safety measures and regulatory legislations may help prevent primary TBI. Prompt and effective management of patients with TBI to reduce secondary brain injury can potentially improve outcomes. Ongoing research on the subject would help us refine our knowledge and management and help improve outcomes.

REFERENCES

1. Johnson WD, Griswold DP. Traumatic brain injury: a global challenge. Lancet Neurol. 2017;16:949-50.
2. Taylor CA, Bell JM, Breiding MJ, et al. Traumatic brain injury-related emergency department visits, hospitalizations, and deaths—United States, 2007 and 2013. MMWR Surveill Summ. 2017;66:1-16.
3. Gururaj G. Epidemiology of traumatic brain injuries: Indian scenario. Neurol Res. 2002;24:24-8.
4. Shekhar C, Gupta LN, Premsagar IC, et al. An epidemiological study of traumatic brain injury cases in a trauma centre of New Delhi (India). J Emerg Trauma Shock. 2015;8:131.

5. Perel P, Roberts I, Bouamra O, et al. Intracranial bleeding in patients with traumatic brain injury: a prognostic study. BMC Emerg Med. 2009;9:15.
6. Smith DH. Neuromechanics and pathophysiology of diffuse axonal injury in concussion. Bridge (Washington, DC: 1969). 2016;46:79.
7. Kinoshita K. Traumatic brain injury: pathophysiology for neurocritical care. J Intensive Care. 2016;4:29.
8. Teasdale G, Jennett B. Assessment of coma and impaired consciousness: a practical scale. Lancet. 1974;304:81-4.
9. Wijdicks EF, Bamlet WR, Maramattom BV, et al. Validation of a new coma scale: the FOUR score. Ann Neurol. 2005;58:585-93.
10. Marshall LF, Marshall SB, Klauber MR, et al. A new classification of head injury based on computerized tomography. Spec Suppl. 1991;75:S14-20.
11. Maas AI, Hukkelhoven CW, Marshall LF, et al. Prediction of outcome in traumatic brain injury with computed tomographic characteristics: a comparison between the computed tomographic classification and combinations of computed tomographic predictors. Neurosurgery. 2005;57:1173-82.
12. Marmarou A, Lu J, Butcher I, et al. IMPACT database of traumatic brain injury: design and description. J Neurotrauma. 2007;24:239-50.
13. Steyerberg EW, Mushkudiani N, Perel P, et al. Predicting outcome after traumatic brain injury: development and international validation of prognostic scores based on admission characteristics. PLoS Med. 2008;5:e165.
14. Collaborators MRC CRASH Trial. Predicting outcome after traumatic brain injury: practical prognostic models based on large cohort of international patients. BMJ. 2008;336:425-9.
15. Carney N, Totten AM, O'reilly C, et al. Guidelines for the management of severe traumatic brain injury. Neurosurgery. 2017;80:6-15.
16. McHugh GS, Engel DC, Butcher I, et al. Prognostic value of secondary insults in traumatic brain injury: results from the IMPACT study. J Neurotrauma. 2007;24:287-93.
17. Kudo D, Yoshida Y, Kushimoto S. Permissive hypotension/hypotensive resuscitation and restricted/controlled resuscitation in patients with severe trauma. J Intensive Care. 2017;5:11.
18. Bullock MR, Chesnut R, Ghajar J, et al. Surgical management of acute subdural hematomas. Neurosurgery. 2006;58:S2-16.
19. Bullock MR, Chesnut R, Ghajar J, et al. Surgical management of traumatic parenchymal lesions. Neurosurgery. 2006;58:S2-25.
20. Cooper DJ, Rosenfeld JV, Murray L, et al. Decompressive craniectomy in diffuse traumatic brain injury. N Engl J Med. 2011;364:1493-502.
21. Hutchinson PJ, Kolias AG, Timofeev IS, et al. Trial of decompressive craniectomy for traumatic intracranial hypertension. N Engl J Med. 2016;375:1119-30.
22. Contant CF, Valadka AB, Gopinath SP, et al. Adult respiratory distress syndrome: a complication of induced hypertension after severe head injury. J Neurosurg. 2001;95:560-8.
23. Berger-Pelleiter E, Émond M, Lauzier F, et al. Hypertonic saline in severe traumatic brain injury: a systematic review and meta-analysis of randomized controlled trials. Can J Emerg Med. 2016;18:112-20.
24. Andrews PJ, Sinclair HL, Rodriguez A, et al. Hypothermia for intracranial hypertension after traumatic brain injury. N Engl J Med. 2015;373:2403-12.
25. Roberts I, Sydenham E. Barbiturates for acute traumatic brain injury. Cochrane Database Syst Rev. 2012;12:CD000033.
26. Myburgh J, Cooper DJ, Finfer S, et al. Saline or albumin for fluid resuscitation in patients with traumatic brain injury. N Engl J Med. 2007;357:874-84.
27. Szaflarski JP, Sangha KS, Lindsell CJ, et al. Prospective, randomized, single-blinded comparative trial of intravenous levetiracetam versus phenytoin for seizure prophylaxis. Neurocrit Care. 2010;12:165-72.
28. Margolick J, Dandurand C, Duncan K, et al. A systematic review of the risks and benefits of venous thromboembolism prophylaxis in traumatic brain injury. Can J Neurol Sci. 2018;45:432-44.
29. McClave SA, Taylor BE, Martindale RG, et al. Guidelines for the provision and assessment of nutrition support therapy in the adult critically ill patient: Society of Critical Care Medicine (SCCM) and American Society for Parenteral and Enteral Nutrition (ASPEN). J Parenter Enteral Nutr. 2016;40:159-211.
30. Hartl R, Gerber LM, Ni Q, et al. Effect of early nutrition on deaths due to severe traumatic brain injury. J Neurosurg. 2008;109:50-6.
31. Wang D, Zheng SQ, Chen XC, et al. Comparisons between small intestinal and gastric feeding in severe traumatic brain injury: a systematic review and meta-analysis of randomized controlled trials. J Neurosurg. 2015;123:1194-201.
32. Rao GS. Biomarkers and prognostication in traumatic brain injury. J Neuroanaesthesiol Crit Care. 2017;4:2.

CHAPTER 19

Encephalitis

Rob Bevan

INTRODUCTION

Encephalitis is common in critical care and has both pathological and clinical definitions.[1-4] It comprises a complex syndrome of neurological symptoms and signs, which overlap other neurological conditions.[4]

PATHOPHYSIOLOGY

Encephalitis is defined pathologically as a global inflammation of the brain parenchyma. The mechanism of inflammation may follow either the direct infection of neuronal cells by microorganisms, resulting in inflammation and eventual necrosis, or as a result of perivascular (usually lymphocytic) inflammation occurring as a result of a systemic reaction to (for example) a viremia. This may further lead to demyelination and eventually gliosis.[2,4,5] The inflammatory process may also involve the meninges, resulting in a "meningoencephalitis." The trigger for the inflammatory process may be infectious, autoimmune, or a combination of the two.

Infectious encephalitis most commonly has a viral etiology, transmitted either directly, or via an arthropod vector. Alternatively, the infectious agent may be amoebic, bacterial, or parasitic. Encephalitis is often a rare manifestation of a common human infection, readily detectable in the population; it is therefore not always straightforward to ascribe causality between a microorganism and encephalitis.[6]

Arboviral viruses that have been shown to cause encephalitis utilize arthropod vectors, with specific infections being prevalent in certain geographical regions. In Asia, viruses are commonly mosquito borne (e.g. dengue, Japanese and West Nile encephalitis) but may also be tick borne. Specific viral etiologies can be missed if nonendemic to the site of presentation, therefore a careful exposure history should be sought.[7]

It is beyond the scope of this chapter to cover all of these viruses in detail, however, the emergence of Zika virus, a *Flavivirus* transmitted by the *Aedes* mosquito deserves mention as a recently reported and emerging viral cause of meningoencephalitis in travelers.[8,9]

Bacterial causes include streptococcal and staphylococcal infections, as well as *Listeria*, syphilis, and tuberculosis.[10]

Autoimmune encephalitis may result from a process of direct and/or indirect cellular damage from antibodies targeting either intracellular antigens, synaptic receptors, ion channels, or other cell surface proteins.[1] There have been significant advances in the classification, identification, and treatment of autoimmune encephalitis. Many of these autoantibodies produce clinical syndromes which have distinct clinical features; not all of which present with fever or cerebrospinal fluid (CSF) pleocytosis.[1]

Pathogenic antibodies may result from the presence of an underlying (and potentially previously undiagnosed) cancer. Indeed the search for the cancer diagnosis may only be initiated by the occurrence of the encephalitis and subsequent identification of a specific neuronal autoantibody profile.[11]

Notwithstanding the increasing knowledge of these uncommon conditions, the specific cause of an individual episode of encephalitis may be elusive in up to 50% of cases—although recent data suggest an etiology can be determined in up to 70% of cases.[12]

EVIDENCE

Definition and Epidemiology

The clinical definition of encephalitis should be considered in any patient presenting with an encephalopathy of at least 24-hour duration, and at least two of fever, seizures, focal neurological deficit, CSF pleocytosis, radiological or electroencephalogram features of encephalitis.[3,6]

The estimated incidence of encephalitis varies widely; however, it is estimated to be between 0.07 cases and 12.6 cases per 100,000 globally.[13] Herpes simplex virus (HSV) (20%) and varicella-zoster virus (VZV) (14%) are the most common viral pathogens in the immunocompetent and immunosuppressed, respectively.[14]

Trends over time in the incidence and prevalence of encephalitis are difficult to interpret given the technological advances which have honed our ability to classify presentations by infectious agent or underlying disease. Autoimmune encephalitis has been estimated to account for approximately 20% of encephalitis presentations,[7] although it is likely that this proportion will increase over time as diagnostic testing improves: polymerase chain reaction (PCR) revolutionized the diagnosis of central nervous system infection at the end of the 20th century, while recent neuroimmunological developments have enabled a reclassification of autoimmune encephalitis.[11]

Investigation and Treatment

The challenge in managing patients with encephalitis on critical care is to identify those who have a treatable condition where there are therapies which can modify the disease trajectory and/or identify a treatable underlying cancer in order to achieve the best possible outcome for the patient.

A suggested approach to investigating the patient with suspected encephalitis is presented in the next section. HSV and VZV encephalitis outcomes improve with antivirals, while some autoimmune encephalitis improves with immunomodulation.[4,14]

Outcome

The outcome of encephalitis depends on the underlying cause, the provision of high-quality supportive intensive care services and to a lesser extent, the development of specific therapies: HSV encephalitis traditionally had a mortality rate of 70%, but with acyclovir this has reduced to between 5% and 20%.[14] The outcomes of VZV encephalitis are similar.[14]

Overall mortality of encephalitis is estimated at between 7% and 18%, with severe disability recorded in between 30% and 60% of survivors.[7,15] Factors reported to be associated with a poor outcome are the need for intubation, autoimmune etiology, age older than 65, an immunocompromised state, and acute thrombocytopenia.[12,15]

Encephalitis occurring in children can also have significant rates of mortality and long-term neurological impairment, with one study reporting up to 80% of patients admitted with encephalitis experiencing some form of long-term impairment at follow-up.[16]

PRACTICE PRESCRIPTION

When to Consider Encephalitis

Encephalitis should be considered in any patient presenting with an altered level of consciousness lasting at least 24 hours, but potentially of up to 3 months. This can include memory loss or psychiatric symptoms.[1] In addition the patient requires at least two of the following to be classified as "possible" encephalitis, and three to be considered "probable":
- Fever >38°C within 72 hours around presentation
- Seizures (generalized or partial)—not explained by previous seizure disorder
- New focal neurological findings
- Cerebrospinal fluid pleocytosis (>5/mm^3)
- Brain imaging abnormality
- Electroencephalogram abnormality

Confirmed encephalitis requires either the gold standard of a brain biopsy demonstrating histological evidence inflammation and microbial infiltration, or more practically confirmation of a microbiological or autoimmune process "strongly associated" with encephalitis.[3]

Of cases, where an underlying etiology is found, infectious causes are thought to be twice as common as autoimmune.[7] The diagnostic workup of the patient with suspected encephalitis is summarized in a comprehensive review by Dubey et al. in 2018,[4] aided by a review of the diagnostic criteria for autoimmune encephalitis by Graus et al. 2 years earlier.[1]

Flowchart 19.1 outlines a suggested initial workup for patients focusing on likely infectious causes, and a screen which would incorporate two of the most common autoimmune etiologies [*N*-methyl-D-aspartate receptor (NMDA-R) encephalitis and acute disseminated encephalomyelitis]. A comprehensive list of potential infectious causes and their links to particular animal or

Encephalitis

FLOWCHART 19.1: Initial workup for patients (Granerod, UK).[4]

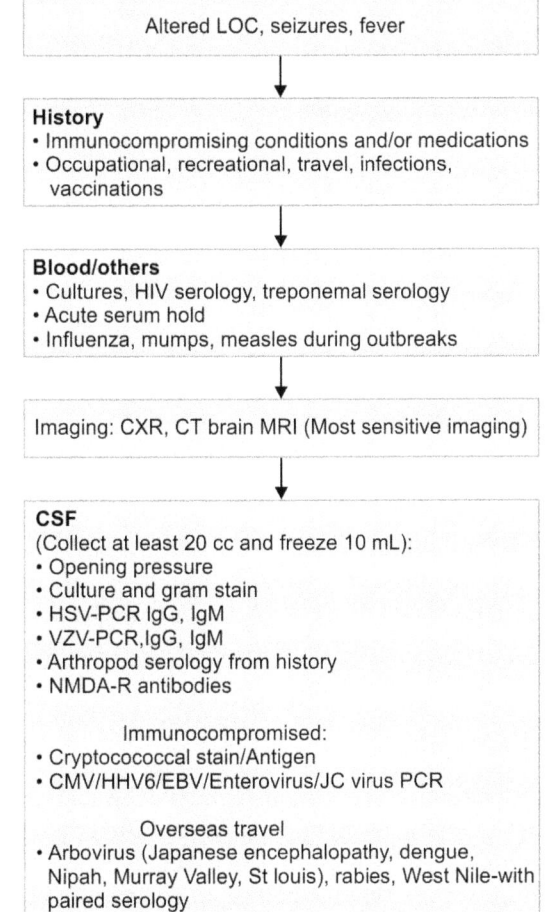

(LOC: level of consciousness; CXR: chest-X-ray; CSF: cerebrospinal fluid; IgM: immunoglobulin; NMDA-R: N-methyl D-aspartate receptor; HSV: herpes simplex virus; VZV: varicella-zoster virus; CMV: cytomegalovirus; EBV: Epstein-Barr virus; PCR: polymerase chain reaction)

travel exposure is outside the scope of this chapter, however, the reader is directed to the 2008 paper by Tunkel et al., which provides an extensive reference resource.[17]

As outlined in Flowchart 19.1 a sizeable sample of CSF should be sent for PCR of the most common viruses. The particular exposures highlighted from the individual patient history may require further testing at this stage.

If the initial diagnostic tests confirm the presence of HSV or VZV then continue acyclovir at 10 mg/kg 8 hourly for 14–21 days (or as per local guidelines). If imaging strongly suspects HSV encephalitis, and initial CSF PCR is negative, then a continuation of acyclovir and repeat examination at 3–7 days is warranted.[17] Confirmation of *Enterovirus* infection should prompt consideration of intravenous immunoglobulin (IVIG), and arboviral infection would warrant supportive treatment.[4]

When to Consider Autoimmune Encephalitis

Table 19.1 outlines some of the symptoms and signs which may be present in addition to those required to consider the initial diagnosis of encephalitis. These features may guide a targeted testing strategy for specific autoimmune encephalitis associated autoantibodies. Magnetic resonance imaging (MRI) should be obtained wherever possible, as the findings can also be helpful in investigating an autoimmune cause (Table 19.2).

Table 19.1: Clinical features linked to autoantibodies.[4]

Symptom/sign	Antibody
Psychosis	NMDA-R, AMPA-R, GABA-B
Movement disorder	NMDA-R, D2-R
Status epilepticus	NMDA-R, GABA-A, GABA-B
Myotonia/spasms/diarrhea	DPPX, CASPR-2
Stiffness	GAD65, GLyR
Cranial neuropathies	Miller-Fisher, Bickerstaff, Ma2, Hu
Limbic encephallitis on MRI	AMPA-R, LGI-1, CASPR-2, Hu/ANNA-1, CRMP-5, Ma 1/Ma2

(NMDA-R: N-methyl-D-aspartate receptor; AMPA-R: amino-3-hydroxyl-5-methyl-4-isoxazolepropenoic; GABA-B: gamma-aminobutyric acid type B; DR-2: dopamine-3 receptor; GABA-A: gamma-aminobutyric acid type A; DPPX: dipeptidyl-peptidase-like protien-6; CASPR-2: contactin-associated protein-like 2; GAD-65: glutamic acid decarboxylase; GlyR: strychnine-sensitive glycine receptor; LGI-1: leucine-rich glioma inactivated-1; ANNA-1: antineuronal nuclear antibody-1; CRMP-5: collapsing response-mediator protein-5)

Table 19.2: MRI findings with autoantibody-associated conditions.[4]

MRI finding	Antibody
Normal	NMDA-R, CASPR-2, GlyR, DPPX, ANNA-1/Hu, CRMP-5
Cortical changes (nonspecific)	NMDA-R, GlyR, DPPX
Cortical atrophy	AMPA-R
Cortical hyperintensity (multifocal)	GABA-A, GAD-65
Medial temporal FAIR hyperintensity	LGI-1, CASPR-2, CRMP-5, Ma1/Ma2
Brainstem FLAIR hyperintensity	ANNA-2, Ma1, Ma2
Demyelination (multifocal)-ADEM	MOG

(NMDA-R: N-methyl-D-aspartate receptor; CASPR-2: contactin-associated protein-like 2; DPPX: dipeptidyl-peptidase-like protein-6; GlyR: strychnine-sensitive glycine receptor; ANNA-1: antineuronal nuclear antibody-1; CRMP-5: collapsing response-mediator protein-5; AMPA-R: amino-3-hydroxyl-5-methyl-4-isoxazolepropenoic; GABA-A: gamma-aminobutyric acid type A; GAD-65: glutamic acid decarboxylase; LGI-1: leucine-rich glioma inactivated-1; MOG: myelin oligodentrocyte glycoprotein)

Confirmation and Treatment of Autoimmune Encephalitis

The mainstay of treatment is immunotherapy in the form of corticosteroids, IVIG, or plasma exchange. The timing of treatment may be prior to confirming the diagnosis if there is a strong clinical suspicion based on presentation/MRI findings and a negative infection screen, and the decision on how and when to treat should involve collaboration with the appropriate teams (e.g. intensive care, infectious diseases, and neurology specialists). The decision on when to treat needs to be balanced with the consideration that the autoimmune encephalitis may be a paraneoplastic phenomenon.

A proposed strategy of treating autoimmune encephalitis is outlined in Flowchart 19.2.[4] The immunotherapy trial may take place while confirmatory tests are awaited and may involve prolonged periods of reassessment and further modification.

Paraneoplastic disorders are autoimmune disorders triggered by underlying cancer, whose symptoms and thus diagnosis may be predated by the emergence of the autoimmune presentation. Autoimmune encephalitis is associated with several underlying neoplastic processes, although these associations may be overemphasized based on their observed frequency (Table 19.3). Prompt identification of the underlying tumor is clinically important for two reasons:[10]

1. Treating the underlying tumor may be required to resolve the encephalitis process (e.g. in the case of NMDA-R).
2. Immunotherapy for the encephalitis may alter the ability to detect the underlying cancer (e.g. lymphoma), or overlap with treatment.

Table 19.3: Association with cancer.[4]

Cancer	Autoantibody	Strength of Association*
Small cell lung cancer	ANNA -1/ Hu, CPRM -5,	Strong
	Ma1/Ma2	Strong
	GABA B, AMPA-R	Moderate
Ovarian teratoma	NMDA-R	Moderate
Thymoma	AMPA-R, LGI-1, CASPR-2	Moderate
	GAD-65, GABA-A	Weak
	GlyR	Rare
Breast adenocarcinoma	AMPA-R	Moderate
Lymphoma	DPPX	Rare

*Strong: >60%, Moderate: 30–60%, Weak: 10–30%, Rare: <10%.

SUMMARY

It is not uncommon to encounter patients with altered levels of consciousness, fever, and seizures in the critical care environment. While the criteria for encephalitis are initially straightforward, a significant level of complexity exists in formulating an appropriate investigation strategy based on their likely infectious exposures. Further complication arises from the fact the underlying etiology may remain elusive, and that common infections can give way to postinfectious processes. Furthermore the broad spectrum of rare, but potentially treatable conditions which make up the autoimmune encephalitides are increasing over time, with rapid advances in diagnostic testing. It is hoped that this chapter will provide a resource in which to remind the reader that there are many causes of "usual" presentation of encephalitis, and that there may be a treatable underlying cause of the "unusual" neurological presentation.

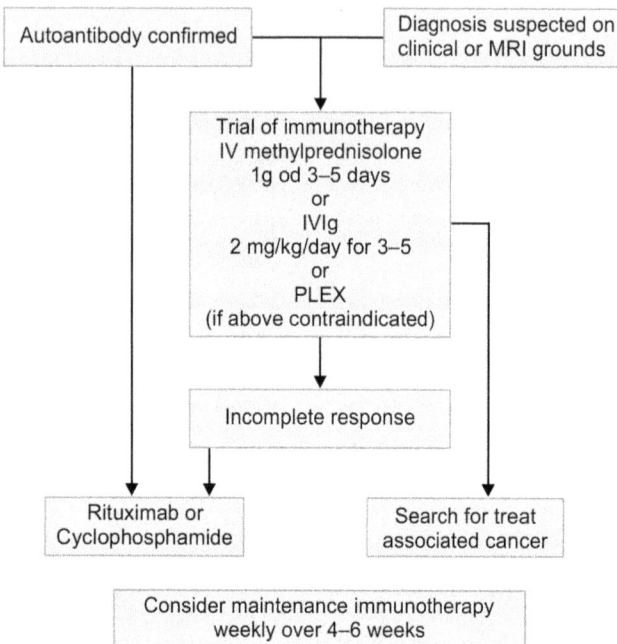

FLOWCHART 19.2: Approach for immunotherapy.

(IVIg: intravenous immunoglobulin; PLEX: plasma exchange)

REFERENCES

1. Graus F, Titulaer M, Balu R, et al. A clinical approach to diagnosis of autoimmune encephalitis. Lancet. 2016;15:391-404.
2. Johnson R. Acute encephalitis. Clin Infect Dis. 1996;23(2):219-24.
3. Venkatesan A, Tunkel AR, Bloch KC, et al. Case definitions, diagnostic algorithms, and priorities in encephalitis: consensus statement of the international encephalitis consortium. Clin Infect Dis. 2013;57(8):1114-28.

4. Dubey D, Tolenado M, McKeown A. Clinical presentation of autoimmune and viral encephalitis. Curr Opin Crit Care. 2018;24:80-90.
5. Whitley R, Gnann J. Viral encephalitis: familiar infections and emerging pathogens. Lancet. 2002;359(9305):507-13.
6. Granerod J, Cunningham R, Zuckerman M, et al. Causality in acute encephalitis: defining aetiologies. Epidemiol Infect. 2010;138:783-800.
7. Granerod J, Ambrose H, Davies N, et al. Causes of encephalitis and differences in their clinical presentations on England: a multicentre, population based prospective study. Lancet Infect Dis. 2010;10:835-44.
8. Carteaux G, Maquart M, Bedet A, et al. Zika virus associated with meningoencephalitis. N Engl J Med. 2016;374(16):595-96.
9. Da Silva I, Frontera J, De Filippis AM, et al. Neurological complications associated with the Zika virus in Brazilian adults. JAMA Neur. 2017;74(10):1190-8.
10. Lancaster E. The diagnosis and treatment of autoimmune encephalitis. J Clin Neurol. 2016;12(1):1-13.
11. Horta E, Lennon V, Lachance D, et al. Neural autoantibody clusters aid diagnosis of cancer. Clin Cancer Res. 2014;20(14):3862-9.
12. Singh T, Fugate J, Rabinstein A. The spectrum of acute encephalitis—causes, management, and predictors of outcome. Neurology. 2015;84(4):359-66.
13. Granerod J, Tam C, Crowcroft N, et al. Challenge of the unknown; a systematic review of acute encephalitis in non-outbreak situations. Neurology. 2010;75:924-32.
14. Kramer A. Viral Encephalitis in the ICU. Crit Care Clin. 2013;29:621-49.
15. Thakur K, Asemota A, Kirsch H, et al. Predictors of outcome in acute encephalitis. Neurology. 2013;81:793-800.
16. Rao S, Elkon B, Flett K, et al. Long-term outcomes and risk factors associated with acute encephalitis in children. J Paediatr Infect Dis Soc. 2017;6(1):20-7.
17. Tunkel A, Glaser C, Bloch K, et al. The management of encephalitis: clinical practice guidelines by the Infectious Diseases Society of America. Clin Infect Dis. 2008;47(3):303-27.

CHAPTER 20

Acute Liver Failure

Lalita Gouri Mitra, Vandana Saluja

INTRODUCTION

Acute liver failure (ALF) is a rare entity, seen in previously healthy adults in their thirties.[1] Reported incidence is one to six cases per million in a year in the developed countries. Hepatotropic viruses, such as hepatitis A and E, are the predominant causes of ALF in the developing world, whereas drug-induced (paracetamol overdose) is the main cause of ALF in the developed countries. Improved vaccination and sanitation measures have reduced the incidence of fecal-oral viral transmission in the United States and Western Europe.[1,2] There is overall female preponderance, especially in regions where viral causes predominate, with pregnant females accounting for 30% of such cases.[3] In 14–20% of patients no etiology can be determined, despite systematic investigation.[4]

Acute liver failure is a life-threatening and rare critical illness. It is a most commonly seen in young adults who do not have pre-existing liver disease.[1]

This syndrome is a manifestation of sudden and severe hepatic injury, due to multiple causes (Box 20.1). Hepatic injury leads to the abrupt loss of metabolic and immunological function of the liver, resulting in encephalopathy, coagulopathy, and multiorgan failure.[2] "Fulminant hepatic failure" was first described in 1970 and is defined as a severe liver injury, potentially reversible in nature, with the onset of encephalopathy within 8 weeks of first symptoms, in the absence of pre-existing liver disease.[5]

BOX 20.1: Etiology of acute liver failure.

Viral
- Hepatitis A, B, D, E
- Cytomegalovirus
- Epstein–Barr
- Herpes simplex
- Parvovirus
- Varicella zoster

Drugs
- Acetaminophen (Paracetamol)
- Nonacetaminophen (e.g. isoniazid, phenytoin, valproate, propylthiouracil, nitrofurantoin)
- Recreational drugs (e.g. cocaine, amphetamine group)
- Ischemic hepatitis
- Budd-Chiari
- Wilson's disease
- Pregnancy
- Mushroom poisoning (*Amanita phalloides*)
- Heat stroke
- Malignant infiltration
- Indeterminate

The key elements of this definition, namely the interval between symptom (most commonly jaundice) and hepatic encephalopathy (HE) (Box 20.2), are still relevant today. The jaundice–encephalopathy (J–E) interval indicates the likely causes, complications, and prognosis of the disease.[6-8]

BOX 20.2: Grading of hepatic encephalopathy (HE).[6]

- Grade 1 HE: Sleep reversal, mild lack of awareness, shortened attention span, and impaired ability to compute
- Grade 2 HE: Lethargy, poor memory, personality change, and asterixis
- Grade 3 HE: Progresses to somnolence, confusion, disorientation, and hyperreflexia, nystagmus, clonus, and rigidity
- Grade 4 HE: Stupor and coma

Depending on the J-E interval, O'Grady et al.[6] have classified fulminant hepatic failure in three groups:
1. *Hyperacute*: J-E interval of up to 7 days
2. *Acute*: J-E interval 8-28 days
3. *Subacute*: J-E interval from 5 weeks to 12 weeks

Clinical encephalopathy can be a late sign in young children; hence, coagulopathy is a commonly used indicator.

Therefore in pediatric patients, it is defined as a multisystem disorder in which severe impairment of liver function with or without encephalopathy, occurring with hepatocellular necrosis in a patient with no underlying chronic liver disease.[9]

PATHOPHYSIOLOGY

Irrespective of etiology (Box 20.1), there is hepatocellular injury, cellular death, and apoptosis with loss of metabolic function. The initiation, propagation, and resolution of the liver injury are determined by monocyte–macrophages. It is thus an innate immune-driven disorder.[10]

Initiation phase: Following an injurious event in the liver, macrophages originate from the Kupffer cells or bone marrow-derived monocytes. Within 12 hours of injury, there is a massive expansion of hepatic macrophages. This is followed by a biphasic macrophage response. The initial tissue destructive "M1" response is followed by resolution "M2" response.[11,12]

Studies have shown that there can be a switching of proinflammatory M1 macrophages to anti-inflammatory M2 macrophages in response to the environment cues.

Propagation phase: Hepatocyte death results in production of large quantities of inflammatory mediators which "spill over" from the injured liver to the systemic circulation. This results in the clinical manifestations of ALF. The M1 response is accompanied by clinical manifestations of systemic inflammatory response syndrome, such as fever, raised leukocyte count, tachycardia, and tachypnea.[13,14] Inflammatory mediators cross the blood–brain barrier and act synergistically with the elevated ammonia levels, resulting in astrocyte swelling.[15]

Resolution phase: The M2 response is mediated by anti-inflammatory mediators, such as interleukin 10 and transforming growth factor β, from the inflamed liver.[16] It opposes the proinflammatory response to limit tissue injury. However, spillover of the M2 response to the systemic circulation predisposes the patient to infection and poor outcomes.[17,18]

Therefore ALF represents an injurious event, followed by either deterioration or recovery due to regeneration.

ETIOLOGY AND OUTCOMES

Identifying etiology helps in determining prognosis and initiates etiology-specific therapies wherever possible. In Asian and African countries, viral illness due to hepatits A, B, and E is the prominent etiology of ALF.[19] In Europe and North America, paracetamol remains the predominant etiology.[20,21] Paracetamol-induced ALF has a higher rate of spontaneous recovery compared to other etiologies.[22]

DIAGNOSTIC APPROACH

History and Physical Findings

Jaundice, coagulopathy, and encephalopathy in patients with no prior liver disease are the sine qua non for diagnosis.[5,23,24]

Risk Factors

Age more than 40 years,[25,26] chronic alcohol use,[25] female sex,[27,28] poor nutritional status,[29] pregnancy,[30] chronic hepatitis B,[31,32] use of paracetamol for chronic pain are risk factors to be considered.[20]

Hyperacute cases seem to have the highest chance of spontaneous recovery, though a higher incidence of cerebral edema. However, this may not always hold true and be prognostically universally relevant, e.g. in countries like India.[33,34]

Exceptions to the definition of ALF, i.e. acute presentations of chronic liver diseases, e.g. autoimmune hepatitis, chronic hepatitis B, and Wilson's disease may present with clinical features of ALF.[35]

Laboratory Findings

Deranged liver function tests with elevated bilirubin, aminotransferases, and international normalized ratio (INR) are present in all cases. However, some specific patterns of derangement may help in etiological diagnosis as follows:[36]

- *Viral hepatitis*: Aminotransferases in the range of 1,000–2,000 IU/L with alanine aminotransferase > aspartate aminotransferase (AST).

Section 2: Organ Dysfunction

- *Acetaminophen:* Low bilirubin, very high AST >3,500 IU/L, and high INR.
- *Acute fatty liver of pregnancy/hemolysis, elevated liver enzymes, and low platelet count syndrome:* Aminotransferases <1,000 IU/L, high bilirubin, low platelet count.
- *Ischemic hepatic injury:* Very high aminotransferases, 25–250 times of upper limit of normal, increased lactic dehydrogenase.
- *Herpes simplex:* Low bilirubin, increased aminotransferases and leukopenia.
- *Valproate/tetracycline toxicity:* Minor to moderate elevation of aminotransferases and bilirubin levels.

List of initial laboratory tests which are helpful is shown in Table 20.1.

Clinical features of ALF are shown in Table 20.2.

MANAGEMENT OF ACUTE LIVER FAILURE IN INTENSIVE CARE UNIT

Recognition of Hepatic Injury

Hyperacute cases of liver injury may present with confusion or agitation with minimal jaundice. Subacute cases may be confused with chronic liver disease.[1]

Acute Liver Failure Versus Liver Injury

Acute liver injury (ALI) represents a milder form or may be a precursor to ALF. It is characterized by the presence of elevated INR >2.0, with the absence of encephalopathy. It has been defined as follows:[42]
- *Acetaminophen induced ALI*
  - Absence of HE

Table 20.1: Laboratory tests important in initial diagnosis of acute liver failure (ALF).

Assessment	Test	Result
Severity	Arterial blood gas	The presence of acidosis is an important prognostic indicator, in paracetamol overdose[37]
	Arterial lactate	Elevated[38]
	Arterial ammonia	High ammonia levels to >200 µmol/L may predict an increased risk of developing intracranial hypertension[39]
	Hemoglobin, leukocytes, platelets	The presence of leukocytosis may suggest infection. Anemia may be present in Wilson's disease in which Coombs-negative hemolytic anemia may occur. Thrombocytopenia may suggest pre-existing advanced liver disease[40]
	Factor V	A low result with hepatic encephalopathy may be predictive of mortality, in viral hepatitis[41]
	Creatinine, urea, sodium, chloride, potassium, calcium	Elevated urea and creatinine, metabolic derangements
Etiology (serum or urine)	HAV IgM, HBsAg, HBc IgM, anti-HCV, anti-HEV, CMV IgM	May be positive
	EBV IgM, HSV IgM, VZV IgM, anti-HIV	May be positive
	Ceruloplasmin, copper	Low ceruloplasmin (<5 mg/dL) in Wilson's disease
	Antinuclear antibody, antismooth muscle antibody, quantitative Ig levels (IgG)	May be positive
	Acetaminophen, toxicology screen	Elevated paracetamol levels, urine positive for paracetamol
	Pregnancy test	May be positive
Imaging studies	Chest X-ray	Possible aspiration pneumonia (due to obtundation with hepatic encephalopathy)
	Abdominal ultrasound with Doppler	Hepatic vessel thrombosis (Budd-Chiari), hepatomegaly, splenomegaly, hepatic surface nodularity

(CMV: cytomegalovirus; EBV: Epstein-Barr virus; HAV: hepatitis A virus; HBc: hepatitis B core; HBsAg: hepatitis B virus surface antigen; HCV: hepatitis C virus; HEV: hepatitis E virus; Ig: immunoglobulin; VZV: varicella-zoster virus)

Table 20.2: Clinical features of acute liver failure.

Brain	Encephalopathy, cerebral edema, intracranial hypertension
Heart	High-output state (due to peripheral vasodilatation), subclinical myocardial injury
Lungs	Acute lung injury, acute respiratory distress syndrome
Liver	Loss of metabolic function, causing hypoglycemia, lactic acidosis, hyperammonemia, and coagulopathy
Pancreas	Pancreatitis (acetaminophen related)
Kidney	Injury or failure
Bone marrow	Suppression (viral and seronegative causes)
Adrenal	Suppression, causing hypotension

- International normalized ratio ≥2.0
- Alanine aminotransferase level ≥10 × upper limit of normal
❑ *Nonacetaminophen induced ALI*
- Absence of HE
- International normalized ratio ≥ 2.0
- Alanine aminotransferase level ≥10 × upper limit of normal
- Bilirubin ≥3.0 mg/dL.

It has been found that in ALI cases due to paracetamol, 93% recover rapidly and fully, whereas non-paracetamol cases with ALI have poor outcome and should be targeted for early referral to a liver transplant center.

Intensive Care Unit Management

All patients with ALF should be managed in the intensive care unit once encephalopathy develops.[43]

Management of Cerebral Edema

Cerebral edema is life-threatening in ALF, especially in those who progress to grade III/IV encephalopathy. Incidence and severity of cerebral edema, cardiovascular complications, and renal failure are the greatest in the hyperacute cohort, which has the greatest chance of spontaneous recovery without a transplant. The subacute cohort is at a lower risk of cerebral edema with more frequent septic complications.[44] In the setting of grade III/IV encephalopathy, patients should be sedated and ventilated.

Other measures for raised intracranial pressure (ICP) which should be initiated include[35,45]

❑ Maintenance of low normal partial pressure of carbon dioxide.
❑ Short-term hyperventilation during raised ICP and hyperemia (seen by elevated jugular bulb oxygen concentration) can be done.
❑ Avoid prolonged hyperventilation.
❑ Aim to maintain a mean arterial blood pressure (MAP) of at least 75 mm Hg, to target a cerebral perfusion pressure (CPP) of at least 50 mm Hg.
❑ Osmotic therapy with 20% mannitol or hypertonic saline. Target serum sodium levels of 145–150 mmol/L.
❑ Intravenous indomethacin can be tried in whom hyperemia is the main contributor.
❑ Head elevation at 45° with avoidance of head turning.
❑ Avoid fever. No proven role of hypothermia currently in this cohort.[46]
❑ Renal replacement therapy (RRT) can be considered for ammonia clearance.[35,47] Continuous modes are better than intermittent modes as they provide hemodynamic and intracranial stability.[48]

Acute Kidney Injury

Incidence of acute kidney injury is around 70% in patients with ALF, and it is associated with a poor prognosis without liver transplant. It is more common with drug-induced (acetaminophen, phenytoin, trimethoprim-sulfamethoxazole, or macrolides) ALF. The need for RRT is dictated as per classical indications, such as acidosis, fluid overload, hyperkalemia. The continuous modes are preferred over intermittent modes of RRT.[35]

Pulmonary Complications

Incidence of pulmonary complications is 30%.[49] Mild acute respiratory distress syndrome (ARDS) is usually a late presentation in the course of the disease coinciding with liver regeneration or development of sepsis.[1] Management of mild ARDS is similar to the conventional management of ARDS with the caveat of careful positive end-expiratory pressure application in presence of raised ICP. However, the presence of lung injury is not considered poor prognostic marker, and the outcomes are similar to those patients who do not have ARDS.[35]

Coagulopathy

In spite of the presence of significant coagulopathy as per laboratory parameters, the incidence of acute bleeding is low. Routine correction of INR is not recommended as it obscures an important prognostic marker of liver function. Coagulopathy correction is advised only in patients who have bleeding or before invasive procedures.[43]

Supportive Care

Fluid and cardiovascular management must address the relationship between MAP and ICP.

- Low arterial blood pressure may be present in absence of sepsis, due to systemic vasodilatation. Restoration of intravascular volume is important to prevent organ failure. Hypotonic intravascular fluids should be avoided due to high risk of cerebral edema.
- Enteral nutrition should be initiated early. Severe protein restrictions should be avoided to prevent catabolism. At least 60 g of protein per day is advisable. Placement of nasogastric tube should be preferably done in intubated and sedated patients to avoid increases in ICP due to gagging.
- *Control of sepsis*: High standards of infection control should be maintained to minimize nosocomial sepsis.[1] Impaired hepatic regeneration may lead to a functional immunosuppression with secondary nosocomial sepsis. Therefore pre-emptive antibiotics have to be administered according to local culture and sensitivity patterns. Prophylactic antimicrobial therapy does not influence survival in this group of patients.[50]

Role of N-Acetylcysteine

N-Acetylcysteine (NAC) is a precursor of glutathione and is the antidote to paracetamol toxicity. The hepatotoxic metabolite of paracetamol and N-acetyl-p-benzoquinone imine is to be inactivated by conjugation with glutathione. NAC is 100% hepatoprotective when given within 8 hours of paracetamol ingestion.

A late presentation should not preclude NAC administration.

Dose: A 140 mg/kg orally as a loading dose, followed by 70 mg/kg every 4 hours; or 150 mg/kg intravenously over 60 minutes as a loading dose, followed by 12.5 mg/kg/h over 4 hours, then 6.25 mg/kg/h.

N-Acetylcysteine has other benefits, such as improved liver oxygenation, and has antioxidant, anti-inflammatory, and immunologic effects. It has beneficial hemodynamic effects and may improve CPP.

In liver failure related to non-paracetamol etiologies, it has been found to be beneficial in patients with HE I and II. It is ineffective in advanced grades of HE. However, NAC may still have a role in mushroom poisoning and drug-induced ALF.[4]

The following therapies are to be initiated simultaneously depending on the etiology of ALF (Table 20.3).[36]

Monitoring

The following monitors help to achieve specific targets with respect to a patient with ALF.
- *Invasive arterial blood pressure*:
  - Mean arterial blood pressure and hence CPP
  - Blood gas analysis

Table 20.3: Specific management of various etiologies of acute liver failure (ALF).

Etiology	Management
Herpes simplex	Acyclovir
Acute fatty liver of pregnancy/HELLP syndrome	Delivery of fetus
Amanita phalloides poisoning	Benzylpenicillin, N acetylcysteine, acitvated charcoal, gastric lavage
Autoimmune hepatitis	Methylprednisone
Acute hepatitis B	Tenofovir, entecavir
Acute Budd-Chiari syndrome	Anticoagulation, TIPSS
Acute Wilson's disease	Measures to reduce serum copper like including plasmapheresis, CVVH, albumin dialysis, or plasma exchange

(CVVH: continuous veno-venous hemofiltration; HELLP: hemolysis, elevated liver enzymes, and low platelet count; TIPPS: transjugular intrahepatic portosystemic shunt)

- *Blood sugar*: Blood sugar monitoring every second hourly for prevention and treatment hypoglycemia.[35]
- *Temperature monitoring*: Avoiding fever is important for controlling ICP.
- *Central nervous system monitoring*:
  - Pupillary size and reaction
  - Optic nerve sheath diameter
  - Transcranial Doppler
- *Intracranial pressure monitoring*: ICP monitoring is controversial and not regarded as standard of care.[44]

Emerging Therapies

Acute liver failure results in the accumulation of ammonia and inflammatory cytokines which result in the development of cerebral edema, circulatory dysfunction, and renal failure.

Extracorporeal liver support (ECLS) devices aim to remove these toxins, improve the pathophysiological features of liver failure, and thus provide a window till native liver recovers or transplant opportunity presents.[51]

An ideal ECLS should perform the functions of detoxification, biosynthesis, and regulation. None of the currently available devices (Table 20.4) satisfy all the criteria.
- *Hepatocyte transplantation*: Hepatocyte transplantation has been shown to improve some biochemical parameters, such as reduction of blood ammonia levels, and improvement of encephalopathy, but patient survival without liver transplantation is rare.[52]

Timing of Liver Transplant

Aim of prognostication is to identify those patients who won't survive with medical therapy alone. Early transplant

Table 20.4: Benefits of Extracorporeal liver support devices in acute liver failure.[52]

Extracorporeal liver support devices	CVS	CNS	Biochemical*	Survival impact
Artificial				
MARS	Yes	Not assessed	Yes	No
SPAD	No	No	No	No
HVP	Yes	Yes	Yes	Yes
Biological/Bioartificial				
Human hepatocytes	Yes	Yes	Yes	No
Porcine hepatocytes	No change	No change	Yes	No

*Biochemical: statistically significant reduction in bilirubin, bile acids, creatinine and ammonia levels

(MARS: molecular adsorbent recirculating system; SPAD: single-pass albumin dialysis; HVP: high volume plasmapheresis; CVS: cardiovascular system; CNS: central nervous system)

referral is advised based on a number of prognostic evaluation systems. Most widely used is the King's College Criteria (Box 20.3).

Liver transplantation: Liver transplant candidacy should be assessed in all patients presenting with ALF, as this may be the only definitive option available for survival. However, higher 3-month mortality has been observed in this group, after a liver transplant.[43] Presence of intracranial hypertension and emergency nature of the disease make the procedure challenging in this group of patients.[1]

Liver transplant surgery is not universally available and less than 10% of liver transplants are performed in ALF.[1] Data from the US Organ Procurement and Transplantation Network indicate that patients with ALF who undergo liver transplantation have survival rates of 87% at 1 year and 78% at 3 years.[43]

BOX 20.3: King's College criteria for selection of recipients for emergency liver transplants.[2]

Paracetamol poisoning–induced ALF
- Arterial pH <7.3 following adequate volume resuscitation
OR *a combination of*
- HE ≥grade 3
- Creatinine ≥300 μmol/L (3.4 mg/dL)
- INR ≥6.5

Non-paracetamol-poisoning etiology of ALF
- Any grade encephalopathy and INR ≥6.5
OR *any 3 of the following*
- INR ≥3.5
- Age less than 10 or more than 40 years
- Jaundice–encephalopathy interval >7 days
- Bilirubin ≥300 μmol/L (17 mg/dL)
- Unfavorable cause (drug induced, liver injury, seronegative disease)

(ALF: acute liver failure; HE: hepatic encephalopathy; INR: international normalized ratio)

REFERENCES

1. Bernal W, Wendon J. Acute liver failure. N Engl J Med. 2013;26(369):2525-34.
2. Bernal W, Auzinger G, Dhawan A, et al. Acute liver failure. Lancet. 2010;17(376):190-201.
3. Acharya SK, Panda SK, Saxena A, et al. Acute hepatic failure in India: a perspective from the East. J Gastroenterol Hepatol. 2000;15:473-9.
4. Donnelly MC, Hayes PC, Simpson KJ. The changing face of liver transplantation for acute liver failure: assessment of current status and implications for future practice. Liver Transpl. 2016;22:527-35.
5. Trey C, Davidson CS. The management of fulminant hepatic failure. Prog Liver Dis. 1970;3:282-98.
6. O'Grady JG, Schalm SW, Williams R. Acute liver failure: redefining the syndromes. Lancet. 1993;342:273-5.
7. Bernuau J, Rueff B, Benhamou JP. Fulminant and subfulminant liver failure: definitions and causes. Semin Liver Dis. 1986;6:97-106.
8. Mochida S, Nakayama N, Matsui A, et al. Re-evaluation of the guideline published by the Acute Liver Failure Study Group of Japan in 1996 to determine the indications of liver transplantation in patients with fulminant hepatitis. Hepatol Res. 2008;38:970-9.
9. Bhaduri BR, Mieli-Vergani G. Fulminant hepatic failure: pediatric aspects. Semin Liver Dis. 1996;16:349-55.
10. Davies LC, Jenkins SJ, Allen JE, et al. Tissue-resident macrophages. Nat Immunol. 2013;14:986-95.
11. Arnold L, Henry A, Poron F, et al. Inflammatory monocytes recruited after skeletal muscle injury switch into antiinflammatory macrophages to support myogenesis. J Exp Med. 2007;204:1057-69.
12. Nahrendorf M, Swirski FK, Aikawa E, et al. The healing myocardium sequentially mobilizes two monocyte subsets with divergent and complementary functions. J Exp Med. 2007;204:3037-47.
13. Possamai LA, Thursz MR, Wendon JA, et al. Modulation of monocyte/macrophage function: a therapeutic strategy in the treatment of acute liver failure. J Hepatol. 2014;6:439-45.
14. Bone RC, Balk RA, Cerra FB, et al. Definitions for sepsis and organ failure and guidelines for the use of innovative therapies

in sepsis. The ACCP/SCCM Consensus Conference Committee. American College of Chest Physicians/Society of Critical Care Medicine. Chest. 1992;101:1644-55.
15. Butterworth RF. The liver-brain axis in liver failure: neuroinflammation and encephalopathy. Nat Rev Gastroenterol Hepatol. 2013;10:522-8.
16. Antoniades CG, Berry PA, Wendon JA, et al. The importance of immune dysfunction in determining outcome in acute liver failure. J Hepatol. 2008;49:845-61.
17. Berry PA, Antoniades CG, Hussain MJ, et al. Admission levels and early changes in serum interleukin-10 are predictive of poor outcome in acute liver failure and decompensated cirrhosis. Liver Int. 2010;30:733-40.
18. Antoniades CG, Quaglia A, Taams LS, et al. Source and characterization of hepatic macrophages in acetaminophen induced acute liver failure in humans. Hepatology. 2012;56:735-46.
19. Lee WM. Etiologies of acute liver failure. Semin Liver Dis. 2008;28:142-52.
20. Larson AM, Polson J, Fontana RJ, et al. Acetaminophen-induced acute liver failure: results of a United States multicenter, prospective study. Hepatology. 2005;42:1364-72.
21. Wei G, Bergquist A, Broome U, et al. Acute liver failure in Sweden: etiology and outcome. J Intern Med. 2007;262:393-401.
22. Lee WM, Squires RH Jr, Nyberg SL, et al. Acute liver failure: summary of a workshop. Hepatology. 2008;47:1401-15.
23. Gimson AE, O'Grady J, Ede RJ, et al. Late onset hepatic failure: clinical, serological and histological features. Hepatology. 1986;6:288-94.
24. Bernuau J, Rueff B, Benhamou JP. Fulminant and subfulminant liver failure: definitions and causes. Semin Liver Dis. 1986;6:97-106.
25. Myers RP, Shaheen AA, Li B, et al. Impact of liver disease, alcohol abuse, and unintentional ingestions on the outcomes of acetaminophen overdose. Clin Gastroenterol Hepatol. 2008;6:918-25.
26. Schmidt LE. Age and paracetamol self-poisoning. Gut. 2005;54:686-90.
27. Russo MW, Galanko JA, Shrestha R, et al. Liver transplantation for acute liver failure from drug induced liver injury in the United States. Liver Transpl. 2004;10:1018-23.
28. Andrade RJ, Lucena MI, Fernandez MC, et al. Drug-induced liver injury: an analysis of 461 incidences submitted to the Spanish registry over a 10-year period. Gastroenterology. 2005;129:512-21.
29. Garfein RS, Bower WA, Loney CM, et al. Factors associated with fulminant liver failure during an outbreak among injection drug users with acute hepatitis B. Hepatology. 2004;40:865-73.
30. Khuroo MS, Kamili S. Aetiology, clinical course and outcome of sporadic acute viral hepatitis in pregnancy. J Viral Hepat. 2003;10:61-9.
31. Chu CM, Liaw YF. The incidence of fulminant hepatic failure in acute viral hepatitis in Taiwan: increased risk in patients with pre-existing HBsAg carrier state. Infection. 1990;18:200-3.
32. Chu CM, Liaw YF. Increased incidence of fulminant hepatic failure in previously unrecognized HBsAg carriers with acute hepatitis independent of etiology. Infection. 2005;33:136-9.
33. Das AK, Ahmed S, Medhi S, et al. Changing patterns of aetiology of acute sporadic viral hepatitis in India—newer insights from north-east India. Int J Curr Res Rev. 2014;6:14-20.
34. Lee WM, Seremba E. Etiologies of acute liver failure. Curr Opin Crit Care. 2008;14:198-201.
35. Cardoso FS, Marcelino P, Bagulho L, et al. Acute liver failure: an up-to-date approach. J Crit Care. 2017;39:25-30.
36. Lee WM, Larson AM, Todd Stravitz R. AASLD position paper: the management of acute liver failure: update 2011. AASLD; 2011. <http://www.aasld.org/practiceguidelines/Documents/AcuteLiverFailureUpdate2011.pdf>.
37. O'Grady JG, Alexander GJ, Hayllar KM, et al. Early indicators of prognosis in fulminant hepatic failure. Gastroenterology. 1989;97:339-45.
38. Bernal W, Donaldson N, Wyncoll D, et al. Blood lactate as an early predictor of outcome in paracetamol-induced acute liver failure: a cohort study. Lancet. 2002;359:558-63.
39. Bernal W, Hall C, Karvellas CJ, et al. Arterial ammonia and clinical risk factors for encephalopathy and intracranial hypertension in acute liver failure. Hepatology. 2007;46:1844-52.
40. Stravitz RT, Ellerbe C, Durkalski V, et al. Thrombocytopenia is associated with multi-organ system failure in patients with acute liver failure. Clin Gastroenterol Hepatol. 2016;14:613-20.
41. Bernuau J, Samuel D, Durand F, et al. Criteria for emergency liver transplantation in patients with acute viral hepatitis and factor V below 50% of normal: a prospective study. Hepatology. 1991;14:49A.
42. Koch DG, Speiser JL, Durkalski V, et al. The natural history of severe acute liver injury. Am J Gastroenterol. 2017;112:1389-96.
43. Gonzalez SA. Acute liver failure. BMJ Best Pract. 2017. <https://bestpractice.bmj.com/topics/en-us/1010> [Accessed December, 2018].
44. Wendon J, Lee W. Encephalopathy and cerebral edema in the setting of acute liver failure: pathogenesis and management. Neurocrit Care. 2008;9:97-102.
45. Clemmesen JO, Hansen BA, Larsen FS. Indomethacin normalizes intracranial pressure in acute liver failure: a twenty-three-year-old woman treated with indomethacin. Hepatology. 1997;26:1423-5.
46. Karvellas CJ, Todd Stravitz R, Battenhouse H, et al. Therapeutic hypothermia in acute liver failure: a multicenter retrospective cohort analysis. Liver Transpl. 2015;21:4-12.
47. Slack AJ, Auzinger G, Willars C, et al. Ammonia clearance with haemofiltration in adults with liver disease. Liver Int. 2014;34:42-8.
48. Davenport A, Will EJ, Davidson AM. Improved cardiovascular stability during continuous modes of renal replacement therapy in critically ill patients with acute hepatic and renal failure. Crit Care Med. 1993;21:328-38.
49. Muñoz SJ. Difficult management problems in fulminant hepatic failure. Semin Liver Dis. 1993;13:395.
50. Karvellas CJ, Cavazos J, Battenhouse H, et al. Effects of antimicrobial prophylaxis and blood stream infections in patients with acute liver failure: a retrospective cohort study. Clin Gastroenterol Hepatol. 2014;12:1942-9.
51. Karvellas CJ, Subramanian RM. Current evidence for extracorporeal liver support systems in acute liver failure and acute-on-chronic liver failure. Crit Care Clin. 2016;32:439-51.
52. UpToDate. Acute liver failure in adults: management and prognosis. [online] Available from https://www.uptodate.com/contents/acute-liver-failure-in-adults-management-and-prognosis#H3. [Accessed December, 2018].

CHAPTER 21

Diarrhea in Intensive Care Unit

Sheetal Gaikwad, Amol Kothekar A, Vijaya Patil

INTRODUCTION

Diarrhea is one of the frequent problems that may complicate or prolong intensive care unit (ICU) course of a critically ill patient. The reported prevalence of diarrhea is 12.9–41%.[1,2] Many conditions and factors lead to diarrhea including infections, enteral feeding, or drugs. It complicates patient's stay by causing fluid losses leading to hemodynamic disturbances, electrolyte losses leading to dyselectrolytemia, malnutrition, and delayed wound healing, increased risk of pressure ulcers due to skin breakdown, etc. Diarrhea also contributes to increased nursing workload and increased ICU length of stay.[1]

PHYSIOLOGY OF THE DIGESTIVE SYSTEM

A normal adult consumes approximately 2–2.5 L fluids in the daily diet. Gut adds another 7 L of fluid from various secretions, such as saliva, gastric juice, biliary and pancreatic fluids, and fluid from the small intestine. Most of this volume, along with digested food, is absorbed back as this chyme (partly digested food with digestive juices) transits through jejunum and ileum, leaving only 1–2 L for colonic absorption. Most of this fluid is reabsorbed by the colon, leaving 100–150 g of stool to be expelled by body. When there is a disturbance in this physiologic process, it results in diarrhea.

DEFINITION OF DIARRHEA

Normal bowel frequency varies from as less as three times per week up to three times per day. In present literature, there is a wide variation in the definition of diarrhea, which is based on criteria of frequency, consistency, 24-hour total stool volume, duration, and a combination of one or more criteria. Realizing this problem, recently a standard definition of diarrhea is proposed where diarrhea is defined as having three or more loose or liquid stools per day with a stool weight greater than 200 g/day and consistency of stools categorized as 5–7 on the Bristol Stool Chart.[3] Working Group on Abdominal Problems (WGAP) of the European Society of Intensive Care Medicine (ESICM) has classified gastrointestinal (GI) injury into four grades according to severity. According to their grading, diarrhea constitutes acute GI injury grade II where digestive and absorptive functions of GI tract are affected, and measures need to be undertaken to prevent further progression to GI failure.[4]

CLASSIFICATION OF DIARRHEA

The causes of diarrhea are multifactorial and variable. Diarrhea can be classified according to the duration, mechanism, and severity.
- *According to duration:* Diarrhea is labeled as acute diarrhea if duration is less than 14 days, persistent diarrhea, if diarrhea is more than 14 days duration, and chronic diarrhea if it lasts for more than 30 days.

Nosocomial or hospital-associated diarrhea is defined as diarrhea developing in a patient hospitalized for more than 3 days.[5]

- *According to mechanism of diarrhea:* Most of the diarrheas are multifactorial, however, based on predominant cause; they can be classified as osmotic, secretary, exudative, and motor diarrheas.
  - *Osmotic diarrhea:* This is due to ingestion of substances that are not absorbed and result in retention and/or secretion of water within the lumen of the intestine. Such substances are either dietary components, such as disaccharides, or poorly absorbable ions, such as magnesium.
    - *Carbohydrate malabsorption:* On ingestion of carbohydrate, the unabsorbed carbohydrate is fermented by colonic bacteria into organic acids which are partly absorbed. Remaining unabsorbed organic acid and unmetabolized carbohydrates in colonic lumen can lead to diarrhea.[6] Similar effect is observed with ingestion of high dose of lactulose. The capacity of the colonic flora for fermentation of carbohydrate is high and so unabsorbed lactose/organic acid will lead to diarrhea only when this capacity is exceeded. Carbohydrate malabsorption is commonly seen in conditions, such as combined small bowel and colon resection, and pancreatic disease. Stool pH with carbohydrate malabsorption is acidic (pH < 6), and an increased osmotic gap may be present (typically >100 mOsm/kg).[7] Stool osmotic gap is calculated as 290−2 × (stool Na$^+$ + stool K$^+$), where 290 is stool osmolality which is constant. Normal stool osmotic gap is 50–100 mOsm/kg.
    - *Poorly absorbed ions, such as magnesium, sulfate, phosphate:* Excessive ingestion of magnesium can lead to diarrhea by increasing stool volume. For each millimole increase in fecal magnesium output, fecal weight increases by approximately 7.3 g.[8] Patients with magnesium-induced diarrhea will have low concentrations of sodium and potassium, a high stool osmotic gap (>50 mOsm/kg), and high concentrations of magnesium. Generally, this is the cause for chronic diarrhea rather than acute diarrhea.
  - *Secretory diarrhea:* This is caused by excessive secretion and/or impaired absorption of fluids and electrolytes across intestinal mucosa. Secretory diarrheas are caused by bacteria, such as *Salmonella, Shigella,* or *Escherichia coli*; viruses such as rotavirus; inflammatory processes; drugs such as human immunodeficiency virus protease inhibitors; endocrinopathies such as Addisons, gastrinoma, pheochromocytoma; and genetic mutations in intestinal proteins.

    Ileal bile acid absorption: Ileal dysfunction or resection results in delivery of a very high concentration of bile acids into the colon (3–5 mmol/L). Bile acid in the colon, in particular the chenodeoxycholate and deoxycholate, stimulates electrolyte and water secretion along with increased colonic motility. This leads to shortening of the colonic transit time and produces diarrhea. This condition can also be seen in patients with abdominal malignancies who may develop radiation-induced ileitis or pancreatitis.[9] These patients respond well to anion exchange resins such as cholestyramine that bind bile acids with high affinity.

    Osmotic and secretary diarrhea can be diagnosed and differentiated based on electrolyte composition and osmotic gap of stool. Secretary diarrhea generally has high electrolyte concentration with low osmotic gap, whereas osmotic diarrhea will have high osmotic gap with low electrolyte concentration.
  - *Exudative diarrhea:* This is mainly caused by the inflammation of intestinal mucosa, which may be infective or noninfective in origin. Here, diarrhea is caused by large quantity of inflammatory materials, such as pus, blood, or proteinaceous material. In these situations, absorption of fluid, electrolytes, and nutrients may also get affected and thus contribute to final stool volume and frequency.
  - *Diarrhea due to altered bowel motility (motor diarrhea):* Increased bowel motility can decrease transit time for intestinal contents and thus decrease absorption. This will result in delivery of large volume of stool to colon. In an adult, normal colonic absorptive capacity is approximately 4 L and person can experience diarrhea when this capacity is exceeded. This is commonly seen in stressful emotional situations but can also be seen in postgastrectomy patients, postnarcotic withdrawal, or with the use of prokinetic drugs, such as metoclopramide or erythromycin.
- *According to the severity of underlying pathophysiology:* Depending on severity of underlying pathophysiology, diarrhea is also classified as life-threatening and non-life-threatening. Life-threatening diarrhea can be noninfective which is mainly due to mesenteric or colonic ischemia or infective due to *Clostridium difficile* (CD) infection (CDI). Non-life-threatening diarrheas are generally caused by drugs, enteral feeding, fecal impaction, etc.

Life-threatening Diarrhea

- *Mesenteric ischemia*: Splanchnic circulation is a key factor that determines digestion and absorption of intraluminal contents and maintenance of the gut mucosal barrier. Blood flow to all intra-abdominal organs including stomach, pancreas, liver, spleen, small intestine, and large intestine comes from splanchnic vessels. Since oxygen requirement of gut fluctuates depending on whether it is in fed state or in fasting state, splanchnic circulation is highly adaptive and splanchnic blood flow varies between 10% and 35% of cardiac output. Out of all the blood received by intestines, approximately 70% blood supply goes to mucosal and submucosal layers. Since oxygen extraction of intestines is relatively low, intestinal ischemia does not occur till blood flow is reduced below 50% of fasting state.

    Occlusive mesenteric ischemia either due to embolism or thrombosis is major cause for mesenteric ischemia accounting to almost 75–80% cases. Non-occlusive mesenteric ischemia due to hypoperfusive states accounts to the remaining 25–30% cases.[10] Overall mortality in acute mesenteric ischemia from any cause is very high with reported mortality of 60–80%.[11] Ischemic colitis has overall mortality of 22% and can be as high as 75% in those requiring surgical intervention.[12]

    These patients typically develop acute abdominal pain that is disproportional to the physical examination, and it is associated with bloody diarrhea. Diagnosis depends on high index of clinical suspicion in patients at risk. Computed tomography (CT) angiography without oral contrast and magnetic resonance angiography are highly sensitive diagnostic tests. Restoration of mesenteric blood supply and surgical intervention in the case of nonviable intestine are main treatment modalities.

- *Neutropenic enterocolitis* is a condition characterized by fever, abdominal pain, neutropenia, and watery or bloody diarrhea in patients with neutropenia (commonly seen in patients with hematological malignancies), and other immunosuppressive conditions, such as acquired immunodeficiency syndrome and organ transplant. Exact pathophysiology is unknown and thought to be multifactorial; however, mucosal injury due to direct cytotoxic effects of chemotherapeutic agent is the most likely mechanism. Histologic features include a paucity of inflammatory and leukemic infiltrates and mucosal and submucosal edema, villous sloughing, and stromal hemorrhage.[13] In adult patients receiving chemotherapy who need hospitalization, incidence of neutropenic enterocolitis is around 5.3%,[14] with mortality of 30–60%.[15] Abdominal ultrasound and CT scan are useful diagnostic modalities which reveal diffuse bowel thickening and mucosal edema. Main treatment modalities are keeping patient nil by mouth to give rest to the bowel, gastric decompression, total parenteral nutrition (TPN), adequate fluid and electrolyte replacement, and use of broad-spectrum antibiotics. Sudden deterioration in patient's condition should prompt clinician to look for bowel gangrene and bowel perforation, since these are known complications and need timely surgical intervention.

- *Clostridium difficile* diarrhea: CD is an anaerobic, spore- and toxin-forming, Gram-positive bacillus present in the bacterial flora of the colon. CDI is the leading and one of the most important causes of nosocomial infection. In present era, CD has replaced methicillin-resistant *Staphylococcus aureus* as the most common causative agent for nosocomial infection.[16] Reported incidence ranges from 3.2/1,000 patient days to 100/1,000 patient days.[17,18]

Risk factors: Systemic review has identified multiple risk factors which are categorized in three main groups.[19]

1. *Pharmacological risk factors* include use of broad-spectrum antibiotics, use of proton pump inhibitors (PPIs), use of histamine 2 receptor antagonists, antacids, nonsteroidal anti-inflammatory drugs, corticosteroids, and use of opiate during the previous episodes of CDI.
2. *Host-related risk factors* include age >65 years, diabetes mellitus, chronic kidney disease, lymphoma or leukemia, solid malignancy, inflammatory bowel disease, congestive heart failure, previous diagnosis of CDI, and chronic obstructive pulmonary disease.
3. *Clinical interventions–related risk factors* include duration of hospitalization, nasogastric tube insertion, stay in ICU, history of surgery, previous GI procedure, low serum albumin, and colonization with vancomycin-resistant enterococci.

Mechanism of action: The virulence of CD is due to the production of enterotoxin A and cytotoxin B. These toxin proteins are internalized by host cells and cause disruption of cytoskeletal structure leading to cell death. This leads to the loss of gut barrier and translocation of bacteria, colonic dilatation, and sometimes bowel perforation. Some strains of CD, in particular NAP1/BI/027, produce another toxin called binary toxin in addition to toxin A and toxin B which enhances virulence. Clinical presentation due to infection with virulent bacilli in high-risk patients may vary from asymptomatic carriage to toxic megacolon.

Diagnosis: CDI should be suspected in patients with acute diarrhea with other abovementioned causes ruled out in the setting of risk factors. Stool should be investigated for glutamate dehydrogenase (GDH) antigen test and toxin A and B assay. GDH has got good sensitivity and rapid turnaround time; it however has poor specificity. The toxin tests have high specificity and rapid turnaround time but have very poor sensitivity, leading to high rate of false negatives.

Non-Life-Threatening Diarrhea

- *Drugs:*
  - *Laxatives and enemas*: Laxative-induced diarrhea is a common problem with incidence varying between 4% and 20% of patients presenting with diarrhea.[20,21] Laxatives are used in ICU prophylactically to prevent constipation, and this may give rise to diarrhea. Also overtreatment of constipation can give rise to diarrhea.
  - *Prokinetic agents* are used commonly in ICU for treating patients with high gastric residual volumes. The use of these agents in the ICU, although common, does not have clear evidence as causative agents for diarrhea. Metoclopramide, erythromycin, and domperidone are the commonly used prokinetic agents and can lead to diarrhea.
  - *Hyperosmolar agents*: Many oral preparations contain lactose, sorbitol, or other osmotically active components (e.g. magnesium) which can induce osmotic diarrhea (Table 21.1).
- *Antibiotic-associated diarrhea (AAD):* AAD is defined as diarrhea, otherwise unexplained, diarrhea that occurs in association with the administration of antibiotics. Incidence of diarrhea depends on the class of antibiotic used; the maximum incidence (10–20%) is seen with cefepime and amoxicillin–clavulanate.[22] AAD due to CDI is associated with more serious consequences as already discussed. AAD can also occur due to suppression of normal intestinal flora and overgrowth of organisms such as *Salmonella, Clostridium perfringens, S. aureus*, or sometimes *Candida albicans*. There are many underlying mechanisms for noninfectious AAD which include:
  - Promotility effects of antibiotics, e.g. erythromycin and azithromycin stimulate motilin receptors and lead to faster gastric emptying;
  - Change in intestinal flora as antibiotics lead to reduction in intestinal anaerobes altering metabolism of intestinal contents, e.g. decreased metabolism of carbohydrates giving rise to osmotic diarrhea; or
  - Decreased metabolism of bile acids giving rise to secretary diarrhea (bile acids are potent secretary agents in colon).
- *Enteral feeding-associated diarrhea:* When GI tract is functional, enteral feeding is the best route to provide nutrition and is shown to favorably affect outcome in critically ill patients.[24-26] Diarrhea is frequent problem in enterally fed critically ill patients with reported incidence ranging from 14% to 78%.[27,28] This large variation in reported incidence reflects the difference in patient population and variety of definitions used.

Mechanisms of Enteral Feeding associated Diarrhea

- *Change in gut hormones:* Enteral feeding route is physiological; however, feeding process is not completely physiological as it lacks cephalic phase of feeding which is essential for stimulating the release of digestive juices. Studies have shown that for stimulation of postprandial physiology, stomach needs at least 530–1,000 kcal load which is not provided by continuous feeds.[29,30] However, postpyloric infusion of 80 kcal/h has been found to be adequate to stimulate postprandial physiology.[31] This may be one of the reasons for diarrhea with continuous intragastric feeding, as the lack of stimulation of gut to postprandial state can lead to decreased digestion and absorption, and thus larger fluid and solute load in colon resulting in diarrhea.
- *Concomitant antibiotic usage*: Bliss et al. in their prospective cohort study found that 93% patients on tube feeds received antibiotics at some point.[32] Use of antibiotics significantly changes colonic flora and may contribute to diarrhea. Also it has been shown that elemental diet can modulate CD growth in gut flora.[33]
- *Contamination of feed in reservoir*: Bacterial contamination of enteral feeds is a likely possibility if proper

Table 21.1: Osmolality of commonly used medications in ICU.[23]

Drug	Osmolality
Acetaminophen suspension	6,425
Potassium chloride	4,225
Aluminum hydroxide gel	1,501
Digoxin solution	5,950
Fluconazole suspension	2,185
Ibuprofen suspension	2,350
Isoniazid solution	8,850
Valproic acid solution	5,010
Voriconazole suspension	2,010
Lactulose solution	4,180

precautions are not taken while preparing feeds or with longer hang times in open system. Study comparing open system versus closed system found lesser incidence of bacterial contamination and diarrhea when using closed system.[34]

- *Hypoalbuminemia:* This has been hypothesized as probable cause as it can lead to intestinal edema and increased secretion leading to secretary diarrhea.
- *Lack of fibers, poorly absorbed fermentable compounds*: Colonic digestion of fibers leads to the production of short-chain fatty acids (SCFAs) which lead to increase in salt and water absorption in the ascending colon. In 20 patients having diarrhea during long-term enteral nutrition, Nako et al. demonstrated an increase in the ratio of anaerobic to aerobic bacteria with fiber supplemented enteral feeds, along with decreased water content of feces, decreased frequency of stools, and improved fecal consistency. They hypothesized that increased anaerobic flora suppressed overgrowth of potential pathogens and thus normalized intestinal flora.

Prevention of enteral feeding–associated diarrhea:

- Since most of these patients also receive concomitant antibiotics which have significant effect on gut, rational use of antibiotics must be the first most important step. Stop antibiotics when no longer needed.
- Stop possible offending agents, such as prokinetics, hyperosmotic drugs, etc.
- Diet modification—use of fibers.
  Dietary fibers are defined as substances that include polysaccharides of plant cell either in its entirety or as a major component. Soluble fiber after undergoing fermentation gives rise to SCFA, mainly butyrate, acetate, and propionate, and are potent promoters of sodium and water absorption. A meta-analysis conducted by Elia et al. suggested a strong effect of fiber-supplemented diet in reducing incidence of diarrhea in patient groups with high incidence of diarrhea.[35]
- Gut microbiota can be modified using probiotics, prebiotics, and synbiotics. Prebiotics are dietary factors that stimulate the growth and/or activity of beneficial microorganisms in gut. The most commonly used prebiotics are inulin-type fructans (inulin, oligofructose, and fructooligosaccharides). No studies have specifically investigated the effect of a prebiotic alone in the prevention of diarrhea during enteral nutrition. Probiotics are "live microorganisms which when administered in adequate amounts confer a health benefit on the host due to mutualistic relationships." Commonly used strains include lactobacilli, bifidobacteria, and *Saccharomyces boulardii* and are available as capsules, powders, yoghurts, and fermented milks. In clinical settings, there is no convincing evidence that any of these combinations work in preventing diarrhea in ICU. *S. boulardii* has been found to be very effective in AAD.[36] However, there are case reports of fungemia in immunocompromised critically ill patients with *S. boulardii* and hence is not recommended in this subgroup.[37,38]

Miscellaneous Diarrheas

Fecal impaction: Sometimes the stools are large and hard and cannot pass out of rectum, leading to constipation due to impaction of stool. It causes rectal distension and increased secretions proximal to obstruction. These secretions pass or leak out around the obstruction giving a sense of diarrhea. A digital examination, followed by stool evacuation and treatment of constipation, is needed.

Fatty Diarrhea or Steatorrhea: It can be because of solubilization of dietary fat due by bile acids or malabsorption by the small intestine. Generally, the causative factors are celiac disease or pancreatic enzyme deficiency, short bowel syndrome, small intestinal bacterial overgrowth, or maldigestion as in post bowel surgery involving extensive bowel resection.

MANAGEMENT OF DIARRHEA

Patients can present to ICU due to severe diarrhea and associated hypovolemia or electrolyte imbalances. Also some ICU patients can develop diarrhea. First step is to assess fluid status and stabilize the patient with adequate fluids resuscitation and correct dyselectrolytemia. Review the ongoing medications and get detailed medical and surgical history. Patients, who present to ICU because of diarrhea, would need urgent attention to rule out life-threatening causes of diarrhea. Management algorithm is presented in Flowchart 21.1.

Prevention is better strategy for managing diarrhea. Rational approach to antibiotics usage may help in reducing incidence of diarrhea. Howell et al. showed association between increasing levels of pharmacological acid suppression and risk of nosocomial CDI.[39] A prospective case–control study by Yearsley et al.[40] also demonstrated a decrease in incidence of diarrhea with judicious use of PPIs. Antimotility agents, such as opioids or loperamide, should not be used routinely, until infective causes and other specific treatable causes, such as pancreatic enzyme deficiency or bile acid malabsorption, have been ruled out. In patients with proved or suspected infectious diarrhea, all precautions should be taken to prevent transmission of infection to other patients and staff in ICU. TPN can be

Section 2: Organ Dysfunction

FLOWCHART 21.1: Diarrhea management algorithm.

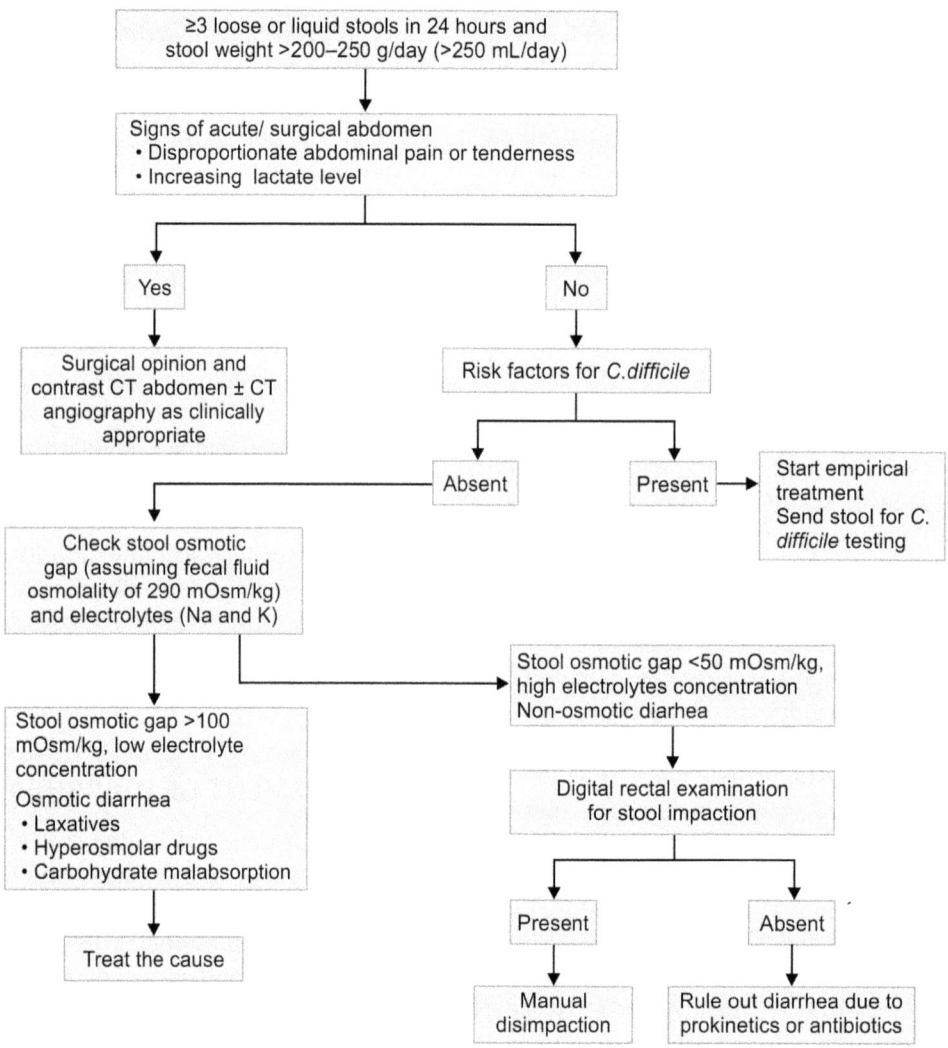

(IV: intravenous)

considered if enteral route cannot be used due to intractable diarrhea.

CONCLUSION

Diarrhea in critically ill patients is common. It is multifactorial, and some of the main causes are change in gut flora, malabsorption of feeds, bacterial overgrowth in gut, CDI, concomitant use of antibiotics, etc. Some of these factors can be modified, whereas others e.g. antibiotics in patients with infection need to continue. It is essential to identify life-threatening diarrheas and diagnose and manage them properly to improve outcomes. Management of non-life-threatening diarrheas is the combination of symptomatic treatment and removal of offending factor when possible. More studies exploring pathogenesis of GI dysfunction and diarrhea in critically ill patients will help in the development of proper management plan and help in reducing incidence of diarrhea.

REFERENCES

1. Tirlapur N, Puthucheary ZA, Cooper JA, et al. Diarrhoea in the critically ill is common, associated with poor outcome, and rarely due to *Clostridium difficile*. Sci Rep. 2016;6:24691.
2. Kelly TW, Patrick MR, Hillman KM. Study of diarrhoea in critically ill patients. Crit Care Med. 1983;11:7-9.
3. Blasera AR, Deanec AM, Fruhwald S. Diarrhoea in the critically ill. Curr Opin Crit Care. 2015;21:142-53.
4. Blaser AR, Malbrain ML, Starkopf J, et al. Gastrointestinal function in intensive care patients: terminology, definitions and management. Recommendations of the ESICM Working Group on Abdominal Problems. Intensive Care Med. 2012;38:384-94.

5. Blasera AR, Deanec AM, Fruhwald S. Diarrhoea in the critically ill. Curr Opin Crit Care. 2015;21:142-53.
6. Hammer HF, Fine KD, Santa Ana CA, et al. Carbohydrate malabsorption: its measurement and its contribution to diarrhoea. J Clin Invest. 1990;86:1936-44.
7. Eherer AJ, Fordtran JS. Fecal osmotic gap and pH in experimental diarrhoea of various causes. Gastroenterology. 1992;103:545-51.
8. Fine KD, Santa Ana CA, Fordtran JS. Diagnosis of magnesium-induced diarrhoea. N Engl J Med. 1991;324:1012-7.
9. Andreyev J. Gastrointestinal symptoms after pelvic radiotherapy: a new understanding to improve management of symptomatic patients. Lancet Oncol. 2007;8:1007-17.
10. Reinus JF, Brandt LJ, Boley SJ. Ischemic diseases of the bowel. Gastroenterol Clin North Am. 1990;19:319.
11. Oldenburg WA, Lau LL, Rodenberg TJ, et al. Acute mesenteric ischemia: a clinical review. Arch Intern Med. 2004;164:1054-62.
12. Diaz Nieto R, Varcada M, Ogunbiyi OA, et al. Systematic review on the treatment of ischaemic colitis. Colorectal Dis. 2011;13:744-7.
13. Scully RE, Mark EJ, McNeely WF, et al. Case records of the Massachusetts General Hospital: weekly clinicopathological exercises: case 3-1997. N Engl J Med. 1997;336:277-84.
14. Gorschluter M, Mey U, Strehl J, et al. Neutropenic enterocolitis in adults: systematic analysis of evidence quality. Eur J Haematol. 2005;75:1-13.
15. Cartoni C, Dragoni F, Micozzi A, et al. Neutropenic enterocolitis in patients with acute leukemia: prognostic significance of bowel wall thickening detected by ultrasonography. J Clin Oncol. 2001;19:756-61.
16. Miller BA, Chen LF, Sexton DJ, et al. Comparison of the burdens of hospital-onset, healthcare facility-associated CDI and of healthcare-associated infection due to methicillin-resistant *Staphylococcus aureus* in community hospitals. Infect Control Hosp Epidemiol. 2011;32:387-90.
17. Rotimi VO, Jamal WY, Mokaddas EM, et al. Prevalent PCR ribotypes of clinical and environmental strains of *Clostridium difficile* isolated from intensive-therapy unit patients in Kuwait. J Med Microbiol. 2003;52:705-9.
18. Lawrence SJ, Puzniak LA, Shadel BN, et al. *Clostridium difficile* in the intensive care unit: epidemiology, costs, and colonization pressure. Infect Control Hosp Epidemiol. 2007;28:123-30.
19. Eze P, Balsells E, Kyaw MH, et al. Risk factors for *Clostridium difficile* infections—an overview of the evidence base and challenges in data synthesis. J Glob Health. 2017;7:010417.
20. Duncan A, Morris AJ, Cameron A, et al. Laxative induced diarrhoea—a neglected diagnosis. J R Soc Med. 1992;85:203-5.
21. Cummings JH, Sladen GE, James OF, et al. Laxative-induced diarrhoea: a continuing clinical problem. Br Med J. 1974;1(5907):537-41.
22. Högenauer C, Hammer HF, Krejs GJ, et al. Mechanisms and management of antibiotic-associated diarrhoea. Clin Infect Dis. 1998;27:702-10.
23. Klang M, McLymont V, Ng N, et al. Osmolality, pH, and compatibility of selected oral liquid medications with an enteral nutrition product: JPEN J Parenter Enteral Nutri. 2013;37 (5):689-94.
24. Khalid I, Doshi P, DiGiovine B. Early enteral nutrition and outcomes of critically ill patients treated with vasopressors and mechanical ventilation. Am J Crit Care. 2010;19:261-8.
25. Doig GS, Heighes PT, Simpson F, et al. Early enteral nutrition reduces mortality in trauma patients requiring intensive care: a meta-analysis of randomised controlled trials. Injury. 2011;42:50-6.
26. Vasken A, Hicham K, Bruno D. Effects of early enteral feeding on the outcome of critically ill mechanically ventilated medical patients. Chest. 2006;129:960-7.
27. Thibault R, Graf S, Clerc A, et al. Diarrhoea in the ICU: respective contribution of feeding and antibiotics. Crit Care. 2013;17:R153.
28. Jack L, Coyer F, Courtney M, et al. Diarrhoea risk factors in enterally tube fed critically ill patients: a retrospective audit. Intensive Crit Care Nurs. 2010;26:327-34.
29. Snape WJ Jr, Matarazzo SA, Cohen S. Effect of eating and gastrointestinal hormones on human colonic myoelectrical and motor activity. Gastroenterology. 1978;75:373-8.
30. Bowling TE. Diarrhoea in the enterally fed patient. Gastroenterology. 2010;1:140-3.
31. Bowling TE, Raimundo AH, Grimble GK, et al. Colonic secretory effect in response to enteral feeding in humans. Gut. 1994;35:1734-41.
32. Bliss DZ, Johnson S, Savik K, et al. Acquisition of *Clostridium difficile* and *Clostridium difficile*-associated diarrhoea in hospitalized patients receiving tube feeding. Ann Intern Med. 1998;129:1012-9.
33. Iizuka M, Itou H, Konno S, et al. Elemental diet modulates the growth of *Clostridium difficile* in the gut flora. Aliment Pharmacol Ther. 2004;20(Suppl 1):151-7.
34. Mickschl DB, Davidson LJ, Flournoy DJ, et al. Contamination of enteral feedings and diarrhoea in patients in intensive care units. Heart Lung. 1990;19:362-70.
35. Elia M, Engfer MB, Green CJ, et al. Systematic review and meta-analysis: the clinical and physiological effects of fibre-containing enteral formulae. Aliment Pharmacol Ther. 2008;27:120-45.
36. McFarland LV. Systematic review and metaanalysis of *Saccharomyces boulardii* in adult patients. World J Gastro-enterol. 2010;16:2202-22.
37. Thygesen JB, Glerup H, Tarp B. *Saccharomyces boulardii* fungemia caused by treatment with a probioticum. Case Reports. 2012;2012:bcr0620114412.
38. Riquelme AJ, Calvo MA, Guzmán AM, et al. *Saccharomyces cerevisiae* fungemia after *Saccharomyces boulardii* treatment in immunocompromised patients. J Clin Gastroenterol. 2003;36:41-3.
39. Howell MD, Novack V, Grgurich P, et al. Iatrogenic gastric acid suppression and the risk of nosocomial *Clostridium difficile* infection. Arch Intern Med. 2010;170:784-90.
40. Yearsley KA, Gilby LJ, Ramadas AV, et al. Proton pump inhibitor therapy is a risk factor for *Clostridium difficile*-associated diarrhoea. Aliment Pharmacol Ther. 2006;24:613-9.

CHAPTER 22

Gastric Stasis in Intensive Care Unit

Amol Kothekar, Nishanth Baliga, Vikas Bhagat

INTRODUCTION

Gastric stasis or gastroparesis is a gastric motility disorder causing delayed gastric emptying (GE) in the absence of mechanical obstruction. Gastric stasis is a common cause of intolerance to enteral nutrition (EN) in critically ill patients. Intolerance to feeds manifests as vomiting or regurgitation of feeds and has potential for development of pneumonia due to aspiration. It may also possibly lead to atrophy of intestinal mucosa, translocation of gut flora, sepsis, and multiorgan failure due to failure in delivery of EN.[1] Gastric stasis is also known to occur outside intensive care unit (ICU) in patients with diabetes mellitus, after gastric surgery, collagen vascular disorders, cirrhosis, etc. In the current chapter, discussion is limited to gastric stasis in critically ill patients.

INCIDENCE

Gastrointestinal (GI) motility disturbances are common occurrence in patients with sepsis, abdominal compartment syndrome, trauma, severe hemodynamic instability, and multiple-organ dysfunction syndrome.[2] Delayed GE has been reported in 50% of mechanically ventilated patients and up to 80% of patients with moderate to severe head injury.[3] Contrary to delayed GE in critically ill patients, small bowel function is relatively preserved creating potential for small bowel feeding.[4]

PHYSIOLOGY OF GASTRIC EMPTYING

Gastrointestinal motility is a complex interplay of myoelectrical activity, contractile activity, tone, compliance, and transit governed by sympathetic, parasympathetic, and enteric nervous system, as well as GI smooth muscle cells. Functionally, stomach is comprised of two distinct motor zones. The proximal motor zone formed by the fundus and proximal third of the corpus of the stomach, acts as a reservoir. The distal zone is formed by the antrum and pylorus of stomach as well as proximal duodenum. Antrum grinds and sieves solid food whereas pylorus along with the proximal duodenum delivers chyme (pulpy food mixed with gastric juice) at a fixed rate into the small intestine.[5] GE follows zero-order kinetics. In other words, rate of GE is fixed irrespective of gastric residual volume (GRV).[6]

Transfer of food bolus from the stomach into the small intestine is carried out by antropyloroduodenal motor activity. Gastric reservoir function and peristalsis occur during and shortly after meals, whereas during fasting the main motility pattern observed is the migrating motor complex (MMC), i.e. a myoelectrical impulse moving caudally from stomach to distal ileum. There are three phases of MMC, phase I—quiescent period, phase II—irregular contraction, and phase III—burst of regular contraction. Likely function of MMC is clearance of luminal contents of stomach and small intestine in preparation of next meal.

The entry of nutrients into the small bowel activates neurohormonal feedback loop which leads to reduction of antral activity, increase in the pyloric tone, and decline in antegrade propagating pressure waves. Hormones involved in this negative feedback mechanism are glucagon, amylin, and glucagon-like peptide-1, cholecystokinin (CCK), and pancreatic polypeptide (PYY). Both CCK and PYY play an important role in the regulation of GE by initiation of negative feedback loop. Plasma levels of both CCK and PYY are elevated in mechanically ventilated, critically ill patients with delayed GE.[7] Cytokines and nitric oxide are known to induce abnormal GI motility in inflammation.[2]

Serotonin (5-hydroxytryptamine, 5-HT), motilin, and ghrelin are the hormones involved in positive feedback mechanism of GE.

- Serotonin stimulates contractions of smooth muscles and gut peristalsis via $5-HT_3$ receptors. On the other hand, it can also inhibit gastric and small bowel motility and colon transit via stimulation of $5-HT_4$ receptors.[2]
- Motilin is secreted by small intestine and is involved in the induction of phase III of MMC during the interdigestive period. In healthy individuals, motilin is probably not released in sufficient quantity to affect gastric motility.[8] However, motilin receptor agonist, erythromycin has shown to be useful in gastric stasis.
- Ghrelin, a motilin-related peptide, promotes GE and small bowel MMCs.[2] Widespread distribution of ghrelin receptors outside the GI tract unlike those for motilin indicates its significant additional non-GI roles in appetite, energy balance, and growth in addition to GE.[8]

PATHOPHYSIOLOGY OF GASTRIC STASIS

Various mechanisms implicated in delayed GE in critically ill patients are:
- Primary motor dysfunction
- Impaired coordination of the proximal and distal stomach
- Inhibitory feedback in the proximal small bowel
- A combination of the above.

In a broad sense, gastric stasis can be looked upon as ileus of stomach in the absence of mechanical obstruction (paralytic/functional ileus).

Causes of paralytic/functional ileus[9] of bowel can be categorized into four types:
1. *Reflectory ileus:* The underlying pathology is abdominal tumor, bleeding, or infection. It is also seen after abdominal and retroperitoneal surgeries.
2. *Drug-induced ileus:* The most common offending agents are opioids.
3. *Metabolic ileus:* Seen in metabolic abnormalities, such as hypokalemia or hyperglycemia (glucose >140 mg/dL).
4. *Vascular ileus:* Due to hypoperfusion of the bowel.

Diagnosis

In conscious patients, gastric stasis usually presents as nausea, vomiting, abdominal pain, or bloating. These signs and symptoms are masked in unconscious patients. Critically ill patients who are enterally fed may develop intolerance to feed, manifesting as vomiting or regurgitation of feeds, abdominal tenderness, increased abdominal girth, etc. In patients with systemic signs, such as worsening of shock, metabolic acidosis, or rising level of lactates, it would be prudent to rule out the presence of gastric stasis.

Tests for Assessment of Gastric Motility

Gastric scintigraphy is considered *the gold standard* for evaluation of GE of both solids and liquids.[2] GE is evaluated directly by measuring the gastric transit time of a radiolabeled test meal by gamma camera. Scintigraphy is noninvasive and has good reproducibility; hence, it is used in research. Its role in bedside decision-making in ICU is limited due to the practical difficulties in transport of critically patient to nuclear imaging suite.

Intermittent measurement of GRV: Intermittent gastric aspiration is the most common practice used for evaluation of GE in critically ill patients. However, it has multiple confounding variable, such as position of tip of feeding tube, tube collapsibility, tube size, volume of syringe used, and operator performing the test.[10] Larger bore feeding tubes generate higher GRVs than smaller bore tubes, silicone feeding tubes are more likely to collapse on aspiration, and percutaneous endoscopic gastrostomy tubes generate lower GRVs than nasogastric tubes in supine position due to anterior location of tip. *GRV* in the supine position can be unreliable as stomach sometimes divides into two separate compartments over the spine.[10] Not surprisingly, correlation between GRV and GE is lacking.[5]

Gastric residual volume does not correlate with GE, and higher GRV does not necessarily mean increased incidence of regurgitation aspiration pneumonia or high mortality. Lowering GRV cutoff offers no advantage as it does not protect patients from aspiration pneumonia, and also it reduces nutrition delivered to patient. Increasing GRV limit to 500 mL is safe as it allows increased nutrient delivery to patients without increasing risk of aspiration pneumonia. However, this may not apply to the patients with recent abdominal surgery or past history of esophageal, duodenal, pancreatic, or gastric surgery and in patients with GI bleed (esophagus, stomach, and small or large bowel) as such patients are generally excluded from these studies.[11]

Pneumonia probably occurs more commonly due to aspiration of contaminated oropharyngeal secretions than due to aspiration of regurgitated gastric contents.[12] Measures, such as 30–45° head end elevation and use of chlorhexidine mouthwash twice a day should be practiced to reduce risk of aspiration and ventilator-associated pneumonia.

Hence, GRV alone should not be used. Guidelines[12] do not recommend automatic cessation of EN for GRVs <500 mL in the absence of other signs of intolerance. Lower cutoff of 300–500 mL may be considered in ethnic groups with average body weights lower than western population.[13]

Ultrasonography (USG) of gastric antrum is a noninvasive method to measure GRV. Cross-sectional image of gastric antrum is obtained with curved low-frequency (2–5 MHz) transducer probe. Antral cross-sectional area (CSA) is calculated from its anteroposterior and craniocaudal diameter. Gastric volume can be predicted from antral CSA and patient's age based on different formulae or prediction models.[14] Use of USG of gastric antrum for assessment of GRV is currently restricted due to limited availability of ultrasound machines and skilled experienced operators; however, this may be extensively used in future (Figs. 22.1A and B).

Other tests, such as 13C-octanoate breath test, 3-*O*-methylglucose absorption test, paracetamol absorption test, and magnetic resonance imaging, can be used for assessment of gastric motility but have limited role in bedside decision-making in critically ill patients.

Bowel sounds are produced due to normal peristaltic activity of small bowel causing movement of its contents.

In critically ill patients, auscultation of bowel sounds is not mandatory for initiation of EN in ICU.[12] EN should not be withheld in the absence of bowel sounds unless bowel ischemia or obstruction is suspected.[15] Bowel sounds do not provide any information about mucosal integrity, barrier function, or absorptive capacity. Bowel sounds do not predict (positive predictive value <25%) tolerance of enteral feeds in patients after major abdominal surgery.[16] However, bowel sounds may have prognostic value in predicting mortality.

TREATMENT

Initial Treatment

Treatment of gastric stasis is mainly supportive or conservative. Reversible causes of paralytic/functional ileus should be addressed first.

If abdominal infection is present, it should be tackled with antibiotics, and source control should be done on priority basis if feasible. Use of opioids should be rationalized.

Reduction of opioids dose with use of nonopioid analgesics may be considered if feasible. Switching from opioid to dexmedetomidine may not improve GE as dexmedetomidine,[17] a selective α2-adrenoceptor agonist, is also known to inhibit GE and GI transit in healthy volunteers. If opioids are mandatory, shorter acting opioids, such as fentanyl, may be considered over longer acting agents, such as morphine; however, there are no studies to support this statement. Inhibitory effect of anticholinergics agents on gastric motility should be kept in mind.[18]

Two most important metabolic abnormalities to look for are hypokalemia and hyperglycemia. Severe hypokalemia

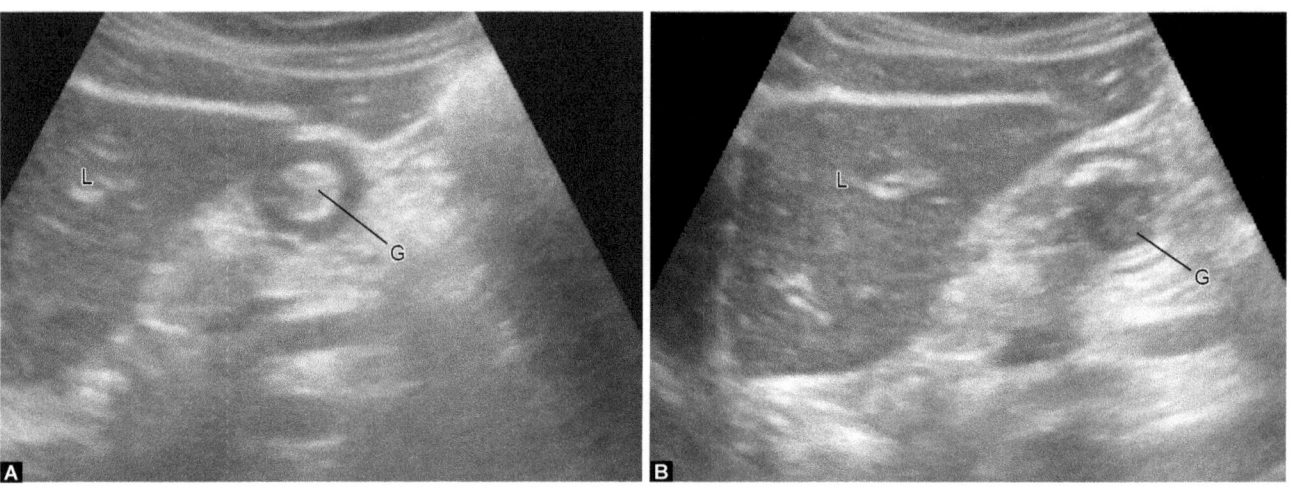

FIGURES 22.1A AND B: USG of stomach in (A) fasting patient (B) patient of clear liquids showing L and G. (G: gastric antrum; L: liver; USG: ultrasonography).

is known to cause intestinal paralysis and normalization of potassium should be done aggressively.

Current evidence does not support intensive insulin therapy (target glucose >110 mg/dL) in critically ill patients; however, association of hyperglycemia (glucose >140 mg/dL) and reduction in GI motility should be kept in mind. A "tighter" control of sugar may be considered in patients with refractory gastric stasis on a case-to-case basis weighing risk of hypoglycemia and benefits of EN; however, evidence is lacking in this regard.

Hypoperfusion of the bowel causes paralytic ileus of bowel, and similar effect may be expected in stomach as well; hence, caution is advocated in patients in shock.

There are some *theoretical concerns* for initiating EN in patients on vasopressors.
- Vasopressors generally divert blood from splanchnic circulation to the vital organs.
- There is always a remote possibility of ischemic bowel with enteral feeding.[12]
- Sympathomimetic vasopressors inhibit motility of bowel including stomach.[5]

However, these "theoretical concerns" do not stand the test of evidence, and the literature actually supports early EN in patients on stable low doses of vasopressors. In a retrospective analysis of prospectively collected multi-institutional medical ICU data of 1,174 patients[19] on ventilation and vasopressors, early EN was associated with decreased ICU and hospital mortality, and beneficial effect of early feeding was more evident in the sickest patients treated with multiple vasopressors.

Enteral nutrition stimulates intestinal growth and function,[20] which probably reduces bacterial translocation. Protective effects of EN can be seen even with lesser volume of feeds. Trophic feeds (10–20 kcal/h or up to 500 kcal/day) have shown to reduce the incidence of GI intolerance and favorably alter clinical outcomes, such as ventilator-free days, mortality, nosocomial infections in patients with acute respiratory distress syndrome requiring vasopressors.[21]

Experts[12] believe in early introduction of trophic feeds (10–20 kcal/h or up to 500 kcal/day) for the initial phase of sepsis and gradual escalation of feeds as tolerated after 24–48 hours (Flowchart 22.1).

Specific Interventions to Prevent and Treat Gastric Dysmotility

- Use of continuous infusions instead of intermittent boluses of enteral feeds
- Use of prokinetic agents
- Postpyloric feeding

Switch from Bolus to Continuous Feeds

Continuous infusion of enteral feed has the theoretical advantage of decreasing the amount of regurgitation and aspiration compared to intermittent boluses. Continuous gastric feeds have demonstrated superior delivery of EN but no significant change in patient outcome.[22] Continuous feeding is recommended in patients intolerant to bolus feeds and also in patients who are high risk for aspiration.[12]

Prokinetic Agents

Prokinetic agents commonly used in clinical practice are dopamine agonists and motilin agonists.

Dopamine Antagonists [23]

Metoclopramide and domperidone are the commonly used dopamine antagonists. Metoclopramide 10 mg four times a day is commonly used. Metoclopramide should be avoided in patients with brain injury due to lack of effect and risk of further increase in intracranial pressure. Domperidone being a peripherally acting dopamine antagonist has little extrapyramidal adverse effects; however, it is not available in parenteral form. Metoclopramide dose needs to be adjusted in patients with renal dysfunction.

Motilin agonists: Erythromycin, a macrolide antibiotic also acts as motilin agonist. At low dose of 3–7 mg/kg/day, erythromycin has been shown to increase both GE and improve feed intolerance in critically ill patients. In a randomized, double-blind trial, erythromycin (200 mg twice a day intravenous) was found to be more efficacious than metoclopramide in improving feed intolerance in critically ill patients.[24]

Clinical Practice Considerations

Either metoclopramide or erythromycin can be used as first-line prokinetic drug. Since erythromycin has antimicrobial properties, there is concern of bacterial resistance when it is used in prokinetic dose, which is suboptimal as an antimicrobial. Availability of parenteral formulation should also be taken into account. Most of the studies of metoclopramide or erythromycin are done with parenteral formulation. Bioavailability of these drugs in critically ill patients may be variable. Moreover, enteral form of erythromycin is available as enteric-coated tablets to prevent inactivation by gastric acid. Crushed or dissolved tablet given through feeding tube may not have the same effect. In addition, erythromycin is incompletely absorbed from small intestine, and food in stomach delays its absorption.[25] However, enteral route is also acceptable for both metoclopramide and erythromycin.[12]

Section 2: Organ Dysfunction

FLOWCHART 22.1: Enteral Nutrition (EN) algorithm for critically ill patients*.

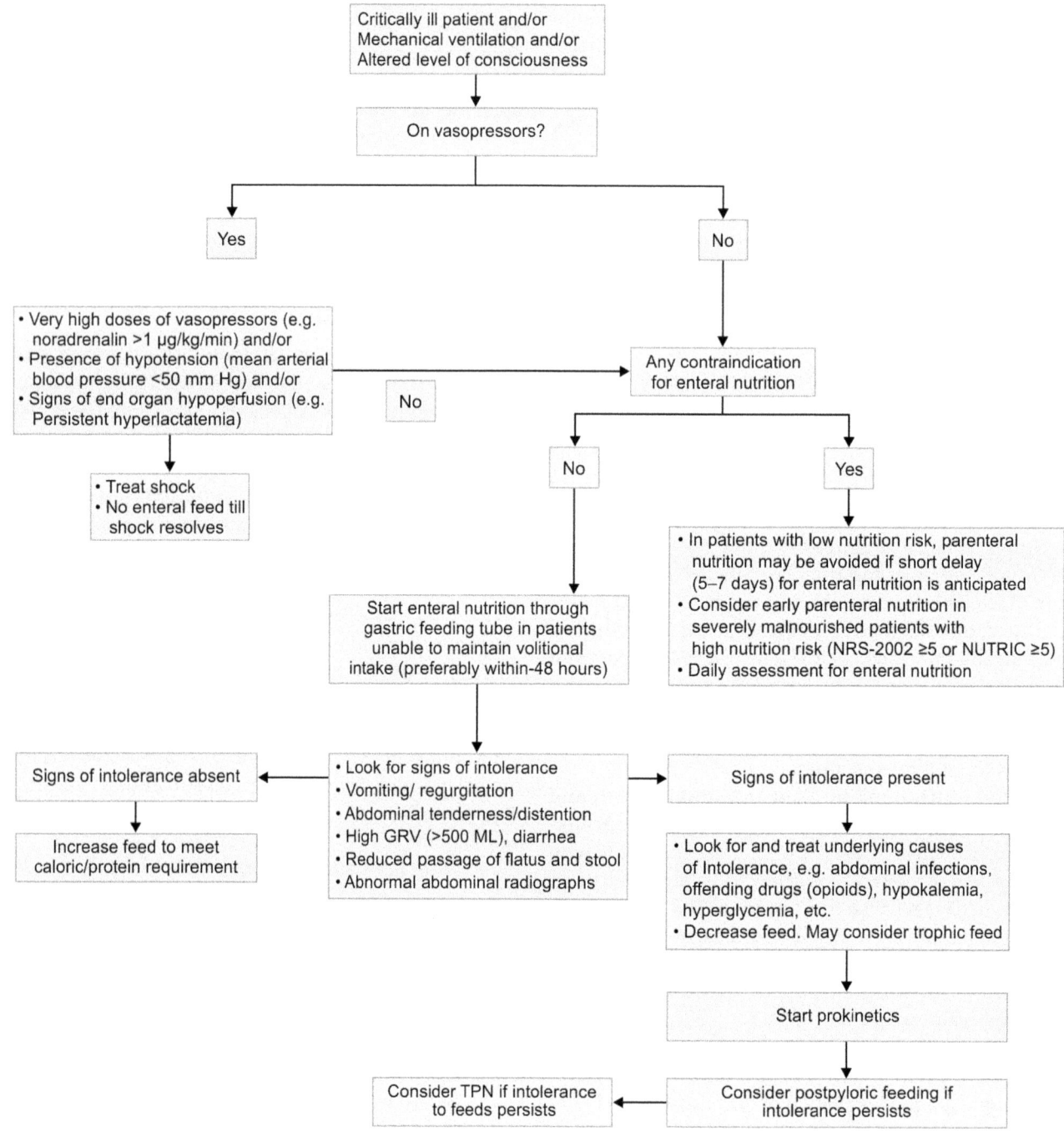

(EN: enteral nutrition; GRV: gastric residual volume; TPN: total parenteral nutrition; NRS: nutritional risk screening; NUTRIC: nutrition risk in critically ill).

* Suggested algorithm based on current literature.

Both metoclopramide and erythromycin are associated with QT prolongation predisposing the patient to cardiac arrhythmias. Similarly, both of them are known for the rapid development of tachyphylaxis within the first 3 days of therapy.[24] The combination therapy of metoclopramide and erythromycin is associated with a lesser degree of drug tachyphylaxis and up to 60% of patients remained responsive at day 7 of treatment without any major adverse effects.[26]

Prokinetic Agents Likely to be Available in Future

Peripherally acting mu-opioid receptor antagonists (PAMORA) reverse inhibitory effect of opiate on small bowel motility without antagonizing the analgesic effects.[23] Alvimopan, a PAMORA, has shown to be effective in bowel recovery and subsequent discharge readiness from hospital in patients with abdominal surgery. CCK-receptor antagonist, loxiglumide, has been shown to improve lower esophageal sphincter function and GE. Motilides are motilin receptor agonists, derived from macrolide structure, have shown to accelerate GE in healthy volunteers.[8] Further studies of these drugs in critical ill patients are warranted.

Postpyloric Feeding

Relative preservation of small bowel function in presence of delayed GE in critically ill patients has led to exploration of postpyloric route as feeding option. Postpyloric tube insertion is technically more difficult than gastric tube insertion, skilled operators are required, and depending on setup, transport out of ICU may be needed. Postpyloric feeding has not shown benefit in terms of mortality, ICU length of stay (LOS), hospital LOS, duration of mechanical ventilation, in spite of reduction in incidence or regurgitation, and aspiration pneumonia.[27,28] Use of postpyloric route is generally restricted to patients at high risk for aspiration. These patients should not be denied benefits of early EN through stomach if postpyloric route cannot be obtained in time.[12] Postpyloric feeding can also be considered in patients in whom caloric goals are not achieved in spite of continuous feeds and use of prokinetic agents.

In patients with prone position, persistent gastric stasis should be aggressively treated with early use of prokinetics, followed by postpyloric feeding if feasible.[15]

Parenteral Nutrition

Patients on EN in whom caloric goals are not met due to feed intolerance should be given trial of prokinetic and postpyloric feeds before considering parenteral nutrition. In patients with low nutrition risk [e.g. Nutritional Risk Screening (NRS-2002) ≤3 or Nutrition Risk in the Critically Ill (NUTRIC) Score ≤5], parenteral nutrition may be avoided in first 7 days even if caloric goals are not met with EN. However, in severely malnourished patients with high nutrition risk (NRS-2002 ≥5 or NUTRIC ≥ 5), early parenteral nutrition should be considered if caloric goals are not met. Patients on parenteral nutrition should undergo daily assessment for feasibility of EN.[12]

The patients who are at high risk for aspiration are listed below:
- Elderly with age >70 years
- Patients on mechanical ventilation
- Patients with reduced level of consciousness, inability to protect the airway or neurologic deficits
- History of gastroesophageal reflux
- Patients on intermittent bolus feeds
- Inadequate nurse-to-patient ratio, poor oral care
- Supine positioning or transport out of the ICU.

Early use of prokinetic agents and postpyloric feeds are advised in these patients, however, there is no data to suggest improved clinical outcome of ICU patients with these measures.

Practical Considerations

- Enteral nutrition should be avoided in patients with uncontrolled shock with inadequate tissue perfusion.
- Caution should be exercised in patients on very high doses of vasopressors (e.g. noradrenalin >1 µg/kg/min) in presence of signs of end-organ hypoperfusion, such as persistent hyperlactatemia.
- Enteral nutrition should be gradually initiated as soon as shock is controlled with fluids and vasopressors/inotropes, and vasopressors requirement is stabilized or decreasing. If patient does not tolerate full enteral feeds, trophic feeds may be given initially.
- All patients should be given head end elevation and chlorhexidine mouth wash unless contraindicated.
- Prokinetic agents and postpyloric feeds should be considered in patients intolerant to feeds.
- Prokinetic agents are known to have tachyphylaxis after 3 days of use.
- Early initiation of prokinetic agents and postpyloric feeds if feasible should be tried in patients who cannot be nursed in propped-up position or patients having risk factors for aspiration.
- Patients having risk factors for aspiration should not be denied EN through stomach if postpyloric feeds cannot be established in time.
- Parenteral nutrition should be considered if full caloric goals are not achieved with EN by 7 days or earlier in severely malnourished patients with high nutrition risk (NRS-2002 ≥5 or NUTRIC ≥5).

REFERENCES

1. Herbert MK, Holzer P. Standardized concept for the treatment of gastrointestinal dysmotility in critically ill patients—current status and future options. Clin Nutr. 2008;27:25-41.
2. Ukleja A. Altered GI Motility in critically ill patients. Nutr Clin Pract. 2010;25:16-25.
3. Kao CH, Changlai SP, Chieng PU, et al. Gastric emptying in head-injured patients. Am J Gastroenterol. 1998;93:1108-12.
4. Marik PE, Zaloga GP. Gastric versus post-pyloric feeding: a systematic review. Crit Care. 2003;7:46-51.
5. Ladopoulos T. Gastrointestinal dysmotility in critically ill patients. Ann Gastroenterol. 2018;31:273-81.
6. Larson JM, Tavakkoli A, Drane WE, et al. Advantages of azithromycin over erythromycin in improving the gastric emptying half-time in adult patients with gastroparesis. J Neurogastroenterol Motil. 2010;16:407-13.
7. Nguyen NQ, Fraser RJ, Bryant LK, et al. The relationship between gastric emptying, plasma cholecystokinin, and peptide YY in critically ill patients. Crit Care. 2007;11:132.
8. Sanger GJ, Wang Y, Hobson A, et al. Motilin: towards a new understanding of the gastrointestinal neuropharmacology and therapeutic use of motilin receptor agonists. Br J Pharmacol. 2013;170:1323-32.
9. Vilz TO, Stoffels B, Strassburg C, et al. Ileus in adults. Dtsch Arztebl Int. 2017;114:508-18.
10. Hurt RT, Mcclave SA. Gastric residual volumes in critical illness: what do they really mean? Crit Care Clin. 2010;26:481-90.
11. Reignier J. Effect of not monitoring residual gastric volume on risk of ventilator-associated pneumonia in adults receiving mechanical ventilation and early enteral feeding. JAMA. 2013;309:249.
12. Mcclave SA, Taylor BE, Martindale RG, et al. Guidelines for the provision and assessment of nutrition support therapy in the adult critically ill patient: Society of Critical Care Medicine (SCCM) and American Society for Parenteral and Enteral Nutrition (A.S.P.E.N.). J Parenter Enteral Nutr. 2016;40:159-211.
13. Mehta Y, Sunavala J, Zirpe K, et al. Practice guidelines for nutrition in critically ill patients: a relook for Indian scenario. Indian J Crit Care Med. 2018;22:263.
14. Putte PVD, Perlas A. Ultrasound assessment of gastric content and volume. Br J Anaesth. 2014;113:12-22.
15. Blaser AR, Starkopf J, Alhazzani W, et al. Early enteral nutrition in critically ill patients: ESICM clinical practice guidelines. Intensive Care Med. 2017;43:380-98.
16. Read TE, Brozovich M, Andujar JE, et al. Bowel sounds are not associated with flatus, bowel movement, or tolerance of oral intake in patients after major abdominal surgery. Dis Colon Rectum. 2017;60:608-13.
17. Iirola T, Vilo S, Aantaa R, et al. Dexmedetomidine inhibits gastric emptying and oro-caecal transit in healthy volunteers. Br J Anaesth. 2011;106:522-7.
18. Aderinto-Adike AO, Quigley EMM. Gastrointestinal motility problems in critical care: a clinical perspective. J Dig Dis. 2014;15:335-44.
19. Khalid I, Doshi P, DiGiovine B. Early enteral nutrition and outcomes of critically ill patients treated with vasopressors and mechanical ventilation. Am J Crit Care. 2010;19:261-8.
20. Seron-Arbeloa C, Zamora-Elson M, Labarta-Monzon L, et al. Enteral nutrition in critical care. J Clin Med Res. 2013;5:1-11.
21. Rice TW, Wheeler AP, Thompson BT, et al. Initial trophic vs full enteral feeding in patients with acute lung injury: the EDEN randomized trial. JAMA. 2012;307:795-803.
22. Macleod JBA, Lefton J, Houghton D, et al. Prospective randomized control trial of intermittent versus continuous gastric feeds for critically ill trauma patients. J Trauma. 2007;63:57-61.
23. Nguyen NQ. Pharmacological therapy of feed intolerance in the critically ills. World J Gastrointest Pharmacol Ther. 2014;5:148.
24. Nguyen NQ, Chapman MJ, Fraser RJ, et al. Erythromycin is more effective than metoclopramide in the treatment of feed intolerance in critical illness. Crit Care Med. 2007;35:483-9.
25. Brunton L, Chabner BA, Knollman B. Chapter 55: Protein synthesis inhibitors and miscellaneous antibacterial agents. In: Goodman & Gilman's the pharmacological basis of therapeutics, 12th ed. New York, NY: McGraw-Hill; 2011. pp. 1529-36.
26. Nguyen NQ, Chapman M, Fraser RJ, et al. Prokinetic therapy for feed intolerance in critical illness: one drug or two? Crit Care Med. 2007;35:2561-7.
27. Heyland DK, Drover JW, MacDonald S, et al. Effect of postpyloric feeding on gastroesophageal regurgitation and pulmonary microaspiration: results of a randomized controlled trial. Crit Care Med. 2001;29:1495-501.
28. Alkhawaja S, Martin C, Butler R, Gwadry-Sridhar F. Post-pyloric versus gastric tube feeding for preventing pneumonia and improving nutritional outcomes in critically ill adults. Cochrane Database of Systematic Reviews. 2015; Aug 4;(8):CD008875.

CHAPTER 23

Mesenteric Ischemia

Subhal Bhalchandra Dixit, Khalid Ismail Khatib

INTRODUCTION

Mesenteric ischemia, i.e. ischemia which affects the small intestine, may be acute or chronic, occlusive or nonocclusive, and arterial or venous. Acute arterial occlusive intestinal ischemia occurs due to embolism to or thrombosis of the superior mesenteric artery (SMA), while thrombosis of superior or inferior mesenteric veins, splenic or portal veins leads to venous occlusive intestinal ischemia. Low cardiac output states or use of high-dose vasopressors may lead to low flow states causing nonocclusive mesenteric ischemia.[1]

PATHOPHYSIOLOGY OF INTESTINAL ISCHEMIA

The intestine is protected from getting ischemic with ill-sustained bouts of low flow due to the presence of collateral circulation. This collateral circulation takes place at the following pathways: (1) superior and inferior pancreaticoduodenal arteries connecting the celiac trunk and SMA; (2) two arteries connect the SMA and inferior mesenteric artery (IMA)—the marginal artery of Drummond (major collateral pathway) and the meandering mesenteric artery (not always present); and (3) rectal collateral circulation between IMA and the systemic circulation.

There are certain areas with proclivity for ischemia. These are the splenic flexure of the colon at the Griffith's point and the rectosigmoid junction at the Sudeck's point.

The resistance of mesenteric arterioles depends upon the prandial state of the intestine, whether it is in the fasting or postprandial state. This can lead to fluctuations in the blood flow of the intestine from 1/10th to almost a third of the cardiac output.[2,3] The intestinal vascular bed is dense, but oxygen extraction is not high, so there is a large margin, before intestinal ischemia will set in. In fact, there needs to be a more than 50% drop in blood flow to the intestines, and it needs to be sustained for more than 12 hours, before intestinal ischemia becomes manifest. The vascular tone of the mesenteric vasculature is regulated by the following factors: (1) postprandial state, (2) systemic hypotension, (3) activity of the sympathetic nervous system, (4) renin-angiotensin-aldosterone system, and (5) vasopressin levels in blood.[3]

INTESTINAL RESPONSE TO ISCHEMIA

Ischemic injury to the intestines will occur if perfusion pressure falls below 30 mm Hg or if the mean arterial pressure falls below 45 mm Hg.[4] The intestine compensates by increased oxygen extraction and dilatation of the blood vessels. However, these compensatory mechanisms fail after a bout of sustained ischemia (approximately 12 hours), and there is progressive constriction of the blood vessels which later become obstructed. There is an increase in the pressure within the obstructed blood vessels and reduced collateral blood flow in the intestines. This will ultimately lead to full thickness necrosis of the intestine and may lead to perforation of the intestine. Another mechanism of injury to the intestine is reperfusion injury, due to free oxygen radical generation and release, associated activation of inflammatory cells and cascade, and may lead to multi-organ dysfunction and failure.

ETIOLOGY OF MESENTERIC ISCHEMIA

- *Mesenteric arterial embolism (50% of cases of mesenteric ischemia)*: From the left atrium and ventricle, cardiac valves, or initial portion of the aorta.[5,6]
- *Mesenteric arterial thrombosis (15–25% of cases of mesenteric ischemia)*: Due to abdominal trauma, intestinal or abdominal infections, thrombosed aneurysm or dissection of the mesenteric artery, and dissection of the aorta.[1] Thrombosis usually occurs on the background of chronic intestinal ischemia due to atherosclerosis.
- *Mesenteric venous thrombosis (5% of cases of mesenteric ischemia)*: Due to hypercoagulable states or secondary to malignancy or previous abdominal surgery.[1]
- *Nonocclusive mesenteric ischemia (20–30% of cases of mesenteric ischemia)*: Due to sustained hypotension and vasoconstriction.[1]
- *Mixed*: It may occur in the cases of volvulus due to adhesions or bands, or obstructed or strangulated hernia, leading to both arterial and venous occlusion. Another cause of mixed (occlusive and nonocclusive) acute mesenteric ischemia is vasculitis, such as polyarteritis nodosa, which affects the small-to-medium arteries.

RISK FACTORS FOR MESENTERIC ISCHEMIA[7]

- *Cardiac disease*: Predisposing to embolism or hypoperfusion or vasoconstriction (due to medications)
- *Aortic intervention*: Either surgery or other aortic interventions, such as aortography, cardiac catheterization, including coronary angiography or endovascular surgery
- Atherosclerotic disease of the celiac axis, SMA or IMA
- Thrombotic disorders (hereditary or acquired)
- Infection of the intestines/inflammation of the intestine or its vasculature
- Hypovolemia
- Hernias (external or internal).

CLINICAL FEATURES

History: (1) Deep vein thrombosis or pulmonary embolism in the past or in the family (50% of patients); (2) past history of vascular embolism (33% of patients); and (3) symptoms of chronic atherosclerotic mesenteric ischemia, such as abdominal pain after food intake, unintentional loss of weight, and an aversion to food.

Symptoms

Abdominal pain: It is the most common presenting symptom and out of proportion to the abdominal signs. The character of the pain (onset, severity) will depend upon the duration of the ischemia and collateral circulation. The onset of the pain is usually sudden, quite severe, periumbilical in location, and associated with nausea or vomiting or both.

Physical Examination

It may vary from normal abdominal examination to mild abdominal distension to grossly distended silent abdomen with signs of peritonitis, depending upon the state of the bowel at presentation. Other signs which may/may not be present are fecal odor to breathe, signs of dehydration, and/or shock.

Laboratory Studies

These are usually nonspecific.
- Leukocytosis, (usually marked), with shift to left (presence/predominance of immature white blood cells) with/without toxic granules
- Hemoconcentration as evidenced by raised hematocrit
- Presence of metabolic acidosis

Radiology

- *Plain X-ray of the abdomen*: It may be completely normal, show signs of intestinal perforation (gas under the diaphragm in upright films), or may show findings suggestive of mesenteric ischemia (distended and/or thickened bowel loops with/without pneumatosis intestinalis).
- *Computed tomography (CT) of the abdomen with intravenous contrast for angiography*: If mesenteric ischemia is suspected, oral contrast should be avoided. It will demonstrate the site of vascular occlusion, intestinal thickening/pneumatosis intestinalis (Fig. 23.1), mesenteric stranding and will also help to rule out other causes of abdominal pain.
- *Magnetic resonance angiography*: It may be useful in patients with allergy to iodinated dyes used for CT.
- *Conventional arteriography of abdominal vessels*: It is performed less often now but is the gold standard.

EVIDENCE

Laboratory Diagnosis in Mesenteric Ischemia

- *Serum lactate level*: It will be raised but is nonspecific for mesenteric ischemia, especially in the presence of other

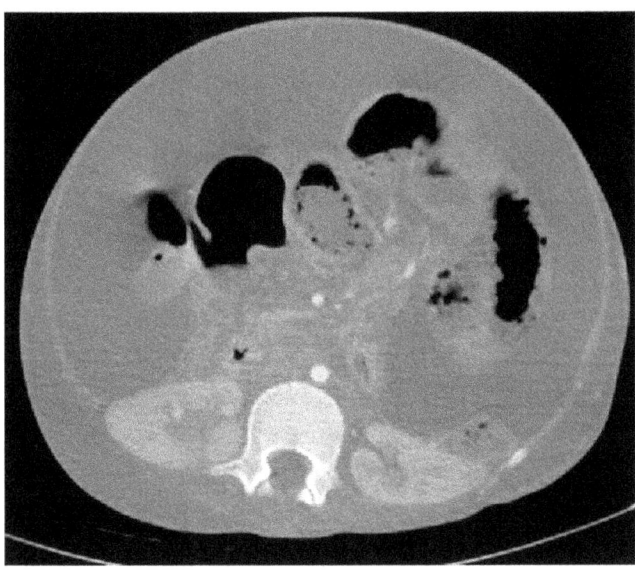

FIGURE 23.1: Thrombosis of superior mesenteric artery.

conditions known to elevate lactate (shock, diabetic ketoacidosis, renal failure, and hepatic failure). A meta-analysis of 23 studies including 1,970 patients presenting to the emergency department with abdominal pain found sensitivity and specificity of L-lactate (isomer of lactate) for acute mesenteric ischemia of 86 [95% confidence interval (CI), 32–55%] and 44% (95% CI, 32–55%).[1] Another study which examined this question found a sensitivity and specificity of 100% and 42%, respectively.[8]
- *Serum amylase*: It was found to be elevated in only 50% of patients.[9]
- *D-Dimer*:[10-12] It has negative predictive value, and patient with abdominal pain and normal D-dimer levels can be confidently said to not have intestinal ischemia. A positive D-dimer may be because of many causes in patients presenting with abdominal pain (acute mesenteric ischemia, pancreatitis, and abdominal aortic aneurysm). A large meta-analysis of patients presenting to the emergency department with abdominal pain found sensitivity and specificity of D-dimer for acute mesenteric ischemia to be 96 (95% CI, 89–99%) and 40% (95% CI, 33–47%).[1]
- *Other laboratory tests*: These are experimental at present and not used in clinical practice. Serum alpha-glutathione S-transferase and intestinal fatty acid binding protein have been studied as biomarkers of mesenteric ischemia.[13,14]

Radiology

- Plain X-ray of the abdomen: It has very low specificity for the diagnosis of acute mesenteric ischemia and may be normal in a quarter of the patients.[15]
- *Computed tomography angiography of abdomen*: A review of six high-quality studies with 619 patients found the sensitivity and specificity of CT angiography of abdomen for the diagnosis of acute mesenteric ischemia to be 93.3 (95% CI, 82.8–97.6%) and 95.9% (95% CI, 91.2–98.2%), respectively.[16] The presence of defined criteria (bowel wall thickening, visualized arterial occlusion, gas in the portomesenteric venous system or intestinal pneumatosis) increases the positive and negative predictive value of CT angiography of abdomen for the diagnosis of acute mesenteric ischemia to 100% and 94%, respectively.[17]

Treatment

Initial management should include measures, such as (1) gastrointestinal (GI) decompression; (2) fluid resuscitation and transfusion in patients with GI bleeding; (3) hemodynamic monitoring and use of ionotropic agents, such as dobutamine, low-dose dopamine and milrinone; (4) correction of electrolyte abnormalities; (5) systemic anticoagulation (except in patients with nonocclusive ischemia); (6) analgesia; and (7) broad-spectrum antibiotics.

Endovascular Thrombolysis

This is less well established than surgery and should be performed in patients without signs of intestinal perforation/infarction or peritonitis. It is particularly useful in patients with significant comorbidities and those with symptoms of shorter duration.[18-20] In a recent series of 34 patients from 12 Swedish hospitals, Alteplase (33 patients) and urokinase infusion (1 patient) were used. The median infusion rate of Alteplase was 0.7 mg/h [interquartile range (IQR), 0.5–1.0 mg/h], and the median total dose was 20 mg (IQR, 11.6–34.0 mg). Successful thrombolysis was achieved in 88% of patients, and it was associated with reduced mortality ($P = 0.048$). At 1 year, 20 patients were alive.[21]

Surgery

Patients with intestinal perforation/infarction should undergo laparotomy. The mortality in patients undergoing surgery for mesenteric ischemia was found to be 47%.[1]

CONCLUSION[22,23]

- Patients presenting with severe pain in abdomen which is out of proportion to the abdominal signs should be suspected to have acute mesenteric ischemia.
- Acute mesenteric ischemia may be due to mesenteric arterial/venous thrombosis, mesenteric arterial embolism, or it can be nonocclusive mesenteric ischemia.

- Plain radiography of the abdomen should not be used in the diagnostic evaluation of acute mesenteric ischemia as it has limited value, although it is able to diagnose patients who have advanced to intestinal perforation.
- Laboratory studies cannot help in identifying patients with acute mesenteric ischemia or patients with infracted intestines, although serum lactate and D-dimer are helpful.
- Computed tomography angiography is the investigation of choice in patients suspected to have acute mesenteric ischemia. Critically ill patients developing abdominal pain/distension with shock requiring vasopressors and/or multiorgan dysfunction/failure should be suspected to have nonocclusive mesenteric ischemia.
- Patients with acute mesenteric ischemia should receive fluid resuscitation, correction of electrolyte abnormalities, especially potassium, broad-spectrum antibiotics, and nasogastric decompression, immediately after diagnosis.
- Anticoagulation with unfractionated heparin should be initiated forthwith, unless contraindicated. It may be the sole treatment required in patients with acute mesenteric ischemia due to venous thrombosis and in some patients with arterial thrombosis/embolism without the signs of peritonitis.
- Laparotomy is urgently required in patients with signs of perforation peritonitis. Occasionally, damage control surgery may be the procedure of choice in critically ill hemodynamically unstable, septic patient with necrotic intestines. Relaparotomy will be required in these patients later.
- Endovascular procedures, such as aspiration embolectomy, vascular stenting, and endovascular thrombolysis with/without stenting, may be feasible in some patients with acute mesenteric ischemia. These have to be performed in centers equipped for such procedures.
- Patients with massive infarction of the intestines should be managed appropriately laparotomy, resection and anastomosis of the bowel when feasible. Such patients will become dependent permanently on total parenteral nutrition.
- Patients in whom none of the treatments are likely to help should be offered comfort care.

REFERENCES

1. Cudnik MT, Darbha S, Jones J, et al. The diagnosis of acute mesenteric ischaemia: a systematic review and meta-analysis. Acad Emerg Med. 2013;20:1087-100.
2. Clair DG, Beach JM. Mesenteric ischemia. N Engl J Med. 2016;374:959-68.
3. Rosenblum JD, Boyle CM, Schwartz LB. The mesenteric circulation. Anatomy and physiology. Surg Clin North Am. 1997;77:289-306.
4. Haglund U, Bergqvist D. Intestinal ischemia—the basics. Langenbecks Arch Surg. 1999;384:233-8.
5. Baddour LM, Wilson WR, Bayer AS, et al. Infective endocarditis in adults: diagnosis, antimicrobial therapy, and management of complications: a scientific statement for healthcare professionals from the American Heart Association. Circulation. 2015;132:1435-86.
6. Baddour LM, Wilson WR, Bayer AS, et al. Infective endocarditis: diagnosis, antimicrobial therapy, and management of complications: a statement for healthcare professionals from the Committee on Rheumatic Fever, Endocarditis, and Kawasaki Disease, Council on Cardiovascular Disease in the Young, and the Councils on Clinical Cardiology, Stroke, and Cardiovascular Surgery and Anesthesia, American Heart Association: endorsed by the Infectious Diseases Society of America. Circulation. 2005;111:e394-434.
7. Fitzgerald T, Kim D, Karakozis S, et al. Visceral ischemia after cardiopulmonary bypass. Am Surg. 2000;66:623-26.
8. Lange H, Jäckel R. Usefulness of plasma lactate concentration in the diagnosis of acute abdominal disease. Eur J Surg. 1994;160:381-4.
9. Wilson C, Imrie CW. Amylase and gut infarction. Br J Surg. 1986;73:219-21.
10. Block T, Nilsson TK, Björck M, et al. Diagnostic accuracy of plasma biomarkers for intestinal ischaemia. Scand J Clin Lab Invest. 2008;68:242-8.
11. Salomone T, Tosi P, Palareti G, et al. Coagulative disorders in human acute pancreatitis: role for the D-dimer. Pancreas. 2003;26:111-6.
12. Adam DJ, Haggart PC, Ludlam CA, et al. Hemostatic markers before operation in patients with acutely symptomatic nonruptured and ruptured infrarenal abdominal aortic aneurysm. J Vasc Surg. 2002;35:661-5.
13. Kanda T, Fujii H, Tani T, et al. Intestinal fatty acid-binding protein is a useful diagnostic marker for mesenteric infarction in humans. Gastroenterology. 1996;110:339-43.
14. Gearhart SL, Delaney CP, Senagore AJ, et al. Prospective assessment of the predictive value of alpha-glutathione S-transferase for intestinal ischaemia. Am Surg. 2003;69:324-9.
15. McKinsey JF, Gewertz BL. Acute mesenteric ischaemia. Surg Clin North Am. 1997;77:307-18.
16. Menke J. Diagnostic accuracy of multidetector CT in acute mesenteric ischaemia: systematic review and meta-analysis. Radiology. 2010;256:93-101.
17. Aschoff AJ, Stuber G, Becker BW, et al. Evaluation of acute mesenteric ischaemia: accuracy of biphasic mesenteric multi-detector CT angiography. Abdom Imaging. 2009;34:345-57.
18. Björck M, Orr N, Endean ED. Debate: whether an endovascular-first strategy is the optimal approach for treating acute mesenteric ischemia. J Vasc Surg. 2015;62:767-72.
19. Ryer EJ, Kalra M, Oderich GS, et al. Revascularization for acute mesenteric ischemia. J Vasc Surg. 2012;55:1682-9.

20. Arthurs ZM, Titus J, Bannazadeh M, et al. A comparison of endovascular revascularization with traditional therapy for the treatment of acute mesenteric ischemia. J Vasc Surg. 2011;53:698-704.
21. Björnsson S, Björck M, Block T, et al. Thrombolysis for acute occlusion of the superior mesenteric artery. J Vasc Surg. 2011;54:1734-42.
22. Expert Panel on Interventional Radiology; Fidelman N, AbuRahma AF, Cash BD, et al. ACR Appropriateness Criteria® radiologic management of mesenteric ischemia. J Am Coll Radiol. 2017;14:S266-71.
23. Bala M, Kashuk J, Moore EE, et al. Acute mesenteric ischaemia: guidelines of the World Society of Emergency Surgery. World J Emerg Surg. 2017;12:38.

CHAPTER 24

Necrotizing Pancreatitis

Pravin Amin, Vinay Amin

INTRODUCTION

Acute pancreatitis (AP) is usually a mild and self-resolving disease in most of the patients (up to 80%), and resolves naturally within a short period of time. In remaining cohort, it rapidly progresses to severe illness which may lead to significant morbidity and mortality.[1,2]

Patients with AP may be hospitalized for a short duration for supportive care or may be subjected to prolonged stay in an intensive care unit (ICU) due to systemic inflammatory response syndrome (SIRS), multiorgan failure, and septic complications. About 15–20% of patients of AP progresses to a severe critical illness with a prolonged course. These critically ill patients may develop organ failure with or without local complications such as pancreatic necrosis. In patients with necrotizing pancreatitis, the mortality is about 17%, with a mortality of 12% in the case of sterile necrosis and up to 30% in infected necrosis.

CLASSIFICATION

The Atlanta Symposium in 1992 set up a global consensus to develop a classification system for AP.[3] This Atlanta classification was useful, though some of these definitions were baffling, because of which it was not uniformly accepted. Over the years clearer concepts of the pathophysiology of organ failure, necrotizing pancreatitis, and the subsequent outcomes, with improved diagnostic imaging, have made it possible to revise the Atlanta Classification. This classification was created by a process initiated by a working group which was a web-based consultation between members of 11 national and international pancreatic societies.[4]

As per the latest Atlanta Classification, AP is split into two groups.[4]
1. Interstitial edematous AP, which is due to inflammatory edema of the pancreatic and peripancreatic tissues, but without evidence of tissue necrosis.
2. Necrotizing AP, 5–10% of patients develop necrosis of the pancreatic parenchyma, the peripancreatic tissues or both.

According to the severity, AP is divided into the following:[4]
- Mild AP, where there is an absence of organ failure and no local and systemic complications.
- Moderately severe AP, where there is an absence of organ failure or a momentary organ failure (<48 hours) with or without local complications.
- Severe AP, where there is enduring organ failure (>48 hours) that may affect one or multiple organs.

According to the local or systemic complications, AP is divided into the following:[4]
- *Local complications*: Acute peripancreatic fluid collections, i.e. pseudocysts of pancreas, acute necrotic collections (ANCs), i.e. walled-off necrosis.
- *Systemic complications*: Exacerbation of pre-existing comorbidity.

ASSESSMENT OF SEVERITY

The severity of AP is evaluated by clinical examination to determine the degree of fluid loss, the severity of organ failure, and the extent of the SIRS score (Box 24.1).[5] Several scoring systems foretell the severity of AP depending on clinical, laboratory, radiologic parameters, and serum markers used in 24–48 hours after the disease presents; such as SIRS, APACHE II score,[6] Modified Marshall scoring system for organ dysfunction (Table 24.1),[7] Ranson signs of severity (Box 24.2),[8] and Balthazar-Ranson CT scoring system (Tables 24.2 and 24.3).[9,10]

ETIOLOGY OF ACUTE PANCREATITIS

The exact etiology of AP permits a clinician to choose the most suitable therapy for each individual patient. Advances in imaging, molecular biology, and genetics have greatly improved the ability to determine etiologies, although in 10–15% of cases of AP, the causes remain unknown.[11]

- *Gallstones*: Mechanical ampullary obstruction can be induced by gallstones.
- *Biliary sludge and microlithiasis*: Most patients with biliary sludge are asymptomatic. However, biliary sludge is commonly found in patients with AP.
- *Alcohol*: It is the second most important of cases of AP.
- *Hypertriglyceridemia*: Serum triglyceride concentrations above 1,000 mg/dL (11 mmol/L) can precipitate attacks of AP.
- *Smoking*: It is an independent risk factor for acute and chronic pancreatitis.
- Post-endoscopic retrograde cholangiopancreatography (ERCP)
- Hypercalcemia
- *Drugs*: Valproic acid, estrogen, HIV (human immunodeficiency virus) drugs, azathioprine, etc.
- *Infections*: Viruses—mumps; bacteria—e.g. *Mycoplasma pneumoniae*;[12] fungi—aspergillus.
- *Trauma*: Blunt or penetrating trauma can damage the pancreas.
- *Pancreatic or pancreas divisum*[13]
- Idiopathic.

CLINICAL MANIFESTATIONS OF ACUTE PANCREATITIS

Most patients with AP have acute onset of severe upper abdominal pain. There may be associated nausea and vomiting. On physical examination, patients have tenderness on palpation, abdominal distension with ileus leading to raised intra-abdominal pressure (IAP), and in severe

BOX 24.1: Defining features of systemic inflammatory response syndrome.

Two or more of the following conditions:
• Temperature >38.3°C or <36.0°C
• Heart rate of >90 beats/min
• Respiratory rate of >20 breaths/min or PaCO$_2$ of <32 mm Hg
• WBC count of >12,000 cells/mL, <4,000 cells/mL, or >10% immature (band) forms

(PaO$_2$: partial pressure of arterial oxygen; WBC: white blood cell)

BOX 24.2: Ranson signs of severity.

At admission:
• Age >55 years
• White blood cell count >16,000/mm³, Glucose >200 mg/dL
• LDH >350 IU/L
• AST >250 U/L
During initial 48 hour:
• Hct decrease of >10% points, BUN increase of >5 mg/dL, Calcium <8 mg/dL
• PaO$_2$ <60 mm Hg
• Base deficit >4 mEq/L
• Fluid sequestration >6 L

(LDH: lactate dehydrogenase; AST: aspartate transaminase; PaO$_2$: partial pressure of arterial oxygen)

Table 24.1: Modified Marshall scoring system for organ dysfunction.

Organ system	0	1	2	3	4
Respiratory (PaO$_2$/FiO$_2$)	>400	301–400	201–300	101–200	≤101
Renal:					
Serum creatinine, μmol/L	≤134	134–169	170–310	311–439	>439
Serum creatinine, mg/dL	<1.4	1.4–1.8	1.9–3.6	3.6–4.9	>4.9
Cardiovascular (systolic blood pressure, mm Hg)	>90	<90 fluid responsive	<90 not fluid responsive	<90 pH <7.3	<90 pH <7.2

(PaO$_2$: partial pressure of arterial oxygen; FiO$_2$: fraction of inspired oxygen)

Section 2: Organ Dysfunction

Table 24.2: Balthazar-Ranson CT scoring system.

Grade	Morphology
A	Normal-appearing pancreas
B	Focal or diffuse enlargement of the pancreas
C	Pancreatic gland abnormalities accompanied by mild peripancreatic inflammatory changes
D	Fluid collection in a single location, usually within the anterior pararenal space
E	≥2 fluid collections near the pancreas or gas either within the pancreas or within peripancreatic inflammation

Table 24.3: Balthazar-Ranson CT scoring system: CT severity index (0-10).

CT grade	Score
A	0
B	1
C	2
D	3
E	4
Necrosis	*Score*
<33%	2
33–50%	4
>50%	6

CT grade (0–4) + necrosis (0–6) = total score

Table 24.4: Complications of pancreatitis.

Type of pancreatitis	Fluid collections
Less than 4 weeks after onset:	
Interstitial edematous pancreatitis (IEP)	Acute peripancreatic fluid collection (APFC)—sterile/infected
Necrotizing pancreatitis	Acute necrotic collection (ANC): *Parenchymal necrosis alone* (sterile/infected)
	Peripancreatic necrosis alone (sterile/infected)
	Pancreatic necrosis with peripancreatic necrosis (sterile/infected)
More than 4 weeks after onset:	
Interstitial edematous pancreatitis (IEP)	*Pancreatic pseudocyst* (sterile/infected)
Necrotizing pancreatitis	*Walled-off necrosis* (sterile/infected)

cases, abdominal compartment syndrome. Patients with severe AP may be febrile, tachycardia, tachypnea, hypoxic, and hypotension leading to shock. In pancreatic necrosis there may be retroperitoneal bleeding to discoloration from ecchymosis in the periumbilical region known as Cullen's sign or in the flanks referred to as Grey Turner's sign.[14]

COMPLICATIONS OF PANCREATITIS

In moderately severe pancreatitis and severe pancreatitis patients can present with complications which can be systemic, local, or both. Acute complications in severe AP may present as severe organ failure involving one or more organs. Shock may be an early manifestation and will need aggressive resuscitation. Systemic complications may involve failure of an organ system (respiratory, cardiovascular, or renal).[4]

The other complications include (Table 24. 4):
1. *Acute peripancreatic fluid collection (APFC)* which is a manifestation of interstitial edematous pancreatitis.[4]
2. *Pancreatic pseudocyst* is a delayed presentation (usually >4 weeks), this is a complication of interstitial edematous pancreatitis.[4]
3. *Pancreatic necrosis* is of two types, ANC seen in the early phase and before demarcation and Walled-off necrosis (WON), which is surrounded by a radiologically identifiable capsule which rarely develops before 4 weeks have elapsed from the onset of pancreatitis.[4]
4. Other local complications of AP include gastric outlet dysfunction, splenic and portal vein thrombosis, and colonic necrosis.

Local complication is suspected when there is a persistence or recurrence of abdominal pain, secondary increase in serum pancreatic enzymes, increasing organ dysfunction, and/or the development of clinical signs of sepsis. Most of the patients with pancreatic necrosis usually have a combination of pancreatic parenchymal necrosis and extrapancreatic necrosis. Rarely, pancreatic necrosis without peripancreatic necrosis has been seen. The associated ileus and necrosis may lead to intra-abdominal hypertension and may subsequently lead to abdominal compartment syndrome.[15]

DIAGNOSIS

Laboratory Data

Serum amylase and lipase are elevated to above three times the upper limit of normal in AP. Levels of lipase remains higher for a longer duration and has a higher specificity when compared to amylase. Serum amylase usually rises by 6-12 hours after the onset of AP. Serum amylase has a half-life of about 10 hours and in milder cases returns to normal levels in 3-5 days. Serum lipase increases within 4-8 hours after the beginning of symptoms and it peaks by 24 hours, and returns to normal levels by 8-14 days.[16,17]

Serum glutamic pyruvic transaminase (SGPT) and serum glutamic oxaloacetic transaminase (SGOT) may be elevated along with leukocytosis along with a high hematocrit due to hemoconcentration because of leakage of intravascular fluid into third space. Low levels of serum calcium are consistent with severe pancreatitis. The level of C-reactive protein (CRP) above 150 mg/dL by 48 hours reflects the severity of pancreatitis.

Imaging

Chest X-ray may demonstrate pleural effusions, atelectasis, pulmonary infiltrates, and even acute respiratory distress syndrome (ARDS). Plain X-ray abdomen may reveal localized ileus of a segment of small intestine known as sentinel loop. The colon cut off sign displays a lack of air in the colon distal to the splenic flexure, this is because of a functional spasm of the descending colon following pancreatic inflammation.

Abdominal Ultrasound

In AP, computerized tomography and magnetic resonance imaging are the most efficient methods of evaluating the etiology. However, in majority of the cases, ultrasound abdomen is still the most common initial investigation in AP as it is cheap, easily accessible, and easily repeatable. Ultrasonography is useful in cases of biliary etiology for gallstones such as cholelithiasis, and can also help in identifying other pathologies which may be unrelated to AP such as abdominal aortic aneurysm.[18] On ultrasound, the pancreas usually appears diffusely enlarged. There may be hypoechoic signals and gallstones may be demonstrated in the gallbladder or in the bile duct. Peripancreatic fluid may be seen on abdominal ultrasound. Endoscopic ultrasonography is a very sensitive test for identifying cholelithiasis and choledocholithiasis.[19]

Contrast-enhanced CT

Not all patients with AP need to undergo contrast-enhanced computed tomography (CECT). However, it should be done in patients who develop or are likely to develop severe AP or complications related to AP. As per the revised Atlanta classification, CECT is the primary tool for assessing the imaging-based criteria for classification such as Balthazar-Ranson CT scoring systems (Tables 24.2 and 24.3). The ideal time for assessing these complications with CT is generally after 72 hours from presentation. CT should be repeated when there is deterioration of clinical status, such as sepsis or hemorrhage.[20]

Computed tomography-guided percutaneous aspiration with Gram stain and culture is recommended when infected pancreatic necrosis is suspected.

Magnetic Resonance Imaging

Magnetic resonance is reserved for detection of choledocholithiasis which is not demonstrated on CECT. Magnetic resonance cholangiopancreatography (MRCP) has become a useful tool to identify stones retained in the common bile duct. Selective use of MRCP can reduce the need for ERCP for patients with suspected gallstone pancreatitis. MR imaging is able to characterize collections to detect the presence of non-liquefied material. MR imaging helps to distinguish walled-off necrosis from a pseudocyst, this is best visualized using T2-weighted imaging.[21,22]

Differential Diagnosis

It includes other causes of upper abdominal pain, such as cholecystitis, cholangitis, acid peptic disease, gastrointestinal perforation, intestinal obstruction, volvulus, and mesenteric ischemia.

COURSE OF THE DISEASE

Generally in most patients AP is mild and the patients recover in 3–5 days. About 20% of patients have moderately severe or severe AP in whom both local and/or systemic complications are seen leading to organ failure. The mortality in AP is about 5% with a much lower mortality in patients with interstitial pancreatitis which is about 3% in comparison to necrotizing pancreatitis which is 17%.[23]

MANAGEMENT OF PANCREATITIS

Supportive Care

Mild AP is treated with supportive care which includes pain control, intravenous fluids, and correction of electrolyte and metabolic abnormalities.

In severe AP, ICU monitoring and support of pulmonary, renal, circulatory, and hepatobiliary function may minimize systemic sequelae. A proton pump inhibitor can be given to decrease gastric acid secretion. Somatostatin receptor agonists are rarely used in patients with pancreatic pseudocysts and may reduce pancreatic secretion in patients with pancreatic fistulae.

Fluid Therapy

During the early phase of AP the risk of hypovolemia secondary to third-space fluid loss has long been recognized, the prevention or early correction of this fluid deficit by intravenous fluid resuscitation is recommended.[24] Only two studies specifically investigated the effect of different fluid types on outcomes in AP. In one study comparing Ringer's lactate alone versus Ringer's lactate plus hydroxyethyl starch (HES), Ringer's lactate plus HES resulted in lower IAP and the requirement for mechanical ventilation when compared with resuscitation with Ringer's lactate alone.[25] The HES group showed a reduced mean peak IAP [mean ± standard deviation (SD) 15 ± 3 cm vs 17 ± 5 cm], significantly lower IAP on days 2–7 ($P <0.05$). By day 5, no patient in the HES group had IAP whereas 33% (7/21) patients in the Ringer's lactate group did.[25] In the other study comparing Ringer's lactate with normal saline, Ringer's lactate reduced systemic inflammation as compared to saline.[26] These two studies did not show a significant difference in the clinical outcomes of organ failure, ICU transfer, pancreatic necrosis, pancreatic infection, length of hospital stay, and in-hospital mortality.

Nine studies reported the effect of the rate of fluid administration on outcomes in AP. The median volume given in the first 24 hours in the aggressive treatment groups was 4.5 L (range, 3.5–5.4 L) and the median volume given in the first 24 hours in the nonaggressive groups was 3.5 L (range, 1.7–4.0 L). Four observational studies provide evidence in favor of aggressive fluid resuscitation.[27-30]

A study found that fluid resuscitation did not prevent pancreatic necrosis. All patients with a persistent hemoconcentration beyond 24 hours went on to develop pancreatic necrosis.[16,27]

However, other studies reported that patients who received less than one-third of the total 72-hour fluid volume in the initial 24 hours of treatment, experienced higher rates of SIRS, organ failure, and mortality.[28] More recent studies (both observational and randomized trials) favor nonaggressive fluid resuscitation.

Five of the seven major international guidelines advise the use of resuscitation goals to guide the rate of fluid therapy and when to cease fluid resuscitation. These goals include mean arterial pressure, heart rate, hematocrit level, urinary output, central venous pressure, blood gas, and electrolyte parameters. For these goals, targets were provided only for MAP (>65 mm Hg) and urinary output (>0.5–1 mL/kg/hr).[31,32]

A study used a protocol-based approach centered around heart rate, blood pressure, urinary output, and hematocrit level. This was associated with less severe pancreatitis [odd ratio (OR) = 11.2; 95% confidence interval (CI) = 1.9–68.7; $P = 0.02$], shorter length of hospital stay (7 vs 3 days; $P = 0.01$), reduced requirement of CT imaging studies (100% vs 15.6%; $P < 0.001$), and reduced use of antibiotics (50% vs 3.1%; $P = 0.01$).[33]

Use of Antibiotics in Acute Pancreatitis

After more than 30 years and at least nine randomized studies and eight meta-analyses, it has been shown there is no benefit of prophylactic antibiotics.[34] Antibiotic therapy is recommended in AP only if there is suspected or confirmed infection.

Host of organisms are identified in various studies, such as Gram-negative isolates (35–55%), Gram-positive isolates (20–35%), anaerobic isolates (8–15%), and fungal isolates (20–25%)[35] (Table 24.5).

Ideally, antibiotic used for treatment of infected pancreatic necrosis should have a good penetration into pancreatic tissue and fluids and should cover most bacterial flora causing the infection. Antimicrobial agents achieving adequate to high tissue concentration in the pancreatic tissue include carbapenems, quinolones, third and fourth generation cephalosporins, chloramphenicol, metronidazole, clindamycin, co-trimoxazole, and fluconazole.[36] Three important issues to be considered before starting empirical antibiotic therapy are: (1) being aware of the prevalent hospital bugs and the local antibiogram; (2) when to initiate therapy, dosing and incorporating pharmacodynamics and pharmacokinetics; and (3) duration of antimicrobial therapy. Duration of therapy is based on clinical or microbiological demonstration of the organism.

Table 24.5: Organisms isolated in patients with acute pancreatitis.

	Gram-negative bacteria	Gram-positive bacteria	Fungal organisms
Aerobe	• Escherichia coli • Klebsiella pneumonia • Enterobacteriaceae • Proteus spp. • Pseudomonas aeruginosa • Citrobacter spp. • Serratia spp.	• Enterococcus spp. • Staphylococcus aureus • Staphylococcus epidermidis • Streptococcus spp.	• Candida albicans • Candida spp.
Anaerobe	Bacteroides spp.	Clostridia perfringens	

Nutritional Support

Most patients with AP have mild disease and do not need additional nutritional support during admission. In mild pancreatitis, oral intake is usually restored within 3-7 days of hospitalization, and nutritional support is not required. Nutritional support is indicated if patients cannot consume normal food after 5-7 days. In general, oral intake of a low-fat diet is usually initiated when abdominal pain has subsided and narcotics are no longer required, abdominal tenderness has markedly decreased, and nausea and vomiting have ceased.[37]

The clear benefit of nutritional support in the management of AP is well established. There are wide-ranging studies on the timing, route, and type of nutrition available to patients with AP. The presence of systemic and local complications of severe pancreatitis can have bearing on the policy employed. This may have an impact on feeding due to the presence of large peripancreatic collections resulting in a mass effect on the upper gastrointestinal system.[37]

Parenteral vs Enteral Nutrition

Over the years, the most debated issue in AP has been the role of enteral nutrition (EN) and total parenteral nutrition (TPN). There have been several prospective randomized trials that have compared EN with TPN, all have relatively few patients that have differed considerably in the entry criteria. EN prevents enteral mucosal atrophy and prevents translocation of bacteria, a possible mechanism of sepsis in patients with AP.[38-40] EN facilitates gastric motility, whereby it is beneficial in patients with ileus, and it is much cheaper option than the parenteral route.[37] TPN though expensive, ensures nutrient delivery however is potentially associated with metabolic and septic complications. In a recent meta-analysis of patients with severe AP, eight studies were used for comparison. EN was associated with a decreased risk of mortality, infectious complications, and organ failure. No difference in hospital stay was noted.[41,42] The Audit of Severe Acute Pancreatitis (ASAP) Study was a prospective observational study of 40 participating sites in Australia and New Zealand. The hospital mortality rate was 15% (95% CI = 8-21%), and there was a tendency toward higher mortality for patients who only received parenteral nutrition than for those who only received EN (28% vs 7%, p = .06).[43] The accompanying editorial however highlighted the following. When mortality was compared between PN and patients who received no nutrition [5 of 18 (28%) vs 3 of 4 (75%), p .01], there was a clear statistical significance, although the numbers in all groups were small. With so much PN bashing over the years, one wonders if the groups compared (EN vs TPN) in previous publications were appropriate.[44]

Timing of enteral or oral nutrition

A low-fat soft or solid diet is safe and associated with shorter hospital stays than a clear-liquid diet with slow advancement to solid foods. No clinical trials evaluating these routines are available.

Oral diets acceptance was evaluated in 274 patients once abdominal pain had resolved and ileus had subsided. About 60 patients (21.9%) experienced pain relapse and 47 of these 60 individuals, pain relapsed within 48 hours of commencement of oral feeding. No pain relapse or pain occurred in those patients randomized to jejunal tube feedings, started a median of 7 days after the onset of symptoms, pain on refeeding was associated with longer duration of initial pain and a higher severity index on CT.[45]

A retrospective study in 1,200 patients with severe AP assessed outcomes of patients treated with early (<48 hours) vs late (>48 hours) EN. A total of 81% of patients in the late EN group developed organ dysfunction as opposed to 21% in the EN group.[46] A recent meta-analysis of eight randomized controlled trials (RCTs) compared early (<24 hour) vs late (>24 hour) EN. In this study, the odds ratio of developing organ failure was decreased in patients who received early EN. Nevertheless, in severe AP there was no benefit in early vs late nutritional support in determining outcomes.[47]

Gastric vs jejunal feeding

A wide range of tolerance to EN exists irrespective of known influences such as mode (continuous or bolus) and level of infusion within the gastrointestinal tract (gastric vs postpyloric). It has been postulated that feeding into the stomach increases pancreatic secretions. In patients operated on for complications of AP, continuous infusion appeared to be safer and reduction in the stimulation of the pancreas was more than bolus infusion. Sufficient data is lacking to validate whether continuous or bolus infusion is superior. In an RCT of early nasogastric vs nasojejunal feeding in severe AP, the investigators found patients tolerated nasogastric feeding well and recommended that nasogastric feeding should be considered a therapeutic option because of its simplicity, averting the need for endoscopic or radiologic interventions.[48] In a recent trial, early enteral feeding through nasogastric was not inferior to nasojejunal in patients with severe AP.[49] A meta-analysis showed no significant differences in mortality rate between nasogastric vs nasojejunal and parenteral feeding. Other outcomes were not different such as length of hospital stay, infectious complications, multiorgan failure, rate of admissions to the ICU, or need for surgery. There was no difference in the recurrence of pain on feeding in the nasogastric vs nasojejunal groups.[50]

Types of Nutrients

Elemental formula is entirely predigested and consists of amino acids, simple sugars, and fat. Semielemental formulas require less digestion than polymeric foods and contain peptides of varying chain length, glucose polymers, and fat primarily as medium chain triglycerides. Polymeric feeds contain nonhydrolyzed proteins, complex carbohydrates, and long chain triglycerides. Few studies compare feeding elemental, semielemental, and polymeric diets to patients with AP and have defined the benefits of semielemental vs polymeric diets.[51] In a meta-analysis there was no difference in outcomes or tolerance with either polymeric or semielemental diets.[52]

The use of glutamine supplementation, immunonutrition, prebiotics, and probiotics sounds attractive but their use is not supported by large-scale studies. The only large-scale multicenter randomized trial in which 298 patients with a predicted severe AP were randomly assigned to receive probiotic preparation or placebo administered enterally. In the probiotic group, the incidence of multiorgan failure and the mortality (16% vs 6%) was significantly higher.[53]

In conclusion, specific nutraceuticals added to EN such as arginine, glutamine, ω-3 polyunsaturated fatty acids, and prebiotics may be associated with some theoretical benefits, but the current studies are insufficient to make recommendations for routine use of these nutrients.[51,54] Probiotics should be avoided in patients with severe AP.

SURGICAL INTERVENTION

In patients with mild AP, found to have gallstones, a cholecystectomy should be performed before discharge to prevent a recurrence of AP. In a patient with necrotizing biliary AP, in order to prevent infection, cholecystectomy is to be deferred until active inflammation subsides and fluid collections resolve or stabilize. Asymptomatic pseudocysts and pancreatic and/or extrapancreatic necrosis do not warrant intervention regardless of size, location, and/or extension.[55] For symptomatic patients with rapidly enlarging pseudocysts, or in the presence of pseudocysts and those who do not improve with medical management, a drainage procedure should be performed. Drainage may be carried out by an interventional radiologist or by a surgeon endoscopically. Drainage of a pancreatic pseudocyst by endoscopy is the preferred modality.[55] Endoscopist use two techniques, a transmural approach by creating a tract between the cyst and gastric or duodenal wall followed by balloon dilatation and placement of stents; or alternatively a transpapillary drainage can be performed, by inserting a pancreatic stent to drain cysts that connects with the pancreatic duct. Percutaneous drainage may be used in an emergency to drain retroperitoneal collections so as to stabilize patients with sepsis prior to definite operative or endoscopic approach.[11] There has been a shift away from urgent surgical debridement of infected necrosis toward more conservative, less invasive approaches. Intervention if needed is preferred to be carried out after 4–6 weeks after the onset of pancreatitis. An ANC which develops into walled-off necrosis may be sterile or may get infected in the course of the illness.[56] An infected pancreatic necrosis and the presence of symptomatic sterile necrosis are clear indications for surgical debridement. Laparoscopic surgery is the preferred modality of therapy in walled-off pancreatic necrosis. Open surgical necrosectomy used to be the gold standard for management of pancreatic necrosis, however this was associated with increased morbidity and mortality. In a multicenter RCT from the Netherlands, a step-up approach to management of infected necrosis was compared with open necrosectomy.[57] The first step was placement of percutaneous drainage catheters in addition to treatment with antibiotics. The catheter was irrigated and upsized as necessary. If the patients did not improve within 72 hours, minimally invasive debridement was performed via a retroperitoneal approach. This approach reduced major complications or death by 29% compared with traditional open necrosectomy.[57]

Endoscopic Retrograde Cholangiopancreatography

Endoscopic retrograde cholangiopancreatography (ERCP) for patients with biliary pancreatitis has a clearly defined role. ERCP in AP patients who have severe acute biliary pancreatitis with signs of cholangitis should undergo ERCP within 24 hours. ERCP should not be used routinely for patients with mild gallstone pancreatitis because it can increase the complications.[58]

Post-ERCP-related pancreatitis is a well-known entity. A meta-analysis of eight RCTs calculated a pooled OR of 0.22 for development of post-ERCP pancreatitis with stent placement.[59] Recently, a large-scale, multicenter RCT showed a 45% reduction in pancreatitis when rectal indomethacin was administered immediately following ERCP to a selected high-risk population.[60]

CONCLUSION

The approach to improve the care of AP is obtaining accurate diagnosis, identifying the causative factors, predicting accurately the early markers of severity, focusing on the appropriate early fluid resuscitation in the initial therapy of severe AP, subsequent monitoring for complications, and appropriate interventions to address these impediments. The two most important markers of severity in AP are organ failure and pancreatic necrosis. Early evidence of organ failure will warrant careful monitoring and suitable therapy in the ICU. Patients who are doubtful to restart oral nutrition within 5 days will require nutritional support. Nutritional support can be delivered by TPN or by enteral feeding, the latter has clear advantages and benefits. In AP caused by gallstones, an ERCP with endoscopic biliary sphincterotomy and stone removal is indicated within the first 24 hours. There is no role for prophylactic antibiotics in necrotizing pancreatitis as recent prospective trials have shown no benefit and prolonged use of these potent antibiotics may lead to the emergence of infection with more resistant organisms. Sterile pancreatic necrosis is largely treated medically during the first few weeks even in the presence of multiorgan failure. CT-guided percutaneous aspiration followed by Gram stain and culture is suggested when pancreatic necrosis with infection is suspected. When infected necrosis is documented surgical debridement is the therapy of choice in sick patients. The timing of surgery is generally left to the judgment of the surgeon, but is preferred 4–6 weeks after the onset of pancreatitis. Surgical debridement may be performed by either surgical, endoscopic, or radiologic techniques. Less invasive procedures are better tolerated and reduce the risk of morbidity and mortality.

REFERENCES

1. Banks PA, Freeman ML, Fass R, et al. Practice guidelines in acute pancreatitis. Am J Gastroenterol. 2006;101:2379-400.
2. Pandol SJ, Saluja AK, Imrie CW, et al. Acute pancreatitis: bench to the bedside. Gastroenterol. 2007;132:1127-51.
3. Bradley EL, 3rd. A clinically based classification system for acute pancreatitis. Summary of the International Symposium on Acute Pancreatitis, Atlanta, Ga, September 11 through 13, 1992. Arch Surg. 1993;128:586-90.
4. Banks PA, Bollen TL, Dervenis C, et al. Classification of acute pancreatitis--2012: revision of the Atlanta classification and definitions by international consensus. Gut. 2013;62:102-11.
5. Annane D, Bellissant E, Cavaillon JM. Septic shock. Lancet. 2005;365:63-78.
6. Dominguez-Munoz JE, Carballo F, Garcia MJ, et al. Evaluation of the clinical usefulness of APACHE II and SAPS systems in the initial prognostic classification of acute pancreatitis: a multicenter study. Pancreas. 1993;8:682-6.
7. Marshall JC, Cook DJ, Christou NV, et al. Multiple organ dysfunction score: a reliable descriptor of a complex clinical outcome. Crit Care Med. 1995;23:1638-52.
8. Ranson JH, Rifkind KM, Roses DF, et al. Prognostic signs and the role of operative management in acute pancreatitis. Surg Gynecol Obstet. 1974;139:69-81.
9. Balthazar EJ, Ranson JH, Naidich DP, et al. Acute pancreatitis: prognostic value of CT. Radiology. 1985;156:767-72.
10. Balthazar EJ, Robinson DL, Megibow AJ, et al. Acute pancreatitis: value of CT in establishing prognosis. Radiology. 1990;174:331-6.
11. Forsmark CE, Baillie J; AGA Institute Clinical Practice and Economics Committee; AGA Institute Governing Board. AGA Institute technical review on acute pancreatitis. Gastroenterology. 2007;132:2022-44.
12. Valdés Lacasa T, Duarte Borges MA, García Marín A, et al. Acute pancreatitis caused by Mycoplasma pneumoniae: an unusual etiology. Clin J Gastroenterol. 2017;10:279-282.
13. Taj MA, Qureshi S, Ghazanfar S, et al. Pancreas Divisum. J Coll Physicians Surg Pak. 2016;26:96-9.
14. Mookadam F, Cikes M. Images in clinical medicine. Cullen's and Turner's signs. N Engl J Med. 2005;353:1386.
15. Marcos-Neira P, Zubia-Olaskoaga F, Lopez-Cuenca S, et al.; Epidemiology of Acute Pancreatitis in Intensive Care Medicine study group. Relationship between intra-abdominal hypertension, outcome and the revised Atlanta and determinant-based classifications in acute pancreatitis. BJS Open. 2017;1:175-81.
16. Yadav D, Agarwal N, Pitchumoni CS. A critical evaluation of laboratory tests in acute pancreatitis. Am J Gastroenterol. 2002;97:1309-18.
17. Tenner S, Baillie J, DeWitt J, et al. American College of Gastroenterology guideline: management of acute pancreatitis. Am J Gastroenterol. 2013;108:1400-15;1416.
18. Working Party of the British Society of Gastroenterology; Association of Surgeons of Great Britain and Ireland; Pancreatic Society of Great Britain and Ireland; Association of Upper GI Surgeons of Great Britain and Ireland. UK guidelines for the management of acute pancreatitis. Gut. 2005;54:iii1-iii9.
19. Morgan DE, Baron TH. Practical imaging in acute pancreatitis. Semin Gastrointest Dis. 1998;9:41-50.
20. Bollen TL, van Santvoort HC, Besselink MG, et al. Update on acute pancreatitis: ultrasound, computed tomography, and magnetic resonance imaging features. Semin Ultrasound CT MR. 2007;28:371-83.
21. Arvanitakis M, Delhaye M, De Maertelaere V, et al. Computed tomography and magnetic resonance imaging in the assessment of acute pancreatitis. Gastroenterology. 2004;126:715-23.
22. Stimac D, Miletic D, Radic M, et al. The role of nonenhanced magnetic resonance imaging in the early assessment of acute pancreatitis. Am J Gastroenterol. 2007;102:997-1004.
23. Triester SL, Kowdley KV. Prognostic factors in acute pancreatitis. J Clin Gastroenterol. 2002;34:167-76.
24. Solanki NS, Barreto SG. Fluid therapy in acute pancreatitis. A systematic review of literature. JOP. 2011;12:205-8.
25. Du XJ, Hu WM, Xia Q, et al. Hydroxyethyl starch resuscitation reduces the risk of intra-abdominal hypertension in severe acute pancreatitis. Pancreas. 2011;40:1220-5.

26. Wu BU, Hwang JQ, Gardner TH, et al. Lactated Ringer's solution reduces systemic inflammation compared with saline in patients with acute pancreatitis. Clin Gastroenterol Hepatol. 2011;9:710-7 e1.
27. Brown A, Baillargeon JD, Hughes MD, et al. Can fluid resuscitation prevent pancreatic necrosis in severe acute pancreatitis? Pancreatology. 2002;2:104-7.
28. Gardner TB, Vege SS, Chari ST, et al. Faster rate of initial fluid resuscitation in severe acute pancreatitis diminishes in-hospital mortality. Pancreatology. 2009;9:770-6.
29. Wall I, Badalov N, Baradarian R, et al. Decreased mortality in acute pancreatitis related to early aggressive hydration. Pancreas. 2011;40:547-50.
30. Warndorf MG, Kurtzman JT, Bartel MJ, et al. Early fluid resuscitation reduces morbidity among patients with acute pancreatitis. Clin Gastroenterol Hepatol. 2011;9:705-9.
31. de-Madaria E, Soler-Sala G, Sanchez-Paya J, et al. Influence of fluid therapy on the prognosis of acute pancreatitis: a prospective cohort study. Am J Gastroenterol. 2011;106:1843-50.
32. Eckerwall G, Olin H, Andersson B, et al. Fluid resuscitation and nutritional support during severe acute pancreatitis in the past: what have we learned and how can we do better? Clin Nutr. 2006;25:497-504.
33. Reddy N, Wilcox CM, Tamhane A, et al. Protocol-based medical management of post-ERCP pancreatitis. J Gastroenterol Hepatol. 2008;23:385-92.
34. Bai Y, Gao J, Zou DW, et al. Prophylactic antibiotics cannot reduce infected pancreatic necrosis and mortality in acute necrotizing pancreatitis: evidence from a meta-analysis of randomized controlled trials. Am J Gastroenterol. 2008;103:104-10.
35. Buchler MW, Gloor B, Muller CA, et al. Acute necrotizing pancreatitis: treatment strategy according to the status of infection. Ann Surg. 2000;23:619-26.
36. Vege SS, Baron TH; Mayo Clinic College of Medicine. Management of pancreatic necrosis in severe acute pancreatitis. Clin Gastroenterol Hepatol. 2005;3:192-6.
37. Meier R, Ockenga J, Pertkiewicz M, et al. ESPEN Guidelines on Enteral Nutrition: Pancreas. Clin Nutr. 2006;25:275-84.
38. Ammori BJ, Leeder PC, King RF, et al. Early increase in intestinal permeability in patients with severe acute pancreatitis: correlation with endotoxemia, organ failure, and mortality. J Gastrointest Surg. 1999;3:252-62.
39. Besselink MG, van Santvoort HC, Renooij W, et al. Intestinal barrier dysfunction in a randomized trial of a specific probiotic composition in acute pancreatitis. Ann Surg. 2009;250:712-9.
40. Fritz S, Hackert T, Hartwig W, et al. Bacterial translocation and infected pancreatic necrosis in acute necrotizing pancreatitis derives from small bowel rather than from colon. Am J Surg. 2010;200:111-7.
41. Yi F, Ge L, Zhao J, et al. Meta-analysis: total parenteral nutrition versus total enteral nutrition in predicted severe acute pancreatitis. Intern Med. 2012;51:523-30.
42. Gianotti L, Meier R, Lobo DN, et al. ESPEN Guidelines on Parenteral Nutrition: pancreas. Clin Nutr. 2009;28:428-35.
43. Davies AR, Morrison SS, Ridley EJ, et al. Nutritional therapy in patients with acute pancreatitis requiring critical care unit management: a prospective observational study in Australia and New Zealand. Crit Care Med. 2011;39:462-8.
44. Amin P. Nutritional support in acute pancreatitis: the saga continues! Crit Care Med. 2011;39:587-8.
45. Petrov MS, van Santvoort HC, Besselink MG, et al. Oral refeeding after onset of acute pancreatitis: a review of literature. Am J Gastroenterol. 2007;102:2079-84; quiz 85.
46. Wu XM, Liao YW, Wang HY, et al. When to initialize enteral nutrition in patients with severe acute pancreatitis? A retrospective review in a single institution experience (2003-2013). Pancreas. 2015;44:507-11.
47. Bakker OJ, van Brunschot S, Farre A, et al. Timing of enteral nutrition in acute pancreatitis: meta-analysis of individuals using a single-arm of randomised trials. Pancreatology. 2014;14:340-6.
48. Eatock FC, Chong P, Menezes N, et al. A randomized study of early nasogastric versus nasojejunal feeding in severe acute pancreatitis. Am J Gastroenterol. 2005;100:432-9.
49. Singh N, Sharma B, Sharma M, et al. Evaluation of early enteral feeding through nasogastric and nasojejunal tube in severe acute pancreatitis: a noninferiority randomized controlled trial. Pancreas. 2012;41:153-9.
50. Zhu Y, Yin H, Zhang R, et al. Nasogastric Nutrition versus Nasojejunal Nutrition in Patients with Severe Acute Pancreatitis: A Meta-Analysis of Randomized Controlled Trials. Gastroenterol Res Pract. 2016;2016:6430632.
51. Marik PE. What is the best way to feed patients with pancreatitis? Curr Opin Crit Care. 2009;15:131-8.
52. Petrov MS, Loveday BP, Pylypchuk RD, et al. Systematic review and meta-analysis of enteral nutrition formulations in acute pancreatitis. Br J Surg. 2009;96:1243-52.
53. Besselink MG, van Santvoort HC, Buskens E, et al. Probiotic prophylaxis in predicted severe acute pancreatitis: a randomised, double-blind, placebo-controlled trial. Lancet. 2008;371:651-9.
54. Thomson A. Nutritional support in acute pancreatitis. Curr Opin Clin Nutr Metab Care. 2008;11:261-6.
55. Tenner S, Baillie J, DeWitt J, et al.; American College of Gastroenterology. American College of Gastroenterology guideline: management of acute pancreatitis. Am J Gastroenterol. 2013;108:1400-15; 16.
56. Freeman ML, Werner J, van Santvoort HC, et al. Interventions for necrotizing pancreatitis: summary of a multidisciplinary consensus conference. Pancreas. 2012;41:1176-94.
57. van Santvoort HC, Besselink MG, Bakker OJ, et al. A step-up approach or open necrosectomy for necrotizing pancreatitis. N Engl J Med. 2010;362:1491-502.
58. Folsch UR, Nitsche R, Ludtke R, et al. Early ERCP and papillotomy compared with conservative treatment for acute biliary pancreatitis. The German Study Group on Acute Biliary Pancreatitis. N Engl J Med. 1997;336:237-42.
59. Choudhary A, Bechtold ML, Arif M, et al. Pancreatic stents for prophylaxis against post-ERCP pancreatitis: a meta-analysis and systematic review. Gastrointest Endosc. 2011;73:275-82.
60. Elmunzer BJ, Scheiman JM, Lehman GA, et al. A randomized trial of rectal indomethacin to prevent post-ERCP pancreatitis. N Engl J Med. 2012;366:1414-22.

CHAPTER 25

Critical Care in Burns

Sunil M Keswani, Shruti Dutta, Pravina Yande

INTRODUCTION

Skin is the outermost covering and the largest organ of the integumentary system of our body. It protects deeper tissues from harsh environment, regulates temperature, and prevents loss of water; the sensory receptors attached to it are involved in detecting pain, pressure, and temperature. Other functions are insulation, vitamin D synthesis, and immunity to protect against pathogen invaders.[1] Hence, skin functions as an overall protection barrier, but burns destroys the protection shield, and our body gets exposed to various external impetuses. Burns is associated with severe skin damage. Therefore serious burns injury needs immediate medical support to prevent further complications and death.

CLASSIFICATION OF BURNS

Burns is a type of injury to the skin caused by various agents scald burn due to spillage of hot liquids, flame burn due to fire, cold burn or frost bite, electrical injury, radiation, friction, sunburn, contact burns with hot objects. Depending upon the thickness of skin injured, burns is classified into four degrees. In first-degree burn, only the superficial layer of the skin is damaged. It appears red in color, and pain lasts not more that 2–3 days, and it heals on its own. When the injury goes beyond the epidermis layer it caused partial-thickness or second-degree burn. Blister formation takes place, and it becomes very painful. Healing takes longer time, up to 2 months, and sometime scarring may occur. In third-degree or full-thickness burn, injury extends up to all the layers of skin. Visible thrombosed capillaries, venules, or other blood vessels are the sign of full-thickness burn. In such type of burns, pain is absent the nerve endings are damaged. Healing does not take place without surgical intervention. In fourth-degree burn the deeper tissues, such as bone, tendon, and muscle, are also affected. It is life-threatening due to huge loss of fluid and more chances of infection of the wound area. It is also associated with amputation or significant functional impairment and often death.[2]

PATHOPHYSIOLOGY OF BURNS

Understanding the burns pathophysiology is prerequisite for appropriate management. As per Jackson's Burn Wound theory the three zones of burns are described in the literature.[3] *Zone of coagulation:* The primary injury site is called the zone of coagulation, where there is an irreversible tissue damage due to coagulation of proteins. *Zone of stasis*: This zone is characterized by reduced tissue perfusion. Here tissue can be salvaged from complete damage by resuscitation. However, prolonged hypotension, infection, edema can lead to complete tissue loss. *Zone of hyperemia*: This is the outermost zone and characterized by increased tissue perfusion. In this zone, tissue can be recouped unless there is sepsis.

CRITERIA FOR HOSPITALIZATION

A child with any burns greater than 10% total body surface area (TBSA); adult with any burn greater than 20% TBSA;

full-thickness burn; inhalational injury; special areas burn—face, eyes, ears, hands, feet, and perineum; chemical/electrical burn; high-pressure steam injury; hydrofluoric acid burn; potentially complex burn—radiation burn; coexisting disease; and associated trauma pregnancy burn are considered critical and need hospitalization.

BURN WOUND ASSESSMENT

Wound Assessment According to Physical Examination

Table 25.1: Physical appearance of burns.[5]

	Superficial	Deep
Appearance	Pink, soft	White, yellow, or brown
Blanches on pressure	Yes	Fixed red or salt and pepper appearance
Hair follicles	Firmly fixed, provide resistance to pull	Pulled easily
Pain	Hyperalgesia to needle touch	Analgesia to needle touch

Clinical burn wound evaluation relies on (Table 25.1).
- *Subjective evaluation*: It is based on the external features of the wound, such as wound appearance, capillary refill, and burn wound sensibility to touch and pinprick.[4]
- Objective evaluation is based on the basis of the wound site, size, and depth and age of the patient (Table 25.2).

Table 25.2: Assessment of burn type and depth.

Depth of burn	Depth of skin involved	Examination finding
Superficial epidermal	The epidermis is affected, but the dermis is intact	Skin is red and painful, but not blistered
Partial thickness—superficial dermal	The epidermis and upper layers of dermis are involved	The skin is pale pink and painful with blistering
Partial thickness—deep dermal	The epidermis, upper and deeper layers of dermis are involved	The skin appears dry or moist, blotchy and red, and may be painful or painless. There may be blisters
Full thickness	The burn extends through all the layers of skin to subcutaneous tissues	The skin is dry and white, brown, or black in color, with no blisters. It may be described as leathery or waxy. It is painless

Wound site is assessed by the injured anatomical part of the body. Size of the burn is usually represented as a percentage TBSA by using Wallace rule of nines, Lund and Browder chart, and rule of palm.[6]

Wound Assessment According to the Anatomical Part

Facial burn: Facial burn impairs anatomical and physiological function and induces swelling, pain, and deformity. Scald burn is the most common cause of facial burn in children, whereas flame and electrical (flash burn) burn is the most common cause of facial burn in adults.[7] Facial and inhalation burn compromise airway and may produce respiratory complications. Eyelid burn is very common in a facial burn. It signifies underlying ocular damage and subsequent blindness.[6] Ophthalmic evaluation is necessary to rule out corneal and conjunctival injury and epithelial loss. One of the postburn deformities of the eyelid is ectropion. Ectropion can lead to keratitis, corneal ulceration, and ultimately loss of vision.[5] Irrigation of eye with copious normal saline and maintenance of adequate lubrication by moisturizing eye drop are done. Nose is more vulnerable to deep burn. In a severe case, there may be soot around the nose and singed hair in a nostril.[7] Nostril splints are often used to prevent stenosis. Nose and ears burn is subsequently a significant reconstructive challenge due to vital tissue and structural support loss. External ear cartilage gets damage in thermal burn and edema, separates the skin from cartilage lead to devascularization of cartilage and chondritis.[5] Chondritis leads to throbbing pain, erythematous swelling, tenderness, and increased cephalo-conchal angle. Chondritis is caused by infection with *Pseudomonas aeruginosa* and *Staphylococcus aureus*. Incision and drainage of pus and regular dressing with sterile vaseline, betadine gauze is recommended management of the chondritis. Majority of ear burn heals without any surgical intervention. Antibiotic creams or ointments, such as mafenide acetate, are recommended to use externally with minimum pressure. In periorral burn, lips and mouth are commonly involved. Local application of lubricant cream or ointment is used for preventing cracking and bleeding.

Wound Assessment According to Etiology of Burn

Based on the etiology of burns, it can be classified into two types: (1) thermal burn and (2) nonthermal burn.

Thermal Burn

Thermal burn is caused by flame, blast, hot liquid, and a hot object. The most common cause of thermal burn is flame burn, and the second most common cause is scald burn.

Flame burn (dry heat): Flame burn is the most common type of burns in the age-group of 16–55 years, and the females are more prone than the males. In India, 80% of flame burn is due to accident, 5% due to suicide, and 10% due to homicide.[8]

Firecracker burn: Hand and eyes are more commonly burn while blasting a firecracker.[9]

Scald burn (wet heat): Burn due to hot liquid is called a scald burn. Scald burn is frequently seen in children in the age-group of 3–5 years. The severity of scald burn depends upon temperature, exposure time, quantity, density of the liquid, age of the victim, and type of the garment.

Steam burn: Steam burn is more dangerous than scald burn. Minor or superficial steam burn can be treated in outpatient department basis; but if face, feet, hand, and genital part are involved then hospitalization is necessary.

Nonthermal Burn

Chemical burn: Chemical burn injury is the most common type of burns in children, adult, and people with disability.[10] They are the main victims because they do not know the handling of the chemicals properly. The chemical burn wound assessment can be done based on pH of chemical agents and concentration, anatomical location, type of wound, duration of exposure. In acid burn, coagulation necrosis takes place as acids can penetrate into deep-lying tissues. In alkali burn, liquefaction necrosis takes place that diffuse and penetrate into deep underlying tissues. Alkali burn is more severe than acid burn because it penetrates the surface and breaks down fat in a process called saponification. The external barrier of the cells is made with fat, so when the fat breaks down, the entire cell falls apart. Common acids which cause burn are hydrofluoric acid, nitric acid, sulfurous acid, hydrochloric acid, sulfuric acid, etc. Substances containing such chemicals include glass polish (hydrofluoric acid), vinegar (acetic acid), and nail polish remover (acetic acid). A car battery can explode and cause a sulfuric acid burn. In acid and alkali burn the first-aid treatment is to irrigate the wounds with water for 20–60 minutes. Water helps to wash out the chemical and also helps to subside the burning sensation, with few exceptions, where water makes the situation more critical. Metallic alkalies, such as metallic lithium, sodium, potassium, and magnesium, react with water and cause serious burns. In such cases the first line of action is to remove the chemical from the affected area, and then water can be used for irrigation.

Electrical burn: Burn injury due to electrocution is called the electrical burn. There are two sources of electrical burn: (1) natural lightning and (2) manmade source—direct current (DC) and alternating current (AC). AC is more dangerous because contact of a person with the power source is prolonged, however, in DC shock the person is thrown away from the power source after shock. Initial assessment of electrical burn is carried out by assessment for entry and exit wound; assessment for trauma injury or fracture of long bone and spine; assessment of tetanic muscle contraction, extremity exploration for presence of 5Ps (pain, pallor, paresthesia, paralysis, and pulselessness), which indicate the development of compartment syndrome (compartment pressure >30 mm Hg);[6] assessment of burn wound, blood investigation for cardiac markers, and electrocardiography monitoring.

Friction burn: Friction burns is also one type of nonthermal burn, which is mostly overlooked and ignored. The most common cause of friction burns is road traffic accident associated with mechanical injury. Upper limb, lower limb, and face are commonly affected with a bone fracture, head injury, nerve and tendon injury. Mechanical injury is always treated as priority, and friction burn is neglected.

Contact burn: This is caused by heat transfer from one object to another object by conduction, convection, and radiation. Contact burn is the example of conduction burn. Children and women are the victims of contact burn. This is found at home and workplace by contact with a saucepan, kettle, cooker, iron, heater, etc.

Silencer burn: Hot muffler pipe or exhaust pipe of a motorcycle or other vehicles can burn skin by slight touch. This type of burn is usually a second-degree burn. If the burns is more than 3 in. in diameter, it is considered major.[11]

PATIENT EVALUATION AFTER BURNS INJURY

As per the acronym *AMPLE*, patient evaluation is carried out. AMPLE stands for: Allergies, Medication, Pre-existing diseases, Last meal and Event of the injury. These include time, location, and incidence. Patient with facial burn should have corneal examination (ophthalmology opinion). Occult injury should be ruled out in all trauma patients. In female, last menstrual period is checked to rule out pregnancy. Routine blood investigations, including complete blood count, serum electrolyte, creatinine, viral makers, blood group, random blood sugar, chest X-ray are also recommended.

Critical Patients are Assessed by Airway, Breathing, Circulation, Disability, Exposure (ABCDE) Approach

Airway and breathing evaluation: Physical signs that indicate an inhalational burn injury include burn to face and neck, singed nasal hair, change in voice with hoarseness or harsh cough, dyspnea, stridor, erythema, or swelling of oropharynx on direct visualization and carbonaceous sputum or soot particles in oropharynx. In such condition, assessment of airway is carried out for any obstruction. After adequate assessment of airway, breathing is assessed.

Circulation and fluid management: Circulatory deficit is evaluated clinically; the evidence of deficit is suggested by the presence of tachycardia, tachypnea, reduced level of consciousness, prolonged capillary refill time, and cooled peripheries.

Disability: After optimization of airway, breathing, circulation, patient's neurological status is assessed.

Exposure: A thorough examination of the whole body is done for any other major associated injuries. All the assessment, treatment administered, and response to the treatment should be documented.

Assessment of burn surface area: The Lund and Browder chart is well accepted for the calculation of percentage of burns (Fig. 25.1).[12] It can be used in children as it takes into account the person's age, and the different proportions of the head and legs in growing children (Table 25.2).[13]

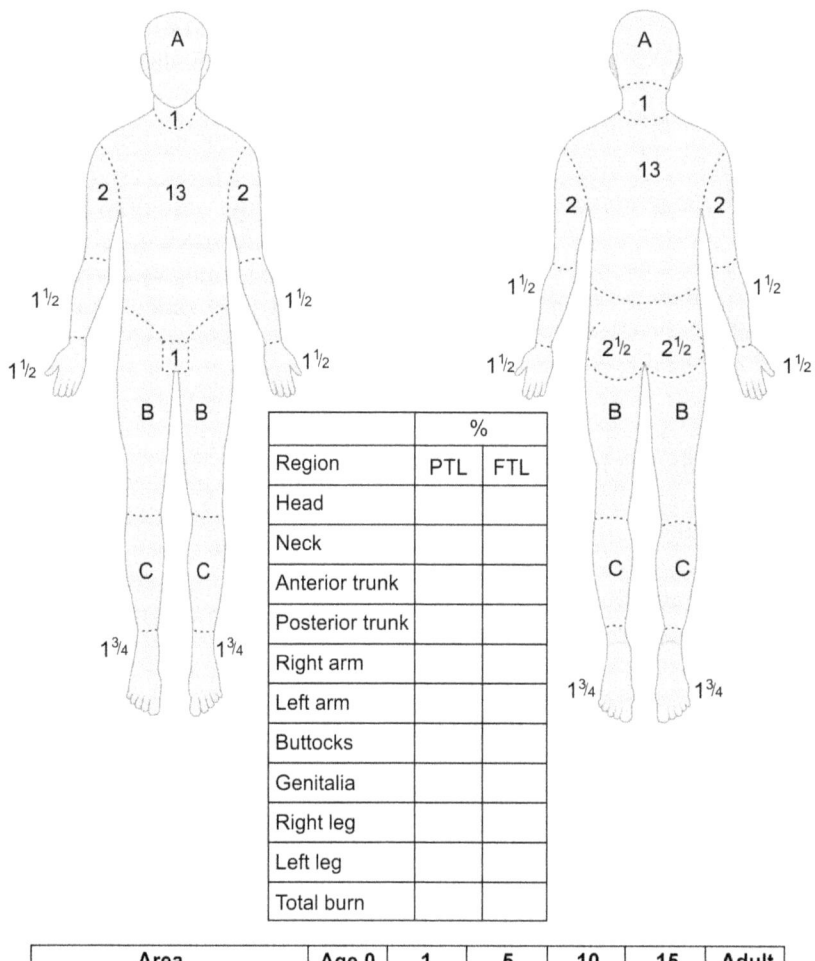

FIGURE 25.1: The Lund and Browder chart.

ACUTE BURNS MANAGEMENT

Fluid resuscitation: Loss of excessive fluid is the major challenge in acute burn. Fluid resuscitation is, therefore, the basis of acute burn management; it maintains the tissue perfusion in the early phase of burn shock. Appropriate fluid management improves survival rate in burns patients.[14] Burns less than 20% is associated with minimum fluid loss, and therefore oral hydration is sufficient, except patients having facial, hand, and genital burns. If the TBSA involved is more than 20%, massive fluid loss is taking place which results in burn shock. In such a situation, administration of fluid is initiated through conventional intravascular route. The "Parkland" formula was introduced in the 1970s and has been accepted worldwide for fluid resuscitation. The formula calculates the volume of fluid required based on TBSA being involved.

Parkland Formula

Initial 24 hours: Ringer's lactated (RL) solution 4 mL/kg/% burn for adults and 3 mL/kg/% burn for children. RL solution is added for maintenance for children:
- About 4 mL/kg/h for children weighing 0–10 kg
- About 40 mL/h + 2 mL/h for children weighing 10–20 kg
- About 60 mL/h + 1 mL/kg/h for children weighing 20 kg or higher.

According to the formula, no colloid should be administered in the initial 24 hours.

Next 24 hours: Colloids are given as 20–60% of calculated plasma volume. No crystalloids should be given. Glucose in water is added in amounts required to maintain a urinary output of 0.5–1 mL/h in adults and 1 mL/h in children.[14]

Modified Parkland Formula

Initial 24 hours: RL 4 mL/kg/% burn (adults) and next 24 hours: colloid infusion of 5% albumin 0.3–1 mL/kg/% burn/16/h is started.[14]

Inhalation Injury

In thermal inhalation injury, airway management and ventilator support is recommended. Incorporation of ventilation is often associated with incidence of ventilator-associated lung injury, which nowadays has been reduced by introduction of lung-protective ventilation strategies using low tidal volumes and permissive hypercapnia.

Tracheostomy

Tracheostomy is a common surgical procedure in severe burn patients with inhalation or face injury. Urgent tracheostomy may be needed when the patient is having airway injuries from smoke, steam, or chemical burns.[15]

Escharotomy and Fasciotomy

Critically ill patients with burns often require emergency surgeries, such as escharotomy and fasciotomy.[16]

Escharotomy: The aim of the escharotomy is to release the pressure over the involved deeper tissues and to restore their circulation. Escharotomies are often performed as part of a burn's resuscitation care, and the decision is made based on clinical assessment of the patient and their response to treatment. Clinical indications for escharotomy include patient complaints of tingling or numbness in limbs. The clinical signs may include hypothermia of the affected areas suggesting poor perfusion, reduced oxygen saturation, delayed or no capillary refill, shallow respiratory effort, restricted chest, and abdominal wall movement. The escharotomy is usually performed within the first 48 hours of injury. The incisions should extend from burnt skin to unburnt skin ideally, or at least into areas of more superficial burns, down to subcutaneous fat, and release any constrictions. In the limbs, incisions should be made in the midaxial line, both medially and laterally, and on the chest and abdominal wall, the incisions are made in the midaxillary lines, which can be joined by a transverse incision below the costal margin to allow adequate release. The wound edges should be adequately parted upon incision; any residual constrictions should be checked by running a finger along the length of the incision. Cautery should be used to control postprocedure bleeding.

Fasciotomy: Compartment syndrome is a painful condition that occurs when pressure in the compartment which holds the muscles build to high levels. This pressure can decrease blood flow, which prevents nourishment and oxygen from reaching nerves and muscles. Fasciotomies are performed when there are circumferential burns. It is a surgical procedure to incise fascia to relieve pressure which otherwise would have resulted in loss of circulation to the tissue. It is a limb-saving method which is done to treat compartment syndrome.

DEBRIDEMENT AND SKIN GRAFTING

If patient is stable, then early excision is done within 48 hours. At a time, 15–20% dead skin is excised, and the wound is covered by autograft or allograft, and sometimes sandwich grafting is used. If patient's condition is not stable, then delayed debridement is done after 15–20 days, after patient becomes stable, followed by skin grafting. In the case of unavailability of autograft, for high percentage of burns, glycerol preserved allograft from cadaver is used as temporary biological dressing material.

Pain Management

Pain is classified into three types: (1) background pain, (2) procedural pain, and (3) surgical pain. Patient's subjective feeling is the key indicator for treatment according to the National Accreditation Board for Hospitals and Healthcare Providers. Pain in burns are classified by depth (first degree, second degree, and third degree) and area (%TBSA). In superficial and shallow dermal burn with large total surface area, severe pain is experienced, whereas in deep dermal burns and full-thickness burns are painless. Assessment of pain in burns is done on the basis of the following points: anatomical location(s), intensity—Wong-Baker Faces Pain Scale (0–10), onset, duration, variation, alleviating and aggravating factors, medication history. The patient feels severe pain during and after dressing, so burn dressing under analgesia is necessary. Before removal of the dressing, it is soaked with 500 mL normal saline containing 15 mL of 2% xylocaine. This helps to remove adherent dressing easily and is less painful. Intravenous analgesia (KTM—Ketamine, Tramadol, and Midazolam) is infused 30 minutes before the dressing procedure. The dose of analgesia is titrated with pain by using pulse oximeter. The composition of the analgesia cocktail for adults is: 50 mL normal saline, 100 mg ketamine, 10 mg midazolam and 100 mg tramadol and the infusion rate start from KTM- 4 mL/hr and titrated according to pain. Whereas the solution composition for children is: 50 mL normal saline, 50 mg ketamine, 5 mg midazolam and 50 mg tramadol and the infusion rate start from 0.5–1 mL/hr and titrated as per pain. Some nonopioid and opioid drugs, such as paracetamol, fentanyl, are also used as part of pain management. Physical interventions, such as heat, cold, and electrical stimulation, exercise, physical or occupational therapy, immobilization, are various strategies used for pain management. Cognitive behavioral strategies include distraction, relaxation, and hypnosis. Patients and families are being educated about some noninvasive methods, which often help to prevent or alleviate pain (e.g. distraction, music, reading, prayer, meditation, massage therapy, etc.).

Antibiotic Protocol in Burns

Patient care is improved by promoting the best practice in antibiotic prophylaxis and therapy. The protocol helps to retard the emergence and spread of multiple antibiotic-resistant bacteria. The use of unnecessary or ineffective antibiotics is eliminated and restricts the use of expensive and powerful ones. Antibiotics will be given only when patient actually requires. Colonized patients who are not actually infected should be avoided antibiotic treatment. If the clinical condition is improving in general then antibiotic strategy should not be changed. However, if there is no clinical response within 72 hours, the clinical diagnosis, the choice of antibiotic, and/or the possibility of a secondary infection should be reconsidered. The antibiotic should be given for the minimum length of time that is effective. The therapy would be reviewed after 10 days. For surgical (early excision or debridement and grafting) prophylaxis the antibiotic should be started intraoperatively just before debridement.[8]

Nutrition in Burns

A burns patient's nourishment depends upon early oral feeding. It should be started within 48–72 hours just after completion of resuscitation. Burn patients find difficulty while chewing the food so special diet has to be prepared for them and administered through nasogastric tube. Small measured quantity is given per hourly basis and monitored continuously. The buttermilk diet is the safe and well-tolerated food for the burns patients, it contains 1 kcal energy per mL. It consists of curd—1 L, eggs—four, banana—four, sugar—four tablespoons. The total volume to be made is 1,760 mL, energy content is 1,760 kcal, protein content is 60 g, and carbohydrate content is 340 g. The starting quantity is 10 mL/h for every 6 hours to reach a maximum of 3–5 mL/kg/h for children and 2 mL/kg/h for adults.[17]

CONCLUSION

Burns is a life-threatening trauma. Understanding the physiology and imparting good critical care is mandatory to improve the survival rate. The recent development of modern techniques with respect to critical care, such as fluid resuscitation protocols, early burn excision, antimicrobial and infection control, nutritional support, have led to the improvement of the rate of morbidity and mortality due to burns.

REFERENCES

1. Kolarsick PAJ, Kolarsick MA, Goodwin C. Anatomy and physiology of the skin. J Dermatol Nurses Assoc. 2011;4:203-13.
2. Garcia-Espinoza JA, Aguilar-Aragon VB, Ortiz-Villalobos EH, et al. Burns: definition, classification, pathophysiology and initial approach. Gen Med (Los Angeles). 2017;5:5.

3. Hettiaratchy S, Dziewulski P. Pathophysiology and types of burns. BMJ. 2004;328(7453):1427-9.
4. Monstrey S, Hoeksema H, Verbelen J, et al. Assessment of burn depth and burn wound healing potential. Burn. 2008;34:762-9.
5. National Programme for Prevention, Management and Rehabilitation of Burn Injuries (NPPMRBI). Practical Handbook of Burns Management. Burns-extent and severity. Chapter 6, Page 19 (dghs.gov.in/WriteReadData/userfiles/file/Practical_ handbook-revised_Karoon.pdf).
6. National Programme for Prevention, Management and Rehabilitation of Burn Injuries (NPPMRBI). Practical Handbook of Burns Management. Burns of special sites. Chapter 10, Page 33 (dghs.gov.in/WriteReadData/userfiles/file/Practical_ handbook-revised_Karoon.pdf).
7. Dziewulski P, Villapalos JL, Barret JP. Adult burn management. In: Handbook of burns acute burn care, acute management of facial burns. 2012;1:291-310.
8. Zatriqi V, Arifi H, Zatriqi S, et al. Facial burn—our experience. Mater Sociomed. 2013;25(1):26-7.
9. Sarabahi S. Chapter 14, Burn wound management. Principle and Practice of burn care. 2010. p.154.
10. Tandon R, Agrawal K, Narayan RP, et al. Firecracker injuries during Diwali festival: the epidemiology and impact of legislation in Delhi. Indian J Plast Surg. 2012;45:97-101.
11. Yin S. Chemical and common burns in children. Clin Pediatr (Phila). 2017;56(5_suppl):8S-12S.
12. [online] Available from http://mclaren.adam.com/content. aspx. Valid URL: http://www.mayoclinic.com/health/first-aid-burns/FA00022. Product Id=117& pid=1& gid=000030.
13. Hettiaratchy S, Papini R. Initial management of a major burn: II—assessment and resuscitation. BMJ. 2004;329(7457):101-3.
14. Murari A. A modified Lund and Browder chart. Indian J Plast Surg. 2017;50(2):220-1.
15. Haberal M, Sakallioglu Abali AE, Karakayali H. Fluid management in major burn injuries. Indian J Plast Surg. 2010;43(Suppl):S29-36.
16. Jones WG, Madden M, Finkelstein J, et al. Tracheostomies in burn patients. Ann Surg. 1989;209(4):471-4.
17. Wong L, Spence RJ. Escharotomy and fasciotomy of the burned upper extremity. Hand Clin. 2000;16(2):165-74.
18. Keswani, SM. In: Udwadia FE (Ed). Management of critically ill burns patients. Principles of critical care. 3rd edition, 2014. pp. 794-804.

CHAPTER 26

Necrotizing Soft Tissue Infections

Rob Bevan

INTRODUCTION

Necrotizing soft tissue infection (NSTI) is the broad term used to describe an acute, rapidly progressing necrosis of the skin, subcutaneous tissues, and muscle as a result of microbial infection. NSTI can in turn progress to sepsis, organ failure, and death.[1]

NSTI can arise as a result of seemingly trivial injury, with either an inoculation source through the epidermis or via hematogenous infiltration. Localized infection can progress in the deeper layers of adipose tissue, fascia, and muscle with little to see on surface inspection, potentially hindering the diagnosis and leading to delays in identification and treatment with significant adverse consequences.[2]

Necrotizing fasciitis (NF) is the term which was used by Wilson in 1952 to describe NSTIs which extend to the fascia, but spare the underlying muscle,[3] although alternative terms such as "gangrene" were described prior to this, notably in a case series by Meleney in 1924.[4]

EVIDENCE

Classification

Necrotizing soft tissue infections can be classified according to their depth (e.g. cellulitis, fasciitis, myositis), or their anatomical location (e.g. Fournier's gangrene involving the perianal area from enteric or urethral entry, or Ludwig's angina affecting the submandibular facial spaces).[5,6]

A classification which is based on microbiological cause was devised in 1977 by Giuliano et al.[7] They divided NF into two main entities, based on whether the infection was poly- or monomicrobial. Although *Group A Streptococcus* (GAS) and *Staphylococcus aureus* were the predominant organisms cultured from patients in these early series, there was conjecture as to the role of the less often cultured growth of Gram-negative bacterial strains.[3,4,7] This led to reporting of three main entities:[2]

1. NF type I: Polymicrobial involving aerobic and anaerobic organisms.
2. NF type II: Monomicrobial, usually from a Gram-positive organisms.
3. NF type III: Monomicrobial, from a Gram-negative organism.

A more recent review has combined types II and III into one entity, returning the nomenclature back to type I "polymicrobial" and type II "mono-microbial," which shall be used for the remainder of this chapter.[6]

Type I Necrotizing Fasciitis

Type I infections have traditionally been thought to be the most prevalent form of NSTI, occurring in 55–75% of cases,[8] although others have reported an equal proportion of mono- and polymicrobial presentations.[9] Polymicrobial infection can involve both aerobic and anaerobic bacteria, with up to ten different organisms cultured in the wounds of some patients.[10]

There are several risk factors which may predispose patients to type I NF: Older age, the presence of comorbidity, immunocompromised, diabetes mellitus, peripheral vascular disease, chronic ulcers, or lower gastrointestinal or urogenital mucosal breaches in particular.[6]

Type II Necrotizing Fasciitis

Type II infections are monomicrobial, with by far the most common organisms in this group being Gram-positive bacteria. GAS predominates, with methicillin-resistant *S. aureus* the next commonest.[2,6]

Type III Necrotizing Fasciitis

Infection with Gram-negative organisms is less common but well described: *Vibrio vulnificus* and *Aeromonas hydrophilia* may be introduced via wounds sustained in salt and freshwater, respectively.[6] Monomicrobial growth of *Clostridium* species (*C. perfringens*, *C. histolyticum*, or *C. novyi*) account for the NSTI previously called "gas gangrene," typically following severe crush or penetrating trauma.[6]

Patients presenting with type II NF are generally younger, healthier, and more likely to have a history of surgery, trauma, or intravenous drug use.[2] The exception to this would be those who present with *Escherichia coli* infection, who tend to be more similar in risk factor profile to type I NF patients.[6]

Epidemiology

Necrotizing soft tissue infection has been described as being "exceedingly rare," with a rate in the US population of 0.04 cases per 1,000 person years.[11] This seems low, given much higher reported rates elsewhere, including in the author's hospital in South Auckland, New Zealand.[12,13] The highest annual rates reported were in Thailand, with 15 cases per 100,000 population—more than three times that of New Zealand.[14]

The incidence of NF had been thought to be increasing; however, our experience in Auckland has been of a gradual decrease in the incidence of NF since an annual peak of 5 cases per 100,000 population in 2004.[9] Trends have been stable in much larger data sets from the United States.[15] Reported mortality for all patients with NF has ranged from 10% to 40%, albeit over numerous studies confounded by improvements over the last four decades in recognition, treatment, and access to critical care services. Notwithstanding, NSTI mortality remains high (up to 70%) for those with established organ failure.[16]

Pathophysiology

There are two main mechanisms by which microorganisms can gain entry to deep tissues and trigger a process which leads to NSTI:[6]

- *Direct portal of entry via a break in the skin or mucosa:* These may be as trivial as minor lacerations, insect bites, or deroofed viral vesicles. The local invasion of microorganism leads to endotoxin release in the dermis, triggering an acute inflammatory reaction presenting as erythema, swelling, and pain. This reaction ultimately results in vascular endothelial activation, platelet aggregation, microvascular occlusion, and necrosis, which in turn manifests macroscopically as bullae and ecchymoses. The "vicious cycle" of localized ischemia, inflammation, vascular occlusion, and necrosis extends the zone of infection deeper until the fascial plane is involved. This is summarized in Figure 26.1.

- *Hematogenous spread to a deep tissue injury in the context of bacteremia:* A trivial injury may result in localized deep tissue inflammation which activates the body's usual repair processes, with the inherent chemotaxis of a host of repair cells interacting with an activated endothelium via the milieu of cytokines and adhesion molecules. A concomitant transient bacteremia—for example, as a result of a streptococcal respiratory tract infection—results in carriage of organisms to the site and subsequent binding of the organism within the deep tissue. Further bacterial proliferation and activation of the same vicious cycle of inflammation, vascular occlusion, and necrosis described above leads to a similar pattern of tissue damage. This is summarized in Figure 26.2.

The local effects of NSTI can rapidly spread to produce systemic inflammation, multiorgan failure, and death, with the precise mechanism depending on the organism.

While a detailed description of the complexities of the inflammatory cascade is outside the scope of this chapter, the mechanism associated with Group A streptococcus (GAS) deserves a special mention: GAS is able to trigger an immune inflammatory response by bypassing the usual mechanism of antigen presentation. Most bacterial antigens would be presented to a tiny fraction of T-lymphocytes, which would then initiate a proportionate inflammatory response. The M-protein expressed on the GAS is able to directly activate up to 20% of all T cells, resulting in a cytokine release which is orders of magnitude higher than would otherwise result from conventional bacterial antigenic

Section 2: Organ Dysfunction

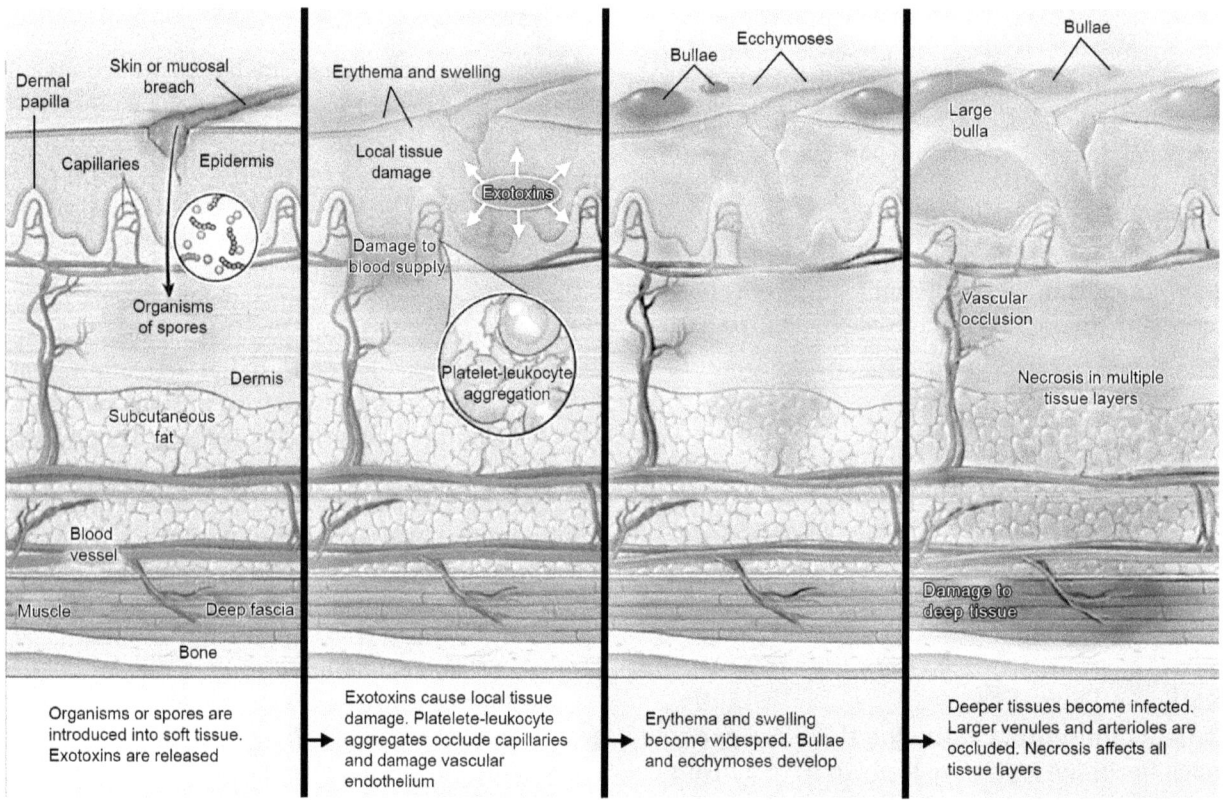

FIGURE 26.1: Infection through a skin or mucosal breach.
Source: Stevens.[6]

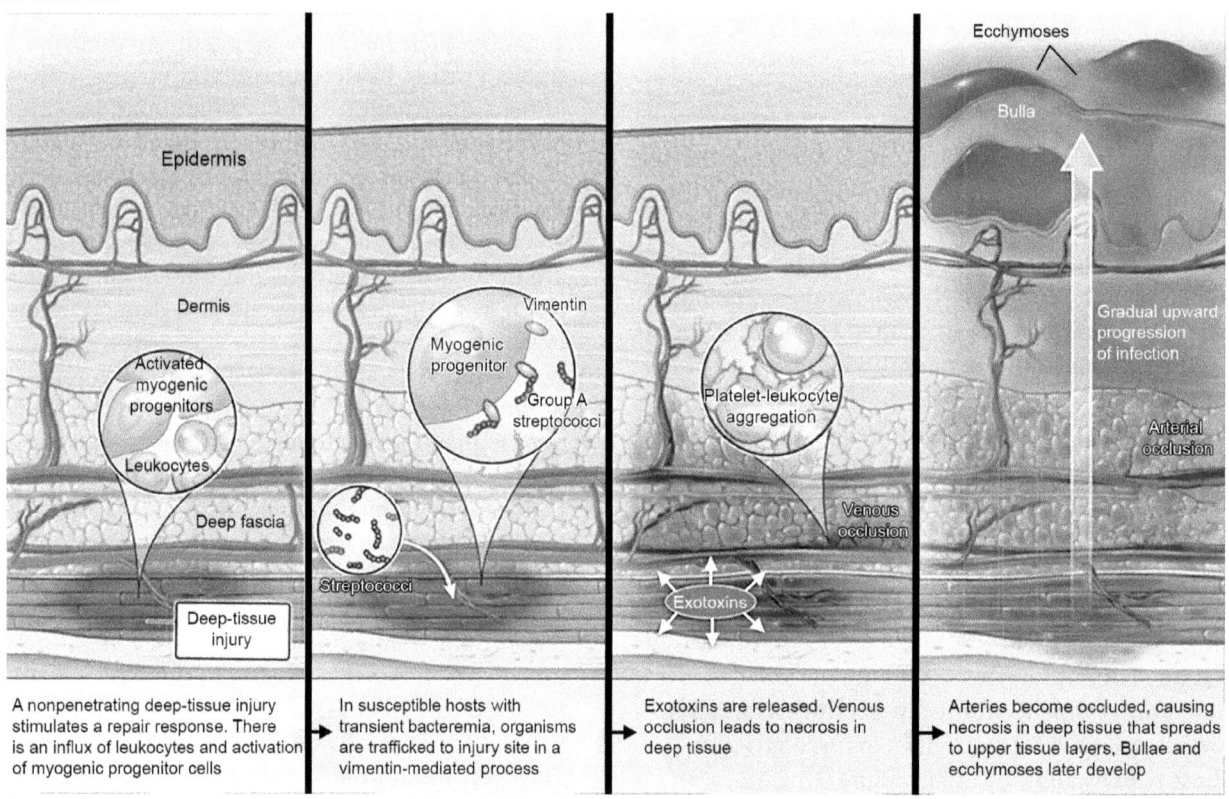

FIGURE 26.2: Hematogenous spread of a transient bacteremia.
Source: Stevens.[6]

presentation.[2] This "superantigen" effect results in the relative disproportionate response of widespread endothelial damage, capillary leak, and intravascular hemolysis which can rapidly lead to end-organ damage, failure, and death.

PRACTICE PRESCRIPTION

Patient Assessment

The most important task when assessing a patient with soft tissue infection is to identify the presence of a necrotizing process.[17] The initial presentation of patients with early NSTI will overlap those with less severe infections, such as cellulitis or a forming abscess. Delineating the patient with emerging NSTI from those with cellulitis is probably the most challenging aspect of management.[1] The postoperative surgical patient provides a further potential source of diagnostic error if NSTI is not considered in the differential of severe pain—especially after abdominal, rectal, or gynecological surgery.[6]

A delay in diagnosis results in an inherent delay to achieving source control, which in this condition is strongly associated with increased morbidity and mortality.[17] *As a result, it has been postulated and remains the protocol within the author's hospital that all STIs are admitted under surgical services in the hope that this may contribute to earlier detection of features suggesting an NSTI.*[9]

A suggested algorithm for the initial workup of patients suspected of having NSTI is presented in Figure 26.3. While pain, erythema, and fever will be common, a low index of suspicion should exist for patients who present with pain out of proportion to the cutaneous signs.[2] The presence of bullae, crepitus from gas in the subcutaneous tissue (either on palpation or imaging), or evidence of acute progression despite appropriate prior antibiotic therapy indicates the patient is potentially entering a late stage of disease, and emergent surgical consultation is warranted.

Necrotizing soft tissue infection should be on the differential for patients presenting with sepsis, even if they do not complain of the classic triad of pain, erythema, and fever: nonsteroidal anti-inflammatory drugs or other antipyretic use may mask fever; opiates, neuropathy, or obtundation may mask pain.[6]

Investigations should be targeted at obtaining the microbiological diagnosis, stratifying risk, and assessing for end-organ complications.

There are scoring systems aimed at discriminating between necrotizing from nonnecrotizing infections; the most well known is the Laboratory Risk Indicator for Necrotizing Fasciitis (LRINEC), which is outlined in Tables 26.1 and 26.2.[18]

Table 26.1: The LRINEC score.

Variable	Score
C-reactive protein (mg/mL)	
<150	0
>150	4
White blood cell count (per mm³)	
<15	0
15–25	1
>25	2
Hemoglobin (g/dL)	
>13.5	0
11–13.5	1
<11	2
Sodium (mmol/L)	
>135	0
<135	2
Creatinine (μmol/L)	
<141	0
>141	2
Glucose	
<10	0
>10	1

(LRINEC: laboratory risk indicator for necrotizing fasciitis)

Table 26.2: Predicting NSTI from LRINEC score [Anaya].

Risk group	LRINEC score	Probability of NSTI (%)
Low	Less than 5	<50
Intermediate	6–7	50–75
High	8 or more	>75

(NSTI: Necrotizing soft tissue infection; LRINEC: laboratory risk indicator for necrotizing fasciitis)

Although, the reported positive predicted value of a LRINEC score of 6 or above is reported to be as high as 92%, it has never been validated. The score performs poorly in children and could be affected by sepsis or inflammation from other sources.[2,6] Although a high LRINEC score has been incorporated into a diagnostic algorithm for NF in a recent review, it is unclear what effect a lower score would have (if any) on the suggested workup.[6] For this reason the LRINEC score is not incorporated into Flowchart 26.1.

Given the potential for the patient to present with organ dysfunction, the investigation of NSTI should occur in parallel with hemodynamic resuscitation, institution of early and appropriately broad-spectrum antimicrobials,

FLOWCHART 26.1: Management algorithm for suspected NSTI. (NSTI: Necrotizing soft tissue infection).

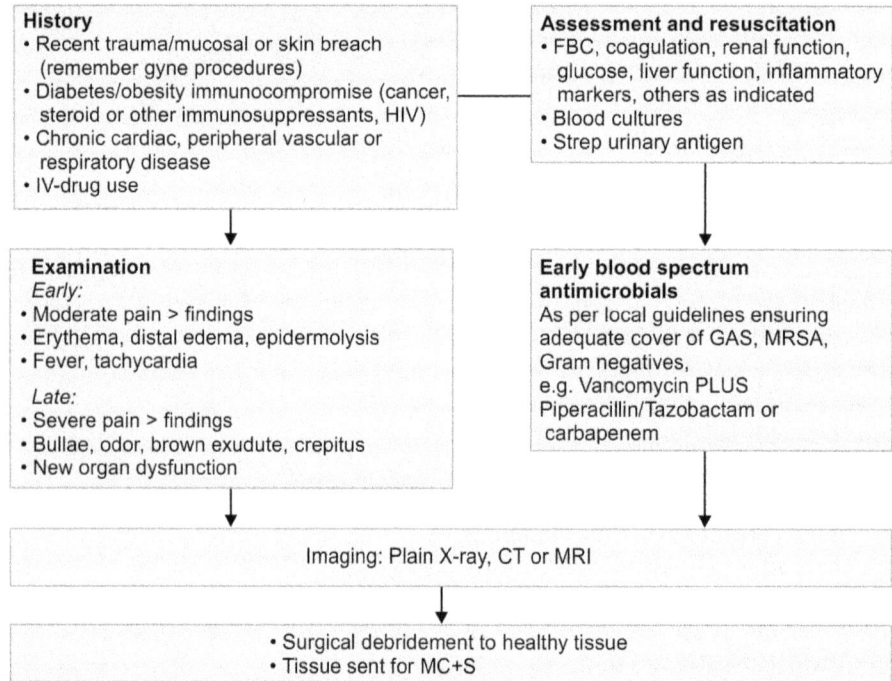

(IV: intravenous; FBC: full blood count; GAS: group A Streptococcus; MRSA: methicillin-resistant staphylococcus; MRI: magnetic resonance imaging)

early involvement of critical care services, and most importantly coordination of an urgent surgical opinion. *Although interim admission to the intensive care unit may be required, this should not delay the patient proceeding to surgery when NSTI is suspected.*

A suspicion of NSTI warrants surgical exploration, which constitutes dissection down to the fascia, a visual inspection (for a transition from shiny white to dull gray), palpation (for the presence of a tan fluid leaking from the tissues), and incision to confirm healthy underlying muscle beneath. *All necrotic tissue must be excised* back to bleeding healthy tissue, and this intervention by itself may markedly improve the patient's condition.[19] There may be a need for more than one operation to ensure the necrosis has not spread.

Patients with NSTI would usually be managed on an intensive care unit following their trip to surgery—usually remaining intubated if a return to surgery is expected, for titration of hemodynamic support, and observation and other organ supports as required. Good supportive care, with attention to adequate nutrition, prevention of thrombotic or bleeding complications, is paramount. So too is the early involvement of the multidisciplinary team in planning rehabilitation.

Adjunctive treatments have been postulated to have a role in the management of NSTI:

❏ *Hyperbaric oxygen (HBO)* involves the therapeutic administration of 100% oxygen at a supraatmospheric pressure, from within a hyperbaric chamber.[20] HBO is postulated to be beneficial in NSTI via the provision of improved partial pressure of oxygen in the necrotic tissue. This is thought to improve antibiotic efficacy and immune cell function—postulated to improve patient outcomes.[20] HBO is however a controversial treatment, as there are significant theoretical risks.[20] The results of the 2015 Cochrane analysis of the role of HBO in NF are easy to summarize—there were no studies whatsoever of sufficient quality to include in the analysis; therefore, there is no reliable data to recommend incorporating HBO into the management of NSTI.[20]

❏ *Intravenous immunoglobulin (IVIG)* has also been postulated as an adjunctive treatment, especially for type II NF due to GAS. Only one multicenter, double-blind randomized control trial has been reported for streptococcal toxic-shock syndrome, which showed a faster resolution in organ failure sequential organ failure assessment score, but no significant mortality benefit.[21] At present, there is no proven role for IVIG in the management of NSTI.

SUMMARY

Necrotizing soft tissue infection is a life-threatening condition which can initially masquerade as a trivial infection or a vague painful illness. If unrecognized and/or appropriate management is delayed, the condition can rapidly escalate to a life-threatening emergency. Even when managed optimally, NSTI has a high mortality. Of those who survive, there is a high burden of morbidity related both to the effects of surgical debridement, and the increasingly apparent effects of prolonged critical illness.

REFERENCES

1. Cainzos M, Gonzales-Rodriguez F. Necrotizing soft tissue infections. Curr Opin Crit Care. 2007;13:433-9.
2. Hakkarainen T, Kopari N, Pham T, et al. Necrotizing soft tissue infections: review and current concepts in treatment, systems of care, and outcomes. Curr Probl Surg. 2014;51(8):344-62.
3. Wilson. Necrotizing fasciitis. Am Surg. 1952;18(4):416-31.
4. Meleney F. Hemolytic streptococcus gangrene. Arch Surg. 1924;9:317.
5. Schwartz M, Pasternack M. Cellulitis and subcutaneous tissue infections. In: Mandell G, Bennett J, Dolin R (Eds). Principles and practice of infectious diseases, 6th edition. Philadelphia, PA: Churchill Livingstone; 2005. pp. 1172-94.
6. Stevens D, Bryant A. Necrotizing soft-tissue infections. N Engl J Med. 2017;377:2253-65.
7. Giuliano A, Lewis F, Hadley K, et al. Bacteriology of necrotizing fasciitis. Am J Surg. 1977;134(1):52-7.
8. Howell G, Rosengart M. Necrotizing soft tissue infections. Surg Infect. 2011;12:185-90.
9. Kulasagaran S, Cribb B, Vandal A, et al. Necrotizing fasciitis: 11-year retrospective case review in South Auckland. ANZ J Surg. 2016;86(10):826-30.
10. McGee E. Necrotizing fasciitis review of pathophysiology, diagnosis and treatment. Crit Care Nurs Q. 2005;28(1):80-4.
11. Simonsen E, Orman E, van Hatch B, et al. Cellulitis incidence in a defined population. Epidemiol Infect. 2006;134(2):293-9.
12. Nisbett M, Ansell G, Lang S, et al. Necrotizing fasciitis: review of 82 cases in South Auckland. Intern Med J. 2011;41(7):543-8.
13. Mitchell A, Williams A, Dzendrowskyj P. Necrotising fasciitis: an 8.5-year retrospective case review in a New Zealand intensive care unit. Crit Care Resusc. 2011;13(4):232-7.
14. Khamnuan P, Chongruksut W, Jearwattanakanok K, et al. Necrotising fasciitis: epidemiology and clinical predictors for amputation. Int J Gen Med. 2015;8:195-202.
15. Arif N, Yousifi S, Vinnard C. Deaths from necrotizing fasciitis in the United States 2003-2013. Epidemiol Infect. 2016;144(6):1338-44.
16. Stevens D, Bisno A, Chambers H, et al. Practice guidelines for the diagnosis and management of skin and soft tissue infections: 2014 update by the Infectious Diseases Society of America. Clin Infect Dis. 2014;59:147-59.
17. Anaya D, Dellinger P. Necrotizing and soft tissue infection: diagnosis and management. Clin Infect dis. 2007;44:705-10.
18. Wong C, Khin L, Heng K, et al. The LRINEC (Laboratory Risk Indicator for Necrotizing Fasciitis) score: a tool for distinguishing necrotizing fasciitis from other soft tissue infections. Crit Care Med. 2004;32:1535-41.
19. Cocanour C, Chang P, Huston J, et al. Management and novel adjuncts of necrotizing soft tissue infections. Surg Infect. 2017;18(3):250-72.
20. Levett D, Bennett M, Millar I. Adjunctive hyperbaric oxygen for necrotizing fasciitis. Cochrane Database Syst Rev. 2015;1:CD007937.
21. Norrby-Teglund A, Ihendyane N, Darenberg J. Intravenous immunoglobulin adjunctive therapy in sepsis, with special emphasis on severe invasive group A streptococcal infections. Scan J Infect Dis. 2003;35(9):683-9.

CHAPTER 27

Metabolic Acidosis

Michael AJ Park, Ross Callum Freebairn

INTRODUCTION

The human body contains and produces acids that are essential for life, including metabolic activity, protein synthesis, and digestion. In human blood the majority of acids are in an aqueous solution (plasma, interstitial fluid, cerebrospinal fluid, or intracellular) and are referred to by their anion. These acids are classified into either "strong acids" or "weak acids." Strong acids almost fully dissociate or ionize (>99%), however, weak acids only partially ionize or dissociate.[1] Acids dissociate in plasma to form a hydrogen ion (H^+) and the acid's anion or conjugate base. Lactic acid acts as a strong acid at physiological pH because it almost fully dissociates in plasma to form H^+ ions and its anion, lactate. Protein, phosphate, and bicarbonate are examples of weak acids that only partially dissociate. Bicarbonate acts as a buffer because the degree of its dissociation is dependent on the current acidity of the solution.

The hydrogen-ion concentration within the plasma is usually maintained within a narrow range with the normal physiological concentration of hydrogen ion of 40 nmol/L or mEq/L that equates to a pH of 7.4.

METABOLIC ACIDOSIS VERSUS ACIDEMIA

The body's ability to regulate hydrogen-ion concentration or pH and maintain a constant level is crucial for cellular metabolism and normal physiology. There is a very large turnover of hydrogen ions every day, and the average adult will produce acids that add approximately 1-1.5 mmol/kg of hydrogen ions.

Acidosis is a clinical disturbance that occurs when the amount of acid in the plasma has increased. This may be due to increased production of acids, reduced metabolism of acids, reduced excretion of acids, or ingestion/administration of exogenous acid. The term "metabolic acidosis" covers all nonvolatile acids and therefore essentially includes all acids in the plasma with the exception of respiratory acid, carbonic acid (H_2CO_3).[2]

When the plasma acidity increases the body will attempt to maintain a normal hydrogen-ion concentration through its buffering and compensatory mechanism. The buffers include the volatile acid, carbonic acid, and the following nonvolatile acids albumin, globulins, and phosphate.

A metabolic *acidosis* can occur despite a normal pH or hydrogen-ion concentration. However, biochemically, there is usually respiratory compensation highlighted by a decrease in both PCO_2 and HCO_3 concentration, and depending on the cause a raised anion gap.

Metabolic *acidemia* occurs when the amount of acid in the blood overwhelms the compensatory mechanism, and the pH falls (below 7.35), or the hydrogen-ion concentration exceeds 40 nmol/L. As with metabolic acidosis, biochemically, there will usually be a decrease in PCO_2 and HCO_3, and depending on the cause a raised anion gap.

GAMBLEGRAM

Due to the law of electrical neutrality, there must be an equal amount of positive (cations) and negative (anions)

Metabolic Acidosis

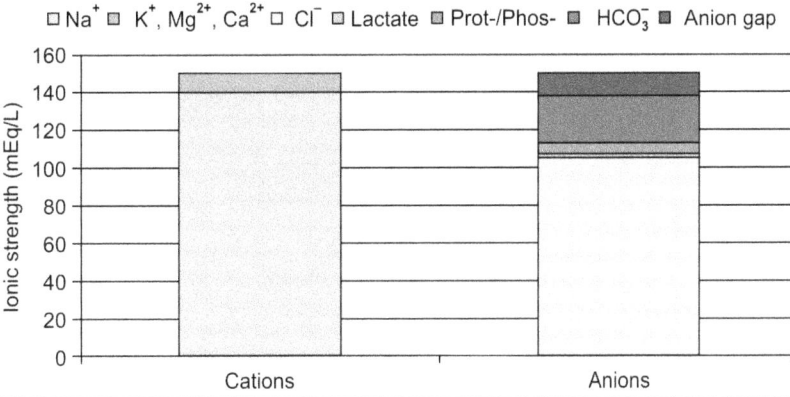

FIGURE 27.1: Gamblegram.

ions. Cations are formed when a metal loses electrons and a nonmetal gains electrons. In the human plasma the commonly measured cations are sodium (Na^+), potassium (K^+), magnesium (Mg^{2+}), calcium (Ca^{2+}), and hydrogen (H^+).[3] The more commonly measured anions are chloride (Cl^-), bicarbonate (HCO_3^-), albumin ion, phosphate (PO_4^-), and lactate.

The gamblegram has two columns, one for cations and one for anions (Fig. 27.1). Each column contains the total amount of either measured cations or anions that are added together according to their ionic strength rather than molar quantity. Hydrogen-ion concentration is on the top of the cation column, but as it is about a million times smaller (nanomoles per liter rather than millimoles per liter) than the other measured cations, it cannot be seen.[4]

BICARBONATE

Bicarbonate is a negatively charged ion that helps maintain electroneutrality. It is essentially a measure of CO_2 in the blood, and it is a dependent variable and influenced by the hydrogen-ion concentration via the carbonic acid/bicarbonate dissociation equilibrium below. It is a physiological buffer and referred as a volatile weak electrolyte because it is in equilibrium with PCO_2.

$$H_2O + CO_2 \leftrightarrow H_2CO_3 \leftrightarrow HCO_3^- + H^+$$

Bicarbonate has a close relationship with chloride, especially in the plasma membrane Cl^-/HCO_3^- exchangers that are located throughout the human body where bicarbonate ions are exchanged with chloride ions to maintain electroneutrality.[5] Due to this relationship and as a result of the difficulty measuring chloride when the Henderson–Hasselbach equation was developed, bicarbonate was seen as the "metabolic" anion rather than chloride.

EVALUATING METABOLIC ACIDOSIS

Metabolic acidosis is not uncommon in patients in the critical care setting, and the degree of metabolic acidosis can be associated with poor outcomes.[6] Compared to respiratory acidosis, the cause of metabolic acidosis can vary depending on the underlying disorder(s) and can be difficult to treat.

There are various ways of evaluating metabolic acidosis. However, the underlying cause can be essentially broken down into three disorders.
1. A relative increase in chloride ion concentration
2. An increase in endogenous acid
3. An increase in exogenous acid

A relative increase in chloride ion concentration is usually associated with a metabolic acidosis with a low or normal anion gap. Any rise in chloride relative to sodium ion will result in an increase of hydrogen ion (HCl).[7] The other two, a rise in either endogenous or exogenous acid, are usually associated with a raised anion gap. The underlying cause of a metabolic acidosis may be due to one, two, or all three disorders.

Two methods will be discussed to evaluate the cause of the metabolic acidosis, the anion gap and the net unmeasured ions (NUI), previously known as the strong ion gap.[8]

ANION GAP METHOD

As stated above, human plasma should contain an equal amount of anions and cations. However, the amount of the routinely measured cations in plasma is always greater than the amount of the measured anions, resulting in an "anion gap." The formula used clinically is shown below.

Anion gap = measured Na^+ - (measured Cl^- + bicarbonate)
= 6–12 mEq/L (see Fig. 27.2)

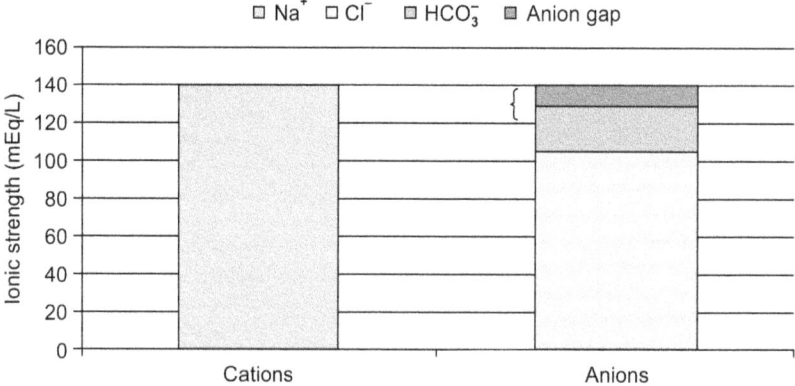

FIGURE 27.2: Anion gap.

Some calculations include the potassium, which effectively adds 4 to the cation total. As potassium does not vary physiological very much (less than ±2 mmol/L), it adds little to the variation in anion gap and is usually omitted. The formula does not include the other major cations, namely magnesium and calcium, however, these cations are tightly maintained by the body and therefore do not vary widely. In effect, magnesium and calcium counterbalance the other major anions that are not included in this calculation, phosphate, and lactate; however, both lactate and phosphate can increase significantly during illness. In health the calculated anion gap is made up of negatively charged proteins with the predominant protein being albumin.

The normal range for the anion gap will vary depending on the reference range for the measured electrolytes and also whether the measured potassium is added to sodium or not before subtracting the major anions. The anion gap can be low, normal, and elevated and can help evaluate the cause of metabolic acidosis. The most common causes of metabolic acidosis are usually due to either a normal anion gap acidosis or a raised gap acidosis.

NORMAL ANION GAP ACIDOSIS

Normal anion gap acidosis often occurs when the acidosis is due to a relative rise in chloride level compared to the sodium level. This was previously known as hyperchloremic acidosis, but this term is a misnomer because the acidosis can occur even if the chloride level is below its normal range.[9] It is the difference between chloride and sodium concentration that is relevant not the actual level of chloride.

A nonraised anion gap acidosis can be due to 0.9% NaCl administration, acetazolamide, and some renal tubular acidosis disorders.[10] These disorders can lead to a relative increase in plasma chloride concentration. Diarrhea, high output stomas, and a pancreatic fistula can also lead to a normal anion gap acidosis. Ileostomy and pancreatic fluids are sodium rich but relatively chloride poor.[11,12] The resulting sodium loss compared to chloride leads to the normal anion gap acidosis.

RAISED ANION GAP ACIDOSIS

In the anion gap method the measured anions are only chloride and bicarbonate. The anion gap can therefore include any other anion that has not been measured, including any endogenous and exogenous acids. Table 27.1 shows the causes of both normal and raised anion gap acidosis.[13,14]

The anion gap method is useful when dealing with one type of metabolic acidosis, but it does not help when dealing with critical care patients that may have a mixed metabolic acidosis.

Albumin contributes to the anion gap, and the reduction in circulating plasma albumin should result in a fall in the anion gap. Correction for the low albumin concentrations commonly present in the critically can be made using the equation of Figge: $AG + (0.25 \times (44 - albumin))$.[15]

THE PHYSIOCHEMICAL OR NET UNMEASURED IONS (STRONG ION GAP) METHOD

As mentioned above, in health the anion gap is mainly made up of proteins with the predominant protein being albumin. During critical illness, however, plasma albumin levels decrease, and the resulting effect is that the anion gap should decrease. This would result in a lowering of the hydrogen-ion concentration if all the other anions and cations remained normal. Hypoalbuminemia in isolation therefore can result in an alkalosis. Hypoalbuminemia is common during critical illness, however, there is usually a simultaneous increase in other anion or anions. An example is septic shock that normally results in hypoalbuminemia and a rise in lactate meaning that the calculated anion gap

Metabolic Acidosis

Table 27.1: Causes of a normal anion gap and raised anion gap acidosis.

Normal anion gap acidosis		Raised anion gap acidosis
Chloride effect	*Endogenous acid*	*Exogenous acid*
• Saline administration • Acetazolamide • Renal tubular acidosis – Chloride channel disturbances • Sodium loss – Diarrhea – High output ileostomy – Pancreatic fistula	• Renal failure – Sulfates – Phosphates – Hippurates – Urates • Lactic acidosis • Ketoacidosis – Diabetic – Starvation – Alcoholic • Pyroglutamic acid • Krebs cycle intermediates – Succinic acid • Acute-phase proteins • Aspartic acid • Homovanillic acid • Hydroxyphenyllactic acid	• Salicylates • Methanol (formate) • Glycolates • Formaldehyde (formate) • Toluene (hippurates) • Paraldehyde (acetate) • Gelatin • Ethylene glycol (oxalate)

may be normal or elevated. In effect the decrease in plasma albumin during illness can mask an underlying increase in an endogenous or exogenous acid.

The anion gap method of evaluating metabolic acidosis can have little diagnostic value when dealing with critically unwell patients. This is accentuated in patients who have multiple reasons for their metabolic acidosis such as a patient with an elevated chloride and low albumin concentration due to intravenous saline administration for their ethylene glycol-induced renal failure. In this case the metabolic acidosis would be due to chloride, an exogenous acid (e.g. oxalic acid), and endogenous acids (e.g. renal failure). The net unmeasured ion (NUI) method is essentially an evolved anion gap method because the calculation uses all the measured cations (hydrogen, sodium, magnesium, potassium, and calcium) and more of the anions (chloride, bicarbonate, lactate, phosphate, proteins, and albumin). The more anions that are measured the more accurate the NUI will be. If lactate is not measured nor used in the calculation then the lactate becomes part of the NUI. In essence, it is similar to base excess but corrected for the strong ions, proteins, phosphate, and PCO_2.

The NUI method is based on Stewart's strong ion difference (SID) but has been adapted by Peter Constable to look at plasma only.[16,17] The calculation is difficult to do without a computer, but the concept is relatively easy using the gamblegram. The equation includes the Henderson's equations, and therefore this method should be seen as an evolution rather than a revolution of the traditional method of interpreting acid–base disturbances.

Remember that the law of electrical neutrality means that each column of the gamblegram must be equal. The cation column can be calculated by measuring the concentration of hydrogen, sodium, calcium, magnesium, and potassium ions and calculating their ionic strength. The ionic strength of the anion column can be calculated by measuring chloride, bicarbonate, protein, albumin, lactate, urate, and phosphate. The ions with one negative or positive charge have an ionic strength of 1 mEq/L; however, magnesium, calcium, monohydrogen phosphate and sulfate have an ionic charge of three rather than 2 mEq/L.[18] If the two columns are not equal then there must be a quantity of unmeasured ions. In the example shown in Figure 27.3 the red portion of the anions column represents the quantity of unmeasured anions that must be present to the allow electrical neutrality.

ESTIMATING NUI USING ANION GAP CORRECTED FOR ALBUMIN AND LACTATE

When there are unmeasured anions contributing toward metabolic acidosis, there is normally marked difference between the calculated anion gaps compared to the measured anion gap. Negatively charged albumin is the predominant anion in the anion gap. Approximately, a quarter of plasma albumin is charged, and therefore the estimated anion gap is the measured albumin divided by 4.[19]

Example:

Na 140 mmol/L − (Cl 105 mmol/L + HCO_3^- 15 mmol/L) = measured anion gap: 20

Albumin 24/4 = estimated anion gap = 6

Lactate: 5 mmol/L

Estimated net unmeasured ions = (6 + 5) − 20 = −9 mEq/L

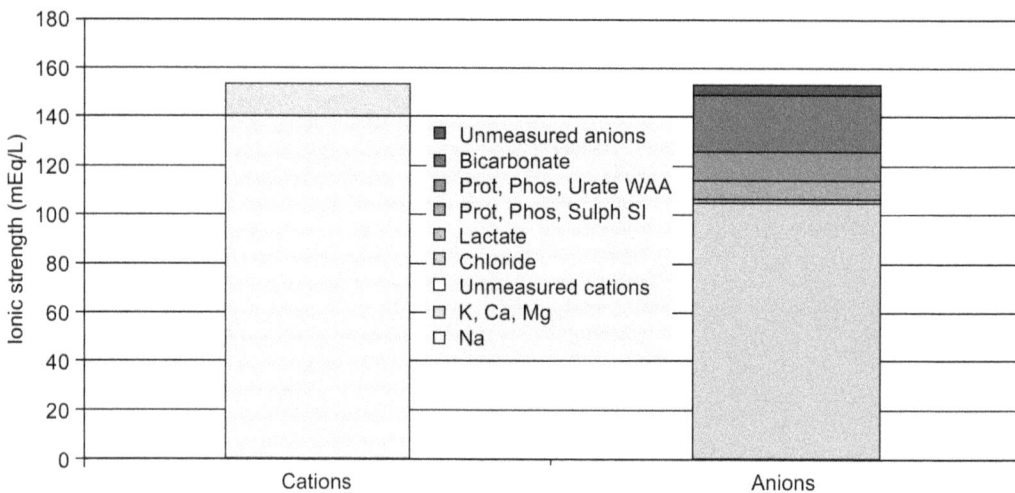

FIGURE 27.3: Net unmeasured ions (strong ion gap).

The estimated NUI becomes more accurate if the anion gap is also corrected for phosphate.[20] Although simple to calculate, this calculation assumes that the cations other than sodium are normal. Both the anion gap and the corrected anion gap will be inaccurate if there is an increase in cations, such as magnesium, calcium, lithium, and some paraproteins.

WHAT ARE THE NET UNMEASURED IONS (NUI)?

Essentially the net unmeasured ions (NUIs) are made up of any anion that has not been measured. In health the amount is ±2 mEq/L. In critical illness the amount increases depending on the underlying cause of the metabolic acidosis. In chloride-related metabolic acidosis (normal or low anion gap metabolic acidosis) the NUI will be close to zero because the chloride is a measured ion. NUI will also be zero if lactate is elevated and it has been used in the calculation. The composition of the NUI will be any unmeasured acid/anion that makes up the list of endogenous or exogenous acids seen in Table 27.1.

WHY MEASURE NUI?

The metabolic acidosis in critically ill patients can be multifactorial in origin and can include the chloride effect from saline administration. However, it is increased lactate and unmeasured ions that have been associated with increased mortality. NUI or strong ion gap is a significant predictor of outcome in critically unwell patients and is usually the main cause of metabolic acidosis.[21] NUI can be helpful to predict whether treatments are effective and also predict mortality in varying subsets of critically unwell patients.[22-24] It is also useful in the management of diabetic ketoacidosis (DKA) and can be used to track the ketones despite the acidifying effect of NaCl 0.9% administration from the increasing chloride levels and the alkalizing effect from the dilution of the plasma albumin concentration.

MANAGEMENT OF METABOLIC ACIDOSIS. IS IT H⁺ OR THE ANION THE PROBLEM?

Metabolic acidosis therefore simply represents a rise in any anion with an accompanying rise in hydrogen ion in order to maintain electroneutrality. Severe acidosis can have a deleterious effect on cellular function, tissue perfusion, and myocardial contractility. However, it remains unknown whether this deleterious effect is purely due to the hydrogen ion level. Sepsis-related metabolic acidemia is certainly associated with myocardial depression; however, patients with DKA do not have the same myocardial depression despite hydrogen ion levels that far exceed the levels associated with sepsis. This question is whether it is the hydrogen ion, the anion, or the reason behind the rise in the anion, and therefore hydrogen ion that causes the harmful effect? The rise in hydrogen-ion concentration may only be a marker of illness rather like a raised white cell count or C-reactive protein. Management of metabolic acidosis therefore requires the correction of the metabolic derangement that led to the anion and hydrogen ion rise (e.g. restoring tissue perfusion) or removal of the anion itself (e.g. dialysis for ethylene glycol ingestion).

EFFECT OF FLUIDS

Commonly prescribed intravenous fluids can have an effect on plasma acid–base balance depending on the fluids electrolyte content and the resulting effective SID (Table 27.2). Sodium chloride 0.9% solution contains equal

Table 27.2: The SID of commonly used intravenous fluids and its effect on the hydrogen ion concentration.					
Solution	0.9% NaCl	Ringer's lactate	PL148	Albumin 4%	5% Glucose
Na^+	150	130	140	140	0
Cl^-	150	109	98	128	0
SID	0	27	50	12	0
Effect on [H^+]	Increase	Slight decrease	Decrease	Increase	Increase

(Cl^-: chloride ion; H^+: hydrogen ion concentration; Na^+: sodium ion; PL148: plasmaLyte 148; SID: strong ion difference)

amounts of sodium and chloride, thus the SID is zero. The solution contains a significantly higher amount of chloride (about 50% higher) compared to human plasma, and the net effect following administration is to increase plasma chloride levels to a higher degree than the sodium. This leads to an elevated chloride anion relative to the sodium cation. In order to maintain electroneutrality the hydronium ion must increase, causing an acidemia. The increase in hydrogen-ion concentration drives the carbonic acid/bicarbonate equation toward CO_2 and H_2O. The acidemia will persist until the CO_2 is removed through ventilation. This phenomenon occurs with any fluid that has an effective SID that is less than the bicarbonate level (usually <25 mmol/L). Acidemia can occur with any fluid that has a SID of zero, including fluids with electrolytes, such as 5% glucose solution. This phenomenon was previously known incorrectly as a "dilutional acidosis."

Intravenous fluids that have an effective SID greater than 25 (e.g. PlasmaLyte 148) will result in a lower plasma chloride compared to sodium, resulting in a lowering of hydrogen ion and therefore an accompanying alkalosis.

Any protein containing fluid, such as albumin and gelatin, will result in an increase of negatively charged protein and will contribute toward the fluids SID. In the case of gelatin containing fluids the negatively charged gelatin can contribute to the rise in the NUI in plasma.[25]

It remains inconclusive at present whether the chloride-induced metabolic acidosis associated with 0.9% NaCl administration causes harm.

ROLE OF SODIUM BICARBONATE

Sodium bicarbonate has an in vitro SID of zero. In vivo, however, the bicarbonate will associate with hydrogen ions to form CO_2. If the body is unable to remove this excess CO_2 then sodium bicarbonate like any other fluid with a SID of zero would have an acidifying effect. However, through ventilation, the CO_2 can be cleared. This results in effectively giving a chloride-free sodium solution. The plasma sodium concentration will therefore increase relative to chloride. Sodium bicarbonate will therefore countereffect any acidosis, resulting from a relative rise in chloride due to the administration of chloride-rich fluids that have an effective SID less than 25. If there is a rise in an endogenous acid other than chloride (e.g. lactate) or a rise in exogenous acid (e.g. formates from methanol), then the administration of sodium bicarbonate will only mask the acidotic effect by lowering the hydrogen-ion concentration. It will not reverse the underlying disorder that led to the acidosis. Sodium bicarbonate to date has shown little mortality benefit in patients with severe metabolic acidosis.[26]

REFERENCES

1. Hamm L, Nakhoul N, Hering-Smith KS. Acid–base homeostasis. Clin J Am Soc Nephrol. 2015;10(12):2232-42.
2. Lloyd P. Strong ion calculator—a practical bedside application of modern quantitative acid–base physiology. Crit Care Resus. 2004;6:285-94.
3. Dias RP, Silvera IF. Observation of the Wigner-Huntington transition to metallic hydrogen. Science. 2017;355(6326):715-8.
4. Gamble JL. Chemical anatomy, physiology and pathology of extracellular fluid; a lecture syllabus, 5th edition. Cambridge: Harvard University Press; 1947.
5. Pfortmueller CA, Uehlinger D, von Haehling S, et al. Serum chloride levels in critical illness-the hidden story. Intensive Care Med Exp. 2018;6:10.
6. Gunnerson KJ, Saul M, He S, et al. Lactate versus non-lactate metabolic acidosis: a retrospective outcome evaluation of critically ill patients. Crit Care. 2006;10(1):R22.
7. Yunos NM, Bellomo R, Story D, et al. Bench-to-bedside review: chloride in critical illness. Crit Care. 2010;14:226.
8. Lloyd P, Freebairn RF. Using quantitative acid–base analysis in the ICU. Crit Care Resus. 2006;8:19-30.
9. Story DA. Hyperchloremic acidosis: another misnomer?. Crit Care Resus. 2004;6:188-92.
10. Constable, PD. Iatrogenic hyperchloremic acidosis due to large volume fluid administration. Int J Intensive Care. 2005;12:111-22.
11. Stevens T, Conwell DL, Zuccaro G, et al. Electrolyte composition of endoscopically collected duodenal drainage fluid after synthetic porcine secretin stimulation in healthy subjects. Gastrointest Endosc. 2004;60(3):351-5.
12. Levitan R, Goulston K. Water and electrolyte content of human ileostomy fluid after d-aldosterone administration. Gastroenterology. 1967;5(3):510-2.
13. Moviat M, Terpstra AM, Ruitenbeek W, et al. Contribution of various metabolites to the "unmeasured" anions in critically ill patients with metabolic acidosis. Crit Care Med. 2008;38(3):752-8.

14. Morgan TJ. What exactly is the strong ion gap, and does anybody care?. Crit Care Med. 2004;6:155-66.
15. Figge J, Rossing TH, Fencl V. The role of serum proteins in acid–base equilibria. J Lab Clin Med. 1991;117:453-67.
16. Stewart PA. Modern quantitative acid–base chemistry. Can J Physiol Pharmacol. 1983;61:1444-61.
17. Constable PD. A simplified strong ion model for acid–base equilibria: application to horse plasma. J Appl Physiol. 1997;83:297-311.
18. Murray JW. Activity Scales and Activity Corrections, Chapter 6, University of Washington. Available from https://www.ocean.washington.edu/courses/oc400/Lecture_Notes/CHPT6.pdf.
19. Constable, PD. Experimental determination of net protein charge and Atot and Ka of nonvolatile buffers in human plasma. J Appl Physiol. 2003;95:620-30.
20. Zampieri FG, Park M, Ranzani OT, et al. Anion gap corrected for albumin, phosphate and lactate is a good predictor of strong ion gap in critically ill patients: a nested cohort study. Rev Bras Intensiva. 2013;25(3):205-11.
21. Masevicius FD, Birri PNR, Vazquez AJ, et al. Relationship of at admission lactate, unmeasured anions, and chloride to the outcome of critically ill patients. Crit Care Med. 2017;45:e1233-9.
22. Kaplan LJ, Kellum JA. Initial pH, base deficit, lactate, anion gap, strong ion difference, and strong ion gap predict outcome from major vascular injury. Crit Care Med. 2004; 32(5):1120-4.
23. Balasubramanyan N, Havens PL, Hoffman GM. Unmeasured anions identified by the Fencl-Stewart method predict mortality better than base excess, anion gap, and lactate in patients in the pediatric intensive care unit. Crit Care Med. 1999;27(8):1577-81.
24. Drolz A, Horvatits T, Roedl K, et al. Acid–base status and its clinical implications in critically ill patients with cirrhosis, acute-on-chronic liver failure and without liver disease. Ann Intensive Care. 2018;8:48.
25. Morgan TJ. Clinical review: the meaning of acid–base abnormalities in the intensive care unit-effects of fluid administration. Crit Care. 2005;9(2):204-11.
26. Jaber S, Paugam C, Futier E, et al. Sodium bicarbonate therapy for patients with severe metabolic acidaemia in the intensive care unit (BICAR-ICU): a multicentre, open label, randomised controlled, phase 3 trial. Lancet. 2018;392(10141):31-40.

CHAPTER 28

Anaphylaxis

B Craig Ellis

INTRODUCTION

Anaphylaxis is a generalized hypersensitivity reaction, characterized by vasodilation ("flare" or erythema, distributive shock), extravasation of fluid (angioedema, hypovolemic shock), and smooth muscle contraction (bronchospasm, cramping visceral, and/or uterine pain). Impaired cardiac function may also occur although the contribution of this effect is difficult to define because of the multiple other pathophysiological changes causing hypotension in anaphylaxis.

The clinical definition of anaphylaxis is a skin rash accompanied by the involvement of at least one of the cardiovascular (e.g. low blood pressure, signs of poor perfusion or collapse), respiratory (e.g. stridor or bronchospasm), or gastrointestinal systems (e.g. abdominal pain, vomiting, or diarrhea), following exposure to an antigen. A consensus clinical definition has been developed that can be used for both research and clinical application (Box 28.1).[1] It is important to note that skin features may be absent in about 20% of cases.[2] Therefore, if an otherwise young and healthy patient presents with sudden cardiovascular collapse or severe bronchospasm, initial treatment as anaphylaxis is warranted even if the typical skin features are absent. A simple pragmatic approach to diagnosis that clinicians can use to trigger the administration of epinephrine is as in Box 28.2.

It is also important to note that bradycardia commonly accompanies hypotension in awake patients,[3] not tachycardia

BOX 28.1: National Institute of Allergy and Infectious Diseases/Food Allergy and Anaphylaxis Network consensus clinical definition of anaphylaxis.

Anaphylaxis is highly likely when any one of the following three criteria are fulfilled:
1. Acute onset of an illness (minutes to several hours) with involvement of the skin, mucosal tissue, or both (e.g. generalized hives, pruritus or flushing, swollen lips-tongue-uvula). And at least one of the following:
    i. Respiratory compromise (e.g. dyspnea, wheeze-bronchospasm, stridor, reduced PEF, hypoxemia)
    ii. Reduced BP or associated symptoms of end-organ dysfunction [e.g. hypotonia (collapse), syncope, incontinence]
2. Two or more of the following that occur rapidly after exposure to a likely allergen for that patient (minutes to several hours):
    i Involvement of the skin-mucosal tissue (e.g. generalized hives, itch-flush, swollen lips-tongue-uvula)
    ii Respiratory compromise (e.g. dyspnea, wheeze-bronchospasm, stridor, reduced PEF, hypoxemia)
    iii. Reduced BP or associated symptoms [e.g. hypotonia (collapse), syncope, incontinence]
    iv. Persistent gastrointestinal symptoms (e.g. crampy abdominal pain, vomiting)
3. Reduced BP after exposure to known allergen for that patient (minutes to several hours):
    i. Infants and children: Low systolic BP (age specific) or greater than 30% decrease in systolic BP
    ii. Adults: Systolic BP of less than 90 mm Hg or greater than 30% decrease from that person's baseline

---

(BP: blood pressure; PEF: peak expiratory function)

as is usually expect. Indeed, a sudden fall in heart rate after an initial tachycardia may herald impending cardiac arrest

Section 2: Organ Dysfunction

BOX 28.2: Pragmatic indications for epinephrine administration.

> *Any acute onset illness with typical skin features* (urticarial rash or erythema/flushing, and/or angioedema), PLUS involvement of *respiratory and/or cardiovascular* systems and/or persistent severe *gastrointestinal* symptoms
>
> OR
>
> *Any acute onset of hypotension or bronchospasm or upper airway obstruction* where anaphylaxis is considered possible, even if typical skin features are not present

and can be triggered by inappropriately placing the patient in an upright or semi-upright (sitting) position.[4]

CAUSES

Overall, the causes of anaphylaxis are roughly equally distributed between drugs (25%), stinging insect (*Hymenoptera*) venoms (25%), foods (25%), and unidentified/other causes (25%), although the relative proportions vary between geographical areas and populations. In urban settings, severe reactions in adults are usually due to drugs.[5] In rural and outdoor settings, severe reactions are predominantly due to *Hymenoptera* stings (venoms) or other insect bites (e.g. March or "Horse" flies), leech bites, snakebites, and marine venoms (e.g. jellyfish stings). Exercise may be a cofactor in some cases leading to so-called summative anaphylaxis where a stimulus (usually a physical one such as exertion, but also heat, cold, and alcohol have been suggested) appears to increase the sensitivity of mast cells to an immunoglobulin E (IgE)-mediated trigger in susceptible people. The main form of summative anaphylaxis is food-dependent, exercise-induced anaphylaxis, where the combination of exercise plus ingestion of the food (usually within 2 hours but sometimes as long as 5 hours) leads to sudden anaphylaxis with cardiovascular collapse during or soon after exercise. The food, despite the presence of specific IgE antibodies, is normally tolerated in the absence of exercise.[6] As well as exercise being a potential cofactor in triggering some reactions, reduced physiological reserve and lactic acidosis from strenuous exercise may significantly reduce physiological reserve and thus increase the severity of any reaction and make it resistant to treatment.

BIOCHEMICAL MEDIATORS

Allergen exposure results in activation of local mast cells. These respond by degranulation and the release of preformed and newly synthesized mediators. More generalized mediator release by other inflammatory cells and possibly also mast cells in areas remote from the allergen exposure then may occur, although the amplification mechanism for this process is poorly understood.[5,7]

Historically, we have focused on histamine as the main mediator involved in anaphylaxis. We now know that a wider spectrum of mediators are involved, including histamine, mast cell tryptase; tumor necrosis factor; a number of interleukins (ILs) (especially IL6, IL10 and tumor necrosis factor receptor I), leukotrienes, and complement breakdown products.[8] Therefore, any attempt at mediator antagonism is likely to be futile, and treatment relies on "physiological antagonism" with epinephrine and fluids to address: (1) dilation of blood vessels, (2) extravasation of fluid into the tissues, (3) impaired cardiac function, and (4) smooth muscle contraction in the lungs (bronchi) and gut.

CLINICAL PRESENTATION

The individual mediators cause specific physiological effects which, in turn, cause the signs and symptoms of anaphylaxis that we see clinically. Box 28.1 summarizes these clinical features in the context of a diagnostic approach to anaphylaxis.

Anaphylaxis is unique in how it produces the pattern of poor perfusion and shock seen clinically.[9] Anaphylaxis has been (and still is, in most teaching material) classified as distributive shock; however, it probably encompasses varying degrees of the four main types of shock mechanisms:

1. Cardiogenic—from a direct myocardial depressive effect from the mediators
2. Hypovolemic—from the loss of circulating volume into the tissues due to leaky blood vessels
3. Distributive—from the vasodilation of vessels resulting in pooling of the circulating volume
4. Obstructive—from vasoconstriction of the pulmonary arteries

Bradycardia may occur suddenly as a reflex response to poor venous return to the heart and a dramatic reduction in ventricular filling. There may be a reflex component to this, perhaps accentuated by anaphylactic mediators. The degree to which one factor contributes to the shock pattern seen varies depending on the allergen and the route of exposure.

Biphasic Response

Classically there have been concerns that there can be a recurrence of the anaphylaxis signs and symptoms 4–12 hours after initial resolution. It has variably been attributed to the effects of the adrenaline on the mediator cells wearing off or a recurrence of the initial triggering process. While biphasic responses do occur, they are rare and unlikely to be worse than the initial response but they may be delayed out to 12–24 hours. Most patients presenting with anaphylaxis do not need to be observed for a prolonged period post event when they have returned to baseline. Those who have presented in a life-threatening or peri-arrest state should be observed for a minimum of 12 hours.[5,10,11]

MANAGEMENT

The evidence on which management is based is extremely sparse, consisting of anecdote, some observational studies, animal studies, pathophysiological principles, and expert opinion. The cornerstones of recommended management are epinephrine and, in the presence of shock, intravenous fluid therapy.

Antihistamines

There is no evidence to support the routine use of antihistamines in anaphylaxis. There have been no randomized or good observational human studies supporting the use of H1 or H2 receptor blocking drugs.[12] There is also animal evidence of harm.[13,14] H1 antihistamines when administered parenterally have also been associated with hypotension.[15]

The administration of oral H1 antihistamines has a role in the treatment of symptomatic itch associated with urticarial rashes seen in hypersensitivity reactions (of which anaphylaxis is a subgroup), but none as a front-line treatment agent.

Glucocorticoid Steroids

There is no evidence to support the routine use of steroids.[16] There are similarities with asthma (where there is clear evidence of benefit from steroid treatment), and it has been proposed that they have a role in attempting to shorten the duration of symptoms and to reduce the incidence and severity of the biphasic response sometimes seen in anaphylaxis.[16] There is no evidence to suggest that steroids do either. We also do not know if there are any long-term effects on allergic reactivity from steroids given around the time of antigen exposure.

Approach to Treatment

The focus of the treatment of anaphylaxis must be one of placing the patient in a supine position, the administration of high flow oxygen, the administration epinephrine and, if required, intravenous fluid resuscitation.

General Measures

It has been demonstrated that rapid changes in posture may precipitate cardiac arrest, and those who remain in a sitting position once they have lost consciousness are at greater risk of cardiac arrest. A relative bradycardia is also seen in some patients following venom-mediated anaphylaxis associated with the onset of hypotension, although the exact mechanism is not known, this may in part explain the positional cardiac arrest that is sometimes seen.[4,9] Therefore, all patients displaying evidence of anaphylaxis should be laid supine early as a basic first aid measure and should not be propped in a sitting or semireclined position.

Epinephrine and Intravenous Fluids

Although there is no high-level evidence for the efficacy of epinephrine,[17] pathophysiological considerations, animal studies,[18] large case series,[19] and a prospective epinephrine infusion study, where reaction features stopped with epinephrine and returned when the infusion was stopped,[3] provide support for its likely usefulness.

The quickest and often effective route of initial administration for epinephrine is by intramuscular (IM) administration. Absorption by this route has been shown to be superior to subcutaneous administration.[20] In most patients, a single dose is all that is required; however, in ~30% of severe reactions, repeated doses can be required.[5]

The lack of response to IM administration is likely attributed to a combination of several effects—poor circulation and hence poor absorption from muscle beds and a need for higher systemic concentrations to reverse the cardiovascular effects of anaphylaxis. This is not infrequently seen in both hospital and prehospital practice and has been demonstrated in an animal model of severe anaphylaxis with cardiovascular collapse.

Bolus intravenous administration of epinephrine has historically been considered a high-risk activity and has not been recommended. It has been suggested that outside of a fully equipped resuscitation environment with monitoring facilities, intravenous epinephrine is not appropriate.[21]

The author has personal experience with the use of a dilute epinephrine infusion (1mg epinephrine in 1,000 mL normal saline titrated to effect) without invasive monitoring, central line access, or a syringe driver, in the place of bolus administration with no apparent loss of efficacy or increase in side effects. While this has not been subjected to a randomized trial, there is good observational evidence of efficacy and safety.[3] In cases where there has been failure to respond to IM dose(s), this option is supported by clinical guidelines produced by both the Therapeutic Guidelines Group (Australia) and the Australasian Society for Clinical Immunology and Allergy.[22,23]

Fluid therapy is the second mainstay of resuscitation behind epinephrine. Large volumes of fluid may be required. The majority of patients will respond to intravenous fluids and epinephrine.

BOX 28.3: Suggested management approach.

1. Lie patient supine
2. Administer 0.5 mg IM epinephrine (into lateral thigh if possible)
3. Administer high flow oxygen
4. Monitor conscious state, heart rate, blood pressure, respiratory rate, and SpO_2
5. Repeat IM 0.5 mg IM if no improvement within 10 minutes
6. Obtain IV access
7. If systolic BP <100 mm Hg and/or additional signs of poor perfusion, administer 1,000–2,000 mL of normal saline (if available)
8. If deteriorating despite IM epinephrine, consider 1:1,000,000 infusion*
    (1 mg into 1,000 mL normal saline or 0.5 mg into 500 mL or 0.25 mg into 250 mL)
    i. Administer at 1–2 mL a minute titrated to clinical effect.
    ii. Infusion can be increased up to "wide open" if required.

(BP: blood pressure; IM: intramuscular; IV: intravenous)

*Individual institutions have their own approaches and concentrations to epinephrine infusions. This approach provides a safe method which does not require invasive monitoring, central access, or a syringe driver or infusion pump to administer

We recommend an initial treatment regimen outlined in Box 28.3. The primary focus needs to continue to be on early IM administration of epinephrine but also recognition that there will be a small number of nonresponders that may require aggressive intravenous fluid resuscitation and intravenous epinephrine. Outside a resuscitation environment, a dilute infusion can be administered safely and efficaciously and is a viable option for health centers or smaller hospitals or clinics.

Other Measures

Some cases of very severe anaphylaxis appear to be resistant to epinephrine and fluids. Advanced procedures, including intubation/ventilation, potent vasoconstrictors (such as vasopressin or metaraminol), and mechanical cardiac support (intra-aortic balloon pump), have been reported as necessary to prevent death. These will be outside the scope of practice for most practitioners.

SUMMARY

Anaphylaxis is a relatively common resuscitative emergency. The diagnosis is usually formulaic but requires the practitioner to consider it as a possibility and initiate treatment aggressively and early. Optimal treatment is based around early IM epinephrine use and consideration of intravenous adrenaline if there is a slow or minimal response to the IM route. Proven adjunct therapy consists of supine positioning and the use of fluids to manage signs of shock.

REFERENCES

1. Sampson HA, Munoz-Furlong A, Campbell RL, et al. Second symposium on the definition and management of anaphylaxis: summary report—second National Institute of Allergy and Infectious Disease/Food Allergy and Anaphylaxis Network symposium. Ann Emerg Med. 2006;47(4):373-80.
2. Brown SGA. Clinical features and severity grading of anaphylaxis. J Allergy Clin Immunol. 2004;114(2):371-6.
3. Brown SGA, Blackman KE, Stenlake V, et al. Insect sting anaphylaxis; prospective evaluation of treatment with intravenous adrenaline and volume resuscitation. Emerg Med J. 2004;21(2):149-54.
4. Pumphrey RS. Fatal posture in anaphylactic shock. J Allergy Clin Immunol. 2003;112(2):451-2.
5. Brown SGA, Stone SF, Fatovich DM, et al. Anaphylaxis: clinical patterns, mediator release, and severity. J Allergy Clin Immunol. 2013;132(5):1141-9.e5.
6. Oyefara BI, Bahna SL. Delayed food-dependent, exercise-induced anaphylaxis. Allergy Asthma Proc. 2007;28(1):64-6.
7. Golden DB. What is anaphylaxis?. Curr Opin Allergy Clin Immunol. 2007;7(4):331-6.
8. Stone SF, Cotterell C, Isbister GK, et al. Elevated serum cytokines during human anaphylaxis: identification of potential mediators of acute allergic reactions. J Allergy Clin Immunol. 2009;124(4):786-92.e4.
9. Brown SGA. The pathophysiology of shock in anaphylaxis. Immunol Allergy Clin North Am. 2007;27(2):165-75.
10. Rohacek M, Edenhofer H, Bircher A, et al. Biphasic anaphylactic reactions: occurrence and mortality. Allergy. 2014;69(6):791-7.
11. Grunau BE, Li J, Yi TW, et al. Incidence of clinically important biphasic reactions in emergency department patients with allergic reactions or anaphylaxis. Ann Emerg Med. 2014;63(6):736-44.e2.
12. Sheikh A, Ten Broek V, Brown SGA, et al. H1-antihistamines for the treatment of anaphylaxis: Cochrane systematic review. Allergy. 2007;62(8):830-7.
13. Silverman HJ, Taylor WR, Smith PL, et al. Effects of antihistamines on the cardiopulmonary changes due to canine anaphylaxis. J Appl Physiol. 1988;64(1):210-7.
14. Felix SB, Baumann G, Niemczyk M, et al. Effects of histamine H1- and H2-receptor antagonists on cardiovascular function during systemic anaphylaxis in guinea pigs. Agents Actions. 1991;32(3-4):245-52.
15. Ellis B Craig BS. Parenteral antihistamines cause hypotension in anaphylaxis. Emerg Med Australas. 2013;25(1):92-3.
16. Choo KJ, Simons FE, Sheikh A. Glucocorticoids for the treatment of anaphylaxis. Cochrane Database Syst Rev. 2010;3:CD007596.
17. Sheikh A, Shehata YA, Brown SGA, et al. Adrenaline for the treatment of anaphylaxis: Cochrane systematic review. Allergy. 2009;64(2):204-12.

18. Mink SN, Simons FE, Simons KJ, et al. Constant infusion of epinephrine, but not bolus treatment, improves haemodynamic recovery in anaphylactic shock in dogs. Clin Exp Allergy. 2004;34(11):1776-83.
19. Fisher MM. Clinical observations on the pathophysiology and treatment of anaphylactic cardiovascular collapse. Anaesth Intensive Care. 1986;14(1):17-21.
20. Simons FE, Gu X, Simons KJ. Epinephrine absorption in adults: intramuscular versus subcutaneous injection. J Allergy Clin Immunol. 2001;108(5):871-3.
21. Harper NJN, Dixon T, Dugué P, et al. Suspected anaphylactic reactions associated with anaesthesia. Anaesthesia. 2009;64(2):199-211.
22. ASCIA. Health professional information paper: anaphylaxis. Sydney: Australasian Society of Clinical Immunology and Allergy; 2013.
23. Emergency Medicine Expert Group. Therapeutic guidelines: toxicology and wilderness. Melbourne: Therapeutic Guidelines Limited; 2008.

CHAPTER 29

Organophosphate Poisoning

Amarja Ashok Havaldar, Carol D'silva, Bhuvana Krishna

INTRODUCTION

Poisoning with organophosphorus (OP) compounds remains a public health problem and a clinical issue that is responsible for as many as 200,000 deaths every year.[1] The case fatality for self-poisoning in developing countries is commonly 10–20%, but for particular pesticides it may be as high as 50–70%.[2]

Majority of the cases are a part of deliberate self-harm, more so in developing countries in the Asia-Pacific region. Some of the common reasons stated for this are lack of regulations for the sale of these compounds, especially the highly toxic classes, and failure to ban toxic compounds.

Treatment over the years continues to focus on atropine and oximes, the only difference, off late being earlier and better resuscitation, and questionable efficacy of oximes.

HISTORY

Lassaigne and Franz Anton Voegeli in the early 1800s were the first to combine alcohol plus phosphoric acid to obtain triethylphosphate (TEP), an OP compound.[3] However, TEP had no anticholinesterase activity up to millimolar concentrations.

Tetraethyl pyrophosphate (TEPP) was the first ever acetylcholinesterase (AchE) inhibitor synthesized by de Clermont. He tasted the compound, and described it as a sticky liquid with a burning taste and a peculiar odor without realizing its toxic potential.[4]

In 1932 Willy Lange and his graduate student also experienced blurred vision, breathlessness and confusion while working on dimethyl and diethyl phosphofluoridate, and fortunately lived to tell the tale. This observation laid the background for developing OP compounds as insecticides and warfare agents.

Gerard Schrader, considered the father of modern OP insecticide toxicology, identified a method to synthesize TEPP, and it was the first OP compound for commercial use. Work on OP compounds soared in the period of the Second World War where its use as nerve agents was identified by the Germans. The nerve agents, tabun, sarin, and soman were developed in that period for potential use as chemical warfare agents. Tabun was used in 1986 in the Iraqi war against Iran and Sarin was recently used in 1995 in the Tokyo subway attack which killed around 12 people and intoxicated 5,000 people.

Parathion was one of the first OP compounds synthesized commercially at the end of the Second World War that had optimal stability and insecticidal activity.

Use of OP compounds has dropped to 33% in the US as per recent data in 2012[5] but its use still remains high in developing countries. About one-eighth of the global $69 billion agrochemical sales in 2012 were for OP compounds consisting of 10.5% glyphosate, 0.89% glufosinate, and 0.81% chlorpyrifos.[6]

CHEMISTRY

Organophosphorus compounds are ester, thiol or amide derivatives of phosphoric acid. OP compounds consist of a pentavalent phosphorus that is attached with a

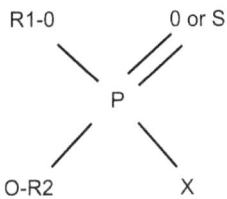

FIGURE 29.1: Basic chemical structure of an organophosphorus (OP) compound.

double bond to a sulfur (phosphorothioate) or an oxygen (phosphate) (Fig. 29.1). The R1 and R2 are commonly alkoxy groups, i.e. OCH_3 or OC_2H_5. OP compounds vary in their chemical structures, the main groups being phosphate, phosphorothioate, O-alkyl phosphorothioate and phosphorodithioate. Most OP compounds used as insecticides are phosphorothioates (i.e. they have a P = S bond), and need to be bioactivated in vivo to their oxygen analogs to exert their toxic action, but some (e.g. dichlorvos, methamidophos, or the nerve agents sarin, soman) have a P = O bond and do not require any bioactivation. Compounds with a P == S bond are referred to as thions (parathion, fenthion) while those with a P == O bond are referred to as oxons.

"X" is the so-called leaving group that is removed when the OP phosphorylates AChE, and is the most sensitive to hydrolysis.

Once phosphorylated, AchE can get hydrolyzed over a period of days to weeks. A loss of one of the two alkyl side groups leads to "aging" of the enzyme following which the enzyme is irreversibly inhibited and synthesis of new enzyme is a must for normal function. OP compounds are lipophilic hence easily absorbed from skin, lungs and gastrointestinal tract.

Absorption from the skin depends on contact time, lipophilicity and additives (solvents/emulsifiers) that can hasten absorption.

Once absorbed they are rapidly stored in the liver, fat, kidney and salivary glands.

Phosphorothiates (diazinon, parathion) being more lipophilic are often stored in fat and can give rise to delayed symptoms after a phase of apparent clinical recovery.

The oxons that inhibit AChE can be deactivated by hydrolases, such as the carboxylesterases and by A-esterases (e.g. paraoxonase).

CLASSIFICATION

Organophosphorus compounds may be classified as diethyl or dimethyl based on the alkoxy groups in R1 and R2 moieties (Table 29.1) and have important clinical implications in treatment and recovery. Dimethyl compounds undergo reactivation much faster when compared to diethyl compounds.

The World Health Organization (WHO) in combination with the Globally Harmonized System of Classification and Labeling of Chemicals, in their new revised update in 2009, have classified pesticides into five classes based on the LD50 (median lethal dose) dose (mg/kg) in rats.[7] A few examples of OP compounds based on this classification are shown in Table 29.2. Eddleston et al., however, showed that OP poisoning should not be treated as a single entity but treated based on the compound consumed, as there is considerable variability in response to treatment and outcomes with different OP compounds.[8] In his paper he also observed that chlorpyrifos had a higher LD50 in rats, but this finding did not translate in human populations. In the 802 patients who had consumed either fenthion, dimethoate or chlorpyrifos, the proportion of mortality was higher in the dimethoate

Table 29.1: Classification of organophosphorus (OP) compounds basis the side chain groups.

Diethyl	Dimethyl
Quinolphos, chlorpyrifos, trizophos, phorate, diazinon, parathion and dichlofenthion	Dichlorvos, monocrotophos, acephate, malathion, fenthion

Table 29.2: Classification of organophosphorus (OP) pesticides as per hazard level—WHO classification 2009 update.

Class	Hazard Level	Lethal dose in rats—oral (mg/kg)	Examples
Ia	Extremely hazardous	<5	• Chlormephos • Parathion • Parathion—methyl • Phorate • Sulfotep
Ib	Highly hazardous	5–50	• Dichlorvos • Dicrotophos • Monocrotophos • Omethoate
II	Moderately hazardous	50–2,000	• Chlorpyrifos • Cyanophos • Diazinon • Dimethoate • Fenthion
III	Slightly hazardous	>2,000	• Chlorpyrifos methyl • Malathion • Temephos • Fosamine
U	Unlikely to present acute hazard	>5,000	–

and fenthion groups. Response to treatment and need for endotracheal intubation were also higher in these groups.

What happens in a case of organophosphorus poisoning?
Organophosphorus compounds bind to acetylcholinesterase (AchE) and phosphorylates it. AchE hydrolyses acetylcholine, a major neurotransmitter in the autonomic and central nervous system. OP compounds additionally bind to butyrylcholinesterase in the plasma. Inhibition of AChE results in accumulation of acetylcholine (ACh) at autonomic (both sympathetic and parasympathetic) preganglionic and some central synapses and at autonomic parasympathetic postganglionic and skeletal afferent nerve endings.

Oxon (P == 0) group phosphorylates the serine hydroxyl group of the active site of AchE. The rate of spontaneous reactivation is faster for dimethoxyphosphoryl than diethoxyphosphoryl enzyme and may be aided with the use of oximes. In dimethyl compounds, the half-life is about 1 hour; if diethyl, the half-life is around 30 hours.[1] Unfortunately, if the organophosphorus is present in high concentrations, newly reactivated acetylcholinesterase will be rapidly re-inhibited.

Partial dealkylation of this serine group of AchE non-enzymatically leads to the so-called "aging" of the enzyme. Once aged, the enzyme is rendered inactive after which no reactivation is possible.

The rate of aging depends on the structure of the OP compound. The half-life of aging of dimethlyphosphorylated and diethylphosphorylated AChE is 3.7 hours and 33 hours, respectively and the therapeutic windows therefore are 13 hours and 132 hours, respectively (4 times the half-life).[9]

The activity of any aged, inhibited enzyme returns to normal only by re-synthesis of new enzyme in the liver.

CLINICAL FEATURES

Clinical features and severity of symptoms often depend on the compound, mode of entry into the body and any added solvents. Ingestion and inhalational routes when compared to dermal routes are associated with a more rapid onset of clinical toxidrome.

Acute clinical features of cholinergic crisis occur within 1–2 hours and are primarily due to muscarinic symptoms, commonly abbreviated as DUMBELS/SLUDGE symptoms (Table 29.3). They rarely occur after 24 hours, however may occur in case of dermal exposure.

Although bradycardia is a common presenting feature, tachycardia may also be an initial manifestation due to bronchospasm and subsequent hypoxia, secondary to nicotinic stimulation in high doses.

Bronchorrhea and bronchospasm can result in hypoxia and respiratory failure, which is an important cause of death following OP poisoning. Many patients in third world countries often die due to respiratory failure before reaching the hospital.

These patients develop acute respiratory failure as a result of reduced central respiratory drive, neuromuscular dysfunction and bronchorrhea.[1]

Nicotinic symptoms like fasciculations usually involve eyelids, tongue, face muscles, and calf muscles before proceeding to respiratory paralysis.

Myocardial injury has also been reported in cases of severe poisoning with a modest rise in Troponin I at a median time of 15 hours postingestion.[10]

Dimethoate poisoning commonly results in cardiovascular shock.

Seizures are relatively uncommon and seen in only 1–3% of patients.

DIAGNOSIS

1. Usually clinical—a history of consumption is usually obtained or else the characteristic smell of OP compounds or the solvent, aids in diagnosis. In any case if the history is not available, a cholinergic toxidrome picture should raise suspicion of OP poisoning.
2. Cholinesterase assays: These include two biochemical assays—serum pseudocholinesterase (also called butyrylcholinesterase) and red cell cholinesterase.

Both these enzymes serve as surrogates for activity of AchE in central and peripheral nervous systems.

Table 29.3: List of muscarinic, nicotinic and central nervous system (CNS) symptoms seen in organophosphorus (OP) poisoning.

Muscarinic receptor stimulation in parasympathetic system	• Salivation • Lacrimation • Bronchospasm, bronchorrhea • Miosis • Urination, diarrhea • Vomiting (emesis) • Bradycardia • Hypotension
Nicotinic receptor stimulation in sympathetic system and neuromuscular junction	• Fasciculations • Muscle cramps, fatigue • Paralysis • Tachycardia • Hypertension • Mydriasis
CNS receptor stimulation (nicotinic and muscarinic)	• Headache • Anxiety • Dizziness • Restlessness • Confusion • Agitation • Coma • Respiratory failure

Butyrylcholinesterases assays do not correlate with severity of poisoning as some OP compounds have a higher affinity for pseudocholinesterase as compared to AchE. Hence they can be used to detect exposure to an organophosphorus or carbamate pesticide but is not reliable in determining the severity of poisoning.[1] If followed up, gradual increase of levels in the blood correlates with decrease in levels of OP compounds and clinical recovery. More studies are needed to assess the utility of the use of butyrylcholinesterase assays to identify clinical recovery to aid in initiating weaning or to stop oxime therapy.

Red cell AchE, on the other hand, measures acetylcholinesterase expressed on the surface of red cells and is a good marker of severity of poisoning. However its correlation with recovery is less as compared to butyrylcholinesterase assays.

This is due to the slow regeneration of red cell AchE by erythropoiesis, around 1% per day. It is far more specific than butyrylcholinesterase for diagnosis.

It is important to remember that postcollection, the serum sample has to be rapidly cooled and diluted, as room temperature can allow the cholinesterase inhibition to continue in vitro and give falsely low values.[1]

In developing countries issues of cost, limited availability, delay in diagnosis, and variability in different biochemical assays limit these tests to being more useful for research purposes.

A new method of gas chromatography or liquid chromatography with mass spectrometry has been employed which helps in quantitative estimation of OP compounds in serum, gastric lavage or urine samples. Singh et al. used gas chromatography with a nitrogen phosphorous detector to identify 6 OP compounds in vitro including phorate, dimethoate, malathion, chlorpyrifos, diazinon and ethion. This was done with a turnaround time of 1–2 hours for extraction and analysis. However, larger studies and validity testing of this method is required.[11]

DELAYED EFFECTS

In 1976, Wadia et al.[12] attempted to study the various neurological manifestations in over 200 patients with diazinon poisoning. He described two types of paralysis—type 1, seen at presentation and attributed to muscarinic overdose. He also noted a type 2 paralysis in 36 patients which occurred after 24 hours and did not respond to atropine or pralidoxime. At that time they were unable to explain the cause of type 2 features and it was attributed to nicotinic manifestations or a possible different site of action other than AchE. Over the years however delayed effects of OP toxicity have been well classified and extensively studied and are as follows.

1. *Intermediate syndrome*: This condition is often seen 24–96 hours post recovery from the initial cholinergic crisis phase. As it occurs prior to delayed neuropathy and post the acute cholinergic syndrome phase it is aptly termed as the "intermediate" syndrome.
   Its incidence is around 20% following oral consumption of OP compounds, with no association between the type of OP compound and its occurrence.[13]
   Patients develop an acute respiratory failure while being conscious and after initial recovery of the cholinergic symptoms. Only a certain group of muscles remain involved, exact cause being unknown.
   The common muscles involved are the muscles of respiration, i.e. diaphragm, intercostals, neck flexors, proximal limb muscles and cranial motor nerves.
   It is believed to be due to persistent excess of acetylcholine at the neuromuscular junction leading to a sustained overstimulation of the neuromuscular junction.
   ENMG studies show a decrement-increment response initially followed by a decremental response, i.e. decrease in twitch height or compound action potential with repetitive nerve stimulation.[13]
   Treatment is mainly supportive and includes ventilatory support with gradual weaning as neuromuscular recovery occurs.
   These patients usually recover within 7–21 days without any sequelae.

2. *Delayed organophosphate encephalopathy (DOPE)*: This is a recently described entity wherein patients present with features of coma with absent brainstem reflexes and is a brainstem death mimic. It is known to occur after approximately 4–5 days of recovery from the cholinergic phase and a period of normal consciousness and may last for days to weeks. The main differentiating feature from brain death is presence of miosis and nonreacting pupils. Computed tomography of the brain and cerebrospinal fluid analysis are usually normal.
   The exact mechanism is still unclear and persistent cholinesterase inhibition due to lipophilic OP compounds which slowly get redistributed from fat stores has been attributed as a possible cause.[14] Recovery usually occurs with no permanent sequelae.

3. *Organophosphorus induced delayed polyneuropathy*: This is a rare delayed neurotoxic effect that occurs around 1–4 weeks post-OP consumption, once signs of acute cholinergic toxicity have subsided. The site of target is postulated to be neuropathy target esterase (NTE), predominantly present in nerve tissues. NTE is a 147-kDa membrane-bound protein of the patatin-like phospholipase family.

Only OP compounds which can cause phosphorylation and aging of at least 70% NTE, similar to that of AchE can give rise to OPIDP.[15]

It leads to a disruption of axonal transport and glial axonal interactions, finally leading to axonal injury and demyelination.

This is commonly seen with poisoning with the following compounds—chlorpyrifos, dichlorvos, isofenphos, methamidophos, mipafox, trichlorfon, trichlornat, phosphamidon/mevinphos and by certain carbamates.

It manifests as a central and distal sensorimotor polyneuropathy wherein symptoms begin with paresthesias in the distal extremities followed by sensory loss, ataxia, and flaccid paralysis.

Treatment remains supportive and unlike intermediate syndrome patients may take as long as 6-12 months to recover and have debilitating residual weakness.

MANAGEMENT

The principles in the management of any toxin include:
- Reducing further absorption of the poison
- Enhancing elimination of the drug
- Use of specific antidote to counteract the effects of already absorbed poison.[16,17]

1. *General supportive therapy*:
   - *Airway and breathing*—respiratory failure is one of the life-threatening complications in OP poisoning. Initial management of OP poisoning includes assessment of airway and possible need for intubation.[18]
   - *Decontamination*:
     i. *Skin decontamination*—removal of contaminated clothes and cleaning of skin with soap and water. During the process of decontamination, protection of healthcare personnel is equally important as OP compounds can easily get absorbed through skin and conjunctiva. Soap containing 30% ethanol is advised.[19]
     ii. *Gastric lavage*:
         Rationale—this is the easiest and most commonly practiced intervention in poisoning. It helps in the elimination of unabsorbed OP compounds.[16,18]
         Being lipophilic, significant amount of OP compounds get absorbed through gastric mucosa. Hence gastric lavage performed within 4 hours of consumption of OP compounds may be useful.
         There are no trials comparing utility of gastric lavage versus no gastric lavage. There was no reported benefit with use of gastric lavage in human studies. It was a usual practice in majority of the studies.[19,20]
     iii. *Activated charcoal*:
         Rationale—it is used in poisoning where ingested poison gets adsorbed, to prevent entry into the circulation.
         In a study by Eddleston et al., comparing multidose activated charcoal versus single dose charcoal in various poisoning cases including pesticide poisoning, no benefit as well as no harm was reported with the use of charcoal in both the groups.[21]
   - *Fresh frozen plasma (FFP)*:
     Rationale—the butyrylcholinesterase present in the FFP helps in neutralization of the poison thereby helps in hydrolysis of acetylcholine and facilitate neuromuscular transmission.
     Two trials compared FFP versus control and FFP versus albumin and saline. FFP use was associated with more complications possibly due to release of bound OP compounds, causing clinical worsening.[22,23]
   - *Benzodiazepines*:
     Rationale—seizures are a relatively uncommon manifestation of OP poisoning, occurring in around 1-3% of cases. As with other toxicological seizures, benzodiazepines are the first-line drugs used to control seizures.[1] They are also useful to allay agitation and anxiety in the poisoned patient.
   - *Magnesium*:
     Rationale—magnesium acts on calcium channels and its blockage leads to reduced release of acetylcholine. Magnesium also has effect on NMDA receptor thereby reduces overstimulation of CNS by OP compounds.
     A phase II study recently done by Basher et al. compared 4 g, 8 g, 12 g and 16 g of magnesium sulfate versus placebo, in 50 patients of OP poisoning, and showed a trend toward decreased mortality with higher doses of magnesium sulfate. No mortality was observed in the 16 g group. However, a larger RCT is definitely warranted to confirm its benefits.[24]

SUPPORTIVE THERAPIES WITH NO PROVEN BENEFIT AS OF TODAY

- *Lipid emulsions*: Lipid emulsion has been advised in the treatment of local anesthetic toxicity.
  The mechanism of action includes cardiomyocyte metabolism and lipid sink mechanism, which depends upon the lipid solubility of local anesthetics.
  Rationale—as some of the OP compounds are lipid soluble it may be considered. At present there is not

enough evidence to recommend the use of this therapy.[18] Further studies are required.

- *Clonidine*—it is a centrally acting α agonist.
  Rationale—clonidine reduces synaptic acetylcholine release.
  There is only a phase II trial which compared three different bolus dosages of clonidine followed by infusion for 24 hours.[25,26] High doses were associated with hypotension. There was no effect on outcome. Routine use of this agent is not yet advised.
- *Sodium bicarbonate*:
  Rationale—increase in pH mediated hydrolysis of OP compound thereby leading to enhance elimination of the compound.
  There is no clear evidence on the use of sodium bicarbonate. Only small RCTs have shown a benefit but till a larger RCT comes along, its practice is not recommended.[27,28]
- *Hemofiltration or hemoperfusion*:
  Rationale—to enhance the elimination of the poison.
  In case of dichlorovas poisoning, use of hemofiltration was shown to be beneficial.[29]
- *Organophosphorus hydrolases*:
  Rationale—these compounds enhance hydrolysis of OP compound. It reduces toxicity and probably it may enhance the effect of oximes. As the concentration of OP compound is reduced, efficacy of oximes may improve.
  It was found to be beneficial in small animal studies. There are no human studies on use of OP hydrolases.[18,30,31]

DEFINITIVE THERAPY

Atropine

Rationale: The effects of OP compounds manifest as a result of muscarinic and nicotinergic actions. Use of atropine as antimuscarinic agent helps in counteracting these effects.

Atropine is used as an initial bolus of 0.6–3.0 mg and doubling the initial dose after 5 minutes till the desired endpoint is achieved. Atropine infusion is to be continued at the rate of 10–20% of the dose required to achieve clinical endpoint. The endpoint for adequate dosing of atropine is HR >80 beats/min and systolic BP >80 mm Hg and clear chest and clear axillae.[1] The use of pupillary dilatation is not the desired endpoint in case of OP poisoning. Atropine infusion is continued for 24–48 hours and gradually tapered over next 3–5 days taking into account individual variability.[18-20,25]

A recent randomized controlled trial invovling 50 patients, comparing the effect of atropine infusion versus intermittent atropine, showed that atropinization was achieved faster with atropine infusion, with early discharge from ICU.[32]

Atropine is indicated to counteract the CNS effects of OP compounds. Sometimes atropine itself can cause toxicity in the form of psychosis and delirium and it becomes difficult to differentiate OP toxicity from atropine toxicity, in such patients glycopyrrolate can be used as an alternative.

An RCT that compared atropine versus glycopyrrolate in OP poisoning showed no significant differences in mortality, with lesser respiratory complications in the glycopyrrolate group.[33]

Oximes

There are several types of oximes available, e.g. pralidoxime (PAM), obidoxime, HI6, HIo7. The most potent oxime is obidoxime.[34]

Among the various oximes PAM is well studied. *Mechanism of action of oximes*—in OP compound poisoning, inhibition of acetylcholinesterase results in accumulation of acetylcholine and impaired neuromuscular transmission. AchE has an active esteric side which OP compounds phosphorylate and an inactive anionic site as shown in Figure 29.2. Oximes bind to this anionic site and causes reactivation of acetylcholinesterase by releasing the phosphate from the serine residue before the enzyme is aged (Figs. 29.3 and 29.4). This reactivation is predominantly observed in the skeletal muscles as compared to CNS.

Use of PAM in OP compound poisoning has been debated and criticized. WHOs recommendation on use of PAM is mainly based on animal studies. The recommended dose is 30 mg/kg bolus followed by more than 8 mg/hr continuous infusion for 7 days.[35]

A study comparing atropine with PAM as a continuous or intermittent bolus has shown that loading dose followed by continuous infusion reduces morbidity and mortality in moderately severe cases of OP poisoning.[36] This study

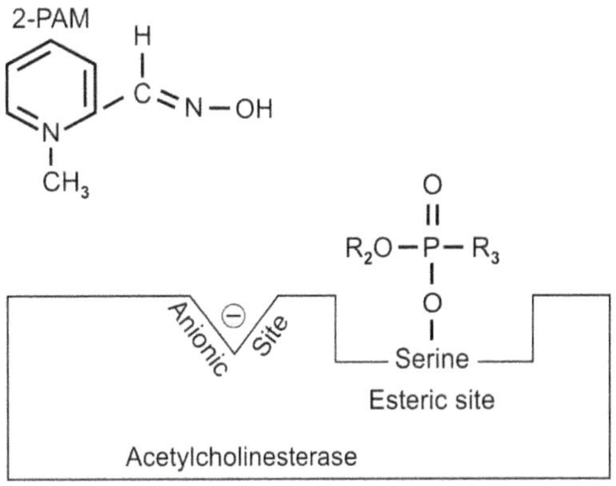

FIGURE 29.2: Structure of pralidoxime (PAM) and binding of an organophosphorus (OP) compound to acetylcholinesterase.

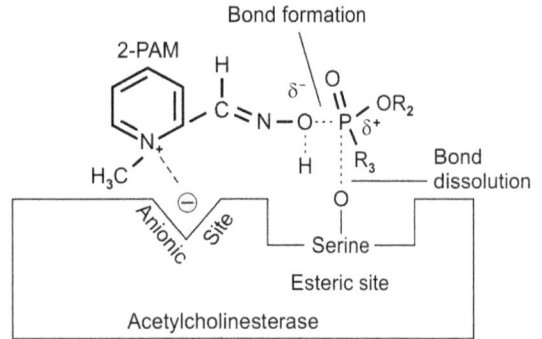

FIGURE 29.3: Binding of pralidoxime (PAM) to anionic site of acetylcholinesterase.

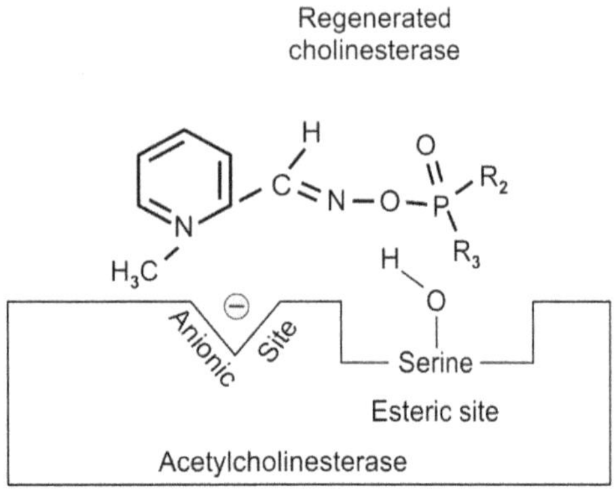

FIGURE 29.4: Oxime phosphate compound diffuses and regenerated acetylcholinestrease is formed.

had several limitations. It was not a double-blind study. Among the baseline characteristics, patients who consumed dimethyl compounds were in PAM infusion group. Study included patients with moderately severe poisoning. The bolus dose of PAM was higher than the WHO recommended dose.

Cherian et al. in his study comparing the 12 g versus 1 g of PAM, i.e. high dose versus low dose of PAM, showed higher incidence of intermediate syndrome and need for ventilator support in the high dose PAM group.[37] Based on the results of this study, a subsequent double blind study was done to compare PAM versus placebo, which showed use of PAM was not beneficial.[38] These two studies contradicted the routine use of PAM in OP poisoning.[39]

Eddleston et al. in the double-blind study comparing bolus of PAM followed by infusion versus saline showed no difference in the survival and need for intubation.[40] As compared to the previous study of high dose PAM,[36] in this trial PAM infusion was given over 7 days. Red cell acetylcholinesterase activity was monitored in this study.

There are several studies comparing atropine with PAM versus atropine alone in OP poisoning. Two meta-analyses published in 2006 had similar results. The meta-analysis of six trials by Rahimi et al. concluded that oximes are not effective in the management of OP compound poisoning, and can be dangerous and worsen patient's clinical condition.[41] A meta-analysis by JV Peter et al., comprising of seven studies, out of which two were RCTs, showed null effect or possible harm with the use of PAM.[42]

In a study comparing atropine alone versus atropine and PAM does not support the use of PAM in moderate to severe poisoning.[43]

The study on two dose regimens of PAM comparing WHO recommended dose of 2 g followed by 8 mg/kg/hr versus 2 g bolus followed by 1 g 6 hourly showed reduced morbidity and mortality in moderate cases of OP poisoning. In the WHO regimen, incidence of intermediate syndrome was less and mean dose of atropine used was also less than the control group. The study had several limitations, there was no blinding and allocation concealment.[44]

Obidoxime—is one of the oximes. Oximes do not cross the blood brain barrier. Hence CNS effects of OPP cannot be completely counteracted by oximes. A recent animal study on intranasal administration of obidoxime along with standard treatment of atropine and PAM has shown possible benefit of addition of obidoxime on CNS toxicity of OP compounds.[45] The study evaluating kinetics of different oximes showed reactivation of acetylcholinesterase was effective with obidoxime.[46]

Oximes are not without side effects. Rapid administration is associated with nausea, vomiting and blurring of vision, diastolic hypertension and dizziness.[35]

The possible reasons proposed for negative trials of oximes are: (1) Nature of OP compound consumed, dimethyl or diethyl, (2) Geographical area and class of OP compund available in that region, (3) Amount of OP compound consumed, (4) Severity of poisoning, as stated by several studies as moderate or severe poisoning, (5) Time to reach hospital, (6) Nonavailability of RBC cholinesterase levels in majority of the studies, (7) Effect of aging on efficacy of oximes, (8) Various dosages of oximes used in different studies with variable results.[47]

CARBAMATE POISONING

Carbamate insecticide poisoning presents as a cholinergic crisis that is clinically indistinguishable from OP poisoning.

Unlike OP compounds they carbamylate the AchE enzyme and the enzyme is reactivated by spontaneous hydrolysis that occurs slowly. This happens as the carbamate—AchE bond is far less stable and does not undergo aging like with OP compounds.

Examples of carbamates include aldicarb, propoxur, aminocarb, carbaryl, dimetan, bendiocarb, etc.

The clinical signs and symptoms are similar to those of OP compounds. Carbamates do not cross the blood brain barrier as easily as OP compounds and thus CNS symptoms are not as severe.[48,49]

The cholinergic symptoms usually resolve within 24-48 hours without much sequelae. The occurrence of intermediate syndrome, delayed polyneuropathy is rare with carbamate poisoning.

Use of plasma cholinesterase essays can be misleading to diagnose carbamate poisoning as they can produce a transient anticholinesterase effect.

TREATMENT

The patient usually recovers quickly with the use of atropine. The dose and mode of administration remains the same as with OP poisoning. The requirement and duration of the infusion maybe lower, due to the spontaneous hydrolysis and early reversal of cholinergic toxicity.

The use of oxime therapy in carbamate intoxication has sparked controversy. Oxime monotherapy has shown to be harmful in carbaryl poisoning in animal studies.

Barring the single case report from Farago[50] which showed increased mortality following oxime therapy, in several case series and reports[51,52] thereafter have shown positive outcomes with respect to mortality when used along with atropine. However, there is no robust evidence to support its use at this time.

Due to the short duration of action of carbamates, PAM is used only when the patient fails to respond adequately to atropine, serious mixed poisonings with both carbamate and organophosphorus compounds, or in serious poisonings by unidentified cholinesterase inhibitors.[53]

REFERENCES

1. Eddleston M, Buckley NA, Eyer P, et al. Management of acute organophosphorus pesticide poisoning. The Lancet. 2008;371:597-7.
2. Eddleston M. Patterns and problems of deliberate self-poisoning in the developing world. QJM. 2000;93(11):715-31.
3. Chambers JE, Levi PE. Organophosphates: chemistry, fate, and effects. San Diego: Academic Press; 1992.
4. Petroianu GA. Toxicity of phosphor esters: Willy Lange (1900–1976) and Gerda von Krueger (1907–after 1970). Die Pharmazie—An International Journal of Pharmaceutical Sciences. 2010;65:776-80.
5. Atwood D, Paisley-Jones C. Pesticides Industry Sales and Usage: 2008–2012 Market Estimates. United States Environmental Protection Agency: Washington, DC, USA. 2017.
6. Casida JE. Organophosphorus xenobiotic toxicology. Ann Rev Pharmacol Toxicol. 2017;57:309-27.
7. WHO. (2009). Who.int. 2009. WHO|The WHO Recommended Classification of Pesticides by Hazard. [online] Available from https://www.who.int/ipcs/publications/pesticides_hazard/en/ [Accessed Dec., 2018].
8. Eddleston M, Eyer P, Worek F, et al. Differences between organophosphorus insecticides in human self-poisoning: a prospective cohort study. The Lancet. 2005;366:1452-9.
9. Worek F, Bäcker M, Thiermann H, et al. Reappraisal of indications and limitations of oxime therapy in organophosphate poisoning. Hum Experiment Toxicol. 1997;16:466-72.
10. Cha YS, Kim H, Go J, et al. Features of myocardial injury in severe organophosphate poisoning. Clin Toxicol. 2014;52:873-9.
11. Singh B, Dogra TD. Rapid method for the determination of some organophosphorus insecticides in a small amount of serum in emergency and occupational toxicology cases. Indian J Occup Environ Med. 2009;13:84-7.
12. Wadia RS, Sadagopan C, Amin RB, et al. Neurological manifestations of organophosphorous insecticide poisoning. J Neurol Neurosurg Psychiatry. 1974;37:841-7.
13. Karalliedde L, Baker D, Marrs TC. Organophosphate-induced Intermediate syndrome. Toxicol Rev. 2006;25:1-4.
14. Peter JV, Prabhakar AT, Pichamuthu K. Delayed-onset encephalopathy and coma in acute organophosphate poisoning in humans. Neurotoxicology. 2008;29:335-42.
15. Jokanović M, Kosanović M, Brkić D, et al. Organophosphate-induced delayed polyneuropathy in man: an overview. Clin Neurol Neurosurg. 2011;113:7-10.
16. Levine M, Brooks DE, Truitt CA, et al. Toxicology in the ICU: Part 1: general overview and approach to treatment. Chest. 2011;140:795-6.
17. Brooks DE, Levine M, O'Connor AD, et al. Toxicology in the ICU: Part 2: specific toxins. Chest. 2011;140:1072-5.
18. Eddleston M, Chowdhury FR. Pharmacological treatment of organophosphorus insecticide poisoning: the old and the (possible) new. Br J Clin Pharmacol. 2016;81:462-70.
19. Sundaray NK, Kumar R. Organophosphorus poisoning: current management guidelines. Med Update. 2010;20:420-5.
20. Palaniappen V. Current concepts in the management of organophosphorus compound poisoning. Med Update. Mumbai, India: The Association of Physicians of India. 2013. pp. 427-3.
21. Eddleston M, Juszczak E, Buckley NA, et al. Multiple-dose activated charcoal in acute self-poisoning: a randomised controlled trial. The Lancet. 2008;371:579-87.
22. Pazooki S, Solhi H, Vishteh HR, et al. Effectiveness of fresh frozen plasma as supplementary treatment in organophosphate poisoning. Med J Malaysia. 2011;66:342-5.
23. Pichamuthu K, Jerobin J, Nair A, et al. Bioscavenger therapy for organophosphate poisoning–an open-labeled pilot randomized trial comparing fresh frozen plasma or albumin with saline in acute organophosphate poisoning in humans. Clin Toxicol. 2010;48:813-9.
24. Basher A, Rahman SH, Ghose A, et al. Phase II study of magnesium sulfate in acute organophosphate pesticide poisoning. Clin Toxicol. 2013;51:35-40.

25. Blain PG. Organophosphorus poisoning (acute). BMJ Clin Evidence. 2011;2011.
26. Perera PM, Jayamanna SF, Hettiarachchi R, et al. A Phase II clinical trial to assess the safety of clonidine in acute organophosphorus pesticide poisoning. Trials. 2009;10:73.
27. Balali-Mood M, Ayati MH, Ali-Akbarian H. Effect of high doses of sodium bicarbonate in acute organophosphorous pesticide poisoning. Clin Toxicol. 2005;43:571-4.
28. Wong A, Sandron CA, Magalhaes AS, et al. Comparative efficacy of pralidoxime vs sodium bicarbonatein rats and humans severely poisoned with OP pesticide (Abstract). J Toxicol Clin Toxicol. 2000;38:554-5.
29. Li Z, Wang G, Zhen G, et al. Application of hemoperfusion in severe acute organophosphorus pesticide poisoning. Turkish J Med Sci. 2017;47:1277-81.
30. Sogorb MA, Vilanova E, Carrera V. Future applications of phosphotriesterases in the prophylaxis and treatment of organophosporus insecticide and nerve agent poisonings. Toxicol Letters. 2004;151:219-33.
31. Raushel FM. Bacterial detoxification of organophosphate nerve agents. Curr Opin Microbiol. 2002;5:288-95.
32. Khan KK, Khanam B, Siddiqui SA, et al. Comparison of atropine intravenous infusion versus intermittent atropine in the management of organophosphorus poisoning in ICU. J Evid Med Healthcare. 2018;5:379-82.
33. Bardin PG, Van SE. Organophosphate poisoning: grading the severity and comparing treatment between atropine and glycopyrrolate. Crit Care Med. 1990;18:956-60.
34. Kassa J. Review of oximes in the antidotal treatment of poisoning by organophosphorus nerve agents. J Toxicol: Clin Toxicol. 2002;40:803-6.
35. Bevan M. Proposal for the inclusion of pralidoxime in the WHO model list of essential medicines. 17th Expert Committee on the Selection and Use of Essential Medicines Geneva. 2009.
36. Pawar KS, Bhoite RR, Pillay CP, et al. Continuous pralidoxime infusion versus repeated bolus injection to treat organophosphorus pesticide poisoning: a randomised controlled trial. Lancet. 2006;368:2136-41.
37. Johnson S, Peter JV, Thomas K, et al. Evaluation of two treatment regimens of pralidoxime (1 g single bolus dose vs 12 g infusion) in the management of organophosphorus poisoning. J Assoc Phys India. 1996;44:529-31.
38. Cherian AM, Peter JV, Samuel J, et al. Effectiveness of pralidoxime in the treatment of organophosphorous poisoning (OPP): a randomized double blind, placebo controlled clinical trial. J Assoc Physic India. 1997;45:22-4.
39. Cherian MA, Roshini C, Peter JV, et al. Oximes in organophosphorus poisoning. Indian J Crit Care Med. 2005;9:155-63.
40. Eddleston M, Eyer P, Worek F, et al. Pralidoxime in acute organophosphorus insecticide poisoning—a randomised controlled trial. PLoS Med. 2009;6:e1000104.
41. Rahimi R, Nikfar S, Abdollahi M. Increased morbidity and mortality in acute human organophosphate-poisoned patients treated by oximes: a meta-analysis of clinical trials. Hum Experiment Toxicol. 2006;25:157-62.
42. Peter JV, Moran JL, Graham P. Oxime therapy and outcomes in human organophosphate poisoning: an evaluation using meta-analytic techniques. Crit Care Med. 2006;34:502-10.
43. Chugh SN, Aggarwal N, Dabla S, et al. Comparative evaluation of atropine alone and atropine with pralidoxime (PAM) in the management of organophosphorus poisoning. J Indian Acad Clin Med. 2005;6:33-7.
44. Mahesh M, Gowdar M, Venkatesh CR. A study on two dose regimens of pralidoxime in the management of organophosphate poisoning. Asia Pacific J Med Toxicol. 2013;2:121-5.
45. Krishnan JK, Arun P, Appu AP, et al. Intranasal delivery of obidoxime to the brain prevents mortality and CNS damage from organophosphate poisoning. Neurotoxicology. 2016;53:64-73.
46. Moyer RA, McGarry Jr KG, Babin MC, et al. Kinetic analysis of oxime-assisted reactivation of human, Guinea pig, and rat acetylcholinesterase inhibited by the organophosphorus pesticide metabolite phorate oxon (PHO). Pesticide Biochem Physiol. 2018;145:93-9.
47. Walton EL. Pralidoxime and pesticide poisoning: A question of severity? Biomed J. 2016;39:373-5.
48. Lima JS, Reis CA. Poisoning due to illegal use of carbamates as a rodenticide in Rio de Janeiro. J Toxicol Clin Toxicol. 1995;33:687-90.
49. Saadeh AM, al-Ali MK, Farsakh NA, et al. Clinical and sociodemographic features of acute carbamate and organophosphate poisoning: a study of 70 adult patients in north Jordan. J Toxicol Clin Toxicol. 1996;34:45-51.
50. Farago A. Fatal suicidal case of Sevin (1-naphthyl-N-methylcarbamate) poisoning. Arch Toxikol. 1969;24:309-15.
51. Burgess JL, Bernstein JN, Hurlbut K. Aldicarb poisoning. A case report with prolonged cholinesterase inhibition and improvement after pralidoxime therapy. Arch Intern Med. 1994;154:221-4.
52. Ekins BR, Geller RJ. Methomyl-induced carbamate poisoning treated with pralidoxime chloride. West J Med. 1994;161:68-70.
53. Kurtz PH. Pralidoxime in the treatment of carbamate intoxication. Am J Emerg Med. 1990;8:68-70.

CHAPTER 30

Snake Envenomation

Srinivas Samavedam, Ganshyam Jagathkar

INTRODUCTION

Mortality due to snakebites is fairly common in India, though frequently underreported. Snakebite is an often unrecognized, mismanaged, life-threatening medical emergency, commonly seen in the rural/semi-urban population.[1] Multiple factors seem to contribute toward increased mortality—lack of awareness, use of traditional remedies, shortage of medical personnel and infrastructure, scarcity of antisnake venom (ASV), etc.[2] There are about 300 species of snakes found in India, 52 amongst them being venomous. The most common venomous snakes causing majority of the deaths belong to the following families—Elapidae family which includes the Indian Cobra (*Naja naja*), Indian Krait (*Bungarus caeruleus*) and Viperidae family which includes the Russell's viper (*Daboia russelii*) and the Saw-scaled viper (*Echis carinatus*).[3]

CLINICAL FEATURES

Snake venom is modified saliva of the animal consisting of peptides and enzymes with cytotoxic, neurotoxic, hemotoxic, and anticoagulant properties. Clinical features of envenomation are dependent on multiple factors—species, amount of venom injected, site of bite, feeding state of the snake, and the time duration between the bite and administration of ASV.[4] Majority of the envenomations can be broadly classified into four clinical syndromes with a possible overlap of symptoms (Flowchart 30.1).[5]
1. Neurotoxic/neuroparalytic—Cobra, Krait
2. Hemotoxic/vasculotoxic—Vipers
3. Myotoxic—Sea snakes
4. Progressive swelling syndrome—Vipers.

Neuroparalytic Syndrome

This is commonly seen with the Elapidae group—Cobra and the Krait—and is usually characterized by descending paralysis starting with ptosis, diplopia, dysphonia, dysarthria, dysphagia, eventually leading to paralysis and respiratory arrest. Onset of symptoms is early in Cobra bites; however, it can be significantly delayed in Krait bites often leading to misdiagnosis. Manifestations may mimic brain death with dilated nonreacting pupils, leading to a whole lot of neurological tests (very common with Krait bites). Victims often present with abdominal discomfort, vomiting, and inability to wake up in the mornings.[6] Krait bite needs a very high index of suspicion, as the fang marks are very indistinct and often invisible.

Significant myocardial involvement with cardiogenic shock and cardiac arrest are also seen in Cobra bites. Cardiac involvement is associated with a very high mortality.[7]

Bedside tests to identify impending respiratory failure include the single-breath count, sustained head elevation, and the breath-holding time. Inability to speak in complete sentences also underlines the severity.[5]

FLOWCHART 30.1: Management of snakebite.

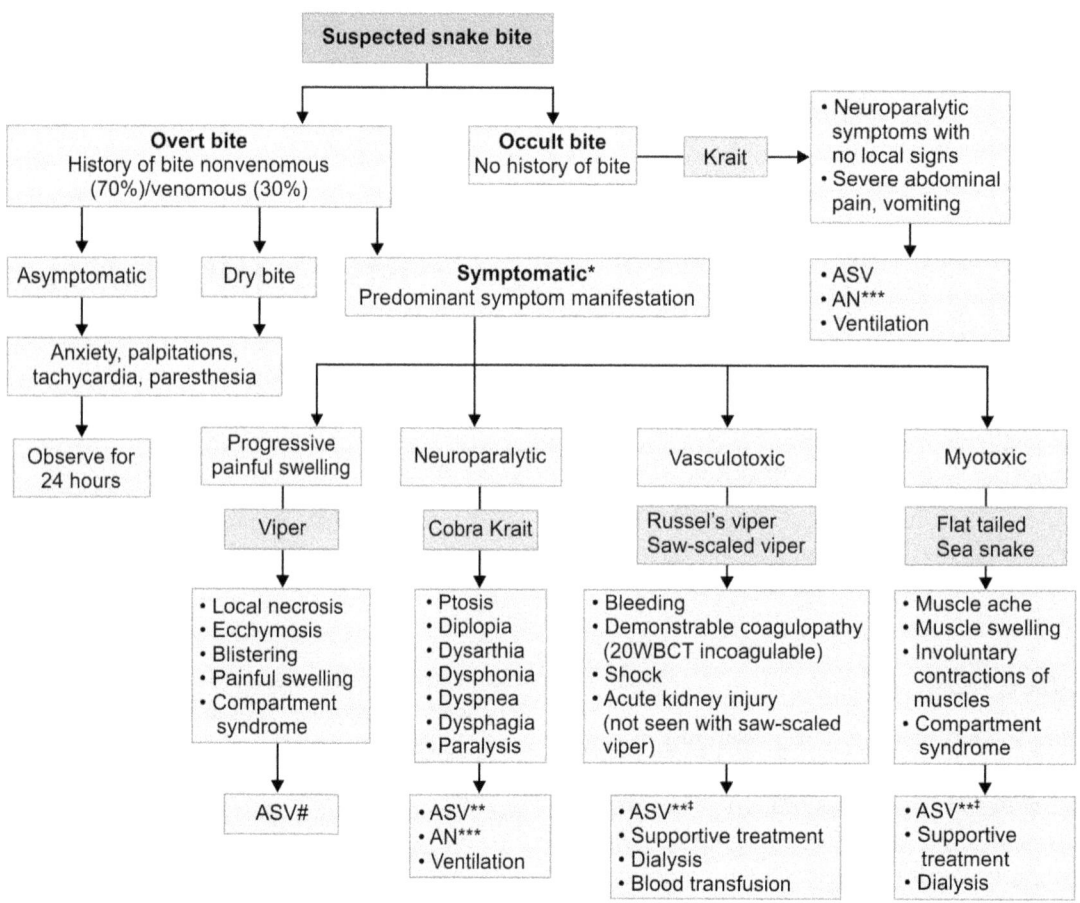

Source: Ministry of Health and Social Welfare, 2017.

* Even though present as predominant manifestation but there may be overlap of syndrome as well
# ASV indicated in rapidly developing swelling only. Purely localized swelling with or without bite marks is not an indication of ASV
** For reaction to antisnake venom (ASV) Dose of adrenaline 0.5 mg IM (in children 0.01 mg/kg)
‡ Specific ASV for sea snake and Pit viper bite is not available in India. However, available ASV may have some advantage by cross reaction.
*** AN injection atropine 0.6 mg followed by neostigmine (1.5 mg) IV stat (in children injection, atropine 0.05 mg/kg followed by injection, Neostigmine 0.04 mg/kg IV). Repeat neostigmine 0.5 mg (in children 0.01 mg/kg) with atropine every 30 minutes for 5 doses. Thereafter taper dose at 1 hour, 2 hour, 6 hour and 12 hour. Positive response is measured as 50% or more recovery of the ptosis in one hour. If no response after 3rd dose stop AN injection. No AN injection in confirmed krait bite.

Note: The snake specie shown above are indicative only. Russell's viper envenoming in Tamil Nadu and some other areas commonly causes paralysis—the venom of this species considerably across its range in India.

Vasculotoxic/Hemotoxic Syndrome

This is commonly seen with the Viperidae bites which usually have local and systemic manifestations. Pain, erythema, swelling, and edema at the bite site with necrosis leading to compartment syndrome are common. Tender regional lymphadenopathy has also reported. Systemic effects manifest as bleeding from various sites—epistaxis, gum bleeding, ecchymotic patches, bleeding from the bite site, and pre-existing conditions (hemorrhoids).[5] Acute kidney injury (AKI) requiring renal replacement therapy is common due to hypovolemia, hematuria, hemoglobinuria, rhabdomyolysis, and direct toxic effects of the venom. Other clinical features, such as subconjunctival hemorrhage, parotid swelling, acute respiratory distress syndrome, and shock, are also seen.

Systemic capillary leak syndrome: It is a life-threatening complication sometimes seen with Russell's viper bite characterized by severe hypotension and shock secondary to endothelial dysfunction and increased capillary leak.[5]

MANAGEMENT OF SNAKEBITE ENVENOMATION

Reassure the victim, as majority of the bites are due to nonvenomous snakes. The victim should be transported to the nearest medical center. Immobilize the limb with the help of a splint as is done in the case of a fracture.[5]

Do not apply tourniquet nor resort to any traditional remedies. There is no role of local ASV injection at the bite site.

ASSESSMENT

Review history thoroughly and estimate the time elapsed in transporting the patient. Assess vital parameters and act accordingly. Immediate intubation may be needed for impending respiratory arrest in neuroparalytic syndromes. Fluid resuscitation and vasopressor therapy should be initiated for hemodynamic compromise.

If the victim is transported with a tourniquet, check for the pulse distal to the tourniquet. If there is a strong suspicion of venomous bite, loading dose of ASV to be given prior to removal of the tourniquet[5] and neostigmine/atropine should be readily available for immediate administration.

Laboratory Workup

The 20-minute whole blood clotting test: The whole blood clotting time is a useful bedside test to assess the coagulation status in vasculotoxic bites. A volume of 2 mL fresh venous blood is taken in a clean glass test tube and left undisturbed at room temperature. After 20 minutes, gently tilt the tube for the presence of a clot—if the blood does not clot it indicates coagulopathy and the need for ASV. The test has to be repeated every hour for the first 3 hours and 6 hourly for 24 hours or longer depending on the clinical situation.

Other routine laboratory workup is needed, including a complete coagulation panel, renal functions, arterial blood gas test, liver function test, complete urine examination, creatine phosphokinase, electrolytes (hyperkalemia common if AKI sets in), ultrasonography abdomen, two-dimensional echocardiography, etc.

ANTISNAKE VENOM

It is the only specific treatment for snake envenomation. In India, polyvalent ASV is available which is effective against the four common species—Russell's viper, Saw-scaled viper, Cobra, and the Krait. The currently available ASV may not effectively treat envenomation by other species. ASV is an expensive and scarce commodity and hence should be used judiciously; at the same time, it is a life-saving therapy and should not be denied to any victim. ASV is available in two forms—freeze-dried and a liquid form, whichever form is available should be used immediately. The average range of venom injected during a bite is around 5–147 mg.[5] Each vial of ASV neutralizes around 6 mg of Russell's viper venom. Hence the average dose usually required to treat snakebite is between 20 and 30 vials. However, in certain situations, additional vials may be needed. If there is no clinical improvement despite adequate dose of ASV, the possibility of envenomation by other species should be considered.

Dosage

Neuroparalytic symptoms: About 10 vials stat over 30 minutes as an infusion, followed by a second dose of 10 vials after 1 hour if there is no improvement.[5]

Atropine/Neostigmine: Administer 0.6-mg atropine along with 1.5-mg neostigmine intravenous (IV) immediately and repeat every 30 minutes for five doses, followed by tapering doses at 1 hour, 2 hours, 6 hours, and 12 hours. Positive response is seen by visible improvement in ptosis. Stop, if there is no improvement after three doses or complete recovery or if side effects occur.[5] Neuroparalytic syndrome due to Krait envenomation may not respond to atropine/neostigmine as it affects presynaptic fibers where Ca^{++} is the neurotransmitter. Injection calcium gluconate 10 mL slow IV every 6 hours can be tried till neuroparalysis recovers (5–7 days).

Vasculotoxic

Two regimens have been proposed:
1. *Low dose:* About 10 vials for Russell's viper or 6 vials for Saw-scaled viper, as stat infusion over 30 minutes, followed by 2 vials every 6 hours till clotting time normalizes or for 3 days whichever is earlier.[5]
2. *High dose:* About 10 vials stat as an infusion over 30 minutes, followed by 6 vials 6 hourly till clotting time normalizes. Some experts suggest the low-dose regimen as it seems to be equally effective and conserves a scarce commodity like ASV.

Patients with capillary leak syndrome may need higher doses of ASV.

Victims with vasculotoxic bites are prone to develop disseminated intravascular coagulation (DIC); check for platelets, prothrombin time/international normalized ratio, activated partial thromboplastin time, and fibrinogen levels. Patients in DIC will need supplementation with fibrinogen/fresh frozen plasma (FFP). There is no role for prophylactic FFP transfusions. FFPs should be transfused only after giving ASV.[5]

Note: The dose of ASV in pregnancy and children is the same as adults (the amount of venom injected doesn't differ).

Antisnake Venom Administration

- No contraindications for ASV administration.
- No test dose should be given.
- To be given only as an IV infusion over 30 minutes to 1 hour.
- Needs close monitoring, as patients can develop life-threatening anaphylactic reactions. In the event of an anaphylaxis, use adrenaline 1 in 1,000–0.5 mg intramuscular (IM) in the deltoid/thigh for adults (can use IV infusion in the cases of shock and hypotension) and 0.01 mg/kg for children. Chlorpheniramine maleate—10 mg for adults and 0.2 mg/kg for children should be used. Hydrocortisone can be used; however, it may not be of much benefit as it takes a few hours to act.
- Restart ASV 10–15 minutes after recovery from the anaphylaxis.[5]

Other Measures

Hemodynamic support—in the form of fluid resuscitation and vasopressor, support is needed for all patients in shock. Forced alkaline diuresis can be tried to prevent pigment nephropathy and AKI.[5] Patients with AKI, metabolic acidosis, and hyperkalemia need renal replacement therapy. The national guidelines recommend the use of broad-spectrum prophylactic antibiotics for the cellulitis.[5]

Surgical Intervention

Antisnake venom helps in reducing edema[8] and prevents surgical intervention. However, if the patient develops severe compartment syndrome, fasciotomy may be needed. Corticosteroids are not effective in decreasing the edema and can increase complications, hence it should be avoided.[9]

SCORPION STING ENVENOMATION

Scorpion sting is the second most common emergency envenomation encountered in India. Annually about 1.5 million envenomations occur all over the world with 2,600 fatalities.[10] The severity and mortality seem to be higher in pediatric population. The distributions of the incidence of scorpion sting across the world and in India are shown in Figures 30.1 and 30.2.

Symptomatic treatment is still the norm in most centers due to lack of easy access to antivenom.

All venomous scorpions belong to the family Buthidae.[11] Scorpions belonging to the genera *Hottentotta*, *Androctonus*, and *Mesobuthus* are encountered in South-East Asia. They are usually seen in dry, hot environments and are nocturnal in habit. Scorpion sting envenomation is not a notifiable disease, which might be the reason for underreporting. The sting of a scorpion rests in its thick tail—the apparatus, including a secreting gland coupled with a sharp semi-curved sting. Systemic effects are more common with stings

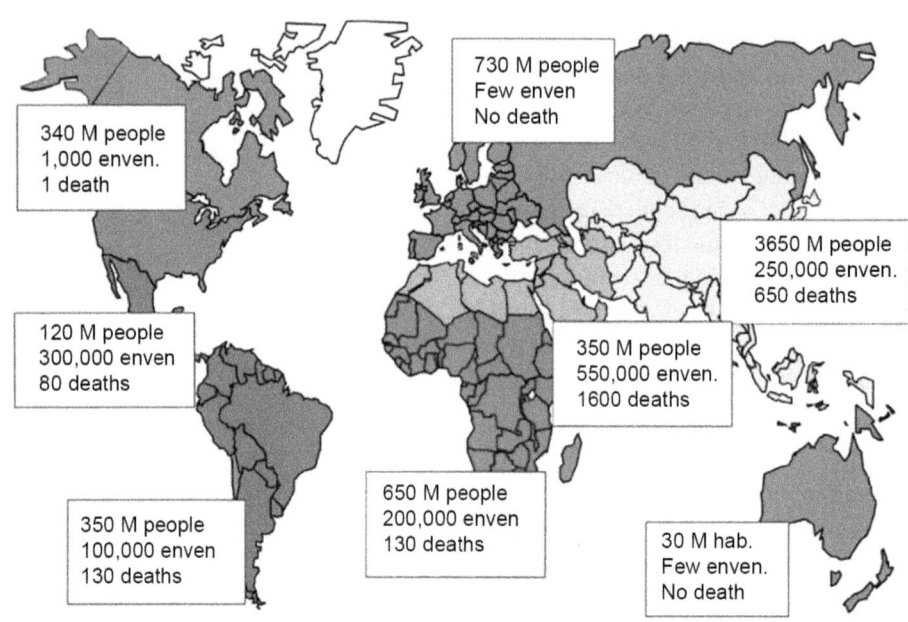

FIGURE 30.1: Distribution and fatalities of scorpion sting in the world.[10]

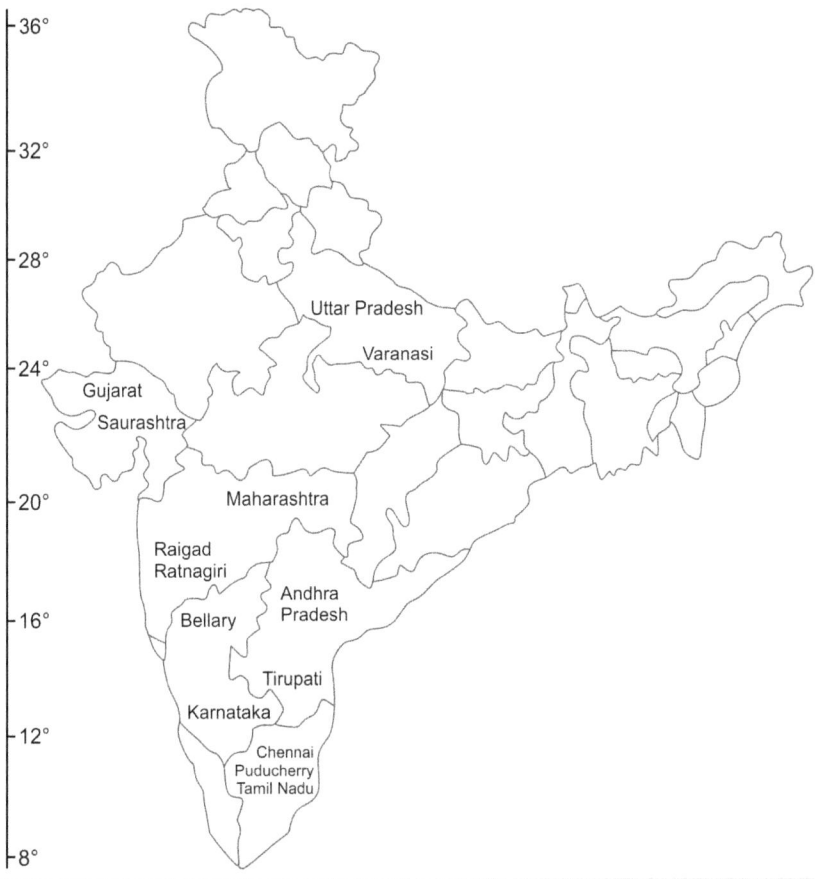

FIGURE 30.2: Endemic distribution of venomous scorpion stings in India.[12]

of the Buthidae family, whereas stings of the Scorpionidae family are associated with local symptoms.[12-14] Usually the venom is deposited in the subcutaneous tissue with an absorption time of 7–8 hours. The venom reaches its maximum concentration within an hour. The venom of scorpion contains multiple low-molecular-weight peptides, neurotoxins, cardiotoxins, nephrotoxins, hemolytic toxins, hyaluronidase, etc., which explains the multisystem effect of scorpion venom. The neurotoxin of scorpion venom is more potent than the neurotoxin in snake venom. The voltage-gated sodium and potassium channels are the main targets for scorpion neurotoxins. The "autonomic storm" associated with scorpion sting envenomation results from the release of neurotransmitters.

Clinical Manifestations

The clinical manifestations depend upon the species of scorpion and the quantity of venom injected. Subsequent stings tend to be less toxic than preceding ones. Children tend to have more severe manifestations. The autonomic storm manifests as vomiting, sweating, bradycardia, ventricular premature contractions, and hypotension, followed by a prolonged sympathetic phase of hypertension, tachycardia, and pulmonary edema. Scorpion sting envenomation can be categorized into four clinical grades (Table 30.1).

Table 30.1: Clinical grading of scorpion sting.

Grade	Manifestations
Grade I	Severe excruciating local pain at the sting site radiating along with corresponding dermatomes, mild local edema with seating at the sting site, without systemic involvement
Grade II	Signs and symptoms of autonomic storm characterized by acetylcholine excess or parasympathetic stimulation and sympathetic stimulation
Grade III	Cold extremities, tachycardia, hypotension, or hypertension with pulmonary edema (respiratory rate >24 per minute, basal rales or crackles in lungs)
Grade IV	Tachycardia, hypotension with or without pulmonary edema with warm extremities (warm shock)

FLOWCHART 30.2: Proposed algorithm for the management of scorpion sting.[11]

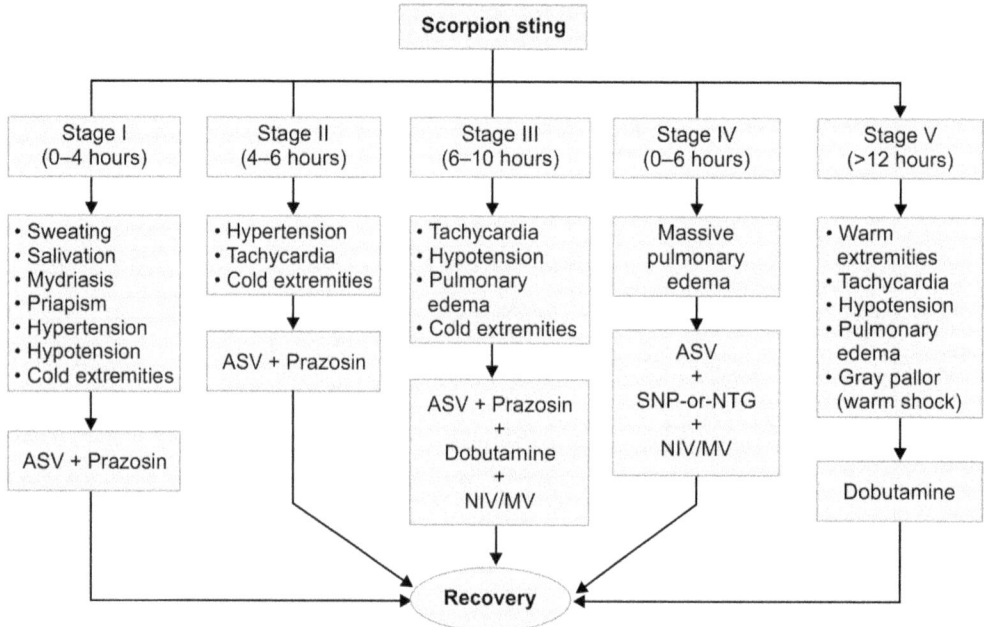

The Rabat Morocco consensus meeting classified scorpion envenomation into three classes.[15]
1. Class I: Local manifestations
2. Class II: Systemic involvement
3. Class III: Cardiogenic failure, hypertension, arrhythmias, bradycardia, respiratory failure, and neurological failure

Management

A proposed algorithm for management of scorpion sting is shown in Flowchart 30.2.

Scorpion antivenom: IV administration of the antivenom is recommended at the earliest. The role of the antivenom is primarily to counter the circulating unbound venom. The sympathetic overstimulation that happens in the later stages can be prevented by the antivenom. Evidence seems to suggest a quick reversal of neurological manifestations with the use of antivenom.[16] In India, a nonspecific F(ab)2 antivenom is available for clinical use. This is currently available as a 10-mL vial. About 1 mL of antivenom is expected to neutralize the effects.

Prazosin: The use of prazosin has been shown to be effective in a prospective randomized controlled trial by Bawaskar et al.[10] Combining prazosin with antivenom seems to be the most effective therapy.[11] The dose of prazosin is 30 µg/kg orally every 6 hours for 48 hours. Cardiovascular manifestations should be managed as for other conditions. Dobutamine has been used for left ventricular dysfunction, but advanced hemodynamic monitoring is essential.

There are isolated case reports of venoarterial extracorporeal membrane oxygenation being used successfully for scorpion sting-related cardiovascular complications.[12]

BEE STING

Bee sting is not uncommon in tropical countries. The severity seems to be higher in adults.[15] Bees belongs to the order Hymenoptera. The family Apidae includes the honey bees which are the most common cause of bee stings worldwide. The female worker bees are equipped with a banded stringed apparatus which is mostly used as a defense mechanism. The sting is usually fatal for the honey bees themselves. African honey bees are known to sting their targets more than once. Each sting releases a large amount of venom (50–140 µg). The composition of the venom includes vasoactive amines, mast cell depolarizing peptides, hyaluronidase, and melittin.[16] The manifestations of bee sting can range from mild-to-severe local reaction extending to various degree of anaphylactic reactions. Multiple stings are associated with severe systemic manifestations. The various manifestations and grades are shown in Tables 30.2 and 30.3.[15] The more severe manifestations include rhabdomyolysis, Guillain-Barre syndrome, and coagulation failure. Professional Bee keepers might benefit from skin prick or intradermal tests. Serum immunoglobulin E levels in conjunction with skin tests also predict the probability of severe reactions to a sting.

Table 30.2: Classification of manifestations of bee sting.

Severity	Representation	Manifestations
Mild	+	Pruritus, erythema, urticaria, nausea, angioedema, rhinitis
Moderate	++	Mild asthma, moderate angioedema, abdominal pain, vomiting, diarrhea, mild and transient hypotensive symptoms
Severe	+++	Laryngeal edema, collapse or loss of consciousness, hypotension, rarely incontinence, seizures

Table 30.3: Mueller grading of bee sting envenomation.

Grade I	Systemic reaction is characterized by generalized urticaria or erythema, itching, malaise or anxiety
Grade II	Reactions may include symptoms associated with grade I reactions as well as generalized edema, tightness in the chest, wheezing, abdominal pain, nausea and vomiting, and dizziness
Grade III	Reactions may include symptoms associated with grade I or II reactions as well as symptoms of dyspnea, dysarthria, hoarseness, weakness, confusion and a feeling of impending doom
Grade IV	Reactions may include symptoms associated with grade I, II or III reactions as well as any two of the following—fall in BP, loss of consciousness, incontinence of urine or feces, or cyanosis

Treatment

Recognition of anaphylaxis on the basis of respiratory and cardiovascular features is crucial. The first drug of choice for anaphylaxis is epinephrine (adrenaline) 0.3 mL of 1:1,000 solution given IM. The earlier the epinephrine is administered, the quicker the resolution. In the hospital, epinephrine may be given as infusion after the initial dose. Antihistamines (H_1 and H_2 blockers) should be added but are not substitute for epinephrine. Patients who are previously beta blocked might need glucagon (1–5 mg IV bolus, followed by 5–15 µg/min infusion). The sting should be gently eased out rather than squeezed out. Antivenom is available in western countries, but its availability in India is unknown.

SUMMARY

Snakebite is a treatable medical emergency. Early transport to a medical facility and institution of ASV along with aggressive organ support can save many lives. It can often be misdiagnosed and mismanaged (especially Krait bite); hence, a high index of suspicion is needed.
- Scorpion envenomation is associated with significant morbidity and mortality if systemic effects cannot be identified and neutralized. Prazosin is a useful part of the treatment algorithm.
- Beestings are likely to produce anaphylaxis which has to be managed aggressively.

REFERENCES

1. Majumder D, Sinha A, Bhattacharya SK, et al. Epidemiological profile of snakebite in South 24 Parganas district of West Bengal with focus on underreporting of snakebite deaths. Indian J Public Health. 2014;58:17-21.
2. Mohapatra B, Warrell DA, Suraweera W, et al.; For the Million Death Study Collaborators. Snakebite mortality in India: a nationally representative mortality survey. PLoS Negl Trop Dis. 2011;5(4):e1018.
3. Bawaskar HS, Bawaskar PH, Punde DP, et al. Profile of snakebite envenoming in rural Maharashtra, India. J Assoc Physicians India. 2008;56:88-95.
4. Alirol E, Sharma SK, Bawaskar HS, et al. Snake bite in South Asia: a review. PLoS Negl Trop Dis. 2010;4(1):e603.
5. Bawaskar HS, Bawaskar PH, Bawaskar Parag H. Premonitory signs and symptoms of envenoming by common krait (Bungarus caeruleus). Trop Doct. 2014;44(2):82-5.
6. Ministry of Health and Social Welfare. Management of snake bite. India: Ministry of Health and Social Welfare; 2017.
7. Bawaskar HS. Aphasia in a farmer after viper bite. Lancet. 2002;360(9346):1703.
8. Toxicology.ucsd.edu.
9. Rojnuckarin P, Chanthawibun W, Noiphrom J, et al. A randomized, double-blind, placebo-controlled trial of antivenom for local effects of green pit viper bites. Trans R Soc Trop Med Hyg. 2006;100:879-84.
10. Nuchprayoon I, Pongpan C, Sripaiboonkij N. The role of prednisolone in reducing limb oedema in children bitten by green pit vipers: a randomized, controlled trial. Ann Trop Med Parasitol. 2008;102:643-9.
11. Chippaux JP. Emerging options for the management of scorpion stings. Drug Des Devel Ther. 2012;6:165-73.
12. Bawaskar HS, Bawaskar PH. Scorpion sting: update. J Assoc Physicians India. 2012;60:46-55.
13. Tarmiz A, Mgarrech I, Kortas C, et al. Successful use of extracorporeal membrane oxygenation for the treatment of cardiogenic shock due to scorpion envenomation. Case Rep Critical Care. 2017;2017:8073989.
14. Golden DB. Stinging insect allergy. Am Fam Physician. 2003;67(12):2541-6.
15. Krishna MT, Ewan PW, Diwakar L, et al. Diagnosis and management of hymenoptera venom allergy: British Society for Allergy and Clinical Immunology (BSACI) guidelines. Clin Exp Allergy. 2011;41(9):1201-20.
16. Burns DA. Diseases caused by arthropods and other noxious animals. In: Burns DA, Breathnach SM, Cox NH, Griffiths CEM (Eds). Rook's textbook of dermatology, 8th edition. Blackwell Publishing. 2009. pp. 38.2-4.

CHAPTER 31

Toxidromes

Chulananda Dias Goonasekera, Lakshman Karalliedde, Lounja Bouikhsaine

INTRODUCTION

Critical care involves scrupulous monitoring and therapy of uncompensated single or multiple organ failure until self-sustainable recovery. The diagnostic clinical features of organ failures and supportive therapies are well established, including the paradigms of therapeutic prioritization of failed organ function in critical care. When clinical features do not match the organ dysfunction at hand, a toxidrome should be suspected. Identification of a toxidrome aids the clinician in directing therapeutic actions, as well as narrowing the differential diagnosis and identification of the class of toxin.

Toxidrome is a toxin-induced syndrome. It is a clinical constellation of signs and symptoms that is very suggestive of a particular poisoning or category of intoxication. Toxidromes may mimic multiorgan failure at presentation but an explicable pathophysiological rationale for the organ failures may be lacking. For example, breathlessness and frothing at mouth may be seen in the absence of heart failure or lung infection. A life-threatening bradycardia may occur in the absence of any cardiac or neurological pathology. In the extreme, they may appear "brain dead" when they are not.[1]

Toxidromes result from chemical or biological external toxins. Each constitutes a group of clinical features found on physical examination and ancillary testing.[2] The pathogenesis is attributed to either receptor blockade or stimulation and/or cellular dysfunction. The management strategies are often determined by the "toxidrome" without precise identification of the specific agent that caused the signs and symptoms. Appropriate antidotes are used if the causative poison is known. Unfortunately, toxidromes are not clinically specific because symptoms from multiple coingestants often occur simultaneously, clouding the clinical picture.

Specific clinical features of a toxidrome may help resolve diagnostic dilemmas. For example, noting the presence of dry axilla in a markedly agitated patient may be the only way of differentiating between toxicity following an anticholinergic agent and a sympathomimetic agent. Similarly, miosis may be the only sign distinguishing opioid toxicity from a benzodiazepine overdose.

When specific antidote is available, its timely use is very important. A few examples are intravenous (IV) acetylcysteine (for acetaminophen toxicity), digoxin-binding antibodies (for digitalis alkaloid toxicity), and hydroxocobalamin (for cyanide). Fomepizole (a competitive inhibitor of alcohol dehydrogenase) is useful for methanol and ethylene glycol toxicity to prevent the formation of toxic acid metabolites.

Sodium bicarbonate has a role in correcting severe acidosis from toxic alcohols and cyanide. It is also used to treat toxicity due to salicylates and sodium channel blocking agents, such as tricyclic antidepressants. It enhances renal elimination of salicylates. Conversely, the priority in sodium channel toxicity is to provide sufficient sodium to overcome the blockade; efficacy of which manifests as a narrowing of the QRS segment in electrocardiogram (ECG).

A "toxidrome" manifests when the dose of a toxin or poison exceeds the capacity of an individual to compensate, or to detoxify and eliminate. Thus, an individual's vulnerability to a poison or toxin becomes an indispensable part of therapeutic planning. The recognition and management of toxidromes are yet evolving. This chapter explores the symptomatology, pathophysiology, and evidence-based therapeutic strategies for established toxidromes that are likely to need critical care at presentation. The poisonings of insidious onset following arsenic and lead are not discussed.

GENERIC PRINCIPLES OF THERAPY

The general supportive measures in toxidromes[3] follow the principles of resuscitation, i.e. ABCs (airway, breathing, and circulation) whilst maintaining cervical spine stability when necessary (following neck trauma). The airway patency is ensured, breathing mechanically assisted if necessary, and the circulation stabilized with IV fluids, and vasopressors or inotropes as required. Prevention of further absorption of the poison from skin, eyes, gut, lungs, or parenteral routes is the next priority. A combination of antidotes, such as thiamine, dextrose, and naloxone, is considered for patients in a coma.

Gastrointestinal decontamination may be considered using emesis, gastric emptying or lavage, whole bowel irrigation, and use of activated charcoal combined with a cathartic if appropriate. Emesis induced by Ipecac is not considered to be of benefit to prevent drug absorption hours after ingestion or when systemic toxicity has manifested.[4] Gastric lavage is used only if the patient has ingested a life-threatening amount of a poison within an hour of seeking treatment,[5] unless the poison itself delayed the gastric emptying (e.g. tricyclic antidepressants, opioids, or salicylates). Gastric lavage is contraindicated in poisoning with caustic or petroleum products, such as kerosene. This is to prevent the risk of aspiration-induced lung injury. Airway protection is paramount before gastric lavage. Cathartic, if used, is limited to a single dose to minimize adverse effects.[6]

Often, activated charcoal is used as the sole method for gastrointestinal decontamination. It is an effective adsorbent but is not effective following intoxications with organophosphates (OPs), carbamates (CBs), alcohols, lithium, hydrocarbons, iron, and acids. Charcoal aspiration can also lead to pneumonia, acute respiratory distress syndrome, and death. Thus, airway protection is crucial in patients with impaired consciousness or in those with convulsions. Multidose activated charcoal significantly enhances drug elimination, especially following life-threatening ingestion of carbamazepine, dapsone, phenobarbital, quinine, or theophylline.[7] Consider whole bowel irrigation only if activated charcoal is not considered to be effective as in iron or lithium overdose.[8] Repeated oral dosing of activated charcoal maintains a concentration gradient across the gut. This promotes poison migration from blood into the intestinal lumen (gut dialysis). In addition, activated charcoal disrupts the enterohepatic circulation of agents that undergo biliary elimination. In salicylate toxicity, activated charcoal decreases its absorption. However, single-dose oral activated charcoal administered in emergency department (ED) has not been shown to significantly affect clinical outcomes of self-poisoned patients.[9]

Intravenous fat emulsion may be useful as a binding agent following poisoning with bupivacaine, verapamil, chlorpromazine, and some tricyclic antidepressants and beta-blockers.[10,11]

Promoting diuresis with urinary alkalinization (pH > 7.5) with IV sodium bicarbonate and volume loading is helpful to eliminate salicylates and phenobarbital. Hypokalemia is the most common complication that follows urinary alkalization. Extracorporeal removal of toxins (hemodialysis, hemoperfusion, or hemofiltration) is reserved for toxins undergoing delayed or insufficient clearance due to organ dysfunction, or when toxic metabolites are produced leading to delayed toxicity.[12] Lithium, ethylene glycol, salicylate, and acetaminophen poisonings often necessitate hemodialysis.[13]

The recognition of the offending poison is important to initiate administration of appropriate antidotes. The antidote can neutralize or counteract the poison or the toxin. For example, after snake envenomation, the antidote is antivenom. Some antivenoms are specific to venoms of some snakes. Often polyspecific antidotes are used when the identity of the snake is uncertain.

Ancillary testing is helpful but not in all toxidromes. Although most laboratories provide screening of urine for the common drugs of abuse, these do not directly influence outcomes. This is because a "positive" screen may not reveal the current intoxication. In general, clinical symptoms are long gone before the screen becomes "negative." Cannabinoids remain positive for weeks or months in urine after exposure. Benzodiazepines may yield false-negative results due to the complexity of their metabolism. Amphetamines are associated with false-positive results due to its structural similarity to other legal medications. However, therapeutic drug level monitoring is useful to avoid toxicity.

Serum or blood level assays are useful to direct patient care in toxidromes following acetaminophen, salicylate, lithium, digoxin, methanol, and ethylene glycol poisoning. For drugs, such as phenytoin, valproic acid, and carbamazepine, the elevated levels only confirm the presence of the drug in the blood. These levels are also unlikely to influence ongoing care as care pathways are often clinically driven.

Toxidromes evolve, and acute, intermediate, and long-term effects may differ requiring constant revision of management strategies. New toxidromes are also recognized following poisoning with newer agents. Therefore, seeking advice from a Regional Poison Control Centre is always prudent.

ANTICHOLINERGIC TOXIDROME

The anticholinergic toxidrome, also referred to as an antimuscarinic toxidrome, is produced by a number of agents that possess antimuscarinic properties. This may occur following the ingestion of Jimson plant seeds (*Datura stramonium*),[14] post anesthesia following the use of atropine, scopolamine, glycopyrrolate, and ingestion of prescription or over the counter medications possessing anticholinergic activity, such as antihistamines, mefloquine, tricyclic antidepressants, and antipsychotics.[15] It is also reported following the use of eye drops containing atropine (Fig. 31.1).[16]

Symptomatology

The diagnosis of anticholinergic toxicity is clinical. Presentations are variable. Central manifestations range from excitatory symptoms including delirium and agitation to depression, stupor, and coma.[17] The clinical features are traditionally summarized as delirium (mad as a hen), poor vision due to mydriasis (blind as a bat), dry skin and mouth (dry as a bone), flushing (red as a beet), and pyrexia (hot as an oven).[18] Added features include tachycardia, hypoactive bowel, and urinary retention.

Pathophysiology

Anticholinergic agents competitively inhibit binding of the neurotransmitter acetylcholine (ACh) to muscarinic receptors located in the central nervous system (CNS), in the target organs of the parasympathetic nervous system, and in the sympathetic nervous system-sweat glands. Large doses may also induce nicotinic and neuromuscular receptor blockade. Muscarinic receptors are found on peripheral postganglionic cholinergic nerves in the smooth muscle (intestinal, bronchial, and cardiac), the secretory glands (salivary and sweat), the ciliary body of the eye, and the CNS. The onset of anticholinergic toxicity is variable. It depends on the toxin but usually occurs within 1–2 hours of oral ingestion. Atropine is rapidly absorbed orally and achieves peak plasma concentrations within 2 hours. Diphenoxylate-

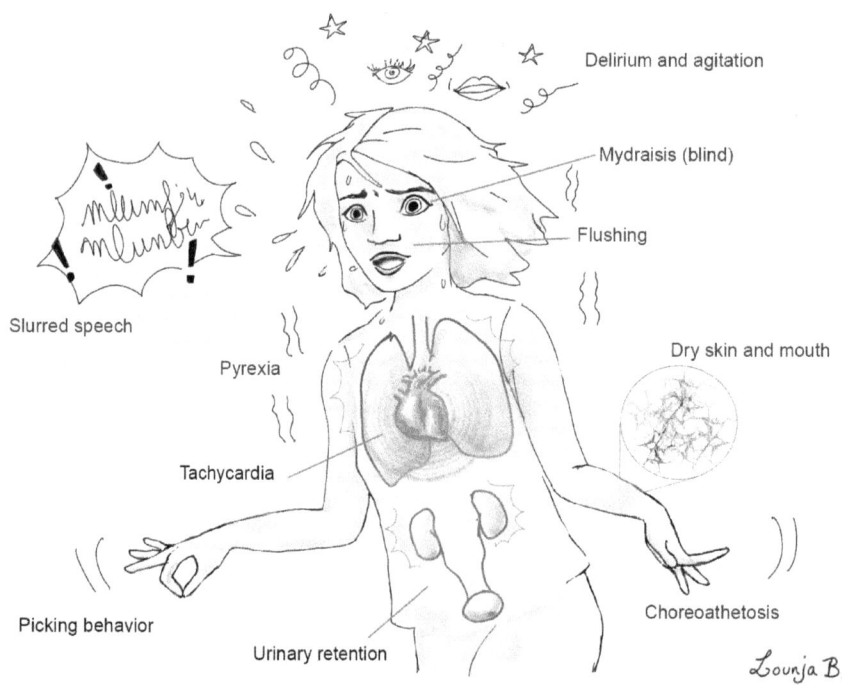

FIGURE 31.1: Anticholinergic toxidrome.

atropine (e.g. Lomotil) is an antidiarrheal agent that may present with toxicity up to 12 hours after ingestion. Scopolamine may persist for over 24 hours.[19]

Practice Prescription

This toxidrome should be considered in the differential diagnosis of altered mental status following general anesthesia.

Provide general supportive and protective therapies. The serum drug levels are neither helpful nor easily available. Measure blood glucose to rule out hypoglycemia as a cause of any alteration in mental status and consider measuring acetaminophen and salicylate levels, as these are common coingestions. Perform an ECG to rule out conduction system abnormalities and dysrhythmias. Do a pregnancy test in all women of childbearing age. Patients with severe psychomotor agitation and seizures should have a serum creatinine kinase level measured to detect rhabdomyolysis.

Because sweating is inhibited in intoxicated patients, treatment of agitation is important to prevent hyperthermia. The first choice is benzodiazepines. Avoid phenothiazines and butyrophenones to sedate patients with anticholinergic toxicity as they are themselves anticholinergic and may exacerbate symptoms. Hyperthermia should be treated using standard guidelines.

If the patient's mental status is intact, consider decontamination with activated charcoal (1 g/kg; maximum 50 g). The use of physostigmine may be useful in patients manifesting with both peripheral and moderate central (moderate-to-severe agitation/delirium) anticholinergic toxicity. Physostigmine promptly reverses anticholinergic syndrome-related altered mental status and respiratory depression.[20]

Asymptomatic patients should be observed in hospital for a minimum of 6 hours. If they remain asymptomatic during this period of observation, they may be discharged.

CHOLINERGIC TOXIDROME

This syndrome is commonly seen following pesticide poisoning is potentially fatal. OP, organochlorine, and CB compounds act as acetylcholinesterase (AChE) inhibitors. It affects peripheral and CNSs, skeletal and smooth muscles, liver, pancreas, and brain. Recently used nerve agents ("Novichok" and "Sarin") are highly purified OPs with very high toxicity.[21-23] "Sarin" exposure is associated with OP-induced delayed neurotoxicity, chronic neurotoxicity, and endocrine disruption. In addition to the effects on the cholinergic system, "Sarin" also indirectly activates several neurotransmitters, including gamma-aminobutyric acid (GABA) and alter other signaling systems. A cholinergic crisis can also result from drug–drug interaction, e.g. donepezil and fluoxetine or similar selective serotonin reuptake inhibitors (SSRIs) that inhibit cytochrome P450 enzymes.[24] OP-induced oxidative stress can also lead to diabetes and other metabolic disorders.[25]

Symptomatology

The onset of symptoms can be acute (within 24 hours), delayed (24 hours to 2 weeks), or late (beyond 2 weeks) and are mostly respiratory, cardiovascular, or neurological. The main routes of exposure are inhalational, dermal, and oral. The fastest onset follows inhalational absorption, usually within a few minutes of exposure.

Traditionally, the clinical features are described upon receptor-specific effects on muscarinic, nicotinic, and CNS receptors.[26] Muscarinic features, such as bradycardia, bronchoconstriction, diaphoresis, pupil constriction predominate, but nicotinic receptor stimulation related clinical features, may occur at the same time.

Neurological clinical features include restlessness, delirium, agitation, miosis, impairment of consciousness, fasciculations, convulsions, and paralysis. Delirium however may also be attributed to treatment with atropine. Extrapyramidal manifestations, ocular signs, ototoxicity, presentation as a Guillain-Barre syndrome and sphincter involvement, and late-onset cerebellar ataxia have been reported.[27,28] Neuropsychiatric disorders may occur following chronic exposure.

Three types of paralysis are described. Type I paralysis, characterized by weakness, fasciculations, cramps, and twitching, occurs acutely with the cholinergic symptoms including impaired consciousness responding to atropine.[29] Type II paralysis, termed "intermediate syndrome," is seen with an insidious onset in more than half of patients, 24-96 hours following poisoning. It mostly involves proximal, neck and respiratory muscles, and cranial nerves and recovers within 1-2 weeks.[30-32] Type III paralysis is characterized by distal weakness observed 2-3 weeks after poisoning. Its recovery is often incomplete and may take weeks to months. This late-onset neuropathy is characterized by distal weakness, cramping pain, and paresthesia of the extremities.[33,34] Weakness of specific muscle groups at sites of dermal exposure, cranial nerve palsies, isolated laryngeal paralysis, and diaphragmatic paralysis has also been reported.[35]

The respiratory paralysis can be fatal even after a variable period of artificial respiration. Patients with early respiratory failure have normal repetitive nerve stimulation in electrophysiological studies suggesting a predominant central muscarinic mechanism. Patients with late respiratory failure show evidence of neuromuscular dysfunction.[36] Electromyography studies during Type II paralysis show a myasthenic response.

Coma is seen in a quarter of patients and can last from hours to days. Some manifest altered consciousness or coma days after poisoning and is termed delayed OP encephalopathy or "CNS intermediate." Coma with absent brainstem reflexes or encephalopathy has been reported 4 days after normal consciousness with subsequent spontaneous resolution. The clinical distinguishing feature between "brain death" and this "mimic" is the presence of "small miosed pupils."[37] Other late effects include poor concentration and memory and posttraumatic stress disorder.

Cardiac manifestations are observed in two-third of patients with OP poisoning. These include QTc prolongation, ST-T segment changes, and T wave abnormalities.[38] Other cardiac manifestations may be sinus bradycardia or tachycardia, hypotension or hypertension, supraventricular and ventricular arrhythmias and ventricular premature complexes and noncardiogenic pulmonary edema. Death may occur either due to arrhythmias[39] or severe and refractory hypotension.[40,41]

Pancreatitis was reported in 12.8%.[42] Metabolic complications, such as hyperglycemia and glycosuria, and diabetic ketoacidosis have been described.[43]

Pathophysiology

An exacerbated cholinergic response is the basis of symptomatology. The clinical features are described by the mnemonic SLUDGE, i.e. S (salivation), L (lacrimation), U (urination), D (diarrhea), G (GI distress), and E (emesis). Other associated common central features include agitation, confusion, lethargy, seizures, and coma. The electroencephalogram in patients with late-onset coma showed features of encephalopathy.

Nerve agents irreversibly inhibit AChE and lead to a buildup of ACh in the CNS that provokes seizures and centrally mediated respiratory arrest. Overstimulation of central receptors may contribute to early death.[23] Focal respiratory center seizures result in an increase in phrenic nerve output initially, followed by sudden cessation of activity.[44] Although respiratory system plays a major role in the pathogenesis of nerve agent toxicity, there appears to be no long-term respiratory sequelae.

Accumulation of ACh at peripheral autonomic synapses leads to peripheral signs of intoxication and overstimulation of the muscarinic and nicotinic receptors, which is described as the "cholinergic crisis" (i.e. diarrhea, sweating, salivation, miosis, and bronchoconstriction). Exposure to high doses of "Sarin" can result in tremors, seizures, and hypothermia. Greater buildup of ACh at neuromuscular junctions can cause paralysis and ultimately peripherally mediated respiratory arrest and death.

Organophosphate compounds bind to AChE in the plasma, red cells, and cholinergic synapses in the central and peripheral nervous system. Red cell cholinesterase activity correlates better with the severity of exposure.[45-47] Once red-cell AChE has aged, it only recovers via erythropoiesis. This contributes to delayed recovery.[48]

Practice Prescription

Pay attention to your own safety. Use personal protective equipment (PPE) when attending to these patients as the contaminated poison may be absorbed via skin, mucous membranes, and by inhalation. Suck out secretions, stabilize the airway, administer oxygen by mask, and intubate and ventilate if necessary. Remove the patient's clothing (place in a double bag, sealed, labeled, and stored securely), shower, wash down or rinse-wipe-rinse with liquid soap and water, or dilute detergent. Remove any contact lenses and irrigate the eyes with lukewarm water or normal saline solution. Activated charcoal may be used. Gastric lavage may have a role. Assess the cause, give antidotes if appropriate, and consult poisoning center.[49]

The choice of anticholinergic antidote depends on the targeted receptor—central, peripheral, or both. Atropine is the logical choice, as it acts on central and peripheral cholinergic receptors.[50] Glycopyrrolate is advocated[51] but it does not cross the blood–brain barrier. Benzodiazepines and scopolamine cross the blood–brain barrier rapidly and are useful to counter central and extrapyramidal effects. With adequate atropinization, the acute cholinergic symptoms abate within a few hours, but watch for delayed effects.[50] Pralidoxime may not offer significant benefit but some disagree.[52,53]

Natural and synthetic antioxidants seem protective against OP-induced histopathological and biochemical alterations. Thus supplementing people with exposure to OPs with antioxidants, such as vitamin E and C, is now recommended.[54] Evaluation of blood oxidative stress parameters are useful for monitoring.

Acute muscarinic effects on the heart (bradycardia, hypotension) can be lifethreatening. Nicotinic effects of muscle weakness contribute to respiratory weakness, while the acute central effects such as restlessness, agitation, confusion, and convulsions further compromise airway and breathing and increase the risk of aspiration and hypoxia. Many of these muscarinic effects are reversed by atropine but nicotinic neuromuscular effects are not.[55] An organ-specific approach is required in the management of neurological syndromes and respiratory failure[56-58] and cardiac and electrocardiographic abnormalities.[39,59,60] Patchy myocardial involvement could be responsible for lethal cardiac complications. Sinus tachycardia, QT interval prolongation, ST-T changes, U waves, and ventricular premature contractions occur.[39,59] Hypoxemia, acidosis, and electrolyte derangements predispose to cardiac abnormalities.[60] Tachycardia and high blood pressure, observed in acute poisoning, is possibly a result of overwhelming cholinergic effects on the CNS, sympathetic ganglionic synapses, and adrenal medulla.[55]

Due to irreversible binding of OP to AChE, prolonged neuromuscular blockade following muscle relaxants may occur. Avoid succinylcholine as its metabolism is impaired due to plasma butyrylcholinesterase (pseudocholinesterase) inhibition.

The standard treatment for "Sarin"-like nerve agent exposure is postexposure injection of atropine, accompanied by an oxime, and diazepam.[21] Some experimental pretreatment with exogenous cholinesterase, monoclonal or catalytic antibodies, and prophylactic gene therapy has been attempted.[61]

Hyperthermia is a serious complication usually observed in hot and humid environments. This may be attributable to atropine therapy. In such cases, active cooling and sedation should be considered using towels soaked with cold water placed at points of maximum heat loss (e.g. axillae, groins) and a fan to maintain a constant airflow.[62]

Small studies suggest benefit from new treatments, such as magnesium sulfate.[63] Since some OP pesticide poisonings are very difficult to treat, bans on pesticides could be the only way to reduce case fatalities after poisoning.[48]

Effective respiratory protection is vital for emergency preparedness against a chemical attack.[64] The emergency preparedness, PPE for first responders, decontamination of exposed individuals, and atropine, oxime, and benzodiazepine therapy offer the best strategy. Aggressive prosecution of suspected terrorists is required to mitigate this threat (Table 31.1).[65]

SYMPATHOMIMETIC TOXIDROME

A prolonged "fight or flight" response resulting from sustained stimulation of sympathetic system leads to this syndrome. Its associated with poisoning from bath salts[67,68] and prescription (asthma and narcolepsy medications) and nonprescription medications.[69] The nonprescription agents include over-the-counter cold preparations (containing ephedrine), illegal street drugs (cocaine, amphetamines, methamphetamine, and mephedrone), dietary supplements (ephedra alkaloids), and drugs of abuse, such as "ecstasy" (3,4-methylenedioxy methamphetamine). Similar features also occur following withdrawal of GABAergic drugs, such as barbiturates, baclofen, bicuculline, and flumazenil that stimulate or block GABA-mediated neurotransmission or inhibit its reuptake (Fig. 31.2).[70]

Table 31.1: OP poisoning pharmacopeia.

	Doses	Remarks
Atropine	0.6–4 mg IV (maximum 20 mg) (child—20 µg/kg IV)	Repeat dose every 10–20 minutes until secretions dry up and the heart rate rises to 80–90 beats/min. Reversal of pinpoint pupils is a poor guide
Pralidoxime	Give 2 g or 30 mg/kg IV over 4 minutes and every 4–6 hours or infuse IV at 8–10 mg/kg/h for 7 days	This prevents bonding between cholinesterase and OP and 12 hours and 36 hours since poisoning is considered a good window of opportunity for pralidoxime
Diazepam	Give 5–10 mg IV for an adult (1–5 mg IV for a child)	Repeat as required[66]

(OP: organophosphate)

Symptomatology

Adults present with typical adrenergic signs and symptoms, some of which are potentially lethal.[70] A confused, agitated, delirious, hallucinating patient with hyperthermia (rash), diaphoresis, piloerection, hypertension, tachycardia, and tremor or myoclonus is common. Epistaxis and visual disturbance due to pupillary dilatation may occur. There is a risk of intracranial hemorrhage. Acute psychosis, paranoia, bruxism, and seizures are recognized features. There could also be associated chest pain, palpitations, muscle pain, and rhabdomyolysis, especially following synthetic cathinone poisoning.[71] Blood biochemistry may reveal increased creatine phosphokinase (CPK) levels and hyponatremia due to sweating.

Patients who smoke crack cocaine may additionally develop bronchospasm, asthma exacerbation, pneumothorax, and lung injury. Sympathomimetic-induced hyperthermia can produce significant morbidity (from end-organ damage) and death. Acute kidney injury may also occur.

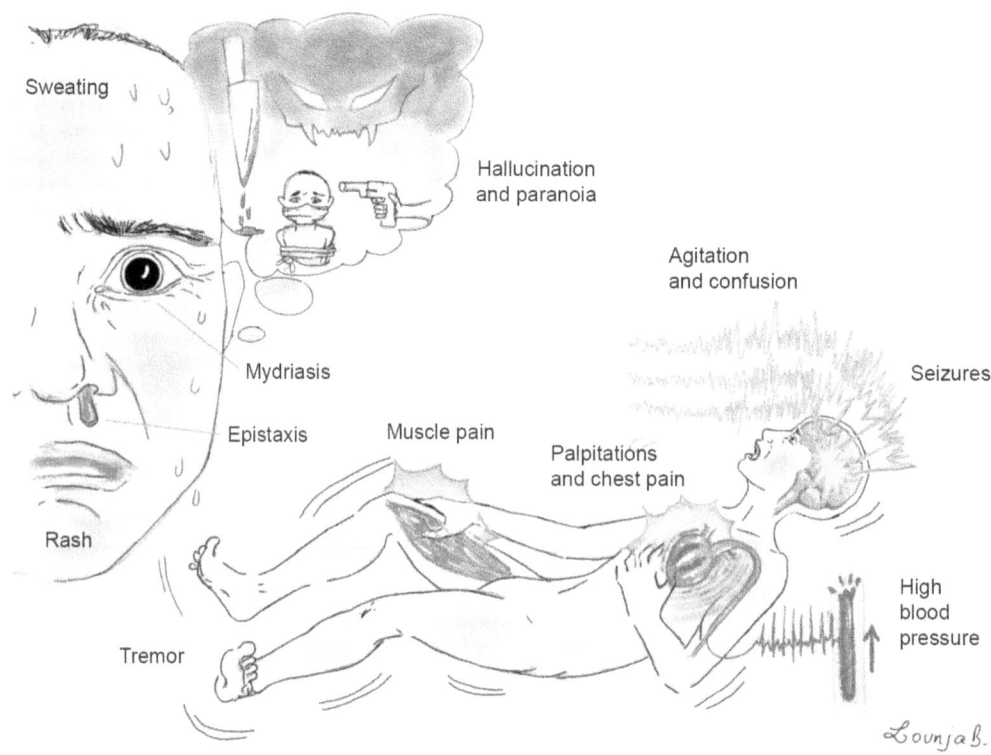

FIGURE 31.2: Sympathomimetic toxidrome

Pathophysiology

Extreme hypertension can result in headache, hypertensive encephalopathy, and intracranial hemorrhage. Sympathomimetic-induced chest pain, myocardial ischemia, myocardial infarction, and cardiomyopathy and cardiac dysrhythmias such as supraventricular tachycardia, atrial or ventricular fibrillation, torsade de pointes and second- or third-degree heart block (as a reflex response to hypertension) are likely.

Hyperthermia results from excessive muscular activity (continuous dancing) and extreme agitation, myoclonus, and seizures. The abuse of sympathomimetic agents in hot, humid environments (e.g. dance clubs, summer evenings) and dehydration can further exacerbate hyperthermia.

Seizures, strokes, and intracerebral bleeds are well-documented complications. Dissecting thoracic aneurysms and mesenteric ischemia are rare but lethal consequences.

Children present with similar signs and symptoms observed in adults along with inconsolable crying, vomiting, and abdominal pain. Since similar features are also the presenting features of many serious pediatric diseases (e.g. sepsis, intussusception, and intracranial lesion), extensive ancillary tests are needed in children to rule out significant disease. Synthetic cathinone can be identified using gas chromatography–mass spectrometry or liquid chromatography.

Practice Prescription

The treatment is primarily supportive. Managing airway and controlling agitation chemically or by physical restraint constitute first aid. Control seizures with IV diazepam or barbiturates and agitation with benzodiazepines or droperidol or olanzapine. Benzodiazepines counteract excessive epinephrine and norepinephrine release and reuptake inhibition. Amphetamine-induced seizures are short lived. Phenytoin should be avoided as its channel-blocking properties can precipitate dysrhythmias.

Hyperthermia needs continuous core temperature monitoring, benzodiazepine, and fluid resuscitation. If body temperature >39.5°C, consider rapid external cooling. This may need paralysis, intubation, and mechanical ventilation.

Consider urgent reduction in blood pressure using titrated doses of benzodiazepine, phentolamine (1 mg IV repeated every 5 minutes) and a vasodilator (glyceryl trinitrate or sodium nitroprusside). Never give beta-blockers as unopposed α-stimulation can lead to severe vasoconstriction.

If there are features of coronary ischemia, treatment with nitroglycerine, morphine, and antiplatelet drugs should be considered. Beta-blockers are contraindicated because they may worsen hypertension and coronary vasoconstriction. The management of hyponatremia may need water restriction. If hyponatremia is profound (<120 mmol/L) and associated with seizures, consider administering hypertonic saline 3% NaCl 4 mL/kg over 30 minutes, followed by further doses to maintain the plasma Na > 120 mmol/L. The goal of raising the serum sodium is kept within an hourly rate of 1-3 mmol/L as faster correction may result in central pontine myelinolysis.

If moderate doses of benzodiazepines are not effective, consider antipsychotics to treat agitation, aggression, or psychosis. Lorazepam, intramuscular (IM) haloperidol, or risperidone have been used successfully. Butyrophenones, such as haloperidol, should be used with caution because they may contribute to hyperthermia or dysrhythmias.

Diazepam, midazolam, ziprasidone, or diphenhydramine may be primarily prescribed for sedation and the treatment of persistent myoclonus. A treatment protocol for the management of "bath salts" related toxidrome has been described.[72]

SYMPATHOPLEGIA TOXIDROME

This results from sympatholytic (or sympathoplegic) drugs inhibiting the downstream effects of the sympathetic nervous system.

Symptomatology

Sympathoplegia reduces heart rate and blood pressure and causes vasodilation. Professional musicians, public speakers, actors, athletes, and dancers consuming beta-blockers to minimize "performance anxiety" are victims of this toxicity. Clonidine overdose may be associated with added CNS depression, bradycardia, miosis, hypotonia, respiratory depression, and seizures.

Pathophysiology

Sympatholytic drugs can be broadly categorized based on their mechanism of action. This includes (1) compounds that cause the release of adrenergic mediators norepinephrine and adrenaline from depots in the sympathetic nerve endings (reserpine, guanethidine); (2) compounds obstructing the release of mediators from the sympathetic nerve endings (bretylium tosylate, alpha-methyldopa); and (3) compounds that block adrenal receptors (phentolamine, propionic acid, dihydroergotamine, and propranolol, and prazosin an α-1-receptor antagonist). α-2-adrenergic receptor agonists, such as clonidine and guanfacine acting presynaptically and centrally, inhibit the release of adrenaline and noradrenaline. Drugs, such as methyltyrosine, inhibit adrenergic receptor signaling by blocking the synthesis of catecholamines.[73,74]

Practice Prescription

Gastric lavage followed by administration of activated charcoal decreases absorption following acute oral ingestion. IV fluid therapy and dopamine infusions are recommended for severe hypotension. Atropine sulfate is used to manage persistent bradycardia. Treatment of hypotension with alpha-adrenergic blocking agents (e.g. tolazoline) is not recommended.[75] Children with clonidine overdose may not need atropine therapy.[76]

Some patients with labetalol overdose may not respond to conventional therapy with glucagon and α-adrenergic receptor-stimulating agents. They may respond to type III phosphodiesterase inhibitors (amrinone) that produce an increase in cardiac output and improved mental status.[77] Severe methyldopa overdose causes prolonged and profound hypotension, sinus bradycardia, and drowsiness. Supportive management may need IV infusion of a large amount of fluids and gelofusine, injections of ephedrine sulfate, and IV infusion of norepinephrine, dopamine for several days.[78]

Overdose of minoxidil causes severe hypotension and tachycardia. Resuscitate with crystalloids, IV dopamine, and phenylephrine to achieve hemodynamic stability. Myocardial infarction is a known complication.[79]

NEUROMUSCULAR BLOCKADE

Partial neuromuscular junction blockade can lead to difficulty in breathing, laryngeal spasm, agitation, and even respiratory arrest. This is often seen following anesthesia recurarization occurring in the postoperative recovery room. Naturally occurring neurotoxins (e.g. botulinum) can also cause deadly neuroparalytic dysfunction.

Assays for rapid and sensitive detection of neurotoxins are yet to be achieved.[80] Thus, the management relies on the clinical diagnosis.

Botulism is recognized in four naturally occurring syndromes: foodborne botulism results from ingestion of foods contaminated with botulinum toxin; wound botulism is caused by *Clostridium botulinum* colonization of a wound; infant botulism is caused by intestinal colonization and toxin production (may be seen in adults also); and inhalational botulism resulting from aerosolization of botulinum toxin. Iatrogenic botulism resulting from injection of toxin is also possible.

All forms of botulism produce the same distinct clinical syndrome of symmetrical cranial nerve palsies, followed by descending, symmetric flaccid paralysis of voluntary muscles, which may progress to respiratory compromise and death.

There are many drugs other than those used in anesthesia, which may interfere with neuromuscular transmission.[81] Awareness of the possibility of such an effect is important, to effectively manage myasthenic syndromes. This minimizes unnecessary morbidity and fatal outcomes in what is potentially a reversible condition.[82]

Myasthenia gravis is a disorder of the neuromuscular junction resulting in weakness of all striated voluntary muscles and could be drug induced. Prednisone, D-penicillamine, and aminoglycosides have been implicated.[83]

Symptomatology

Neuromuscular blocking drugs used in anesthesia are also known as muscle relaxants. Patients who have received a neuromuscular blocking drug should always have their respiration assisted or controlled until the drug has been inactivated or reversed. They should also receive adequate inhalational or IV anesthetic or sedative drugs during surgery to prevent awareness.

Nondepolarizing neuromuscular blocking drugs have a slower onset of action than the depolarizing blocker-suxamethonium chloride. Drugs with a shorter or intermediate duration of action, such as atracurium besilate and vecuronium bromide, are more widely used than those with a longer duration of action, such as pancuronium bromide.

Pathophysiology

Nondepolarizing neuromuscular blocking drugs compete with ACh for receptor sites at the neuromuscular junction, and their action can be reversed with anticholinesterases, such as neostigmine. Nondepolarizing neuromuscular blocking drugs include pancuronium bromide, rocuronium bromide, and vecuronium bromide, atracurium besylate, cisatracurium, and mivacurium.

Practice Prescription

In botulism, the mainstays of therapy are meticulous intensive care including mechanical ventilation, when necessary and timely treatment with antitoxin.[84]

Anticholinesterases reverse the effects of the non-depolarizing (competitive) neuromuscular blocking drugs, such as pancuronium bromide, but they prolong the action of the depolarizing neuromuscular blocking drug suxamethonium chloride.

Neostigmine is used specifically for the reversal of nondepolarizing (competitive) blockade. It acts within 1 minute of IV injection, and effects last for 20–30 minutes; a second dose may then be necessary. Glycopyrronium bromide, or alternatively atropine sulfate, is given before or with neostigmine to prevent the muscarinic effects of neostigmine, such as bradycardia and excessive salivation.

Sugammadex (the first selective relaxant binding agent) is a modified gamma cyclodextrin that can be used for rapid reversal of neuromuscular blockade induced by rocuronium bromide or vecuronium bromide. In practice, sugammadex is used for rapid reversal of neuromuscular blockade in an emergency.

OPIOID TOXIDROME

The most common opioids contributing to opioid toxidrome, also known as "Knockdown toxidrome," are codeine, heroin, propoxyphene, and oxycodone/hydrocodone.

The use and misuse of prescription opioid analgesics, street pills, such as "Norco," containing fentanyl, and various amounts of acetaminophen and hydrocodone contribute to the outbreaks of morbidity and mortality. Illicitly manufactured novel synthetic opioids such as U-47700 and W-18[85] and fentanyl are highly potent and can cause severe toxicity even in the opioid-tolerant patient.

Symptomatology

Opioids cause a well-recognized toxidrome including respiratory depression, decreased level of consciousness, pinpoint pupils, hypotension, unresponsiveness, and death. Sedative hypnotics are like opioids, but pupillary changes are not observed. For example, meperidine and tramadol, despite their classification as opioids, do not cause miosis.

Pathophysiology

Toxicity is determined by the amount ingested and speed of absorption. Some opioids, such as dextropropoxyphene, methadone, and tramadol, have additional properties that account for their toxicity.

Practice Prescription

Apply general supportive measures including endotracheal intubation and ventilation if needed. Ancillary tests, such as urine opiate screening, may not identify some of the above agents; and hence, clinicians cannot rely on these tests to rule out opioid intoxication.

Naloxone is the opioid antagonist of choice, and its dose should be titrated to the clinical response. The duration of action of naloxone is relatively short; and therefore, repeated doses or infusion may be required. Paradoxical increase in toxicity may be seen with naloxone promoting gut motility and absorption of any remaining drug in the gut. Certain fentanyl analogs may require repeated doses of naloxone for reversal of effects of opioids.[86]

SEROTONINERGIC (SEROTONERGIC) TOXIDROME

Serotonin toxicity syndrome (toxidrome) is likely amongst patients who take multiple serotonergic drugs, particularly coadministered with monoamine oxidase inhibitors (MAOIs) or 5-hydroxytryptamine (5-HT) reuptake blockers. The toxidrome can vary from mild to severe.

Tramadol overdose associated seizures and raised CPK levels are also linked to a potential serotonin syndrome.

Symptomatology

Serotonin syndrome is often described as a clinical triad of mental status changes, autonomic hyperactivity, and neuromuscular abnormalities. Thus clinical features associated with serotonin toxicity are numerous. Confusion, hypomania, agitation, altered mental state, myoclonus, hyperreflexia, tremor, shivering, diaphoresis, and fever are the main features. However, clonus (inducible, spontaneous, or ocular), agitation, diaphoresis, tremor, and hyperreflexia are considered salient and contributed to the development of Hunter Serotonin Toxicity Criteria.[87] In life-threatening serotonin toxicity, hypertonicity and fever >38°C are universal.

Pathophysiology

A striking number of drugs and drug combinations have been associated with the serotonin syndrome. These include MAOIs, tricyclic antidepressants, SSRIs, opiate analgesics, over-the-counter cough medicines, antibiotics, weight-reduction agents, antiemetics, antimigraine agents, drugs of abuse, and herbal products. The withdrawal of medications has also been associated with the syndrome.

Animal experiments suggest that $5\text{-}HT_{1A}$ receptors were involved in the hypothermic response, while $5\text{-}HT_{2A}$ and N-methyl-D-aspartic acid receptors mediated head shakes, hyperthermia in this toxidrome. The time frame of using antidotes in the treatment of the 5-HT toxidrome is important to prevent death.[88] Tramadol overdose related impaired consciousness, ECG changes, and convulsions may be opioid and/or serotonin induced.

Practice Prescription

Apply generic supportive measures. No laboratory tests confirm the diagnosis of the serotonin syndrome. In tramadol overdose, mydriasis or tachycardia appears to indicate a higher risk for seizures. Management may need to be focused on both μ-opioid agonism and potential serotonin syndrome.[89]

The management involves the removal of the precipitating drugs, provision of supportive care, control of agitation, administration of $5\text{-}HT_{2A}$ antagonists, control of autonomic instability, and the control of hyperthermia. Many cases of the serotonin syndrome typically resolve within 24 hours after the initiation of therapy and the discontinuation of serotonergic drugs.

Supportive care along with administration of IV fluids and correction of vital functions remain the mainstay of therapy. Hyperthermia patients (>41.1°C) are severely ill and should receive the above therapies as well as immediate sedation, neuromuscular paralysis, and endotracheal intubation. Clinicians should avoid succinylcholine because of the risk of arrhythmia from hyperkalemia associated with rhabdomyolysis. Control agitation with benzodiazepines. Physical restraint is ill advised and may contribute to mortality as enforcing isometric muscle contractions are associated with severe lactic acidosis and hyperthermia. Administer $5\text{-}HT_{2A}$ antagonist. Cyproheptadine is the recommended drug. Sublingual olanzapine is useful. If a parenteral agent is needed, consider IM chlorpromazine.

Control of autonomic instability involves stabilization of fluctuating pulse and blood pressure. Hypotension arising from MAOI interactions should be treated with low doses of direct-acting sympathomimetic amines (e.g. norepinephrine, phenylephrine, and epinephrine). Direct agonists do not require intracellular metabolism to generate a vasoactive amine.[90]

CYANIDE TOXIDROME

Cyanide poisoning may result from exposure to cyanide, its salts, or cyanogenic compounds in residential fires, industrial accidents, and drug and plant intoxication. It can present in multiple ways. Following a chemical disaster, hydrocyanic acid and its derivatives are the usual toxins. Relief or control of symptoms and mortality is highly dependent on quick treatment with a cyanide antidote sodium thiosulfate and hydroxocobalamin.[91]

In victims of fires, recognition of the cyanide toxidrome is hampered by its short half-life in blood and the poor stability of cyanide. In contrast, carboxyhemoglobin, as a marker of carbon monoxide poisoning, is easily measured and lasts long in the blood. There is no evidence to support the arbitrary fixed lethal thresholds of 50% for carboxyhemoglobin, and 3 mg/L for cyanide, in victims after fires. Comparison of pure carbon monoxide and pure cyanide poisonings suggest that a cyanide toxidrome can be defined considering signs and symptoms induced by cyanide and carbon monoxide. Cyanide can induce life-threatening poisoning from which a full recovery is possible. A number of experimentally efficient antidotes to cyanide exist, whose clinical use has been hampered due to serious side effects.[92]

Symptomatology

Signs of cyanide poisoning include headache, vertigo, agitation, confusion, coma, convulsions, respiratory arrest, cardiovascular collapse, and death. The onset of symptoms is rapid or quick usually within 30 minutes of exposure, leading to an altered neurological status (82%), including coma (66%), dilated pupils (78%), and abnormal respiratory pattern (93%) (hyperpnea, polypnea, and bradypnea). Cyanide sometimes is described as having a "bitter almond" smell, but it does not always give off an odor, and not everyone can detect this odor. Seizures were witnessed in 26% of poisonings, premature ventricular contractions in 16%, and pulmonary edema in 5%. The mortality rate was 28%.[92,93]

The biochemical hallmark is lactic acidosis. A plasma lactate concentration ≥10 mmol/L in victims following fires without severe burns and ≥8 mmol/L in pure cyanide poisoned patients are sensitive and specific indicators of cyanide intoxication.

Pathophysiology

Cyanide is rapidly reacting and causes arrest of aerobic metabolism. The symptoms are diffuse and lethal and require high clinical suspicion.

The primary target of toxicity is mitochondrial cytochrome oxidase. The onset and severity of poisoning depend on the route, dose, physicochemical structure, and other variables. Common features of poisoning include dyspnea, altered respiratory patterns, abnormal vital signs, altered mental status, seizures, and lactic acidosis.

The diagnosis of cyanide poisoning is challenging. Most patients at presentation are unresponsive, hypotensive, and in respiratory failure or in cardiac arrest. Seizures, cyanosis, cherry red skin, and presence of a bitter almond body odor are some other clinical features. Management includes cyanide antidotes, sodium thiosulfate, and hydroxocobalamin. Most cases require intubation with mechanical ventilation. A substantial number of patients develop refractory hypotension requiring vasopressor support. Most present with a metabolic acidosis with significant lactic acidosis.[94]

With inhalational poisoning, carbon monoxide (colorless, odorless, and tasteless), a product of incomplete combustion, binds to hemoglobin with a much greater affinity than oxygen and reduces oxygen delivery, aggravating the severity of cyanide poisoning. With no signature clinical symptom, diagnosis depends on the patient's history of exposure, elevated carboxyhemoglobin levels, and alterations in mental status.

Cyanide intoxication is often a comorbid disease with carbon monoxide inhalation injury from an enclosed fire but may be the predominant toxin. It acts synergistically with carbon monoxide increasing the risk of fatality. The best diagnostic guides are the presence of high lactate levels, carboxyhemoglobin concentrations greater than 10%, history of smoke inhalation from an enclosed fire, and alterations in levels of consciousness. Treatment with hydroxocobalamin is the standard care.[95]

Practice Prescription

Conventional treatment of cyanide poisoning includes decontamination, supportive and specific treatment, followed by hydroxocobalamin. Provision of 100% normobaric oxygen decreases the half-life of carboxyhemoglobin from 5 hours to 1 hour. Hyperbaric oxygen is a useful adjunct to reduce the half-life of carboxyhemoglobin rapidly and the incidence of delayed neurologic sequelae.

Institute immediate treatment with 100% oxygen, assisted ventilation, decontamination, correction of acidosis, and maintenance of blood pressure. Antidotes include oxygen, hydroxocobalamin, dicobalt EDTA (ethylenediaminetetraacetic acid), and methemoglobin-inducers. Hydroxocobalamin is a useful antidote due to its rapid cyanide binding and lack of serious side effects, even in the absence of cyanide intoxication. Sodium thiosulfate acts more slowly than the other antidotes and is indicated in subacute cyanogen poisoning and as an adjunct to acute cyanide poisoning.[96]

Basic life support includes immediate administration of high flow of oxygen, airway protection, and cardiopulmonary resuscitation. Advanced life support includes mechanical ventilation, catecholamine, and sodium bicarbonate infusion. Oxygen counteracts efficiently the adverse action of cyanide at the mitochondrial level. Sodium thiosulfate, methemoglobin-forming agents, and cobalt compounds act efficiently by forming nontoxic complexes or transforming cyanide into nontoxic stable derivatives.

Cyanide poisoning treatment is based on excellent supportive care with adjunctive antidote therapy. Multiple antidotes exist and vary in availability in different regions.

All currently marketed antidotes appear effective. The mechanism of action of antidotes include chelation, formation of stable, less toxic complexes, promoting the formation of methemoglobin, and provision of sulfur for detoxification by endogenous rhodanese (also known as rhodanase). Each antidote has advantages and disadvantages. For example, hydroxocobalamin is safer than the methemoglobin inducers in patients following smoke inhalation.[96,97]

The efficacy among antidotes seems similar except for the slower onset of action of sodium thiosulfate (administered alone) compared to other antidotes. The potential for serious toxicity limits or prevents the use of the cyanide antidote kit (sodium nitrite),[98] dicobalt edetate, and 4-dimethylaminophenol in prehospital empirical treatment of suspected cyanide poisoning. Hydroxocobalamin on the other hand has not been associated with clinically significant toxicity. Its rapid onset of action neutralizes cyanide without interfering with cellular oxygen use and is well tolerated. Its safety profiles are conducive to prehospital use, safe for use with smoke-inhalation victims, and not harmful when administered to nonpoisoned patients, and is easily administered.[99]

When treating cyanide poisoning associated with smoke inhalation, we should consider not only the efficiency of antidotes but also their safety. Sodium thiosulfate is both efficient and safe but has a delayed onset of action. These methemoglobin-forming agents are potent, but due to the transformation of hemoglobin into methemoglobin, they also impair delivery of oxygen to tissues. Cobalt EDTA and hydroxocobalamin are efficient and act immediately. Cobalt EDTA is more potent on a molar basis; however, numerous side effects limit its use.

In cyanide-poisoned patients, the use of hydroxocobalamin is recommended as the first-line antidote, owing to its safety. In massive cyanide poisoning, due to the limited potency of hydroxocobalamin, continuous infusion of sodium thiosulfate should be considered.[93]

SALICYLATE TOXIDROME

Salicylate poisoning is common and sometimes fatal. Excessive application of topical preparations containing methyl salicylate, or its accidental ingestion, may result in salicylate poisoning. Severe cases could be fatal.[100,101]

Symptomatology

The salicylate toxidrome includes nausea, vomiting, dyspnea, diaphoresis, dizziness, and altered hearing. The development of tinnitus and/or hearing loss has been heralded as an early marker of salicylate toxicity. However, this principle has only been demonstrated in patients receiving escalating doses of salicylates as a therapeutic measure. Poisoned patients typically suffer from mixed respiratory alkalosis and anion-gap metabolic acidosis. Independent predictors of worst outcomes include older age, malnutrition, impaired liver function, and increased respiratory rate, as well as initial serum lactate. The initial salicylate concentration alone was not predictive of mortality.[102]

Pathophysiology

Serum salicylate therapeutic levels range from 15 mg/dL to 30 mg/dL. Toxicity is due to tissue distribution and is not directly related to the blood levels. Thus serum levels and toxicity do not necessarily correlate.

Practice Prescription

Management of salicylate toxicity is difficult. Toxicity is resolving if serial salicylate levels are decreasing and the patient's symptoms are decreasing. If a salicylate-toxic patient is intubated, the patient must be hyperventilated to maintain a compensatory respiratory alkalosis. IV sodium bicarbonate is indicated in patients with clinical symptoms. Urine alkalinization enhances salicylate elimination by "trapping" the salicylate ion in the renal tubules and enhancing its renal excretion. Hemodialysis is indicated when the salicylate level is 100 mg/dL or greater, the significant metabolic derangements do not rapidly clear with fluids, or there is renal insufficiency.

In poisoned children too, urine alkalization therapy has been successfully and safely implemented using bicarbonate bolus of 1 mEq/kg for over an hour and a continuous bicarbonate–potassium–dextrose combination infusion. A urine output of 1.5–2 mL/kg/h and a urine pH of 7.5–8.5 were achievable.[103]

ENVENOMING

Envenoming is a disease of poverty.[104] Envenoming by snakes, scorpions, wasps, ants, and spiders is an occupational hazard frequently encountered by farmers, farm laborers, hunters, and shepherds of tropical and subtropical countries. Venomous snake bite is a common acute life-threatening medical emergency (Fig. 31.3).[105]

Toxins are the poisonous products of organisms that serve defensive and offensive functions, e.g. sanguinary snakes, stinging scorpions, pesticidal plants, fearless

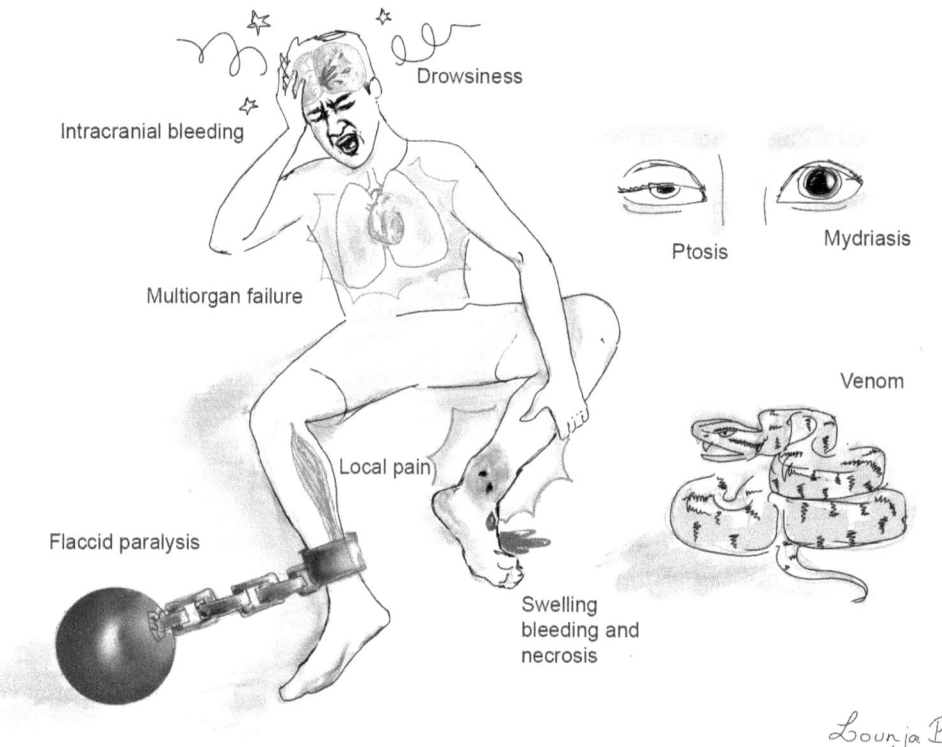

FIGURE 31.3: Envenoming.

frogs, sliming snails, noxious newts, and smarting spiders. These toxins with astonishing molecular specificity are integral component of the self-defensive chemical armor of animals.[106] The toxidromes that result from envenoming depend on the targeted toxic effects of its molecules, e.g. neurotoxicity, nephrotoxicity, and hematoxicity.

Symptomatology

Envenoming can be rapidly life-threatening. It results in local pain and tissue damage, characterized by swelling, blistering, bleeding, and extensive necrosis at the bite site. Viperid venoms can also induce coagulopathy and platelet dysfunction, leading to spontaneous systemic hemorrhages and persistent bleeding from fang marks, wounds, or gums. Intracranial bleeding, including anterior pituitary hemorrhage, and multiorgan failure are common causes of death.[107]

The most important toxic components of venom are those that affect the nervous, cardiovascular, and hemostatic systems and cause tissue necrosis. Venom neurotoxins block or excite peripheral neuromuscular junctions by acting at different sites.

A common symptom of snakebite is drowsiness, suggesting the possibility of a CNS-depressant effect associated with a small nonprotein toxin (found in King cobra). Paralysis following envenoming begins with ptosis, external ophthalmoplegia, and mydriasis, descending to involve muscles innervated by the other cranial and spinal nerves and leading to bulbar and respiratory paralysis, and if ventilation is supported, eventually to total flaccid paralysis.

Marine envenoming may result from bristle worms, crown-of-thorns starfish, sea urchins, venomous fish, stingrays, cone snails, stonefish, blue-ringed octopus, and sea snakes.

Pathophysiology

Scorpion stings are significantly associated with pro-inflammatory cytokine levels in the blood that indicate the severity of scorpion envenoming. These cytokines increase the severity of the visceral damage induced by the direct action of the venom and activation of both the sympathetic and parasympathetic nervous systems.[108]

Snake venoms are rich in protein and peptide toxins that have specificity for a wide range of tissue receptors, making them clinically challenging and scientifically fascinating.[109] Snake venoms are the most complex mixture of toxins and enzymes, each of which may be responsible for one or more distinct toxic actions. It might contain many different toxic and nontoxic proteins and peptides, and nonprotein toxins, carbohydrates, lipids, amines, and other small molecules.

Viper venoms are a large source of proteolytic enzymes causing clotting, bleeding, edema, necrosis, hemorrhage, pain at the bite site, and systemic changes. These severe hematological and hemostatic changes may lead to local and systemic hemorrhages and coagulopathies that are the main cause of death.[110]

Most venom neurotoxins bind to their receptors with high affinity, making reversal of paralysis by antivenom alone virtually impossible. However, rapid improvement in neurotoxicity following antivenom is noted when postsynaptic toxins are implicated (Asian cobras and Australasian death adder). By prolonging the effect of ACh, anticholinesterases sometimes reverse postsynaptic neurotoxicity in such patients. The initial ptosis as seen in botulism, myasthenia gravis, and Graves' disease might be attributable to muscular vulnerability to NM junction blockade.[107]

Hypotension after snakebite is attributed to various constituents including permeability factors that cause hypovolemia from extravasation of plasma and to toxins acting directly or indirectly on cardiac muscle, vascular smooth muscle, and other tissues. Venoms can activate bradykinin, potentiating hypotensive effects. Sarafotoxins, with similarities to endothelin in activity, can potently vasoconstrict coronary and other arteries and delay atrioventricular conduction. Natriuretic peptides found in many snake venoms reduce blood pressure by several mechanisms. Venoms may contain procoagulant enzymes leading to a coagulopathy through the activation of prothrombin, factors V, X, and XIII, and endogenous plasminogen. Toxins bind to a range of platelet receptors, inducing or inhibiting aggregation. Anticoagulant venom phospholipases inhibit the prothrombinase complex. Spontaneous systemic bleeding is caused by hemorrhagins which damage vascular endothelium.[107]

A range of venom myotoxic and cytolytic factors might contribute to local tissue necrosis, rhabdomyolysis leading to myoglobinuria and renal failure. Snakebite-related acute kidney injury is common.[111] Acute interstitial nephritis is one result.[112]

Black widow spider envenomation generally results in self-limiting pain that can be treated in the ED with analgesics and benzodiazepines, usually with no further need for interventions.[113]

Envenoming can result in significant local tissue damage, thrombocytopenia, coagulopathy, neurotoxicity presenting with weakness, and respiratory paralysis. Treatment revolves around general supportive care and antivenom administration.[114]

Practice Prescription

Snakebite victims should be transported as quickly as possible to a medical center. The bite victim should be reassured, the bitten limb immobilized with a makeshift splint or sling, for transport. Walking should be avoided as muscular contractions promote venom absorption. Tourniquets are not recommended because of the risk of severe local damage including ischemia, necrosis, and gangrene if left for long. Instead the bitten limb should be bound firmly with a crepe bandage, starting distally around the toes or fingers and moving proximally. This method is, however, contraindicated for viper and cobra bites as it may increase local tissue damage.[115]

Supportive care, antivenom administration, and treatment of anaphylaxis encompass lifesaving therapy.[116] Immunotherapy is the only specific treatment for snakebite envenoming. Antivenoms are produced by fractionation of plasma obtained from immunized animals, usually horses. Several new antivenoms are in production. Fresh frozen plasma appears to aid restoration of clotting factors more rapidly in snakebite associated with a venom-induced consumption coagulopathy. This mitigates the risk of hemorrhage and reduces the number of antisnake venom vials needed.[117] Protocols for therapy may be region specific.[118]

PLANT TOXIDROMES

Our ancestors used plant poisons to make their hunting weapons more lethal. These poisonous plants thrive near our homes—parks, gardens, hedgerows—and woodlands and sometimes indoor as decorative house plants. For example, Foxgloves (*Digitalis*) look sorcerous but their seeds can kill.[119] The charming blue flowers of monkshood (*Aconitum napellus*) are deceiving and its roots are deadly.[120] Sadly, a majority of (>2/3) plant poisoning victims (fatality 0.9%) are children, mostly due to unintentional exposure.[121,122] Adolescents may experiment with hallucinogenic plants and foragers, and trekkers may misidentify these as edible.[123]

In general, the principles of therapy discussed at the beginning of this chapter apply for plant poisonings too.[124] However, over the years, specific compounds responsible for several plant-induced toxidromes have been identified. The clinical features broadly fall into groups; anticholinergic, cholinergic, mucosal inflammation, gastroenteritis, acute or delayed multisystem organ failure, cardiac dysrhythmia, hepatotoxicity, dermatitis, seizures, and dyspnea.[125] More recently, a simple rapid toxidrome classification system categorized highly toxic plant ingestions into four specific toxidromes: cardiotoxic, neurotoxic, cytotoxic, and gastrointestinal hepatotoxic. This is to permit rapid diagnosis of highly toxic versus less toxic and nontoxic plant ingestions and direct early clinical management to improve outcomes. This rapid classification system, however, is based on chemical nomenclatures and pharmacological effects, and not on clearly presenting toxidromes.[123] We have discussed this large arena of plant poisoning in a summary table to assist attending clinician rapidly deploy relevant specific therapies where available (Table 31.2).

MISCELLANEOUS DRUG OVERDOSES

This chapter is not complete without referring to other common drug over dosages, which may not mimic a toxidrome but need more specific approach. Some common issues are described here.

ACETAMINOPHEN

Acetaminophen is a significant problem. Its toxicity has no early symptoms. A level is obtained in all cases of possible intentional overdoses. Most of the acetaminophen ingested is metabolized to inactive compounds but 5–10% is oxidized by the P-450 system to the hepatotoxic N-acetyl-p-benzoquinoneimine. This is detoxified by conjugation with glutathione and eliminated in the urine. In acetaminophen overdose, the glutathione supply is rapidly used, resulting in free hepatotoxic N-acetyl-p-benzoquinoneimine and subsequent hepatotoxicity that may lead to acute liver failure and death without treatment.

The Rumack–Matthew nomogram guides the use of IV N-acetylcysteine (NAC) in acute (single exposure) overdoses when the time of ingestion is known. Unlike salicylates, there is a limited role for repeat of acetaminophen levels. Traditionally, a toxic level is treated with oral NAC for 72 hours.

NEUROLEPTIC MALIGNANT SYNDROME

Neuroleptic malignant syndrome (NMS) is a potentially fatal complication following the use of neuroleptic drugs. It was initially known as the "akinetic hypertonic syndrome."[126]

The underlying pathology seems to relate to neuroleptic-induced alteration of central neuroregulatory mechanisms and an abnormal reaction of predisposed skeletal muscle

Table 31.2: Plant toxidromes.

	Pathophysiology/pharmacology	Plants	Vital signs	Specific therapy
Cardiac	• Cardiac glycosides • Plants contain a variety of cardiac glycosides, including neriifolin, thevetin A, thevetin B, and oleandrin	*Digitalis lanata* (foxglove)		• Atropine • DigiFab
		Cascabela thevetia (yellow oleander)		• C-P bypass if severe shock

Contd...

Contd...

	Pathophysiology/ pharmacology	Plants	Vital signs	Specific therapy
	<ul><li>Na channel activator</li><li>Binds to sodium channels (nerves, cardiac, skeletal muscle) and creates a persistent depolarized state</li></ul>	*Aconitum* (monkshood) 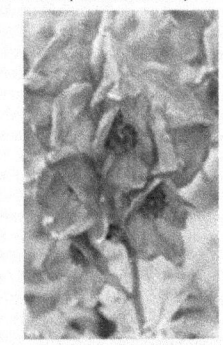 *Veratrum* (false hellebore) 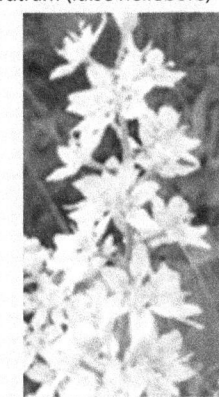 *Zigadenus* (death camas) 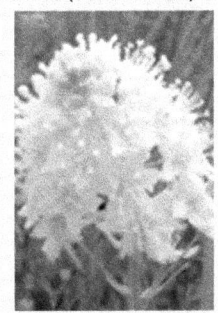 *Rhododendron* (rhodo, azalea) 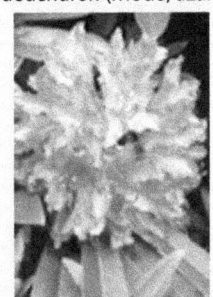	<ul><li>Bradycardia</li><li>Hypotension</li><li>Heart block</li><li>QT widening</li><li>Ventricular dysrhythmias</li><li>Drowsiness</li><li>Confusion</li><li>Paresthesia</li><li>Convulsions</li><li>Muscle weakness</li><li>Fasciculations</li></ul>	

Contd...

Section 2: Organ Dysfunction

Contd...

	Pathophysiology/ pharmacology	Plants	Vital signs	Specific therapy
	• Na/Ca channel blocker. • Taxine A and taxine B are the toxic alkaloids	*Taxus baccata* (English yews)	• Tachycardia and bradycardia • Convulsions • Acidosis • Loss of consciousness • Shock • Widened QRS complex • Ventricular dysrhythmias • Asystole	
	• K channel blocker • Contains ibogaine and indole alkaloids	*Tabernanthe iboga* (Iboga)	• QTc prolongation • Dysrythmias	
Neurotoxic	Anticholinergic	*Atropa belladonna* (deadly nightshade) *Datura stramonium* (Jimson weed)	• Hyperthermia • Coma • Seizures • Ventilatory failure	• Consider GI decontamination even late as seeds ingested slows gastric emptying • Benzodiazepines for agitation, seizures • Physostigmine (cholinesterase inhibitor)

Contd...

Toxidromes 223

Contd...

	Pathophysiology/ pharmacology	Plants	Vital signs	Specific therapy
		Datura aureua (angel's trumpet)		
Cytotoxic	Contains coniine (similar to nicotine)	*Conium maculatum* (poison hemlock) Mistaken for wild carrot and parsley	• Confusion • Seizures • Coma • Hypertension • Tachycardia • Bradycardia • Muscle fasciculations • Myoclonus • Weakness • Paralysis	
	• Contains cicutoxin • Inhibits GABAergic activity	*Cicuta* (water hemlock) Mistaken for wild parsnip, wild carrot	• Seizures often intractable • Cardiovascular decompensation	Avoid phenytoin
	• Cyanogenic • Blocks aerobic metabolism.	*Prunus* (cherries, peaches, plums, apricots, almonds), apples, cassava, hydrangeas, cotoneaster, *Sambucus* spp. (elderberry)	• Lethargy • Altered mental status • Seizures • Shortness of breath, tachypnea • Initial hypertension, then hypotension and CVS collapse • Lactic acidosis	Hydroxocobalamin

Contd...

Section 2: Organ Dysfunction

Contd...

Pathophysiology/pharmacology	Plants	Vital signs	Specific therapy
• Mitosis inhibitors • Contains colchicine • Inhibits microtubule formation	*Colchicum autumnale* (autumn crocus)	• Cardiovascular collapse • Multiorgan system failure • Initial leukocytosis followed by bone marrow failure	No antidote
Protein synthesis inhibitors. Contain toxalbumins (ricin, abrin, robin) that inhibits ribosomes, halts protein synthesis and cause cell death	*Ricinus communis* (castor bean) *Abrus precatorius* (rosary pea) *Robinia pseudoacacia* (black locust or false acacia)	• Minimal toxicity if seeds swallowed intact • GI toxicity if chewed	No antidote

Contd...

Contd...

	Pathophysiology/pharmacology	Plants	Vital signs	Specific therapy
Dermatitis	• Local irritants • Ejection of raphides and other irritant into mucosa causes local irritation	Oxalate plants (sorrel)	• Oropharyngeal inflammation may lead to airway obstruction • Ocular exposure can lead to severe irritation	
	• Phototoxic • Furocoumarin derivatives in the plant causes photodermatitis resulting in blisters and scars • Bergapten (5-methoxypsoralen) is a psoralen (furocoumarin) found in bergamot essential oils, citrus essential oils, and in grapefruit juice that absorb UV light, leading to DNA damage, and phototoxicity	Heracleum mantegazzianum (Giant hogweed) Citrus (lime, grapefruit)	Initial redness turning to blisters and scars may take years to heal. Ocular injury may be sight threatening and hyperpigmentation may take months to fade	• No specific treatments • Prevent, decontaminate, and avoid sunlight exposure
	• Phorbol esters • Various esters of phorbol may act as tumor promoters through activation of protein kinase C. These are irritant and ribosome inhibitors	Euphorbia (spurge)		

(CVS: cardiovascular system; DNA: deoxyribonucleic acid; GI: gastrointestinal; UV: ultraviolet)

possibly resulting from induced abnormal calcium availability in muscle cells causing muscle rigidity, rhabdomyolysis, and hyperthermia.

Dopamine reduces core temperature possibly via central thermoregulation. Neuroleptic drugs block dopamine receptor sites and result in hyperthermia. Dopamine depletion or blockade can both lead to abnormal central thermoregulation and NMS. In addition, blockade of dopamine receptors in the corpus striatum is thought to cause muscular rigidity, generating heat leading to hyperthermia. The peripheral anticholinergic effects of neuroleptics which reduce sweating may be contributory. Dopamine-function-enhancing drugs, such as bromocriptine or amantadine, have shown efficacy in treating neurolept malignant syndrome.

Hyperthermia, rigidity, and elevated creatine kinase concentration are features of NMS and malignant hyperthermia. Both have a mortality rate of 10–30%. Sodium dantrolene, a peripheral muscle relaxant, has been used successfully in both syndromes.

Neuroleptic malignant syndrome typically develops over a period of 24–72 hours but can occur 10–20 days after oral neuroleptics are discontinued.

Muscle rigidity consists of a generalized "lead pipe" increase in tone, which may result in decreased chest-wall compliance with resulting tachypneic hypoventilation, and pulmonary infection secondarily. This increase in muscle tone may be accompanied by extrapyramidal symptoms including dyskinesia, dysarthria, or Parkinsonism. The CPK concentration is always elevated (>1,000 IU/L), reflecting myonecrosis secondary to intense muscle contracture. This often results in acute myoglobinuric renal failure.

Diaphoresis, tachycardia, and abnormally high arterial pressure are signs of autonomic dysfunction. Altered consciousness ranges from agitation to stupor or coma.

Renal failure is a strong predictor of mortality, representing a mortality risk of approximately 50%.

A wide variety of antipsychotic agents is associated with this syndrome, including phenothiazines, butyrophenones, thioxanthenes, benzamides, and miscellaneous novel antipsychotic agents, such as clozapine and risperidone. Other circumstances, such as abrupt discontinuation of neuroleptic or antiparkinsonian agents, and the use of dopamine-depleting agents, have also been reported to produce NMS.

Young adult males predominate among reported cases.

Successful treatment depends on early clinical recognition and prompt withdrawal of the neuroleptic agents. Neuroleptics cannot be removed by dialysis, and blood concentrations decline only slowly. General symptomatic treatment, such as hydration, nutrition, and reduction of fever, is essential. Secondary complications, such as hypoxia, acidosis, and renal failure, must be treated aggressively. Low-dose heparin seems to be indicated to prevent venous thrombosis in an immobilized patient. Other dopamine antagonists, such as metoclopramide, should be avoided. Supportive therapy was the predominant treatment modality.

The benefit of adding specific therapies to supportive measures is still debated. Additional therapies include dantrolene, bromocriptine, and benzodiazepine. Another dopamine agonist, amantadine hydrochloride, has been used successfully in some cases.

KEY POINTS

- The management of toxidromes is founded on supportive care including those of vital function, timely use of antidotes and extracorporeal support in extreme cases.
- Emesis with ipecac or gastric lavage is not of much benefit to patients and may cause harm.
- Activated charcoal may be considered in a patient presenting within 1 hour of ingestion if the risks of further poison absorption outweigh the risks of charcoal administration.
- Multi-dose activated charcoal may be useful in potentially lethal poisoning with carbamazepine, dapsone, phenobarbital, quinine, or theophylline.
- Whole bowel irrigation is limited to poisoning with certain specific substances.
- Accurate interpretation of urine screens and serum drug levels may be helpful.
- Urinary alkalinization is recommended in the presence of salicylate toxicity.
- Watch for delayed onset of life-threatening complications.

REFERENCES

1. Agarwal S, Kaeley N, Khanduri S, et al. Brain dead presentation of snake bite. Indian J Crit Care Med. 2018;22:541-3.
2. Holstege CP, Borek HA. Toxidromes. Crit Care Clin. 2012;28:479-98.
3. Mokhlesi B, Leiken JB, Murray P, et al. Adult toxicology in critical care: part I: general approach to the intoxicated patient. Chest. 2003;123:577-92.
4. Vale JA, Meredith TJ, Proudfoot AT. Syrup of ipecacuanha: is it really useful?. Br Med J (Clin Res Ed). 1986;293:1321-2.
5. Vale JA. Position statement: gastric lavage. American Academy of Clinical Toxicology; European Association of Poisons Centres and Clinical Toxicologists. J Toxicol Clin Toxicol. 1997;35:711-9.
6. Barceloux D, McGuigan M, Hartigan-Go K. Position statement: cathartics. American Academy of Clinical Toxicology; European Association of Poisons Centres and Clinical Toxicologists. J Toxicol Clin Toxicol. 1997;35:743-52.
7. Vale JA, Krenzelok EP, Barceloux GD. Position statement and practice guidelines on the use of multi-dose activated charcoal

in the treatment of acute poisoning. American Academy of Clinical Toxicology; European Association of Poisons Centres and Clinical Toxicologists. J Toxicol Clin Toxicol. 1999;37:731-51.
8. Tenenbein M. Position statement: whole bowel irrigation. American Academy of Clinical Toxicology; European Association of Poisons Centres and Clinical Toxicologists. J Toxicol Clin Toxicol. 1997;35:753-62.
9. Merigian KS, Blaho KE. Single-dose oral activated charcoal in the treatment of the self-poisoned patient: a prospective, randomized, controlled trial. Am J Ther. 2002;9:301-8.
10. Jamaty C, Bailey B, Larocque A, et al. Lipid emulsions in the treatment of acute poisoning: a systematic review of human and animal studies. Clin Toxicol (Phila). 2010;48:1-27.
11. Muller SH, Diaz JH, Kaye AD. Intralipid emulsion rescue therapy: emerging therapeutic indications in medical practice. J La State Med Soc. 2016;168:101-3.
12. Panzeri C, Bacis G, Ferri F, et al. Extracorporeal life support in a severe *Taxus baccata* poisoning. Clin Toxicol (Phila). 2010;48:463-5.
13. Tyagi PK, Winchester JF, Feinfeld DA. Extracorporeal removal of toxins. Kidney Int. 2008;74:1231-3.
14. Mikolich JR, Paulson GW, Cross CJ. Acute anticholinergic syndrome due to Jimson seed ingestion. Clinical and laboratory observation in six cases. Ann Intern Med. 1975;83:321-5.
15. Speich R, Haller A. Central anticholinergic syndrome with the antimalarial drug mefloquine. N Engl J Med. 1994;331:57-8.
16. Hoefnagel D. Toxic effects of atropine and homatropine eyedrops in children. N Engl J Med. 1961;264:168-71.
17. Henry G, Morton MD, Durham NC. Atropine intoxication: its manifestations in infants and children. J Pediatr. 1939;14:755-60.
18. Ramjan KA, Williams AJ, Isbister GK, et al. 'Red as a beet and blind as a bat' Anticholinergic delirium in adolescents: lessons for the paediatrician. J Paediatr Child Health. 2007;43:779-80.
19. McCarron MM, Challoner KR, Thompson GA. Diphenoxylate–atropine (Lomotil) overdose in children: an update (report of eight cases and review of the literature). Pediatrics. 1991;87(5):694-700.
20. Brown DV, Heller F, Barkin R. Anticholinergic syndrome after anesthesia: a case report and review. Am J Ther. 2004;11(2):144-53.
21. Abou-Donia MB, Siracuse B, Gupta N, et al. Sarin (GB, O-isopropyl methylphosphonofluoridate) neurotoxicity: critical review. Crit Rev Toxicol. 2016;46:845-75.
22. Koelle GB. Organophosphate poisoning—an overview. Fundam Appl Toxicol. 1981;1:129-34.
23. Vale JA, Marrs TO, Maynard RC. Novichok: a murderous nerve agent attack in the UK. Clin Toxicol (Phila). 2018:56(1)1-5.
24. Marshall K, Fritz K, Thom W, et al. Toxic interaction between fluoxetine and donepezil: a case of cholinergic toxidrome. J Neuropsychiatry Clin Neurosci. 2012;24:E50.
25. Lukaszewicz-Hussain A. Role of oxidative stress in organophosphate insecticide toxicity—short review. Pestic Biochem Physiol. 2010;98:145-50.
26. Peter JV, Cherian AM. Organic insecticides. Anaesth Intensive Care. 2000;28:11-21.
27. Michotte A, Van Dijck I, Maes V, et al. Ataxia as the only delayed neurotoxic manifestation of organophosphate insecticide poisoning. Eur Neurol. 1989;29:23-6.
28. Brahmi N, Gueye PN, Thabet H, et al. Extrapyramidal syndrome as a delayed and reversible complication of acute dichlorvos organophosphate poisoning. Vet Hum Toxicol. 2004;46:187-9.
29. Wadia RS, Sadagopan C, Amin RB, et al. Neurological manifestations of organophosphorous insecticide poisoning. J Neurol Neurosurg Psychiatry. 1974;37:841-7.
30. Senanayake N, Karalliedde L. Neurotoxic effects of organophosphorus insecticides. An intermediate syndrome. N Engl J Med. 1987;316:761-3.
31. Sedgwick EM, Senanayake N. Pathophysiology of the intermediate syndrome of organophosphorus poisoning. J Neurol Neurosurg Psychiatry. 1997;62:201-2.
32. Jayawardane P, Dawson AH, Weerasinghe V, et al. The spectrum of intermediate syndrome following acute organophosphate poisoning: a prospective cohort study from Sri Lanka. PLoS Med. 2008;5:e147.
33. Jokanovic M, Stukalov PV, Kosanovic M. Organophosphate induced delayed polyneuropathy. Curr Drug Targets CNS Neurol Disord. 2002;1:593-602.
34. Aygun D, Onar MK, Altintop BL. The clinical and electrophysiological features of a delayed polyneuropathy developing subsequently after acute organophosphate poisoning and it's correlation with the serum acetylcholinesterase. Electromyogr Clin Neurophysiol. 2003; 43:421-7.
35. Rivett K, Potgieter PD. Diaphragmatic paralysis after organophosphate poisoning. A case report. S Afr Med J. 1987;72:881-2.
36. Jayawardane P, Senanayake N, Buckley NA, et al. Electrophysiological correlates of respiratory failure in acute organophosphate poisoning: evidence for differential roles of muscarinic and nicotinic stimulation. Clin Toxicol (Phila). 2012;50:250-3.
37. Peter JV, Prabhakar AT, Pichamuthu K. In-laws, insecticide—and a mimic of brain death. Lancet. 2008;371(9612):622.
38. Yurumez Y, Yavuz Y, Saglam H, et al. Electrocardiographic findings of acute organophosphate poisoning. J Emerg Med. 2009;36:39-42.
39. Karki P, Ansari JA, Bhandary S, et al. Cardiac and electrocardiographical manifestations of acute organophosphate poisoning. Singapore Med J. 2004;45:385-9.
40. Munidasa UA, Gawarammana IB, Kularatne SA, et al. Survival pattern in patients with acute organophosphate poisoning receiving intensive care. J Toxicol Clin Toxicol. 2004;42:343-7.
41. Mdaghri YA, Mossadeq A, Faroudy M, et al. Cardiac complications associated with organophosphate poisoning. Ann Cardiol Angeiol (Paris). 2010;59:114-7.
42. Hamaguchi M, Namera A, Tsuda N, et al. Severe acute pancreatitis caused by organophosphate poisoning. Chudoku Kenkyu. 2006;19:395-9.
43. Akyildiz BN, Kondolot M, Kurtoglu S, et al. Organophosphate intoxication presenting as diabetic keto-acidosis. Ann Trop Paediatr. 2009;29:155-8.
44. McDonough JH, Jr., Clark TR, Slone TW, Jr., et al. Neural lesions in the rat and their relationship to EEG delta activity following

seizures induced by the nerve agent soman. Neurotoxicology. 1998;19:381-91.
45. Brahmi N, Mokline A, Kouraichi N, et al. Prognostic value of human erythrocyte acetyl cholinesterase in acute organophosphate poisoning. Am J Emerg Med. 2006;24:822-7.
46. Bobba R, Venkataraman BV, Pais P, et al. Correlation between the severity of symptoms in organophosphorus poisoning and cholinesterase activity (RBC and plasma) in humans. Indian J Physiol Pharmacol. 1996;40:249-52.
47. Eddleston M, Eyer P, Worek F, et al. Predicting outcome using butyrylcholinesterase activity in organophosphorus pesticide self-poisoning. QJM. 2008;101:467-74.
48. Eddleston M, Buckley NA, Eyer P, et al. Management of acute organophosphorus pesticide poisoning. Lancet. 2008;371(9612):597-607.
49. Bateman DN, Good AM, Laing WJ, et al. TOXBASE: poisons information on the internet. Emerg Med J. 2002;19:31-4.
50. Eddleston M, Buckley NA, Checketts H, et al. Speed of initial atropinisation in significant organophosphorus pesticide poisoning—a systematic comparison of recommended regimens. J Toxicol Clin Toxicol. 2004;42:865-75.
51. Robenshtok E, Luria S, Tashma Z, et al. Adverse reaction to atropine and the treatment of organophosphate intoxication. Isr Med Assoc J. 2002;4:535-9.
52. Syed S, Gurcoo SA, Farooqui AK, et al. Is the World Health Organization-recommended dose of pralidoxime effective in the treatment of organophosphorus poisoning? A randomized, double-blinded and placebo-controlled trial. Saudi J Anaesth. 2015;9:49-54.
53. Banerjee I, Tripathi SK, Roy AS. Efficacy of pralidoxime in organophosphorus poisoning: revisiting the controversy in Indian setting. J Postgrad Med. 2014;60:27-30.
54. Soltaninejad K, Abdollahi M. Current opinion on the science of organophosphate pesticides and toxic stress: a systematic review. Med Sci Monit. 2009;15:RA75-90.
55. Namba T. Cholinesterase inhibition by organophosphorus compounds and its clinical effects. Bull World Health Organ. 1971;44:289-307.
56. Peter JV, Sudarsan TI, Moran JL. Clinical features of organophosphate poisoning: a review of different classification systems and approaches. Indian J Crit Care Med. 2014;18:735-45.
57. Eddleston M, Mohamed F, Davies JO, et al. Respiratory failure in acute organophosphorus pesticide self-poisoning. QJM. 2006;99:513-22.
58. Noshad H, Ansarin K, Ardalan MR, et al. Respiratory failure in organophosphate insecticide poisoning. Saudi Med J. 2007;28:405-7.
59. Anand S, Singh S, Nahar Saikia U, et al. Cardiac abnormalities in acute organophosphate poisoning. Clin Toxicol (Phila). 2009;47:230-5.
60. Saadeh AM, Farsakh NA, al-Ali MK. Cardiac manifestations of acute carbamate and organophosphate poisoning. Heart. 1997;77:461-4.
61. Ci YX, Zhou YX, Guo ZQ, et al. Production, characterization and application of monoclonal antibodies against the organo-phosphorus nerve agent Vx. Arch Toxicol. 1995;69:565-7.
62. Eddleston M, Dawson A, Karalliedde L, et al. Early management after self-poisoning with an organophosphorus or carbamate pesticide—a treatment protocol for junior doctors. Crit Care (London, England). 2004;8:R391-7.
63. Pajoumand A, Shadnia S, Rezaie A, et al. Benefits of magnesium sulfate in the management of acute human poisoning by organophosphorus insecticides. Hum Exp Toxicol. 2004;23:565-9.
64. Niven AS, Roop SA. Inhalational exposure to nerve agents. Respir Care Clin N Am. 2004;10:59-74.
65. Wiener SW, Hoffman RS. Nerve agents: a comprehensive review. J Intensive Care Med. 2004;19:22-37.
66. Dickson EW, Bird SB, Gaspari RJ, et al. Diazepam inhibits organophosphate-induced central respiratory depression. Acad Emerg Med. 2003;10:1303-6.
67. Olives TD, Orozco BS, Stellpflug SJ. Bath salts: the ivory wave of trouble. West J Emerg Med. 2012;13:58-62.
68. Prosser JM, Nelson LS. The toxicology of bath salts: a review of synthetic cathinones. J Med Toxicol. 2012;8:33-42.
69. Henry JA, Jeffreys KJ, Dawling S. Toxicity and deaths from 3,4-methylenedioxymethamphetamine ("ecstasy"). Lancet. 1992;340(8816):384-7.
70. Dyer JE, Roth B, Hyma BA. Gamma-hydroxybutyrate withdrawal syndrome. Ann Emerg Med. 2001;37:147-53.
71. O'Connor AD, Padilla-Jones A, Gerkin RD, et al. Prevalence of rhabdomyolysis in sympathomimetic toxicity: a comparison of stimulants. J Med Toxicol. 2015;11:195-200.
72. Mas-Morey P, Visser MH, Winkelmolen L, et al. Clinical toxicology and management of intoxications with synthetic cathinones ("bath salts"). J Pharm Pract. 2013;26:353-7.
73. Khan ZP, Ferguson CN, Jones RM. Alpha-2 and imidazoline receptor agonists. Their pharmacology and therapeutic role. Anaesthesia. 1999;54:146-65.
74. Johnston GD, Smith AM. Management of overdose due to antihypertensive agents. Adverse Drug React Acute Poisoning Rev. 1990;9:75-89.
75. Conner CS, Watanabe AS. Clonidine overdose: a review. Am J Hosp Pharm. 1979;36:906-11.
76. Mathew PM, Addy DP, Wright N. Clonidine overdose in children. Clin Toxicol. 1981;18:169-73.
77. Kollef MH. Labetalol overdose successfully treated with amrinone and alpha-adrenergic receptor agonists. Chest. 1994;105:626-7.
78. Chan TY, Joynt GM. Prolonged profound hypotension complicating severe methyldopa overdose. Int J Clin Pharmacol Ther. 2014;52:628-30.
79. MacMillan AR, Warshawski FJ, Steinberg RA. Minoxidil overdose. Chest. 1993;103:1290-1.
80. Cai S, Singh BR, Sharma S. Botulism diagnostics: from clinical symptoms to in vitro assays. Crit Rev Microbiol. 2007;33:109-25.
81. D'Ambra MN, Dedrick D, Savarese JJ. Kearns-Sayer syndrome and pancuronium—succinylcholine-induced neuromuscular blockade. Anesthesiology. 1979;51:343-5.
82. Argov Z, Mastaglia FL. Drug therapy: disorders of neuromuscular transmission caused by drugs. N Engl J Med. 1979;301:409-13.

83. Barrons RW. Drug-induced neuromuscular blockade and myasthenia gravis. Pharmacotherapy. 1997;17:1220-32.
84. Sobel J. Botulism. Clin Infect Dis. 2005;41:1167-73.
85. Armenian P, Olson A, Anaya A, et al. Fentanyl and a novel synthetic opioid U-47700 masquerading as street "Norco" in Central California: a case report. Ann Emerg Med. 2017;69:87-90.
86. Watson WA, Steele MT, Muelleman RL, et al. Opioid toxicity recurrence after an initial response to naloxone. J Toxicol Clin Toxicol. 1998;36:11-7.
87. Dunkley EJ, Isbister GK, Sibbritt D, et al. The hunter serotonin toxicity criteria: simple and accurate diagnostic decision rules for serotonin toxicity. QJM. 2003;96:635-42.
88. Ma Z, Zhang G, Jenney C, et al. Characterization of serotonin-toxicity syndrome (toxidrome) elicited by 5-hydroxy-l-tryptophan in clorgyline-pretreated rats. Eur J Pharmacol. 2008;588:198-206.
89. Tashakori A, Afshari R. Tramadol overdose as a cause of serotonin syndrome: a case series. Clin Toxicol (Phila). 2010;48:337-41.
90. Boyer EW, Shannon M. The serotonin syndrome. N Engl J Med. 2005;352:1112-20.
91. Meillier A, Heller C. Acute cyanide poisoning: hydroxocobalamin and sodium thiosulfate treatments with two outcomes following one exposure event. Case Rep Med. 2015;2015:217951.
92. Baud FJ. Cyanide: critical issues in diagnosis and treatment. Hum Exp Toxicol. 2007;26:191-201.
93. Megarbane B, Delahaye A, Goldgran-Toledano D, et al. Antidotal treatment of cyanide poisoning. J Chin Med Assoc. 2003;66:193-203.
94. Parker-Cote JL, Rizer J, Vakkalanka JP, et al. Challenges in the diagnosis of acute cyanide poisoning. Clin Toxicol (Phila). 2018;56:609-17.
95. Culnan DM, Craft-Coffman B, Bitz GH, et al. Carbon monoxide and cyanide poisoning in the burned pregnant patient: an indication for hyperbaric oxygen therapy. Ann Plast Surg. 2018;80:S106-12.
96. Borron SW, Baud FJ. Acute cyanide poisoning: clinical spectrum, diagnosis, and treatment. Arh Hig Rada Toksikol. 1996;47:307-22.
97. Borron SW, Baud FJ. Antidotes for acute cyanide poisoning. Curr Pharm Biotechnol. 2012;13:1940-8.
98. Kirk MA, Gerace R, Kulig KW. Cyanide and methemoglobin kinetics in smoke inhalation victims treated with the cyanide antidote kit. Ann Emerg Med. 1993;22:1413-8.
99. Hall AH, Saiers J, Baud F. Which cyanide antidote?. Crit Rev Toxicol. 2009;39:541-52.
100. Anderson A, McConville A, Fanthorpe L, et al. Salicylate poisoning potential of topical pain relief agents: from age old remedies to engineered smart patches. Medicines. 2017;4:30.
101. Robinson K, Rauch A, Hannan L. Salicylate poisoning following topical administration of methylsalicylate. Emerg Med Australas. 2015;27:374-5.
102. Shively RM, Hoffman RS, Manini AF. Acute salicylate poisoning: risk factors for severe outcome. Clin Toxicol (Phila). 2017;55:175-80.
103. Ong GY. A simple modified bicarbonate regimen for urine alkalinization in moderate pediatric salicylate poisoning in the emergency department. Pediatr Emerg Care. 2011;27:306-8.
104. Bawaskar HS, Bawaskar PH, Bawaskar PH. Snake bite in India: a neglected disease of poverty. Lancet. 2017;390:1947-8.
105. Bawaskar HS, Bawaskar PH. Snake bite poisoning. J Mahatma Gandhi Institute Med Sci. 2015;20:5-14.
106. Sack JT. The envenomation of general physiology throughout the last century. J Gen Physiol. 2017;149:975-83.
107. Warrell DA. Snake bite. Lancet. 2010;375(9708):77-88.
108. Bahloul M, Regaieg K, Chabchoub I, et al. Severe scorpion envenomation: pathophysiology and the role of inflammation in multiple organ failure. Med Sante Trop. 2017;27:214-21.
109. Karalliedde L. Animal toxins. Br J Anaesth. 1995;74:319-27.
110. Fahmi L, Makran B, Boussadda L, et al. Haemostasis disorders caused by envenomation by *Cerastes cerastes* and *Macrovipera mauritanica* vipers. Toxicon. 2016;116:43-8.
111. Aye KP, Thanachartwet V, Soe C, et al. Clinical and laboratory parameters associated with acute kidney injury in patients with snakebite envenomation: a prospective observational study from Myanmar. BMC Nephrol. 2017;18:92.
112. Priyamvada PS, Shankar V, Srinivas BH, et al. Acute interstitial nephritis following snake envenomation: a single-center experience. Wilderness Environ Med. 2016;27:302-6.
113. Bush SP, Davy JV. Troponin elevation after black widow spider envenomation. CJEM. 2015;17:571-5.
114. Corbett B, Clark RF. North American snake envenomation. Emerg Med Clin North Am. 2017;35:339-54.
115. Alirol E, Sharma SK, Bawaskar HS, et al. Snake bite in South Asia: a review. PLoS Negl Trop Dis. 2010;4:e603.
116. Hornbeak KB, Auerbach PS. Marine envenomation. Emerg Med Clin North Am. 2017;35:321-37.
117. Holla SK, Rao HA, Shenoy D, et al. The role of fresh frozen plasma in reducing the volume of anti-snake venom in snakebite envenomation. Trop Doct. 2018;48:89-93.
118. Mohammad Alizadeh A, Hassanian-Moghaddam H, Zamani N, et al. The protocol of choice for treatment of snake bite. Adv Med. 2016;2016:7579069.
119. Barrueto F, Jr., Kirrane BM, Cotter BW, et al. Cardioactive steroid poisoning: a comparison of plant- and animal-derived compounds. J Med Toxicol. 2006;2:152-5.
120. Moritz F, Compagnon P, Kaliszczak IG, et al. Severe acute poisoning with homemade *Aconitum napellus* capsules: toxicokinetic and clinical data. Clin Toxicol (Phila). 2005;43:873-6.
121. Dayasiri MB, Jayamanne SF, Jayasinghe CY. Plant poisoning among children in rural Sri Lanka. Int J Pediatr. 2017;2017:6187487.
122. Sriapha C, Tongpoo A, Wongvisavakorn S, et al. Plant poisoning in Thailand: a 10-year analysis from Ramathibodi Poison Center. Southeast Asian J Trop Med Public Health. 2015;46:1063-76. [Erratum appears in Southeast Asian J Trop Med Public Health. 2016;47:334].
123. Diaz JH. Poisoning by herbs and plants: rapid toxidromic classification and diagnosis. Wilderness Environ Med. 2016;27:136-52.
124. de Silva HA, Fonseka MM, Pathmeswaran A, et al. Multiple-dose activated charcoal for treatment of yellow oleander poisoning: a single-blind, randomised, placebo-controlled trial. Lancet. 2003;361(9373):1935-8.
125. Lin TJ, Nelson LS, Tsai JL, et al. Common toxidromes of plant poisonings in Taiwan. Clin Toxicol (Phila). 2009;47:161-8.
126. Adnet P, Lestavel P, Krivosic-Horber R. Neuroleptic malignant syndrome. Br J Anaesth. 2000;85:129-35.

SECTION 3

Specific Syndromes

Outlines

32. Influenza in the Intensive Care Unit
33. Middle East Respiratory Syndrome Coronavirus
34. Tetanus
35. Intensive Care Management of Leptospirosis
36. Dengue in Intensive Care Unit
37. Scrub Typhus
38. Malaria in Intensive Care Unit
39. Tuberculosis in Intensive Care Unit
40. Meliodosis

CHAPTER 32

Influenza in the Intensive Care Unit

Michael Toolis, John Botha

INTRODUCTION

Influenza viruses are an important cause of severe respiratory illness, and during pandemics this may have profound implications for patients, health-care workers, and the provision of appropriate health-care facilities.[1] In 2017, annual global influenza related mortality has been estimated to be 292,000–646,000 total deaths annually.[2]

Influenza viruses belong to the Orthomyxoviridae family and are enveloped negative-sense ribonucleic acid (RNA) viruses which contain seven to eight gene segments.[3] Four types of influenza virus exist: influenza A, B, C, and the recently discovered influenza D. Influenza A and B cause most human disease and are responsible for regular winter seasonal epidemics and occasional pandemics.[4]

Influenza A viruses can be further classified according to the surface glycoprotein antigens hemagglutinin (HA) and neuraminidase (NA). There are 18 HA subtypes and 11 NA subtypes.[5]

Influenza A tends to cause the most severe forms of disease and was responsible for the 1918–1919 Spanish influenza pandemic which killed at least 20 million people.[6] Influenza B tends to cause more mild disease and is sometimes responsible for seasonal endemics. Influenza C is known to cause only mild disease and influenza D is almost entirely confined to cattle.[7]

The World Health Organization (WHO) has published guidelines on the naming of influenza viruses which describes the virus type (A, B, C, or D), the host, location of isolation, isolation number, and year of isolation. For example, the 2009 influenza pandemic is named A/California/7/2009(H1N1)pdm with the suffix "pdm" to indicate that this was a pandemic strain.[8]

TRANSMISSION AND REPLICATION

Influenza viruses are generally spread over short distances via the airborne aerosolized route which occurs mainly via coughing and sneezing.[9] The viruses can also be spread from surfaces. Transmission usually occurs in the first week of the clinical illness and peaks on day 2.

Influenza viral infections tend to occur in annual winter outbreaks known as seasonal epidemics. This may be a result of increased stability of the virus in colder temperatures and because people spend more time confined indoors which may facilitate transmission.[10] In tropical regions, the disease is less confined to winter outbreaks.

Influenza viruses first bind to host cells via the viral HA proteins to sialic acid found on host cells. Viruses then enter host cells by endocytosis predominantly in the epithelial cells of the nasopharynx and to a lesser extent in the lower respiratory tract. After the virus has entered the host cell, viral RNA enters the host nucleus where viral replication occurs, which results in host cell necrosis.[3] An important feature of influenza viral replication is that the viral RNA polymerase does not provide proof reading to prevent mutations. This occurs at an error rate of approximately 2.0×10^{-6} and 0.6×10^{-6} mutations per site per infectious cycle.[11] This causes the virus to acquire spontaneous point mutations, which results in antigen drift and antigen shift which subsequently render viruses unrecognizable to the host immune system and allows for annual epidemics and occasional pandemics to occur.

Antigen drift refers to more subtle antigen mutations in influenza A, B, and C which are responsible for seasonal variations in influenza virus strains and results in local seasonal epidemics. Antigen shift occurs only amongst influenza A viruses and refers to major changes in viral strains which tend to be responsible for irregular and unpredictable pandemics.[12]

The first recognized influenza pandemic was probably in 1510 with the subsequent 1918–1919 Spanish influenza having profound global consequences.[6,13] Further pandemics have been attributed to antigenic shifts in both the HA (H1) and NA (N1) of influenza A, and pandemics have been described in most decades.[14]

Human cases of novel avian influenza A H7N9 were reported to the World Health Organization in 2013 with subsequent waves in 2016 and 2017. In this outbreak, some of the affected patients had exposure to poultry before becoming ill raising significant concerns about the emergence of particularly novel and pathogenic viral strains emerging.[15] Furthermore, an outbreak of swine flu was described in 2009, caused by the H1N1 influenza A virus, and this led to widespread community transmission.[16]

PATHOGENESIS AND PATHOLOGY

Influenza infection rapidly causes constitutional symptoms as a result of the host inflammatory response which involves interleukins (ILs) (IL-2, IL-7, IL-6, and interferon-inducible protein-10), cytokines, interferons, and tumor necrosis factor which are produced by infected host cells.[17] This characteristically results in fever, chills, fatigue, headaches, and myalgia although vomiting and diarrhea is also relatively common.

Mild cases of influenza are self-limiting and typically limited to the upper respiratory tract in the form of pharyngitis, coryza, and tracheitis. This occurs as a consequence of influenza viruses binding to epithelial cells of upper respiratory tract which results in host cell necrosis, macrophage phagocytosis, and submucosal edema.[3]

More severe cases involve the lower respiratory tract which manifests as viral pneumonia and potentially acute respiratory distress syndrome. Histologically, the lower airway demonstrates a congested interstitium with inflammatory infiltrates and air spaces filled with neutrophils and fibrin.[3] Submucosal capillary thrombi and congestion also develops. Later stages of influenza viral pneumonia may also be complicated by a healing fibrotic stage with the development of hyaline membranes within alveoli. Viral pneumonia may also be complicated by secondary bacterial infection due to *Streptococcus pneumoniae*, *Staphylococcus aureus*, and *Haemophilus influenza*.[3,18]

The net effects of severe influenza viral pneumonia include an increased alveolar–arterial gradient, pulmonary shunting, decreased lung compliance, and an increased patient work of breathing which may result in respiratory failure.[19]

It is postulated that particular strains of highly virulent influenza viruses, such as H5N1, have an increased affinity for cells of lower airway. This is thought to contribute to more severe disease episodes, but reduced transmission and lower overall incidence compared to milder disease.[20]

Rarely, severe influenza disease may result in rhabdomyolysis, acute renal failure, myocarditis, encephalitis, and hemophagocytic syndromes; however, the underlying pathogenesis of these processes is less well defined.[21,22]

CLINICAL MANIFESTATIONS

Despite similarities in the presenting signs and symptoms of different viral strains, much has been learnt in recent years about the manifestations of viral strains. Avian influenza A H7N9 infection was noted to cause life-threatening infection in many cases. Studies on hospitalized patients with avian influenza have found that many patients were admitted to the intensive care unit (ICU) with a high mortality.[23] There was also a considerable number of these patients who had an associated bacterial infection diagnosed through blood and sputum cultures. The most common complication was acute respiratory distress syndrome (ARDS) and shock. During this outbreak when many patients were critically ill, data also emerged of mild-to-moderate disease attributed to the influenza A H7N9 virus. This cohort of patients was generally younger and had no underlying medical conditions. Laboratory findings in influenza A H7N9 infected patients revealed that lymphopenia and thrombocytopenia were common and some patients had derangements in liver functions. The most common radiological abnormalities noted on chest radiography and computed tomography scanning in patients with pneumonia were diffuse ground glass opacities and patchy multilobar consolidation.

A pandemic of H1N1 influenza A virus was detected in early 2009 in Mexico, and this was subsequently known as swine flu with transmission over many continents.[24] These patients had symptoms of influenza with a cough and sore throat and confirmed H1N1 influenza A virus detection by real-time reverse transcription-polymerase chain reaction or culture. Swine influenza virus is common throughout pig populations worldwide and transmission of the virus from pigs to humans is uncommon and does not always lead to human influenza. The signs and symptoms of influenza caused by pandemic H1N1 influenza A virus resembled seasonal influenza although gastrointestinal manifestations appeared to be more common. Furthermore, pandemic H1N1 influenza A was associated with pneumonia more frequently than seasonal H1N1 influenza A. In young adults the most common findings of the 2009 H1N1 influenza A pandemic were cough, fever, headache malaise, and sore throat.

Numerous complications of H1N1 influenza A have been described, and pregnant women and neonates are more likely to have severe infection.[25] Young children and immunocompromised hosts were at increased risk for complications and severe disease. The most feared complications related to H1N1 influenza A were severe respiratory manifestations. During the 2009–2010 H1N1 influenza A pandemic, severe cases developed pneumonia, respiratory failure, and ARDS. Significant hypoxemia despite mechanical ventilation was a recognized complication in patients admitted to ICU with respiratory failure. In mechanically ventilated patients, numerous strategies were initiated to improve oxygenation. These included neuromuscular blockade, inhaled nitric oxide, high-frequency oscillatory ventilation, extracorporeal membrane oxygenation, and prone positioning.[26]

Various neurological complications have also been reported in patients with H1N1 influenza A. The most frequently described neurological manifestations have been seizures, encephalopathy or encephalitis with paralysis occurring in a small percentage of cases.

The most commonly observed laboratory findings were deranged liver enzymes, anemia, leukopenia or leukocytosis, thrombocytopenia or thrombocytosis, and hyper bilirubinemia. Imaging in hospitalized patients has revealed a high percentage of pulmonary infiltrates with computer tomography scan findings revealing patchy consolidation or ground glass opacities.

DIAGNOSIS

It is important to consider influenza in the differential diagnosis of a patient presenting with compatible symptoms and to confirm influenza rapidly with the appropriate laboratory investigations. Influenza virus should be considered when patients present with community acquired pneumonia, hospital acquired pneumonia, acute respiratory failure, sepsis, myocarditis, rhabdomyolysis, and encephalopathy. Upper respiratory tract samples should be obtained (nasopharyngeal swabs and throat swabs) and lower respiratory samples if clinically indicated in non-intubated patients and in intubated patients.

Polymerase chain reaction is the most widely available and the preferred method for detecting influenza virus because of its high sensitivity and specificity.[27] Rapid antigen tests can be performed at the bedside but are not often used because of low sensitivity and specificity. Virus culture has a limited role in guiding routine clinical care due to the time it takes to isolate virus and serological assays that detect virus antibody are not useful in diagnosing acute influenza.

TREATMENT

There are two classes of antiviral agents used for the treatment and prevention of influenza: the NA inhibitors and the adamantanes. The recommendations are that antiviral therapy should be administered to patients at risk for complications or those with severe disease requiring hospitalization. The major risk factors for influenza complications are age over 65 years, pregnant women, and patients with chronic medical conditions such as chronic pulmonary conditions and cardiovascular disease. Organ dysfunction, immune-compromised states, and morbid obesity are further risk factors. Young adults less than 65 without high-risk conditions do not require testing or treatment.

Once a decision is made to initiate therapy, this should be expedited as soon as possible.[28] If indicated, therapy should be initiated prior to the results of diagnostic testing. In patients screened with rapid antigen testing for influenza, therapy should be started where clinically indicated even if the rapid antigen test is negative as this test lacks sensitivity.

The influenza A viruses have developed higher rates of resistance to the adamantanes as opposed to the NA inhibitors. For this reason, the NA inhibitors are recommended for the treatment of influenza and oseltamivir is recommended if resistance to this agent is not suspected. In cases where enteral agents are not tolerated intravenous (IV) peramivir may be considered even though this agent has not been universally approved for use in cases of complicated influenza. The usual dose of oseltamivir for the treatment of influenza is 75 mg orally twice daily, and the recommended dose of peramivir is 600 mg IV as a single dose.[29] There have been suggestions that doubling the dose of oseltamivir to 150 mg twice daily in severely ill patients with H5N1 avian influenza may be beneficial, but there appears to be limited evidence to support this practice. Antiviral therapy should be administered for 5 days and consideration given for a more prolonged course in patients who are profoundly ill are immune compromised.

In pregnant patients, influenza is known to cause more severe disease and oseltamivir should be administered despite there being no clinical studies to reflect safety during pregnancy. When administered orally, oseltamivir has good bioavailability and is widely distributed. This agent has been shown to decrease the duration of influenza symptoms and reduces the duration of viral shedding. There are also studies to show that the length of hospitalization and complication rates may decrease with oseltamivir administration. There have also been observational studies that have found an association between oseltamivir use and mortality reduction in patients.[30]

Antiviral resistance is a potential explanation for clinical deterioration and should be considered. Superimposed bacterial infections should also be excluded and if implicated, treated. Fortunately, the NA inhibitors have few side effects with the most commonly reported being diarrhea and there have been reports of delirium in children who have received this agent.

Other agents have also been trialed as therapy for influenza viruses. Nitazoxanide is an antiparasitic agent that has been shown to have activity against influenza viruses, but despite some studies showing benefit, more data are required before this agent can be strongly recommended.[31] Antiviral prophylaxis may be appropriate in individuals at increased risk of complications, in health-care workers, and where housing circumstances predispose to viral transmission.

There have been many adjunctive agents that have also been suggested in the management of influenza. These include clarithromycin, glucocorticoids, and statins. Currently there is insufficient evidence to support their use.

Infection Prevention and Control

Because influenza virus is transmitted by droplet contact and airborne routes, droplet and contact precautions are required at all times.[32] Patients with suspected or confirmed influenza should be nursed in single rooms appropriate for respiratory isolation. Hand hygiene should be adhered to and rooms should be cleaned at least once a day and immediately if visibly contaminated. Personal protective equipment should be used according to hospital policy. Consideration should be given to aerosol generation by devices including ventilators and high flow humidified oxygen systems, and manufacturers' recommendations should be sought.

Intensive Care Unit Response to a Pandemic

The avian and swine flu pandemics placed a significant demand on ICU resources in the affected countries with significant implications for subsequent ICU response planning for pandemics. Numerous recommendations have arisen that include hospital wide strategies, increasing ICU bed capacity and optimizing ICU staffing requirements.[33] Hospitals and ICUs should develop policies and procedures pertaining to pandemics, and these should be activated where indicated. Surveillance and early detection of influenza patients is required with the necessary infection control measures to reduce the spread of virus to other patients and hospital staff. Antiviral prophylaxis should be provided to health-care workers, guided by local policy. During pandemics, ICU bed capacity should be optimized and numerous strategies may facilitate this. They include deferring elective surgery, opening additional beds in noncommissioned critical care spaces, using alternative clinical areas such as recovery units and coronary care units, discharging noncritically ill patients and where appropriate transferring patients to private ICUs. Intensive care staffing can be increased by manipulating shift lengths, limiting leave, and seconding additional medical and nursing staff from nonintensive care areas such as anesthesia and coronary care.[34]

REFERENCES

1. Dewar B, Barr I, Robinson P. Hospital capacity and management preparedness for pandemic influenza in Victoria. Aust N Z J Public Health. 2014;38(2):184-90.
2. Iuliano A, Roguski A, Chang H, et al. Estimates of global seasonal influenza-associated respiratory mortality: a modelling study. Lancet. 2018;391(10127):1285-300.
3. Taubenberger JK, Morens DM. The pathology of influenza virus infections. Annu Rev Pathol. 2008;3:499-522.
4. Azziz Baumgartner E, Dao CN, Nasreen S, et al. Seasonality, timing, and climate drivers of influenza activity worldwide. J Infect Dis. 2012;206:838.
5. Szretter KJ, Balish AL, Katz JM. Influenza: propagation, quantification, and storage. Curr Protoc Microbiol. 2006;Chapter 15:Unit 15G.
6. Taubenberger JK, Reid AH, Krafft AE, et al. Initial genetic characterization of the 1918 "Spanish" influenza virus. Science. 1997;275:1793.
7. Nesmith N, Williams JV, Johnson M, et al. Sensitive diagnostics confirm that influenza C is an uncommon cause of medically attended respiratory illness in adults. Clin Infect Dis. 2017;65:1037.

8. World Health Organization. (2014). Standardization of terminology for the influenza virus variants infecting humans: update. Geneva: World Health Organization. [online] Available from http://www.who.int/influenza/gisrs_laboratory/terminology_variant/en/. [Cited July 30, 2018].
9. Brankston G, Gitterman L, Hirji Z, et al. Transmission of influenza A in human beings. Lancet Infect Dis. 2007;7:257.
10. Reichert TA, Simonsen L, Sharma A, et al. Influenza and the winter increase in mortality in the United States, 1959-1999. Am J Epidemiol. 2004;160(5):492-502.
11. Nobusawa E, Sato K. Comparison of the mutation rates of human influenza A and B viruses. J Virol. 2006;80(7):3675-8.
12. Centers for Disease Control and Prevention (US). How the flu virus can change: "drift" and "shift". [online] Available from https://www.cdc.gov/flu/about/viruses/change.htm. [Cited August 30, 2018].
13. Morens DM, Taubenberger JK, Folkers GK, et al. Pandemic influenza's 500th anniversary. Clin Infect Dis. 2010;51:1442.
14. Bresee J, Hayden FG. Epidemic influenza—responding to the expected but unpredictable. N Engl J Med. 2013;368:589.
15. Li Q, Zhou L, Zhou M, et al. Epidemiology of human infections with avian influenza A(H7N9) virus in China. N Engl J Med. 2014;370(6):520-32.
16. Reed C, Chaves SS, Perez A, et al. Complications among adults hospitalized with influenza: a comparison of seasonal influenza and the 2009 H1N1 pandemic. Clin Infect Dis. 2014;59:166.
17. Sládková T, Kostolanský F. The role of cytokines in the immune response to influenza A virus infection. Acta Virol. 2006;50(3):151-62.
18. Chertow DS, Memoli MJ. Bacterial coinfection in influenza: a grand rounds review. JAMA. 2013;309:275.
19. Traylor ZP, Aeffner F, Davis IC. Influenza A H1N1 induces declines in alveolar gas exchange in mice consistent with rapid post-infection progression from acute lung injury to ARDS. Influenza Other Respir Viruses. 2013;7(3):472-9.
20. van Riel D, Munster VJ, de Wit E, et al. H5N1 virus attachment to lower respiratory tract. Science. 2006;312(5772):399.
21. Sellers SA, Hagan RS, Hayden FG, et al. The hidden burden of influenza: a review of the extra-pulmonary complications of influenza infection. Influenza Other Respir Viruses. 2017;11(5):372-93.
22. Abe M, Higuchi T, Okada K, et al. Clinical study of influenza-associated rhabdomyolysis with acute renal failure. Clin Nephrol. 2006;66:166.
23. Gao HN, Lu HZ, Cao B, et al. Clinical findings in 111 cases of influenza A (H7N9) virus infection. N Eng J Med. 2013;368:2277-85.
24. Perez-Padilla R, de la Rosa-Zamboni D, Ponce de Leon S, et al. Pneumonia and respiratory failure from swine-origin influenza A (H1N1) in Mexico. N Eng J Med. 2009;361:680-9.
25. Siston AM, Rasmussen SA, Honein MA, et al. Pandemic 2009 influenza A(H1N1) virus illness among pregnant women in the United States. JAMA. 2010;303:1517.
26. Davies A, Jones D, Bailey M, et al.; Australia and New Zealand Extracorporeal Membrane Oxygenation (ANZ ECMO) Influenza Investigators. Extracorporeal membrane oxygenation for 2009 influenza A(H1N1) acute respiratory distress syndrome. JAMA. 2009;302:1888.
27. Landry ML, Cohen S, Ferguson D. Real-time PCR compared to Binax NOW and cytospin-immunofluorescence for detection of influenza in hospitalized patients. J Clin Virol. 2008;43:148.
28. Louie JK, Yang S, Acosta M, et al. Treatment with neuraminidase inhibitors for critically ill patients with influenza A (H1N1). Clin Infect Dis. 2012;55:1198.
29. Yu Y, Garg S, Yu PA, et al. Peramivir use for treatment of hospitalized patients with influenza A(H1N1) under emergency use authorization, October 2009-June 2010. Clin Infect Dis. 2012;55:8.
30. Lee EH, Wu C, Lee EU, et al. Fatalities associated with the 2009 H1N1 influenza A virus in New York city. Clin Infect Dis. 2010;50:1498.
31. Haffizulla J, Hartman A, Hoppers M, et al. Effect of nitazoxanide in adults and adolescents with acute uncomplicated influenza: a double-blind, randomised, placebo-controlled, phase 2b/3 trial. Lancet Infect Dis. 2014;14(7):609-18.
32. Horvath JS, McKinnon M, Roberts L. The Australian response: pandemic influenza preparedness. Med J Aust. 2006;185(Suppl. 10):S35-8.
33. Gomersall CD, Loo S, Joynt GM, et al. Pandemic preparedness. Curr Opin Crit Care. 2007;13(6):742-7.
34. Sprung CL, Zimmerman JL, Christian MD, et al.; European Society of Intensive Care Medicine Task Force for Intensive Care Unit Triage during an Influenza Epidemic or Mass Disaster. Recommendations for intensive care unit and hospital preparations for an influenza epidemic or mass disaster: summary report of the European Society of Intensive Care Medicine's Task Force for intensive care unit triage during an influenza epidemic or mass disaster. Intensive Care Med. 2010;36(3):428-43.

CHAPTER 33

Middle East Respiratory Syndrome Coronavirus

Sandeep Kantor, Juhi Chandwani

INTRODUCTION

Middle East respiratory syndrome coronavirus (MERS-CoV) is a novel coronavirus discovered in 2012, in Arabian Peninsula and is a cause of severe respiratory infection in humans, specifically the elderly and people with comorbidities. The disease is severely endemic in dromedary camel populations of East Africa and the Middle East. There is evidence that the MERS-CoV outbreak in human population is sustained by zoonotic transmission from dromedary camels, since closely related viruses have been isolated from the camels but not from any other animal species.[1,2]

Human coronaviruses usually cause mild to moderate flu-like illnesses. Yet, MERS-CoV is unique due to its singular ability to undergo rapid genetic rearrangement and profound molecular variation in its single-stranded ribonucleic acid (ssRNA). Modified viral genome results in new antigenic subtypes, which makes it a challenging task to develop vaccines and therapeutic interventions. Consequently, MERS-CoV infections remain a serious threat not only to the Middle East region, but to the world population at large. This review focuses on the current information of MERS-CoV, with special reference to the genomic structure, clinical features, diagnosis of infection, treatment, and vaccine development. We also look at prospects for MERS-CoV spread and prevention.

EPIDEMIOLOGY

First patient diagnosed of MERS-CoV died of severe pneumonia and renal failure in Jeddah, Saudi Arabia in June 2012.[3] Thereafter cases occurred sporadically with intermittent spurts during the year because of hospital outbreaks and international travels, although the incidence remains low.

As per World Health Organization (WHO) statistics,[4] between 2012 and 30 June 2018, 2,229 laboratory-confirmed cases of MERS-CoV infection have been reported, 83% of whom were reported by the Kingdom of Saudi Arabia (Fig. 33.1). Altogether, cases have been reported from 27 countries in the Middle East, North Africa, Europe, the United States of America, and Asia (Table 33.1). Males above the age of 60 years, with comorbid conditions, such as diabetes, hypertension, renal failure, and immune suppression, are at a higher risk of severe disease, including death. Younger and previously healthy individuals appear more likely to exhibit mild symptoms or be asymptomatic. To date, 791 individuals have died [case fatality rate (CFR) 35.5%].[4]

The true incidence of MERS-CoV is uncertain. Mild and asymptomatic cases may be missed, which can lead to underreporting and information bias about the disease. Human-to-human transmission of MERS-CoV has been demonstrated not only amongst close contacts at home but also in healthcare workers looking after hospitalized patients.[5] However, community outbreaks

Middle East Respiratory Syndrome Coronavirus

Middle East respiratory syndrome coronavirus (MERS-CoV) Summary of Current Situation August 2018

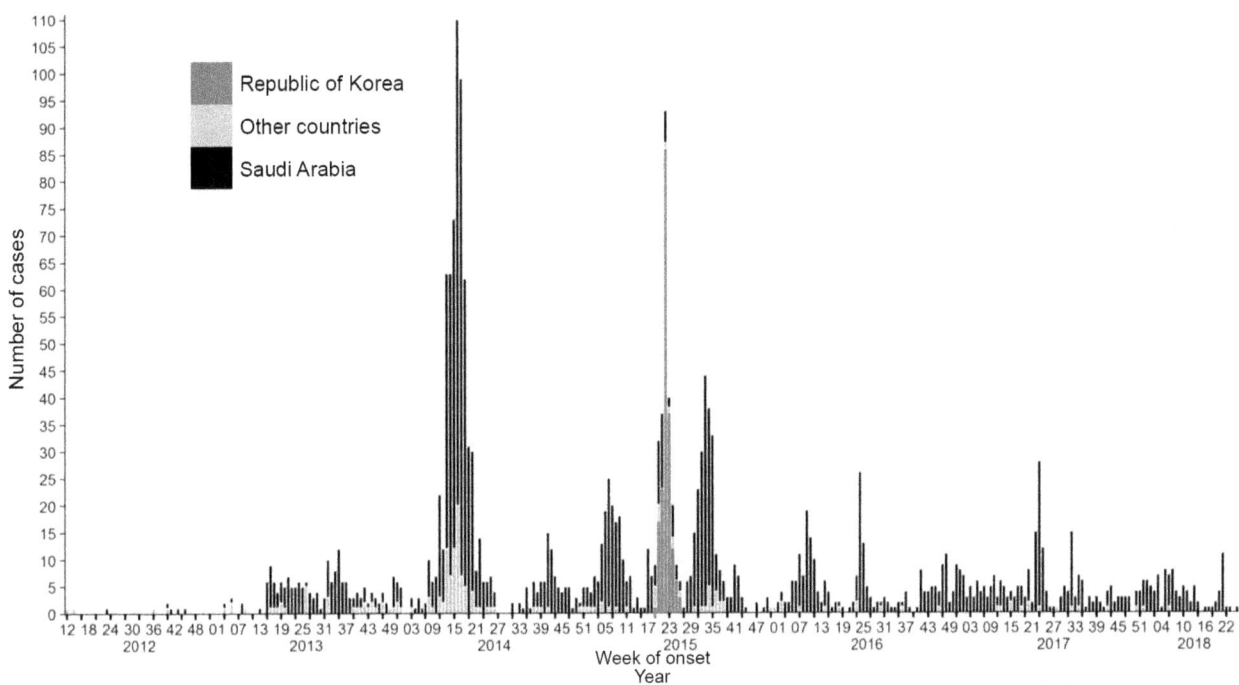

FIGURE 33.1: Epidemic curve of Middle East respiratory syndrome coronavirus (MERS-CoV) human cases as of 30th June 2018.[4]
*Symptomatic cases are plotted by date of symptom onset; asymptomatic cases are plotted by date of notification to WHO.
**Dark gray = Republic of Korea; Black = Kingdom of Saudi Arabia; Light gray = all other countries reporting MERS-CoV cases to date including Algeria, Austria, Bahrain, China, Egypt, France, Germany, Greece, Iran, Italy, Jordan, Kuwait, Lebanon, Malaysia, the Netherlands, Oman, the Philippines, Qatar, Thailand, Tunisia, Turkey, United Arab Emirates, the United Kingdom, the United States, Yemen
Source: World Health Organization

Table 33.1: Number of laboratory-confirmed MERS cases reported by countries, by year, since 2012.[4]

Country reporting	Number of laboratory-confirmed MERS-CoV cases reported	Country reporting	Number of laboratory-confirmed MERS-CoV cases reported
Algeria	2	Oman	11
Austria	2	Philippines	2
Bahrain	1	Qatar	19
China	1	Republic of Korea	185
Egypt	1	Saudi Arabia	1854
France	2	Thailand	3
Germany	3	Tunisia	3
Greece	1	Turkey	1
Iran	6	United Kingdom	4
Italy	1	United Arab Emirates	86
Jordan	28	United States of America	2
Kuwait	4	Yemen	1
Lebanon	2	Total	2,229
Malaysia	2		
Netherlands	2		

*Data as of June 2018
(MERS-CoV: Middle East respiratory syndrome coronavirus)

are rarely seen. This is likely to be mediated by inadequate infection prevention and control (IPC) measures and the augmentation of cases amidst nosocomial outbreaks.[6,7] Virulent corona virus strains like MERS-CoV and severe acute respiratory syndrome coronavirus (SARS-CoV) has changed the way we view coronaviruses, but with little success in developing specific treatment options or vaccine production.

Dromedary camels are the main suspected link as per available evidence for animal-to-human transmission of MERS-CoV. This is based on similarity of both their genomes. Future research addressing the modes of transmission will help to develop strategies to prevent zoonotic transmission of MERS-CoV.

The virus seems to be immutable environmentally at low temperature or low humidity than at higher temperature or higher humidity conditions. MERS-CoV aerosolization does not decrease its stability at 20°C/40% relative humidity condition which makes it easily transmittable through contacts and fomites.[8] Therefore, proper contact precautions have been recommended for health care workers who are involved in care of MERS-CoV patients.

PATHOGENESIS

Coronaviruses are a family of enveloped, ssRNA viruses with tendency for cross transmission between infected animals and humans. Full spectrum of illness varies from common cold to severe respiratory illness.[8] The SARS-CoV belongs to lineage B of the beta-coronavirus, whereas MERS-CoV belongs to lineage C of the same genus.[9] It has a positive-sense ssRNA genome about 30 kb in size. The MERS-CoV genomes share more than 99% sequence identity, indicating a low mutation rate and low variance among the genomes. MERS-CoV genomes are roughly divided into two clades: clade A, which contains only a few strains, and clade B, to which most strains belong.[10] MERS-CoV enters cells via a common receptor, the dipeptidyl peptidase-4 (DPP4), also known as CD26, and replicates in bronchial, bronchiolar, and type I and II alveolar epithelial cells.[11,12] The virus is predominantly seen in respiratory secretions, with the highest viral loads in the lower respiratory tract.[13]

CLINICAL FEATURES AND PROGRESS OF THE DISEASE

In the acute stage of the MERS-CoV infection, there is a severe viremia, leading to multiorgan failure, ultimately ending in coma and death. Patients with severe illness have acute, rapidly progressive viral pneumonia and pneumonitis, progressing to hypoxic lung injury and acute respiratory distress syndrome (ARDS). Acute kidney injury or failure occurs frequently in patients[14,15] as DPP4 is expressed at high levels in the kidney.[16] Viral shedding has also been detected in the urine and stool of infected patients.[17] Secondary bacterial infections due to *Staphylococcus aureus*, group A *Streptococcus*, *Streptococcus pneumoniae*, and *Haemophilus influenzae* type b further augment the pathogenic potential of MERS-CoV, in humans. These bacteria reside in upper airways which makes it easier to collect swabs for rapid diagnostic polymerase chain reaction (PCR) testing. Viral particles in lung alveoli stimulate a host response but alveolar macrophages fail to contain the spread of infection. The strong host cellular immune response and cytokine release lead to inflammation and fluid accumulation in lungs resulting in the characteristic symptoms of MERS-CoV manifesting as high fever, chills, rigors, severe cough, dyspnea, and hypovolemic shock.[18] Different age groups show variable response with increasing incidence, morbidity, and mortality (80%) in the age group of 35–45 years. Strangely the severity of MERS-CoV is lower (40%) in the older age groups, particularly above 55 years.[19] Currently, among all patients, the morbidity rate is approximately 36%, with the median time from the onset of symptoms to death 11.5 days.[20] Chest radiography shows unilateral or patchy pneumonia whereas computed tomography findings are generally consistent patchy consolidation to bilateral ground glass attenuation in more severe cases suggesting ARDS. Laboratory findings include lymphopenia, thrombocytopenia with some cases showing consumptive coagulopathy and derangements of renal and liver functions.

Mechanism of protective immune response that enables the patients to recover remains elusive, however literature from other coronaviruses including SARS-CoV epidemic, says that coordinated innate and adaptive immune responses are required for recovery to take place.[21,22] Innate immune responses is diminished in patients with MERS-CoV along with delayed proinflammatory cytokine induction in cell culture and in vivo,[23-25] which impairs host immune response.

Middle East respiratory syndrome coronaviruses isolated from single outbreaks are closely related[26] as proven by genomic studies accompanied by periodic reintroduction of the virus into human populations. The basic reproduction rate (R_0) for MERS-CoV remains uncertain.[27] Breban et al. reported R_0 of 0.60 and 0.69 using data from two outbreaks.[28] Cauchemez et al. cautioned that in the presence of poor infection control measures R_0 may increase (0.8–1.3) and could lead to a self-sustaining transmission.[29] This observed limited transmission is attributed to the ability of

MERS-CoV to multiply in the lower respiratory tract.[30] The United States Centers for Disease Control and Prevention (CDC) recommends standard contact and airborne precautions with the use of an N-95 mask when caring for an infected patient.[31]

Almost 50% of patients require critical care admission with 40–70% requiring invasive mechanical ventilation. Many develop severe ARDS requiring lung protective ventilation, including prone ventilation and extracorporeal membrane oxygenation. The course of illness may be complicated with multiple organ failure which includes renal failure and circulatory shock.

Middle East respiratory syndrome coronavirus cases have mainly been reported in adults,[32] with children rarely affected.[33,34] Neuromuscular complications are not rare during MERS-CoV infections and are characterized by varying degrees of disturbed consciousness, ataxia, focal motor deficit,[35] and seizure activity.[36]

CASE DEFINITIONS

Case definitions of suspected, confirmed, and probable MERS were developed by WHO, the US CDC, and have been revised since 2013.[37]

Confirmed Case

A person with laboratory confirmation of MERS-CoV infection (a), irrespective of clinical signs and symptoms.

Probable Case

Definition 1
- A febrile acute respiratory illness with clinical, radiological, or histopathological evidence of pulmonary parenchymal disease (e.g. pneumonia or ARDS); and
- Direct epidemiologic link (b) with a laboratory-confirmed MERS-CoV case; and
- Testing for MERS-CoV is unavailable, negative on a single inadequate specimen (c) or inconclusive (d).

Definition 2
- A febrile acute respiratory illness with clinical, radiological, or histopathological evidence of pulmonary parenchymal disease (e.g. pneumonia or ARDS) that cannot be explained fully by any other etiology; and
- The person resides or travelled in the Middle East, or in countries where MERS-CoV is known to be circulating in dromedary camels or where human infections have recently occurred; and
- Testing for MERS-CoV is inconclusive (d).

Definition 3
- An acute febrile respiratory illness of any severity; and
- Direct epidemiologic link (b) with a confirmed MERS-CoV case; and
- Testing for MERS-CoV is inconclusive (d).

  (a) A case may be laboratory confirmed by detection of viral nucleic acid or serology. The presence of viral nucleic acid can be confirmed by either positive results for nucleic acid amplification assays, such as reverse transcription PCR, for at least two specific genomic targets or a single positive target with sequencing of a second target. A case confirmed by serology requires demonstration of seroconversion in two samples ideally taken at least 14 days apart, by a screening [enzyme-linked immunosorbent assays (ELISA), immunofluorescence assays (IFA)] and a neutralization assay.

  (b) A direct epidemiological link with a confirmed MERS-CoV patient may include:
   - Healthcare associated exposure, including providing direct care for MERS-CoV patients, working with healthcare workers infected with MERS-CoV, visiting patients or staying in the same close environment of an individual infected with MERS-CoV.
   - Working together in close proximity or sharing the same environment with individuals infected with MERS-CoV.
   - Traveling together with individuals infected with MERS-CoV in any kind of conveyance.
   - The epidemiological link may have occurred within a 14-day period before or after the onset of illness in the case under consideration.

  (c) An inadequate specimen would include a nasopharyngeal swab without an accompanying lower respiratory specimen, a specimen that has had improper handling, is judged to be of poor quality by the testing laboratory, or was taken too late in the course of illness.

  (d) Inconclusive tests may include: A positive test by nucleic acid amplification assay for a single target without further testing. Evidence of seroreactivity by a single convalescent serum sample ideally taken at least 14 days after exposure by a screening assay (ELISA or IFA) and a neutralization assay, in the absence of molecular confirmation from respiratory specimens.

TREATMENT AND PREVENTION OF INFECTION (VACCINE)

Up until now, no vaccines or specific antiviral drugs are available during an outbreak. Therefore, nonspecific therapeutic interventions are often introduced to prevent severe morbidity and mortality. However, in the case of MERS-CoV, it is necessary to monitor epidemic patterns and investigate the spread of infections to efficiently identify, control, and prevent possible epidemics.

Management includes appropriate support of all organs until patient improves with fluids, vasopressors, and other therapies as indicated.

For secondary bacterial, fungal, and other infections with opportunistic organisms appropriate antibiotics, antiviral, and antifungal may be needed. Therapy with ribavirin and interferon has been shown to suppress MERS-CoV replication in vitro and thus improve the prognosis in MERS-CoV-infected animals.[38] However, it was observed that the therapy needs to be started soon after viral exposure (~8 hours), which resulted in decreased disease severity. This is challenging in human cases due to different time period when patient may present and hence the application of these results from animal studies to humans may not produce similar outcomes.[38,39] Until now no effective antiviral agent has been shown to counter the cytopathic effect of virus. Supportive therapy, as per guidelines developed for SARS-CoV, remains the mainstay of MERS-CoV treatment.

Human vaccine development remains challenging due to highly sophisticated immune evasion mechanisms of viral pathogens.[40] Various vaccines against MERS-CoV have been designed, which are currently being tested in clinical trials. Camel vaccination may be a novel approach to preventing human infection.[41,42]

CONCLUSION

The persistence of MERS due to MERS-CoV, makes it unique. Unlike SARS epidemic, which fortunately disappeared within a year, MERS has remained with us for more than 3 years. The high fatality rate of more than 30%[10] is a cause of major concern and although this number is low, the virus remains a serious threat due to high fatality in patients with comorbidities and the risk of cross transmission in hospital environment. Moreover, the spread of MERS-CoV lineage coincides with the movement of infected livestock or animal products[25] and there is enough epidemiological evidence suggesting its appearance in human populations at periodic intervals,[43] which makes it a potential contender for future pandemic making it a cause of concern for entire population.

To mitigate these risks, professional bodies like WHO and CDC have released various case definitions which will enable to reduce impact of a pandemic threat. Flu-like symptoms with features of lower respiratory tract infections in patients with travel history to the Arab Peninsula should raise the suspicion for diagnosing a MERS-CoV infection. Due to the risk of acquisition in hospital settings, healthcare workers are also educated to be vigilant and aware of any upper respiratory tract infections and possible exposure to MERS-CoV-positive individuals. The measures are recommended to prevent nosocomial outbreaks include good compliance with appropriate personal protection equipment by healthcare workers when managing patients with suspected and confirmed MERS-CoV infection, prompt isolation of infected patients, early laboratory diagnosis, and improvement of ventilation in healthcare facilities.[44,45]

REFERENCES

1. Hemida MG, Elmoslemany A, Al-Hizab F, et al. Dromedary Camels and the Transmission of Middle East Respiratory Syndrome Coronavirus (MERS-CoV). Transbound Emerg Dis. 2017;64:344-53.
2. Reusken C, Haagmaans BL, Koopmans MP. Dromedary camels and Middle East respiratory syndrome: MERS coronavirus in the 'ship of the desert'. Ned Tijdschr Geneeskd. 2014;158:A7806.
3. Zaki AM, van Boheemen S, Bestebroer TM, et al. Isolation of a novel coronavirus from a man with pneumonia in Saudi Arabia. N Engl J Med. 2012;367:1814-20.
4. WHO. (2018). WHO MERS-CoV Global Summary and Assessment of Risk, August 2018 (WHO/MERS/RA/August18). Geneva, Switzerland: World Health Organization; 2018. Licence: CC BY-NC-SA 3.0 IGO. [online] Available from https://www.who.int/csr/disease/coronavirus_infections/risk-assessment-august-2018.pdf?ua=1 [Accessed November 2018].
5. Memish ZA, Zumla AI, Al-Hakeem RF, et al. Family cluster of Middle East respiratory syndrome coronavirus infections. N Engl J Med. 2013;368:2487-94.
6. Memish ZA, Zumla AI, Assiri A. Middle East respiratory syndrome coronavirus infections in health care workers. N Engl J Med. 2013;369:884-6.
7. Saad M, Omrani AS, Baig K, et al. Clinical aspects and outcomes of 70 patients with Middle East respiratory syndrome coronavirus infection: a single-center experience in Saudi Arabia. Int J Infect Dis. 2014;29:301-6.
8. Abdel-Moneim AS. Middle East respiratory syndrome coronavirus (MERS-CoV): evidence and speculations. Arch Virol. 2014;159:1575-84.
9. van Boheemen S, de Graaf M, Lauber C, et al. Genomic characterization of a newly discovered coronavirus associated with acute respiratory distress syndrome in humans. MBio. 2012;3:1-9.

10. Wernery U, Lau SK, Woo PC. Genomics and zoonotic infections: Middle East respiratory syndrome. Rev Sci Tech. 2016;35:191-202.
11. Hocke AC, Becher A, Knepper J, et al. Emerging human middle East respiratory syndrome coronavirus causes widespread infection and alveolar damage in human lungs. Am J Respir Crit Care Med. 2013;188:882-6.
12. Chan RW, Chan MC, Agnihothram S, et al. Tropism of an innate immune responses to the novel human betacoronavirus lineage C virus in human ex vivo respiratory organ cultures. J Virol. 2013;87:6604-14.
13. Guery B, Poissy J, el Mansouf L, et al. Clinical features and viral diagnosis of two cases of infection with Middle East Respiratory Syndrome coronavirus: a report of nosocomial transmission. Lancet. 2013;381:2265-72.
14. Arabi YM, Arifi AA, Balkhy HH, et al. Clinical course and outcomes of critically ill patients with Middle East respiratory syndrome coronavirus infection. Ann Intern Med. 2014;160:389-97.
15. Al-Abdallat MM, Payne DC, Alqasrawi S, et al, and the Jordan MERS-CoV Investigation Team. Hospital-associated outbreak of Middle East respiratory syndrome coronavirus: a serologic, epidemiologic, and clinical description. Clin Infect Dis. 2014;59:1225-33.
16. Lambeir AM, Durinx C, Scharpé S, et al. Dipeptidyl-peptidase IV from bench to bedside: an update on structural properties, functions, and clinical aspects of the enzyme DPP IV. Crit Rev Clin Lab Sci. 2003;40:209-94.
17. Drosten C, Seilmaier M, Corman VM, et al. Clinical features and virological analysis of a case of Middle East respiratory syndrome coronavirus infection. Lancet Infect Dis. 2013;13:745-51.
18. Lin MH, Chuang SJ, Chen CC, et al. Structural and functional characterization of MERS coronavirus papain-like protease. J Biomed Sci. 2014;21:54.
19. Lei J, Mesters JR, Drosten C, et al. Crystal structure of the papain-like protease of MERS coronavirus reveals unusual, potentially druggable active-site features. Antiviral Res. 2014;109:72-82.
20. Bergmann CC, Lane TE, Stohlman SA. Coronavirus infection of the central nervous system: host-virus stand-off. Nat Rev Microbiol. 2006;4:121-32.
21. Channappanavar R, Zhao J, Perlman S. T cell-mediated immune response to respiratory coronaviruses. Immunol Res. 2014;59:118-28.
22. Chu H, Zhou J, Wong BH, et al. Productive replication of Middle East respiratory syndrome coronavirus in monocyte-derived dendritic cells modulates innate immune response. Virology. 2014;454:197-205.
23. Faure E, Poissy J, Goffard A, et al. Distinct immune response in two MERS-CoV-infected patients: can we go from bench to bedside? PLoS One. 2014;9:e88716.
24. Lau SK, Lau CC, Chan KH, et al. Delayed induction of proinflammatory cytokines and suppression of innate antiviral response by the novel Middle East respiratory syndrome coronavirus: implications for pathogenesis and treatment. J Gen Virol. 2013;94:2679-90.
25. Cotten M, Watson SJ, Zumla AI, et al. Spread, circulation, and evolution of the Middle East respiratory syndrome coronavirus. MBio. 2014;5:e01062-13.
26. Milne-Price S, Miazgowicz KL, Munster VJ. The emergence of the Middle East respiratory syndrome coronavirus (MERS-CoV). Pathog Dis. 2014;71:121-36.
27. Breban R, Riou J, Fontanet A. Interhuman transmissibility of middle east respiratory syndrome coronavirus: Estimation of pandemic risk. Lancet. 2013;382:694-9.
28. Cauchemez S, Fraser C, Van Kerkhove M, et al. Middle East respiratory syndrome coronavirus: quantification of the extent of the epidemic, surveillance biases, and transmissibility. Lancet Infec Dis. 2014;14:50-6.
29. de Wit E Rasmussen AL, Falzarano D, Bushmaker T, et al. Middle east respiratory syndrome coronavirus (MERS-CoV) causes transient lower respiratory tract infection in rhesus macaques. Proc Natl Acad Sci, USA. 2013;110:16598-603.
30. Center for Disease Control and Prevention CDC. (2015). Interim infection control and prevention recommendations for hospitalized patients with MERS-CoV. [online] Available from http://www.cdc.gov/coronavirus/mers/infection-prevention-control.html [Accessed November 2018].
31. Senga M, Arabi YM, Fowler RA. Clinical spectrum of the Middle East respiratory syndrome coronavirus (MERS-CoV). J Infect Public Health. 2017;10:191-4.
32. Hui DS, Memish ZA, Zumla A. Severe acute respiratory syndrome vs. the Middle East respiratory syndrome. Curr Opin Pulm Med. 2014;20:233-41.
33. Al-Tawfiq JA, Kattan RF, Memish ZA. Middle East respiratory syndrome coronavirus disease is rare in children: An update from Saudi Arabia. World J Clin Pediatr. 2016;5:391-6.
34. Memish Z.A, Al-Tawfiq JA, Assiri A, et al. Middle East respiratory syndrome coronavirus disease in children. Pediatr Infect Dis J. 2014;33:904-6.
35. Arabi YM, Harthi A, Hussein J, et al. Severe neurologic syndrome associated with Middle East respiratory syndrome corona virus (MERS-CoV). Infection. 2015;43:495-501.
36. Saad M, Omrani AS, Baig K, et al. Clinical aspects and outcomes of 70 patients with Middle East respiratory syndrome coronavirus infection: A single-center experience in Saudi Arabia. Int J Infect Dis. 2014;29:301-6.
37. WHO. (2017). Middle East Respiratory Syndrome Corona Virus: Case definition for reporting to WHO; interim case definitions as of 26 July 2017. [online] Available from http://www.who.int/csr/disease/coronavirus_infections/case_definition/en/ [Accessed November 2018].
38. Omrani AS, Saad MM, Baig K, et al. Ribavirin and interferon alfa-2a for severe Middle East respiratory syndrome coronavirus infection: A retrospective cohort study. Lancet Infect Dis. 2014;14:1090-5.
39. Falzarano D, deWit E, Rasmussen AL, et al. Treatment with interferon-alpha2b and ribavirin improves outcome in MERS-CoV-infected rhesus macaques. Nat Med. 2013;19:1313-7.
40. Kaufmann SH, McElrath MJ, Lewis DJ, et al. Challenges and responses in human vaccine development. Curr Opin Immunol. 2014;28:18-26.

41. Perlman S, Vijay R. Middle East respiratory syndrome vaccines. Int J Infect Dis. 2016;47:23-8.
42. Haagmans BL, van den Brand JM, Raj VS, et al. An orthopox virus-based vaccine reduces virus excretion after MERS-CoV infection in dromedary camels. Science. 2016;351:77-81.
43. Borucki MK, Lao V, Hwang M, et al. Middle East Respiratory Syndrome Coronavirus Intra-Host Populations Are Characterized by Numerous High Frequency Variants. PLoS ONE. 2016;11: e0146251.
44. Hui DS. Super-spreading events of MERS-CoV infection. Lancet. 2016;388:942-3.
45. Zumla, A, Hui DS. Infection control and MERS-CoV in health-care workers. Lancet. 2014;383:1869-71.

CHAPTER 34

Tetanus

Gentle Sunder Shrestha, Saurabh Pradhan, Subhash Prasad Acharya, Jeffrey Lipman

INTRODUCTION

Tetanus is a disease of the nervous system characterized by generalized muscle rigidity, spasms, and autonomic dysfunction that occurs due to the toxins from *Clostridium tetani*. Tetanus is now very rare in the developed countries, but it is still prevalent in the most developing countries.[1,2] Though mortality due to tetanus has much decreased after the advent of modern intensive care management, cardiovascular instability as well as hospital-acquired infections remain important causes of death worldwide.[3]

BIOLOGICAL PLAUSIBILITY

Pathogenesis

Clostridium tetani is a ubiquitous bacterium widely present in the soil, as well as gut of mammals.[4] It is a motile, spore-forming obligate anaerobe. *C. tetani* produces two exotoxins—tetanolysin and tetanospasmin. The clinical significance of tetanolysin is unknown, but the clinical effects are produced by tetanospasmin, which is an extremely potent exotoxin.[2]

The *C. tetani* spores get inoculated into the wound during a penetrating injury. However, the spores germinate only when they receive a favorable environment, which may be provided by a combination of factors, such as the presence of devitalized tissue, a foreign body, localized ischemia, or coinfection with other bacteria. Once the spores germinate into vegetative forms, they secrete the exotoxins. These toxins travel by retrograde axonal transport within the motor neuron to reach the spinal cord and the brainstem. There it enters adjacent inhibitory interneurons, where it blocks neurotransmission, resulting in inactivation of inhibitory neurons. This disinhibition of motor neurons and autonomic neurons results in the typical symptoms of painful spasms and autonomic instability.[5]

Clinical Features

Clinical features of tetanus are usually preceded by an injury, which may be trivial enough to be considered harmless and in 15–25% of the times, patients do not report an antecedent injury.[3] Common injuries include contaminated wounds (soil, manure, and rusty metal), burns, ulcers, gangrene, snakebites, septic abortions, childbirth, and surgery. In the developing countries, tetanus commonly occurs in the neonates in whom the umbilical stump gets infected. The unsanitary practice of using unsterilized tools for cutting the umbilical cord and cultural rituals, such as the use of manure to cover the stump, in some countries are considered important causes of tetanus.[6]

The natural history of tetanus is defined with certain time intervals. The incubation period is the time from injury to the onset of first symptom. This period averages 7–10 days, with a range of 3–21 days.[7] The onset time is defined as the time from first symptom to onset of the first spasm. This period varies between 1 day and 7 days. Shorter incubation and onset times are associated with more severe disease.[3]

The clinical triad of tetanus includes muscle rigidity, spasms, and autonomic dysfunction (if severe). The differences in host immunity, toxin load, the portal of entry, and the primary site of toxin action result in variable presentations of tetanus, which are classified as localized, cephalic, and generalized tetanus. Neonatal tetanus is a special form that occurs in neonates.

Localized tetanus occurs when the toxin load is lower, the injury occurs peripherally or there is partial immunity. It is characterized by muscle spasms in the associated limb. The symptoms may progress to become generalized. Spasms may persist for several weeks to months, and prognosis is comparatively favorable.[3]

Cephalic tetanus is a type of localized tetanus that occurs following trauma to the head or face region. It is characterized by a short incubation period of only 1–2 days, followed by the development of trismus, cranial nerve palsies, weakness in the areas innervated by the facial nerve, and weakness of the extraocular muscles.[3]

Generalized tetanus is the most common form of tetanus accounting for 85–90% of the cases.[3] The nerves with the shortest course from the neuromuscular nerve endings are the first to be affected. Thus most patients present with trismus or lockjaw that occurs due to spasms of the masseter muscles innervated by the trigeminal nerve. The muscle rigidity progresses caudally causing difficulty in swallowing, salivation, and stiffness in the neck, shoulders, and back. A typical sardonic smile described as risus sardonicus is characteristic of tetanus and occurs due to persistent masseter spasm. Tonic spasms of the back muscles causes backward arching of the head, neck, and spine described as opisthotonus. Tonic contractions of the whole body may occur that may be spontaneous or triggered by touch, visual, auditory, or emotional stimuli. Spasms if prolonged can lead to respiratory arrest.[8] Spasms of the oropharyngeal and laryngeal muscles can cause aspiration as well as acute airway obstruction.

Autoimmune dysfunction usually begins in the second week after onset of symptoms, which corresponds to the time it takes for the toxins to reach the brain stem. The toxins cause an enormous release of catecholamines, up to 10 times that of normal.[9] This is clinically manifested as labile hypertension, tachycardia, and sweating. Bradycardia, hypotension, and cardiac arrest may also occur but less frequently. Manifestation of autonomic dysfunction is considered the most severe form of the disease, and the various scoring systems rate its presence as having a poorer prognosis.[10,11]

Neonatal tetanus occurs as a result of the failure to use aseptic techniques in managing the umbilical stump after delivery of mothers who are poorly immunized against tetanus. It is now extremely rare in the developed countries. It typically occurs after 5–7 days of life.[12] The proportionately shorter length of axons in neonates leads to a more rapid progression of the disease than in adults. Symptoms include poor feeding, difficulty in opening the mouth, clenching of hands, and dorsiflexion of feet. Opisthotonus and risus sardonicus may also appear (Table 34.1).[12]

Table 34.1: Ablett classification of severity of tetanus.[11]

Grade	Clinical features
I (mild)	Mild trismus, general spasticity, no respiratory embarrassment, no spasms, no dysphagia
II (moderate)	Moderate trismus, rigidity, short spasms, mild dysphagia, moderate respiratory involvement, respiratory rate >30, mild dysphagia
III (severe)	Severe trismus, generalized spasticity, prolonged spasms, respiratory rate >40, severe dysphagia, apneic spells, pulse >120
IV (very severe)	Grade III plus severe autonomic disturbances involving the cardiovascular system

Diagnosis and Differentials

The diagnosis of tetanus is purely clinical. The typical symptoms with a history of preceding injury strongly suggest tetanus. Investigations are not helpful and, including cerebral spinal fluid analysis, are mostly normal. Localized tetanus, especially limited to facial territory, occasionally may be confused with other conditions causing trismus, such as dental infection. Other mimics include dystonic drug reactions, hypocalcemia, strychnine poisoning, stiff-person syndrome, and hysteria.

Management

There are three principle management strategies. They include the removal of source of infection, neutralization of unbound toxin, and control of symptoms, which include both spasms and autonomic dysfunction.

Removal of Source of Infection

To remove the source of infection, it requires proper wound management and antimicrobial therapy. *C. tetani* germinates in the presence of anaerobic environment; thus, any devitalized tissue needs immediate surgical debridement. However, the spores can survive in tissues without overt necrosis, so debridement must be extensive even if the tissue does not look necrotic. The antimicrobial of choice to treat tetanus has long been intravenous (IV) benzylpenicillin. However, as penicillin with its gamma-aminobutyric acid (GABA) antagonistic effects could potentially worsen muscle spasms,[13] metronidazole has now been considered the preferred antibiotic.[14] Other alternatives include erythromycin, tetracycline, chloramphenicol, and clindamycin.[3]

Neutralization of Unbound Toxin

Since tetanus toxin is irreversibly bound to tissues, only the unbound toxin can be neutralized. The human tetanus immune globulin is the preferred preparation of choice; however, in countries where this preparation is not available, equine antitoxin can also be used. Equine antitoxins have the disadvantage of causing hypersensitivity reactions and thus require an intradermal test dose before full-dose administration. Studies have investigated the role of intrathecal immunoglobulin therapy, and despite a meta-analysis, quality of evidences remains low.[15]

Control of Rigidity and Spasms

These patients are commonly nursed in an isolated room maintaining low light and a quiet environment to avoid unnecessary stimulus for spasms. More severe forms necessitate airway protection with endotracheal intubation or tracheostomy. The mainstay of treatment of tetanus is benzodiazepines. Benzodiazepines bind to $GABA_A$ receptors and facilitate the GABA-mediated opening of chloride channels and subsequent hyperpolarization.[16] Diazepam is the most common benzodiazepine used. It can be used as boluses or as continuous infusions. Doses as high as 100 mg/h have been reported.[17] Due to its longer half-life, and the effect of its active metabolites, prolonged infusions may predispose to delayed awakening. Furthermore, because of the presence of preservative, propylene glycol in diazepam solutions, hefty doses result in high anion gap metabolic acidosis.[18] With no preservative and shorter half-life, midazolam may be preferred. Continuous infusions of benzodiazepines require close respiratory monitoring for those not under mechanical ventilation.

Magnesium sulfate has also been used for the treatment of tetanus. It has several properties that are useful in managing tetanus. It provides sedation, muscle relaxation, vasodilatation and also decreases the release of catecholamines from synapses and adrenal medulla. It also seems to decrease the responsiveness to catecholamines.[19] Magnesium sulfate has been tested as an adjunct to benzodiazepines as well as the sole therapeutic agent in tetanus.

Drugs that could be useful in uncontrolled spasms include propofol and muscle relaxants. Propofol is a potent anesthetic agent and requires careful hemodynamic monitoring. Prolonged infusions can cause propofol infusion syndrome, a serious side effect characterized by metabolic acidosis and hemodynamic instability. Commonly used muscle relaxants include vecuronium and atracurium. Pancuronium, a long-acting agent, is nowadays not preferred as it inhibits catecholamine reuptake and thus could worsen autonomic instability.[20] Continuous infusions of neuromuscular-blocking agents, especially the aminosteroid variety, are avoided as they predispose to critical illness, neuropathy and myopathy. Various other drugs have also been used to control spasms, but many of which are still experimental due to paucity of quality evidences. These include dantrolene, intrathecal baclofen, and antiepileptic agents.[3,21,22]

Control of Autonomic Dysfunction

Benzodiazepines used for sedation are also the mainstay agent for reducing autonomic dysfunction. It may be supplemented with opioids, especially morphine that preserves hemodynamic stability. Beta blockers, such as propranolol, can control episodes of hypertension and tachycardia, but incidences of profound hypotension, pulmonary edema, and cardiac arrests due to persistent beta blockade and unopposed alpha-mediated vasoconstriction have decreased its preference.[23-25] Short-acting agents, such as esmolol, or those with both alpha- and beta-blocking properties, such as labetalol, may be safer.[26] Alpha-2 adrenergic agonists, such as clonidine and dexmedetomidine, can reduce central sympathetic outflow preventing the catecholamine surges that occur in autonomic dysfunction. Other drugs that could be effective for controlling autonomic dysfunction include phenothiazines,[19] antiepileptics, such as sodium valproate,[27] atropine,[28] as well as bupivacaine used via epidural[29] or spinal routes.[30] Hypotensive crises can also occur, which need treatment with dopamine or noradrenaline.[31]

Active Immunization

As natural immunity to tetanus does not occur, all patients with tetanus require tetanus toxoid (TT) vaccine. A full immunization course consists of three doses followed with booster doses every 10 years. In many countries where tetanus is prevalent, it is commonly administered as an infant immunization schedule in combination with diphtheria and/or pertussis.[32] Since neonates have immunity from maternal antibodies, two doses of the vaccine may be administered to childbearing females over 14 years of age or in the second trimester of pregnancy to protect the neonates from neonatal tetanus.[33]

EVIDENCE BASE

Antibiotics

Several studies have compared metronidazole with penicillin. One study found a greater reduction in mortality in the metronidazole group (7% vs 24%).[14] In contrast, two other studies reported no difference in mortality in between the patients treated with either agent.[34,35] Patients receiving metronidazole, however, may require fewer muscle relaxants and sedatives than penicillin group of drugs as these compounds have a GABA antagonistic property that may exacerbate muscle rigidity and spasms.[13]

Magnesium Sulfate

Magnesium sulfate has been used for the treatment of tetanus as early as 1906.[36] A preclinical study found magnesium sulfate to decrease pulse rate, systemic vascular resistance, as well as stroke volume.[19] Magnesium sulfate when used as an adjunct to diazepam decreases the dose requirement as well as its associated side effects.[37,38] It has also been found to be effective as a sole agent.[39] However the largest evidence, a randomized controlled trial (RCT) from Vietnam, reports that while magnesium sulfate may reduce sedation requirements and cardiovascular instability, it could not decrease the need for mechanical ventilation.[40]

Alpha-2 Adrenergic Agonists

Data evaluating the efficacy of alpha-2 agonists are scarce and conflicting. Clonidine has been found to be effective in controlling autonomic dysfunction,[41,42] but some have also reported its failure to control blood pressure. Another study also found that neither clonidine nor dexmedetomidine was able to decrease catecholamine levels in tetanus patients.[43]

Tetanus Immunoglobulins

A meta-analysis of 12 trials and 942 patients has evaluated the efficacy of intrathecal immunoglobulin to reduce mortality and morbidity of tetanus. Though the results from this study show a relative risk of mortality in intrathecal group to be 0.71 (0.62–0.81), the methodological quality of the individual studies has not been scrutinized.[15] There is an ongoing RCT Intrathecal Tetanus Immunoglobulin to Treat Tetanus trial that may answer some of these questions.

Intrathecal Baclofen

Baclofen is considered a GABA agonist that acts by selectively binding to $GABA_B$ receptors.[44] One of the earliest documentations of its application in tetanus was by Muller et al.[44] As baclofen has poor penetration of the blood–brain barrier, intrathecal route is required for it to be effective.[44] A literature search only reveals case reports and small series regarding its use in tetanus, but all available evidences suggest it to be efficacious in controlling tetanic spasms when used either as a continuous infusion or as intermittent boluses.[21,45-47] Intrathecal baclofen may be advantageous to other agents in preserving respiratory drive and allowing voluntary movements.[21] Common complications include hypotension, bradycardia, hypotonia, and meningitis.[45]

PRACTICE PRESCRIPTION

- *Wound care:*
  - Surgical debridement of devitalized tissue as necessary
- *Immunotherapy:*
  - Human tetanus immunoglobulin (HTIG) 500 U intramuscular (IM)/IV as soon as possible.
  - Tetanus toxoid:
    - If patient has completed the course of immunization (≥3 doses) within a 5-year period—TT not required.
    - If patient has completed the course of immunization but has not had a booster within a 5-year period—0.5 mL of TT IM should be injected at a site separate from that for HTIG.
    - If patient has not completed the course of immunization, three doses of TT should be administered at least 4 weeks apart.
- *General measures:*
  - Nurse in an isolated, dark, and quiet room.
  - Intensive care unit admission required for severe spasms, airway protection, or cardiovascular instability.
- *Control of spasms:*
  - Benzodiazepines:
    - Diazepam: About 5 mg IV; incremental doses or continuous infusion given titrated to effect OR
    - Lorazepam: 2 mg IV; incremental doses or continuous infusion given titrated to effect OR
    - Midazolam: 5 mg IV; incremental doses or continuous infusion given titrated to effect.
  - Magnesium sulfate: 75 mg/kg (5 g) IV load then 2–3 g/h; titrate to effect. Monitor—patellar reflex, urine output, and magnesium level (target 2–4 mmol/L).
  - Other agents:
    - Intrathecal baclofen: 40–200 µg bolus, followed by 20 µg/h (maximum dose 2 mg/24 h).
    - Dantrolene: 1–2 µg/kg q4 hours.
    - Chlorpromazine: 50–150 µg IM q4–8 hours.

- Propofol: 10–20 mg boluses repeated to effect or 25–75 µg/kg/min (limit to 48 hours or 4 mg/kg/h).
- *Control of autonomic dysfunction:*
  - Benzodiazepines as above OR/AND
  - Magnesium sulfate as above OR/AND
  - Morphine 5 mg IV boluses; titrate to effect OR/AND
  - Labetalol: 5–20 mg IV repeat every 20 minutes or follow with 1–2 mg/min infusion OR/AND
  - Esmolol: 0.5 mg/kg IV OR/AND
  - Clonidine: 100–200 µg per os q8 hours OR/AND
  - Dexmedetomidine: 0.1–1 µg/kg/h.

REFERENCES

1. Bleck TP. Tetanus: pathophysiology, management and prophylaxis. Dis Mon. 1991;37(9):556-603.
2. Lipman J. Tetanus. In: Bersten AD, Soni N (Eds). Oh's intensive care manual, 7th edition. Beijing: Elsevier; 2014. pp. 607-10.
3. Cook TM, Protheroe RT, Handel JM. Tetanus: a review of literature. Br J Anaesth. 2001;87:477-87.
4. Wilkins CA, Richter MB, Hobbs WB, et al. Occurrence of *Clostridium tetani* in soil and horses. S Afr Med J. 1988;73:718-20.
5. Lalli G, Bohnert S, Deinhardt K, et al. The journey of tetanus and botulinum neurotoxins in neurons. Trends Microgiol. 2003;11:431-7.
6. Idema CD, Harris BN, Ogunbanjo GA, et al. Neonatal tetanus elimination in Mpumalanga Province, South Africa. Trop Med Int Health. 2002;7:622-4.
7. Centers for Disease Control and Prevention. Epidemiology and prevention of vaccine-preventable diseases. In: Tetanus. [online] Available from http://www.cdc.gov/vaccines/pubs/pinkbook/tetanus.html. [Accessed September 8, 2015].
8. Bunch TJ, Thalji MK, Pellikka PA, et al. Respiratory failure in tetanus: case report and review of a 25-year experience. Chest. 2002;122:1488-92.
9. Kelty SR, Gray RC, Dundee JW, et al. Catecholamine levels in severe tetanus. Lancet. 1968;2:195.
10. Wood MJ. Toxin-mediated disorders: tetanus, botulism and diphtheria. In: Cohen J, Powderly WG (Eds). Infectious diseases, 2nd edition. Edinburgh: Mosby; 2004. pp. 289-96.
11. Ablett JJL. Analysis and main experiences in 82 patients treated in the Leeds Tetanus Unit. In: Ellis M (Ed) Symposium on tetanus in Great Britain. Boston Spa, UK: National Lending Library. 1967. pp. 1-10.
12. Thwaites CL, Beeching NJ, Newton CR. Maternal and neonatal tetanus. Lancet. 2015;385:362-70.
13. Johnson HC, Walker A. Intraventricular penicillin. JAMA. 1945;127:217-9.
14. Ahmadsyah I, Salim A. Treatment of tetanus: an open study to compare the efficacy of procaine penicillin and metronidazole. Br Med J. 1985;291:648-50.
15. Kabura L, Ilibagiza D, Menten J, et al. Intrathecal *vs.* intramuscular administration of human antitetanus immunoglobulin or equine tetanus antitoxin in the treatment of tetanus: a meta-analysis. Trop Med Int Health. 2006;11:1075-81.
16. Stahmer SD. Pharmacodynamics of bensodiazepines. S Afr Med J. 1985;68(Suppl.):14-22.
17. Leitch AG. The hypoxic drive to breathing in man. Lancet. 1981;i:428-30.
18. Kapoor W, Carvey P, Karpf M. Induction of lactic acidosis with intravenous diazepam in a patient with tetanus. Arch Intern Med. 1981;141:944-5.
19. James MFM, Beer RE, Esser JD. Intravenous magnesium sulfate inhibits catecholamine release associated with tracheal intubation. AnesthAnalg. 1989;68:772-6.
20. Buchanan N, Cane RD, Wolfson G, et al. Autonomic dysfunction in tetanus: the effects of a variety of therapeutic agents, with special reference to morphine. Intensive Care Med. 1979;5:65-8.
21. Dressnandt J, Konstanzer A, Weinzierl FX, et al. Intrathecal baclofen in tetanus: four cases and a review of reported cases. Intensive Care Med. 1997;23:896-902.
22. Tidyman M, Prichard JG, Deamer RL, et al. Adjunctive use of dantrolene in severe tetanus. Anesth Analg. 1985;64:538-40.
23. Edmondson RS, Flowers MW. Intensive care in tetanus: management, complications and mortality in 100 cases. Br Med J. 1979;1:1401-4.
24. Kerr JH, Corbett JL, Prys-Roberts C, et al. Involvement of the sympathetic nervous system in tetanus. Studies on 82 patients. Lancet. 1968;ii:236-41.
25. Prys-Roberts C, Kerr JH, Corbett JL, et al. Treatment of sympathetic overactivity in tetanus. Lancet. 1969;i:542-6.
26. King WW, Cave DR. Use of esmolol to control autonomic instability of tetanus. Am J Med. 1991;91:425-8.
27. Foca A, Rotiroti D, Mastroeni P, et al. Effects of tetanus toxin after intracerebral microinjection are antagonised by drugs enhancing GABAergic transmission in adult fowl. Neuropharmacology. 1984;23:155-8.
28. Dolar D. The use of continuous atropine infusion in the management of tetanus. Intensive Care Med. 1992;18:26-31.
29. Southorn PA, Blaise GA. Treatment of tetanus-induced autonomic nervous system dysfunction with continuous epidural blockade. Crit Care Med. 1986;14:251-2.
30. Shibuya M, Sugimoto H, Sugimoto T, et al. The use of continuous spinal anesthesia in severe tetanus with autonomic disturbance. J Trauma. 1989;29:1423-9.
31. Corbett JL, Spalding JMK, Harris PJ. Hypotension in tetanus. Br Med J. 1973;3:423-28.
32. Bhatia R, Prabhakar S, Grover VK. Tetanus. Neurol India. 2002;50:398-407.
33. Park K. Park's textbook of preventive and social medicine, 15th edition. India: M/s Banarsidas Bhanot Publishers; 1997. pp. 237-40.
34. Saltoglu N, Tasova Y, Midikli D, et al. Prognostic factors affecting deaths from adult tetanus. Clin Microbiol Infect. 2004;10:229-33.
35. Yen LM, Dao LM, Day NPJ. Management of tetanus: a comparison of penicillin and metronidazole. In: Symposium of antimicrobial resistance in southern Viet Nam; 1997.
36. Blake JA. The use of magnesium sulphate in the production of anaesthesia and in the treatment of tetanus. Surg Gynecol Obstet. 1906;2:541-50.
37. Attagylle D, Rodrigo N. Magnesium sulphate for the control of spasms in severe tetanus. Anaesthesia. 1999;54:302-3.

38. Pokharel K, Tripathi M, Bhattarai B, et al. Large versus small dose magnesium sulfate infusion in tetanus. J Nepal Med Assoc. 2014;52:791-7.
39. Attygalle D, Rodrigo N. Magnesium sulphate for control of spasms in severe tetanus. Can we avoid sedation and artificial ventilation?. Anaesthesia. 1997;52:956-62.
40. Thwaites CL, Yen LM, Loan HT, et al. Magnesium sulfate for treatment of severe tetanus: a randomized controlled trial. Lancet. 2006;368:1436-43.
41. Sutton DN, Tremlett MR, Woodcock TE, et al. Management of autonomic dysfunction in severe tetanus: the use of magnesium sulfate and clonidine. Intensive Care Med. 1990;16:75-80.
42. Gregorakos L, Kerezoudi E, Dimopoulos G, et al. Management of blood pressure instability in severe tetanus: the use of clonidine. Intensive Care Med. 1997;23:893-5.
43. Freshwater-Turner D, Udy A, Lipman J, et al. Autonomic dysfunction in tetanus—what lessons can be learnt with specific reference to alpha-2 agonists?. Anaesthesia. 2007;62:1066-70.
44. Muller H, Borner U, Zierski J, et al. Intrathecal baclofen for treatment of tetanus-induced spasticity. Anesthesiology. 1987;66:76-9.
45. Santos ML, Mota-Miranda A, Alves-Pereira A, et al. Intrathecal baclofen for the treatment of tetanus. Clin Infect Dis. 2004;38:321-8.
46. Demaziere J, Saissy JM, Vitris M, et al. Intermittent intrathecal baclofen for severe tetanus. Lancet. 1991;337:427.
47. Engrand N, Guerot E, Rouamba A, et al. The efficacy of intrathecal baclofen in severe tetanus. Anesthesiology. 1999;90:1773-6.

CHAPTER 35

Intensive Care Management of Leptospirosis

Elizabeth Jane Bennett, Maika Vuli Seru

INTRODUCTION: EPIDEMIOLOGY AND RISK FACTORS

Leptospirosis is a zoonotic infection caused by corkscrew-shaped bacteria from the genus *Leptospira*.[1,2] A large number of mammals, including rodents, cattle, dogs, horses, sheep, goats, and skunks, are animal hosts of this infection, which chronically infects the kidneys. Leptospires are excreted in urine of infected animals and survive, remaining contagious for weeks or months in warm and humid conditions.[2] Transmission to humans occurs incidentally when food, soil, or water contaminated by infected urine comes in contact with human mucous membranes and/or broken skin.[1-4]

Risk factors for infection include any activity which may bring humans into contact with infected animal urine. They include:
- Occupational exposure (farmers, abattoir workers, veterinarians, rice farmers, laboratory workers, etc.)
- Recreational activities (rafting, potholing, caving, swimming, adventure sports, trekking, walking barefoot through surface water, and contact with wild rodents)
- Household exposure (pet dogs, domesticated livestock, rainwater catchment systems, and gardening)

Epidemics may occur when contact with infected animals is enhanced, such as monsoon seasons, heavy rainfall and flooding, and rodent-infested urban slums with poor housing and sanitation.[4] The most common group affected is of young males who are commonly in the above risk groups. Human-to-human transmission is exceptionally rare but has been documented through sexual intercourse or breastfeeding.[1]

Whilst reported worldwide, infection is endemic in many tropical and subtropical countries, many of which are also developing countries.[1] Center for Disease Control and Prevention (CDC) estimates that more than a million cases of leptospirosis occur annually worldwide with an estimated 60,000 deaths.[1] The World Health Organization (WHO) (Leptospirosis Burden Epidemiology Reference Group) estimates that 0.1–1 per 100,000 per annum people living in temperature climates, with the number increasing to 10 or more per 100,000 people living in tropical climates. In epidemics the incidence can increase to 100 or more per 100,000 people per annum.[4] The true incidence of leptospirosis is unknown, but it is thought to be at least double the reported incidence owing to underdiagnosis and underreporting.[4,5]

PRESENTATION: ASSESSMENT AND DIAGNOSIS

Leptospirosis infection in humans can range in presentation from mild to lethal multisystem disease.[1,5] It is important to understand the varied nature of presentations in order to recognize possible leptospirosis and institute timely treatment which needs to commence before laboratory confirmation can occur. It is also important to know and recognize danger signs of severe disease so patients can be monitored and treated in high dependency unit or intensive care unit (ICU).

Clinical Manifestations

Following exposure, the incubation period is usually about 5–14 days but ranges from 2 days to 4 weeks.[1] According to CDC, the majority of infections with leptospirosis are thought to be asymptomatic. Of the patients who do present with clinical disease, most (90%) present with a nonspecific acute febrile illness.[1] Approximately 10% of clinical illness can progress to severe life-threatening multisystem disease[1,2] primarily affecting brain, liver, lungs, heart, and kidneys.

Common symptoms include abrupt onset fever, severe myalgia (particularly lower limbs), headache, vomiting, abdominal pain, diarrhea, jaundice, rash, cough, and red eyes. Since conjunctival suffusion is not a common finding in other differentials of nonspecific fever, this last sign is particularly helpful in signaling the diagnosis of leptospirosis.[6]

Antibodies to leptospires appear in the blood from 5 days to 7 days after onset of illness. Classically, leptospirosis is described as a biphasic illness, with an early acute phase, followed by brief recovery then development of more severe illness suggesting immune-mediated element to this stage of the illness. However, acute monophasic illness is also commonly described.

Severe disease was first described by Weil in 1885 as biphasic illness with a triad of hemorrhage, jaundice, and renal failure in the late phase of illness.[6,7] This is one presentation of severe leptospirosis, but this presentation may be accompanied or replaced by other complications, including dehydration or septic shock, aseptic meningitis, myocarditis and cardiac arrhythmias, rhabdomyolysis and thrombocytopenia and hemorrhage into various organs.[7]

The most life-threatening complication of leptospirosis, respiratory failure from pulmonary hemorrhage, and acute respiratory distress syndrome (ARDS) is an increasingly recognized complication, particularly in countries where leptospirosis is endemic.[1,7-12,21,22] A recent paper debated reasons for this emerging severe presentation, such as possible emergence of new or more virulent serovars, immune reaction to second infection from a different serovar (similar to dengue hemorrhagic fever), or perhaps better recognition.[13] This complication has a high mortality even with good intensive care.

Rarer presentations include pancreatitis or acalculous cholecystitis. Delayed complications, such as uveitis or Guillian-Barre syndrome, may also occur.[7,8]

Laboratory Findings

Laboratory investigations may reveal elevations in creatine phosphokinase, creatinine, and urea. In icteric leptospirosis, bilirubin is elevated and may be accompanied by modest elevations of aspartate aminotransferase and alanine aminotransferase and gamma-glutamyl transferase. Platelets may be normal in patients with mild-to-moderate disease, but thrombocytopenia is often seen in severe cases.[14] Anemia may be present and can occur late, whilst elevation in white cell count (with neutrophilia) is variable.[5,14]

An understanding of the specific diagnostic tests available for leptospirosis is useful. Tests can be divided into supportive and confirmatory (Box 35.1).[3,7] Supportive tests (both detecting immunoglobulin M) are the most frequently used and easy to perform but become positive only after a week into the illness. They also lack sensitivity and specificity and may remain positive for a few years after infection so may be difficult to interpret if the patient is presenting after 5 days. Gold standard test is the microscopic agglutination testing but is only available in reference laboratories and still requires acute and convalescent serum. Culture may take weeks to months. Polymerase chain reaction (PCR) is the only method to confirm infection during the first week but is not always available.[3,7]

Diagnosis

Many diseases can present with similar symptoms and signs to leptospirosis; hence the differential diagnosis is broad, including typhoid, viral hepatitis, malaria, dengue, severe sepsis, hemorrhagic fever, and rickettsial infection, depending on the setting. Initial diagnosis of suspected leptospirosis is made based on clinical findings since with the exception of PCR, laboratory tests must rely on antibody production in the second week. Following supportive and confirmatory laboratory tests and cases can later be redefined as suspected, probable, or confirmed. In Fiji where leptospirosis infection is endemic, sometimes epidemic, evidence-based management guidelines have been recently published to promote better outcomes by earlier recognition, treatment, and referral for tertiary care if required. Box 35.1 discuss these guidelines outlines case definition criteria.[7]

TREATMENT EVIDENCE AND PRACTICE RECOMMENDATIONS

Treatment for leptospirosis involves early appropriate antibiotic treatment and supportive care for complications.

BOX 35.1: Case definitions for leptospirosis, clinical leptospirosis guidelines.[7]

A. **Suspected case:** All three of the following criteria fulfilled. (Note that a suspected case is defined by clinical assessment alone)
Criteria 1: Acute onset of fever (≥38°C), headache, and myalgia
+
Criteria 2: At least one of the following clinical features:
- Conjunctival suffusion (red eyes)
- Jaundice (yellow eyes)
- Acute renal failure (increased or decreased urine output)
- Bleeding (blood-stained sputum, hemoptysis, epistaxis, GI bleed, petechiae)

+
Criteria 3: At least one of the following epidemiological risk factors:
- Occupation: Farmer, abattoir worker, outdoor worker, cleaning streams, exposure to sewage, and garbage
- Contact with animals: Livestock (especially pigs), rodents, pets, wildlife
- Contact with freshwater, soil, or mud: Floodwaters, rivers, lakes, waterfalls, gardens
- Living conditions: Live in rural area or village, no metered water at home
- Live or work in areas with high risk of leptospirosis, e.g. recent cases or outbreaks
- Epidemiological link to a probable or confirmed case, e.g. household member or coworker

B. **Probable case:** Suspected case with at least one of the following:
- Positive rapid diagnostic test (SD Leptospira IgM)
- Positive Leptospira ELISA IgM (Panbio)

C. **Confirmed case:** Suspected case with at least one of the following:
- Positive Leptospira PCR
- MAT: Single sample titer of ≥1:400, or a fourfold rise in titers between samples taken 14 days and 60 days apart
- Isolation of leptospirosis by culture
- Identification of leptospires in tissues

(ELISA: enzyme-linked immunosorbent assay; GI: gastrointestinal; IgM: immunoglobulin M; MAT: microscopic agglutination test; PCR: polymerase chain reaction; SD: standard deviation)
Source: Ministry of Health, Fiji 2016.[7]

Patients with severe leptospirosis may deteriorate extremely rapidly. Intensive care admission is needed for dehydration, hypotension and shock, bleeding, and renal or respiratory failure. Whilst patients often manifest jaundice, liver involvement is often self-limiting, and liver failure is seldom seen.[7,14] Mortality in ICU relates to renal failure or severe pulmonary hemorrhage, and these will be specifically addressed. Many studies have looked for prognostic indicators to flag at risk cases. Factors related to worse outcome, including serum creatinine >200 mmol/L, platelet count <50,000 µmol/L, lactate >2.5 mmol/L, and serum amylase >250 IU/L, delay in initiating antibiotic treatment greater than 2 days from symptom onset[15] and respiratory involvement.[11] To ensure earlier referral of high-risk cases in Fiji, patients are stratified into levels of care by identifying danger for deterioration highlighted in Table 35.1 from recent guidelines.[7]

Antibiotics

Current evidence suggests that early effective antibiotic treatment, commenced in the first 2–3 days of leptospirosis, may reduce both duration of illness and progression to severe disease. WHO recommends rapid presumptive antibiotic treatment prior to the fifth day of illness.[2] It is highly recommended therefore that treatment be started on clinical suspicion since laboratory confirmation is seldom available at this early stage.[7] A study in new Caledonia showed delay in greater than 2 days in antibiotic treatment was a risk factor for more severe disease,[15] whilst another study in Japan found delay in treatment or more than 5 days was correlated with an increased risk of dying.[14]

Whether antibiotic treatment is effective or beneficial when started later in the illness during the immune phase is matter of some controversy in the literature. A Cochrane analysis published in 2012 did not show clear benefit from antibiotics, although there was nonstatistically significant decreased duration of clinical illness.[16] It is important to remember that the presentation of leptospirosis is often nonspecific, confirmation of leptospirosis is usually not available early, and antibiotics are usually required anyway for other differential diagnoses entertained such as severe typhoid.

Many antibiotics have been shown to be effective in vitro against leptospires, including penicillins, macrolides, carbapenems, cephalosporins, and aminoglycosides. Chloramphenicol is not effective.[10] Recommendations in the literature commonly suggest oral doxycycline as the drug of choice for mild infections with azithromycin or amoxicillin as alternatives in pregnant or pediatric cases,[1,7,9] whilst intravenous penicillin or amoxicillin or third-generation cephalosporins are recommended for more severe cases.[1,7,9] Both penicillins and cephalosporins may precipitate Jarisch–Herxheimer reaction in the first 2 days of treatment presenting as rigors, fever, and hypotension as leptospires are killed.[7,8]

Choice of the antibiotic is influenced not only by severity of the illness but also by the presence of renal failure and differential diagnoses being entertained. In Fiji, severe dengue, typhoid fever, and *Klebsiella* sepsis are common infections presenting a similar clinical picture of shock, high temperature, thrombocytopenia, and respiratory failure. Ceftriaxone is chosen once the patient requires intensive care since this antibiotic will also cover the latter two infections. Similarly, if intracellular organism,

Table 35.1: Levels of medical care recommended based on clinical assessment and investigations, clinical leptospirosis guidelines, Ministry of Health, Fiji 2016.[7]

		Danger signs	
Level 1: Outpatient care if patient fulfills all of the following criteria	Level 2: Inpatient care at subdivisional hospital if	Level 3: Inpatient care at divisional hospital if any of the following	Level 4: ICU management if any of the following
No cough or other respiratory symptoms	No cough or other respiratory symptoms	• Cough • Shortness of breath • RR >28 per minute	• RR > 20 per minute • PaO_2 < 60 mm Hg on air • Hemoptysis or blood-stained sputum • Abnormal CXR
Normal BP	Normal BP	Systolic BP < 90 mm Hg	• Systolic BP <90 mm Hg despite adequate fluid replacement
No signs of bleeding	No signs of bleeding	• Any signs of bleeding • Platelets <100,000 per mm³ • Increased prothrombin time and/or INR	• Hemoptysis or blood-stained sputum • Gastrointestinal bleeding • Platelets <50,000 per mm³
Normal urine output	Normal urine output	• Acute renal failure (oliguria or polyuria) • Electrolyte imbalance	• Hemodialysis if any of: – Urea >30 mmol/L – pH <7.2 – Potassium >5.5 mmol/L – Anuria or severe oliguria – Volume overload with pulmonaryedema
No jaundice	No jaundice	Jaundice	
Normal heart rate and rhythm	Normal heart rate and rhythm	Cardiac arrhythmias	
Normal consciousness	Normal consciousness	Altered consciousness	• Glasgow Coma score ≤12 • Seizures
No vomiting	Vomiting and needs IV antibiotics or fluids		
Ambulatory	Not ambulatory for other reasons		

(BP: blood pressure; CXR: chest X-ray; ICU: intensive care unit; INR: international normalized ratio; IV: intravenous; RR: respiratory rate)

such as rickettsia, is a consideration then doxycycline or azithromycin should be considered.

Supportive Care

General supportive care includes the treatment of dehydration or shock, correction of electrolyte abnormalities, and blood or blood products for bleeding complications.

Renal failure is a common complication of leptospirosis needing ICU admission and may be anuric, nonoliguric, or polyuric.[5,7] Polyuric renal failure may be accompanied by hyponatremia and hypokalemia which requires correction.[5] Leptospires in the kidney cause an interstitial nephritis,[2,6] although hypovolemia, rhabdomyolysis, and acute tubular necrosis can also contribute to acute renal failure. In settings where dialysis is not available, renal failure can be fatal. In contrast, with full supportive care, renal function usually recovers rapidly. Supportive treatment includes adequate resuscitation and volume replacement, adjustment of drug doses, and renal replacement therapy for the features outlined in Table 35.1.[7] Dialysis is considered earlier if the patient is bleeding and urea is rising. One study showed better outcomes with daily rather than second daily dialysis but failed to pinpoint optimum timing for commencement.[17]

Respiratory failure, particularly hemorrhage into the lungs, is the recognized major life-threatening complication in leptospirosis ICU admissions and may occur in 20–70%.[9] Patients present with the usual symptoms (febrile illness, headache, myalgia, and red eyes) accompanied by cough, dyspnea, and thrombocytopenia. Chest X-ray shows bilateral pulmonary filtrates. Hemoptysis signals hemorrhage into the lung which ranges from self-limiting to massive, catastrophic, and rapidly fatal.[8] This latter complication, coined severe pulmonary hemorrhage syndrome (SPHS), is associated with a high mortality reported 50% or more for those who require ventilatory support.[1,10-12,18,19] Respiratory failure may also result from

ARDS or acute pulmonary edema secondary to arrhythmias or renal failure.

All patients with signs of impending respiratory failure should be monitored closely. Milder cases may be treated with noninvasive ventilation (NIV) if able to protect their airways, but more severe cases or patients with tachypnea despite NIV should be intubated and ventilated with standard protective-lung ventilation strategies.

In our hospital, platelets are transfused to maintain platelets >50,000 µmol/L aiming to limit ongoing pulmonary bleeding given the increased risk of dying documented with lower platelet counts.[14,15]

Use of high-dose corticosteroids for respiratory complications has been advocated by some authors, given the possible immune-mediated pathogenesis of this respiratory failure. Many case studies are published reporting potential benefit from high-dose steroids,[10,11,12] but some also document potential harm.[18] The 2014 systematic review of this topic found five studies, the one randomized controlled trial showed corticosteroids were ineffective, whilst four studies showing benefit of early steroids in severe pulmonary disease had methodical flaws. They concluded no current supportive evidence exists to recommend the use of high-dose steroid in leptospirosis.[20] Current practice in our unit is to consider steroids only if hydrocortisone replacement therapy is indicated for severe shock as per severe sepsis guidelines.

Other studies have considered plasmapheresis or intravenous immunoglobulin therapy in severe cases of leptospirosis, but more work is required to support these practices. No studies were found regarding the use of tranexamic acid for SPHS.[11,14]

CONCLUSION

Leptospirosis is a globally recognized emerging zoonosis which may require intensive care for complications, particularly acute renal failure or acute respiratory failure, secondary to hemorrhage. Whilst mortality for severe leptospirosis is quoted as 5–15% overall, in patients with SPHS, mortality is in excess of 50%.[1,21,22] Treatment entails prompt recognition, timely antibiotics, and supportive care.

REFERENCES

1. Centres for Disease Control and Prevention. Leptospirosis fact sheet for clinicians. Centres for Disease Control and Prevention; 2018. [online] Available from https://www.cdc.gov/leptospirosis/pdf/fs-leptospirosis-clinicians-eng-508.pdf. [Accessed June, 2018].
2. Goarant C. Leptospirosis: risk factors and management challenges in developing countries. Res Rep Trop Med. 2016;7:49-62.
3. WHO. WPRO fact sheet on leptospirosis. [online] Available from http://www.wpro.who.int/mediacentre/factsheets/fs_13082012_leptospirosis/en/. [Accessed June, 2018].
4. WHO. Leptospirosis Burden Epidemiology Reference Group (LERG). [online] Available from http://www.who.int/zoonoses/diseases/lerg/en/. [Accessed May, 2018].
5. World Health Organization. (2003). Human leptospirosis: guidance for diagnosis, surveillance and control. Geneva: World Health Organization; International Leptospirosis Society. [online] Available from http://whqlibdoc.who.int/hq/2003/WHO_CDS_CSR_EPH_2002.23.pdf.
6. Day N. (2017). Epidemiology, microbiology, clinical manifestations, and diagnosis of leptospirosis. UpTodate. [online] Available from http://www.uptodate.com. [Accessed June 27, 2018].
7. Levett PN. Leptospirosis. Clin Microbiol Rev. 2001;14(2):296-310.
8. Lau C. Clinical guidelines for diagnosis and management of leptospirosis. Leptospirosis Guideline. Ministry of Health, Fiji Islands; 2016;1(1):1-18.
9. Lau C, Human leptospirosis in Oceania. In: Nelgected tropical diseases—Oceania. doi: 10.1007/978-3-319-43148-2_7.
10. Day N. (2017). Treatment and prevention of leptospirosis. UpTodate. [online] Available from http://www.uptodate.com. [Accessed June 27, 2018].
11. Jayakrishnan B, Abid FB, Balkhair A, etal, Severe pulmonary involvement in leptospirosis alternate antibiotics and systemic steroids. Sultan Qaboos Univ Med J. 2013;13(2):318-22.
12. Gulati S, Gulati A. Pulmonary manifestations of leptospirosis. Lung India. 2012;29(4):347-53.
13. Paganin F, Bourdin A, Borgherini G, et al. Pulmonary manifestations of leptospirosis. Rev Mal Respir. 2011;28(9):131-9.
14. Truong KN, Coburn J. The emergence of severe pulmonary hemorrhagic leptospirosis: questions to consider. Front Cell Infect Microbiol. 2012;1:24.
15. Yuzuru K. Clinical observation and treatment of leptospirosis. J Infect Chemother. 2001;7:759-68.
16. Tubiana S, Mikulski M, Becam J, et al. Risk factors and predictors of severe leptospirosis in New Caledonia. PLoS Negl Trop Dis. 2013;1(7):1-8.
17. Brett-Major DM, Coldren R. Antibiotics for the treatment of leptospirosis. Cochrane Database Syst Rev. 2012;(2):CD008264. doi: 10.1002/14651858.CD008264.pub2.
18. Andrade L, Cleto S, Seguro AC. Door-to-dialysis time and daily hemodialysis in patients with leptospirosis: impact on mortality. Clin J Am Soc Nephrol. 2007;2(4):739-44.
19. Rodrigo C, de Silva NL, Goonaratne R, et al. High dose corticosteroids in severe leptospirosis: a systemiatic review. Trans R Soc Trop Med Hyg. 2014;108(12):743-50.
20. Hingorani RV, Kumar R, Hegde AV, et al. Is it time to rethink the use of steroids for pulmonary leptospirosis?. J Assoc Physicians India. 2016;64:78-79.
21. Segura E, Ganoza CA, Campos K, et al. Clinical spectrum of pulmonary involvement in leptospirosis in region oif endemicity, with quantification of leptospirla burden. Clin Infect Dis. 2005;40(3):343-51.
22. Gouvela E, Metcalfe J, Carvalho L, et al. Leptospirosis-associated severe pulmonary hemorrhagic síndrome, salvador, Brazil. Emerg Infect Dis. 2008;14(3):505-8.

CHAPTER 36

Dengue in Intensive Care Unit

Madiha Hashmi

INTRODUCTION

Dengue is a mosquito-borne viral disease. The number of reported dengue cases have risen dramatically and more than half of the world's population is currently at risk of developing dengue. The worst hit regions are the Americas, South-East Asia and Western Pacific.[2] More than 500,000 people with severe dengue are admitted to hospitals each year in the endemic regions and about 2.5% of those affected die.[3] As most of the developing countries do not have the infrastructure or the commitment to collect data, and the WHO classification of dengue lacks universal adoption,[4] there is a high probability that actual number of people inflicted with the dengue disease is even higher and severity of disease is not reported accurately. Unplanned urbanization, inadequate vector control services in affected areas and poor monitoring of climatic conditions like rainfall and humidity encourages spread of infection in developing countries.[3]

TRANSMISSION

The virus: Dengue virus (DEN), from the genus *Flavivirus*, and family *Flaviviridae* is known to have four serotypes (DEN-1, DEN-2, DEN-3 and DEN-4).[2] Infection caused by one serotype confers lifelong immunity against that serotype but cross-immunity to the other serotypes is not complete.[3,5] Subsequent infection by other serotypes increases the risk of developing *severe* dengue.[3] DENV-5 discovered in 2013 is a sylvatic strains unlike the previously known serotypes that follow the human cycle and it is feared that discovery of more sylvatic strains in future will impede the Dengue Vaccine Initiative.[6] Each serotype has several genotypes indicating extensive genetic variability.[7] The "Asian" genotypes of DEN-2 and DEN-3 are known to cause severe dengue disease.[8]

The vector: Female Aedes aegypti mosquito acquires the virus when it bites an infected human and becomes the vector to transmit infection to other people.

The humans: The virus circulates in the blood of the person for 2–7 days before causing fever. This infected human becomes the source of the dengue virus for uninfected mosquitoes.

CLASSIFICATION

Dengue is defined by experts[2] as "one disease entity with different clinical presentations and an unpredictable clinical course and outcome". Dengue was initially classified[9] as undifferentiated fever, dengue fever (DF), and dengue hemorrhagic fever (DHF). Severity of DHF was graded (I–IV) and grades III and IV were grouped as dengue shock syndrome (DSS). There was a need to revise this classification because dengue disease has become more common in adults rather than children and many cases of severe DHF do not fulfill all the given criteria thus making it difficult for clinicians to categorize dengue cases accurately.[4] The new classification suggested by a Geneva based group[2] is more practical and makes the initial triage

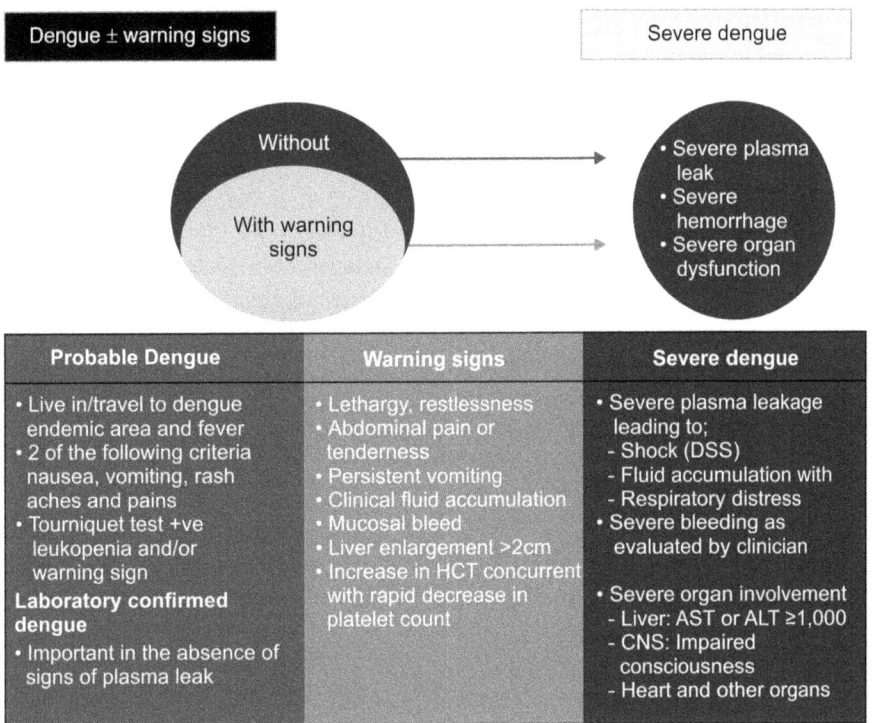

FIGURE 36.1: Classification of dengue. (DSS: dengue shock syndrome; HCT: hematocrit)
Source: Adapted from WHO. (2009). World Health Organization. Guidelines for diagnosis, treatment, prevention and control. Geneva: World Health Organization. [online] Available from http://www.who.int/tdr/publications/training-guideline-publications/dengue-diagnosis-treatment/en/ [Accessed Dec., 2018].

of patients easy by identifying patients that are stable and can be sent home or who may need urgent treatment of life-threatening conditions and close monitoring in the intensive care unit. Universal adoption of this classification will also facilitate consistent reporting of dengue disease for surveillance and research purpose (Fig. 36.1).

Dengue patients without warning signs may progress to severe dengue in a short span of time, a fact that emphasizes the need for vigilant monitoring throughout the course of the disease to improve outcomes.

CLINICAL PRESENTATIONS

Dengue +/- Warning Signs

Asymptomatic seroconversion or minimal symptoms are seen in children and first infections with dengue virus. Patients with moderate to severe disease however progress through three phases (Fig. 36.2).[2]

Febrile Phase

Patients experience sudden onset of high-grade fever, 3–14 days after being bitten by an infected mosquito. This acute febrile phase usually lasts 2–7 days. Classic dengue fever is also known as "break bone fever" as patients experience

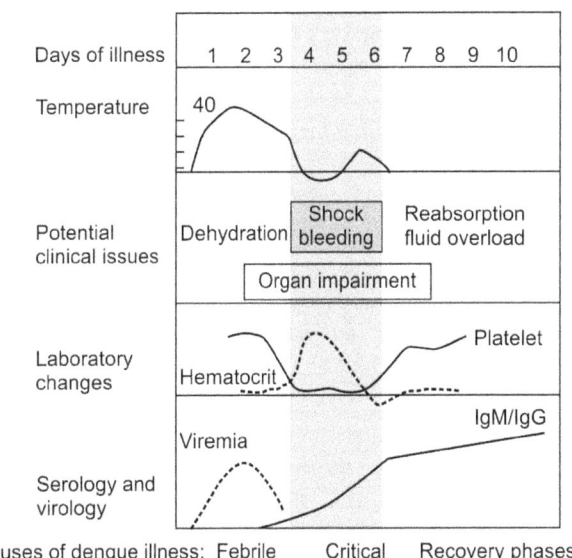

FIGURE 36.2: Clinical course of dengue illness.
Source: Handbook for Clinical Management of dengue @ World Health Organization, 2012.[24]

severe generalized body pain, myalgia, and arthralgia.[10] Facial flushing, skin rash, anorexia, nausea and vomiting are also common. Some patients may present with mucosal membrane bleeding from nose or gums, petechiae and easy bruising.[11] Heavy vaginal bleeding in women of child-bearing age and gastrointestinal bleeding may also occur during this phase although this is not common.[12]

Diagnosis: At this stage it is difficult to diagnose dengue clinically. A *progressive decrease in total white cell count* ($\leq$5,000 cells/mm^3) and a *positive tourniquet test* in this phase are highly suggestive of dengue.[11,13]

At the end of this febrile phase, patients *without* an increase in capillary permeability improve and do not progress to the next phase. However patients *with* increased capillary permeability deteriorate as the fever subsides and manifests the *"warning signs"*. *Monitoring for warning signs is critical in order to recognize progression of disease to the critical phase despite resolution of fever at this stage.*

Critical Phase

The warning signs mark the beginning of the critical phase (Fig. 36.1). This usually coincides with the time of defervescence, i.e. when the temperature goes down and remains below 37.5–38°C.[2] Patients become lethargic but are usually mentally alert. Persistent vomiting and severe abdominal pain are early signs of plasma leakage and get worse if measures are not taken to prevent shock. It is easier to detect fluid accumulation in the chest, abdomen, or gall bladder wall by a portable chest radiograph or ultrasound before clinical signs and symptoms become obvious.

Diagnosis: Following the progressive leukopenia *a sudden fall in platelet count to more than or equal to 100,000 cells/mm^3 and an increase in the hematocrit above the baseline may be the earliest indicators of plasma leakage.*[14] The degree of hemoconcentration above the baseline hematocrit is often directly related to the severity of plasma leakage and is seen before changes in blood pressure and pulse volume.

Cases of dengue with warning signs usually improve if fluid resuscitation is started promptly, but will deteriorate to DSS if the volume of plasma lost through capillary leakage is not replaced adequately.

Recovery Phase

If the patient survives the critical phase that usually lasts 24–48 hours, the fluid lost to the extravascular compartment is reabsorbed and spontaneous diuresis ensues. Gastrointestinal symptoms improve, hemodynamic status stabilizes and patients gradually regain appetite and general vigor. However, if patients receive too much fluid during the febrile or critical phases of illness, worsening pleural effusions, ascites, or pulmonary edema will cause respiratory compromise, complicating the recovery process.

Diagnosis: The hematocrit stabilizes at this stage or the dilutional effect of reabsorbed fluid may lower it. The white blood cell count usually recovers as the fever settles but the recovery of the platelet count usually lags behind.

Severe Dengue

- *Severe plasma leak*: The DSS is a type of hypovolemic shock that results from plasma leakage secondary to increased vascular permeability in patients who receive delayed or inadequate fluid resuscitation. It presents as a physiologic continuum (Fig. 36.3).

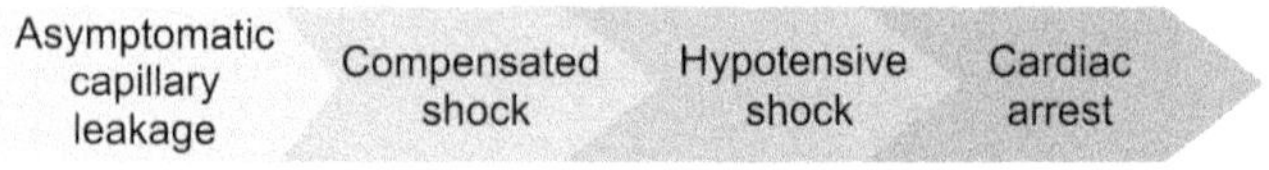

| Asymptomatic capillary leakage | Compensated shock | Hypotensive shock | Cardiac arrest |

FIGURE 36.3: Dengue shock—a physiologic continuum.

- *Compensated shock*: As shock sets in, the compensatory mechanisms maintain a normal systolic blood pressure and may only increase the heart rate and respiratory rate without difficulty in breathing.[15] The increased peripheral vascular resistance raises the diastolic pressure and the difference between the systolic and diastolic pressures known as the pulse pressure narrows. *The hallmarks of compensated shock are: a normal or slightly above normal systolic pressure, narrow pulse pressure ($\leq$20 mm Hg) and signs of poor peripheral perfusion like cold extremities, delayed capillary refill time of more than 2 seconds, and weak peripheral pulses in an alert patient.*
- *Hypotensive or decompensated shock*: When physiologic compensatory mechanisms fail, both systolic and diastolic blood pressures fall. Intense peripheral vasoconstriction leads to cold, clammy and mottled extremities and peripheral pulses disappear. Tachycardia worsens and breathing becomes more rapid and deep indicating onset of metabolic acidosis (Kussmaul's breathing). *A distinguishing feature of this deterioration is an altered mental state as brain perfusion gets compromised* resulting in agitation, confusion, or seizures.

  Long duration of hypotensive shock leads to severe metabolic acidosis, multiple organ failure and a complicated clinical course ending in cardio-respiratory collapse and cardiac arrest.
- *Severe hemorrhage*: The coagulation abnormalities seen in severe dengue are usually not severe enough to cause massive hemorrhage.[16] Severe bleeding is most commonly the consequence of prolong hypotensive shock which, along with thrombocytopenia, hypoxia and metabolic acidosis, leads to multiple organ failure and *disseminated intravascular coagulation*. Massive hemorrhage in the absence of shock is seen in patients who have received acetylsalicylic acid (aspirin), ibuprofen, or corticosteroids

or have a history of peptic or duodenal ulcers.[17] *As DIC sets in the hematocrit decreases and the total white cell count usually increases due to the stress response to massive bleeding.*
- *Multiple organ failure*: Sometimes severe hepatitis, myocarditis, cardiomyopathy, encephalitis[18-20] or severe bleeding develops in dengue disease without obvious plasma leakage or shock though multiple organ failure is more commonly associated with DSS secondary to severe plasma leakage.

LABORATORY DIAGNOSIS

High index of suspicion of dengue in patients from the endemic areas is required for clinical diagnosis of dengue but laboratory confirmation is indicated to confirm the diagnosis, in atypical disease presentation, or to provide information for epidemiological surveillance.[2,21]
- *Isolating the virus or its products*: An acute-phase serum specimen collected *within 5 days of symptom onset* is required to isolate the virus or detect DENV-RNA in the serum by serotype-specific, real-time reverse transcriptase polymerase chain reaction (RT-PCR). Enzyme-linked immunosorbent assay (ELISA) and other commercial kits are also available to detect nonstructural protein 1 (NS1-Ag) in the acute phase of dengue disease.[2]
- *Detecting dengue-specific antibodies*: A convalescent-phase serum specimen collected at *least 6 days after the onset of symptoms* is required to detect IgM antibodies to dengue using an IgM antibody-capture enzyme-linked immunosorbent assay (MAC-ELISA). *Primary infections are characterized by high levels of IgM and low levels of IgG, whereas secondary infections are characterized by low levels of IgM and high levels of IgG*[22] *(Fig. 36.4)*.

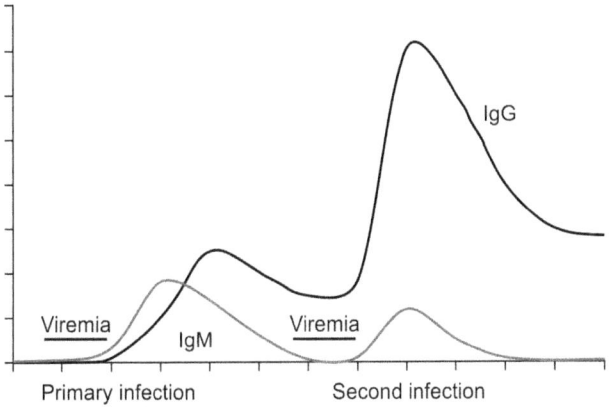

FIGURE 36.4: Virological and serological markers of dengue infection according to time of illness.
Source: Handbook for Clinical Management of dengue @ World Health Organization, 2012.[24]

MANAGEMENT

There is no specific antiviral treatment for dengue disease.[23] Appropriate management of dengue rests on two important decisions made by the frontline clinicians, whether they are general physicians, emergency medicine physicians, or intensivists. Firstly to determine the phase of dengue disease (febrile, critical or recovery), and/or recognize the presence of warning signs based on clinical assessment and simple laboratory tests like white blood cell count and hematocrit. Secondly where and how intensively the patients should be monitored.[2]

Group A: Patients can be sent home and monitored on outpatient basis, if their oral fluid intake is adequate, they are passing urine at least once every 6 hours and do not show any of the "warning signs of dengue".

Group B: If patients show warning signs or have major comorbidities they should be admitted to the hospital for close observation and intravenous hydration.

Group C: Patients with severe dengue should be admitted to an intensive care unit on urgent basis. The unit should have access to blood bank to manage severe hemorrhage, and adequate facilities to manage shock, respiratory distress, or severe organ impairment.

World Health Organization has published comprehensive guidelines for diagnosis, prevention and control of dengue and management algorithms.[2,24] Some important points for the intensivist are highlighted below.

Antipyretics and Analgesics

Paracetamol (acetaminophen) is the drug of choice to treat pain and fever. Aspirin and nonsteroidal anti-inflammatory medications should be avoided as they may exacerbate the bleeding tendency in dengue patients.

Fluid Therapy

Volume resuscitation is the cornerstone of treatment of plasma leak, the pathognomonic feature of dengue.[10,25] *Fluid replacement should be primarily guided by hematocrit* and should be reduced or discontinued when:
- Hematocrit starts decreasing (Box 36.1)
- Urine output is more than or equal to 0.5 mL/kg/hour
- Hemodynamic stability is achieved indicated by decreasing tachycardia, increasing systolic BP, warm extremities, and capillary refill time of less than or equal to 2 seconds.
- Normothermia for more than 24–48 hours without antipyretics

BOX 36.1: Interpretation of hematocrit.[2]

> *Interpretation of hematocrit:*
> - *A rising or persistently high hematocrit together with unstable vital signs* (such as narrowed pulse, tachycardia, metabolic acidosis and poor urine output) indicates active plasma leakage and the need for continuing fluid replacement.
> - *A rising or persistently high hematocrit together with stable hemodynamic status and adequate urine output* indicates that plasma leakage has stopped and intravenous fluid should be withheld. Hematocrit usually starts to fall within 24 hours.
> - *A decrease in hematocrit* (for example, from 50% to 40% or below the patient's known baseline) together with unstable vital signs may indicate major hemorrhage and need for urgent blood transfusion. Concealed bleeding may take several hours to become apparent and the patient's hematocrit will continue to decrease without achieving hemodynamic stability.
> - *A decrease in hematocrit together with stable hemodynamic status and adequate urine output* indicates hemodilution and/or reabsorption of extravasated fluids. Intravenous fluids must be discontinued immediately to avoid pulmonary edema.

Source: Adapted from WHO Guidelines 2009.[2]

- Gastrointestinal symptoms resolve
- Conscious level improves
- Metabolic acidosis resolves indicated by arterial blood gas analysis and/or serum lactate measurements if available.

Isotonic solutions are preferred but the choice of fluid to use in dengue shock is still controversial.[26,27] Colloids should not be used in patients with compensated shock[23] but may be indicated if hematocrit continues to drop in a hemodynamically unstable patient who has no obvious signs of bleeding or if bleeding is obvious but blood is not readily available.

Width of the pulse pressure at presentation predicts the clinical response to resuscitation in dengue shock. Children with a pulse pressure of less than 10 mm Hg and adults with a pulse pressure less than 20 mm Hg on admission are more likely to have prolonged shock than those presenting with higher pulse pressures.[26]

Management of Severe Bleeding

Transfusion of platelets and fresh frozen plasma in dengue does not maintain the platelet numbers and coagulation profile and therefore should be avoided in hemodynamically stable patients with no evidence of active bleeding.[28,29] However, transfusions of platelets and fresh frozen plasma is indicated in the presence of risk factors like uncontrolled hypertension, recent stroke, recent head injury or surgery, anticoagulant treatment, or in anticipation of bleeding in obstetrical deliveries or other surgeries.

Timely blood transfusion can save lives but unnecessary blood transfusions can lead to fluid overload and the rise in hematocrit after transfusion may be misinterpreted as hemoconcentration and severe plasma leakage. Use of H-2 blockers and proton pump inhibitors in gastrointestinal bleeding is of unproven benefit. Nasogastric tube and bladder catheters should be inserted carefully, especially central venous cannulation should be done by experienced physicians and under ultrasound guidance.

Glucose Control

Neuroendocrine stress response causes hyperglycemia in addition to diabetes mellitus or glucose-fluids administered during resuscitation. The increased urine output due to osmotic diuresis caused by hyperglycemia may be misinterpreted as adequate urine output and may also worsen the hypovolemia. Intravenous insulin therapy is preferred to control hyperglycemia as absorption of subcutaneous insulin will be unreliable in the shock state. Hypoglycemia may result from starvation in children, oral hypoglycemic agents in diabetic patients and severe liver failure leading to seizures, mental confusion and unexplained tachycardia. Hypoglycemia should be managed with a bolus of 0.1–0.5 g/kg of glucose, rather than with a glucose-containing maintenance fluid.2

Electrolyte and Acid-base Imbalances

Hyponatremia and hypokalemia may be present in severe dengue secondary to vomiting and diarrhea. Use of isotonic solutions for resuscitation will prevent and correct hyponatremia and potassium supplements in the parenteral fluids may be required to correct hypokalemia. Hyperkalemia may occur secondary to acute renal injury or severe metabolic acidosis. Adequate fluid replacement is required to reverse both metabolic acidosis and hyperkalemia. Renal replacement therapy is an option to manage life-threatening hyperkalemia not responding to medical treatment. Massive transfusion can cause hypocalcemia that should be corrected.

Use of Adjuvants

Corticosteroids and intravenous immunoglobulins are not recommended in the treatment of DSS.[2]

Vasopressor and Inotropic Therapy

Hypovolemia secondary to plasma leakage and/or massive hemorrhage is responsible for dengue shock and appropriate fluid replacement is the first-line of treatment.

However, vasopressors and inotropic agents are indicated in the following situations:
- As a temporary measure to prevent life-threatening hypotension while correction of intravascular volume depletion is in progress, maintaining the mean arterial BP ≥ 65 mm Hg in adults.
- In cardiogenic shock secondary to myocarditis or ischemic heart disease.
- Concomitant septic shock.

Surviving sepsis campaign guidelines[30] should be followed to manage septic shock, although blood transfusion may be warranted at a higher hematocrit than the target hematocrit of less than 30% recommended by SSC guidelines.

Acute Respiratory Distress and Failure

Acute respiratory insufficiency in severe dengue may be the consequence of:
- Severe metabolic acidosis resulting from dengue shock
- Fluid overload leading to large pleural effusions and free fluid in the abdomen
- Acute pulmonary edema
- Acute respiratory distress syndrome (ARDS).

Awake, cooperative and hemodynamically stable patients with mild metabolic acidosis can be given a short trial of noninvasive ventilation (NIV) if hypoxemia does not respond to oxygen supplementation.[31] Invasive mechanical ventilation is indicated if the patient fails the NIV trial, becomes restless, combative or confused or when hypoxemia is accompanied by shock. If the plasma leakage phase has ended and the patient is hemodynamically status, diuretic therapy can be commenced cautiously along with discontinuing intravenous fluid therapy.

IMMUNIZATION

First dengue vaccine, dengvaxia (CYD-TDV), was introduced in 2015. WHO recommends to use dengue vaccine only if epidemiological data from the country indicates a high burden of disease.[32]

DENGUE IN THE ELDERLY

About 10% of elderly dengue patients do not present with fever,[33] therefore it is very important to search for other signs, symptoms and laboratory abnormalities associated with plasma leakage and hemorrhage in this group of patients if coming from dengue-endemic areas. Elderly patients are at an increased risk of gastrointestinal bleeding, acute renal failure, and pleural effusion. Risk of progression to severe dengue and a higher death rate is also reported in the elderly.[34]

DENGUE IN PREGNANCY

High index of suspicion is required to diagnose dengue during pregnancy as the pathognomonic features of the disease may be masked by the physiological changes of pregnancy (increased hematocrit, thrombocytopenia, and leukopenia) or the clinical and laboratory features may point toward more common conditions associated with pregnancy, i.e. eclampsia, hemolysis elevated liver enzymes and low platelet count (HELLP) syndrome, pulmonary embolism, and obstetric causes of vaginal bleeding. Dengue serology should be part of the workup of unexplained fever in pregnancy in the endemic areas.[35]

Dengue in pregnancy may be responsible for adverse outcomes such as preterm birth, low-birth weight and cesarean deliveries, along with the risk of vertical transmission.[36] Severe bleeding may complicate delivery therefore surgical intervention in patients with suspected severe dengue should be carefully planned, and timely referral to healthcare centers equipped with intensive care units and transfusion facilities may prove life-saving.

REFERENCES

1. Brady OJ, Gething PW, Bhatt S, et al. Refining the global spatial limits of dengue virus transmission by evidence-based consensus. PLoS Negl Trop Dis. 2012;6:e1760.
2. WHO. (2009). World Health Organization. Guidelines for diagnosis, treatment, prevention and control. Geneva: World Health Organization. [online] Available from http://www.who.int/tdr/publications/training-guideline-publications/dengue-diagnosis-treatment/en/ [Accessed Dec., 2018].
3. WHO. (2018). Dengue and severe Dengue. [online] Available from http://www.who.int/news-room/fact-sheets/detail/dengue-and-severe-dengue [Accessed Dec., 2018].
4. Bandyopadhyay S, Lum LC, Kroeger A. Classifying dengue: a review of the difficulties in using the WHO case classification for dengue haemorrhagic fever. Trop Med Intern Health. 2006;11(8):1238-55.
5. Halstead SB. Etiologies of the experimental dengues of Siler and Simmons. Am J Trop Med Hyg. 1974;23:974-82.
6. Mustafa MS, Rasotgi V, Jain S, et al. Discovery of fifth serotype of dengue virus (DENV-5): A new public health dilemma in dengue control. Med J Armed Forces India. 2015;71(1):67-70.
7. Leitmeyer KC. Dengue virus structural differences that correlate with pathogenesis. J Virol. 1999;73(6):4738-47.
8. Messer WB. Emergence and global spread of a dengue serotype 3, subtype III virus. Emerg Infect Dis. 2003;9(7):800-9.
9. WHO. (1997). World Health Organization. Dengue haemorrhagic fever: Diagnosis, treatment, prevention and control. Geneva: World Health Organization.
10. Rigau-Pérez JG, Clark GG, Gubler DJ, et al. Dengue and dengue haemorrhagic fever. Lancet. 1998;352:971-7.
11. Kalayanarooj S, Vaughn DW, Nimmannitya S, et al. Early clinical and laboratory indicators of acute dengue illness. J Infect Dis. 1997;176:313-21.

12. Balmaseda A, Hammond SN, Pérez MA, et al. Assessment of the World Health Organization scheme for classification of dengue severity in Nicaragua. Am J Trop Med Hyg. 2005;73:1059-62.
13. Cao XT, Ngo TN, Wills B, et al. Evaluation of the World Health Organization standard tourniquet test in the diagnosis of dengue infection in Vietnam. Trop Med Int Health. 2002;7:125-32, 5.
14. Srikiatkhachorn A, Krautrachue A, Ratanaprakarn W, et al. Natural history of plasma leakage in dengue hemorrhagic fever: a serial ultrasonic study. Pediat Infect Dis J. 2007;26(4):283-90.
15. Pediatric Advanced Life Support (PALS) Provider Manual, Dallas, American Heart Association, 2006.
16. Wills BA, Oragui EE, Stephens AC, et al. Coagulation abnormalities in dengue hemorrhagic fever: Serial investigations in 167 Vietnamese children with dengue shock syndrome. Clin Infect Dis. 2002;35:277-85.
17. Chiu YC, Wu KL, Kuo CH, et al. Endoscopic findings and management of dengue patients with upper gastrointestinal bleeding. Am J Trop Med Hyg. 2005;73(2):441-4.
18. Martinez-Torres E, Polanco-Anaya AC, Pleites-Sandoval EB. Why and how children with dengue die? Revistacubana de Medicina Tropical. 2008;60(1):40-7. 10.
19. Miagostovich MP, Ramos RG, Nicol AF. Retrospective study on dengue fatal cases. Clin Neuropathol. 1997;16:204-8. 24.
20. Solomon T. Neurological manifestations of dengue infection. Lancet. 2000;355:1053-105.
21. Shu PY, Huang JH. Current advances in dengue diagnosis. Clin Diagn Lab Immunol. 2004;11(4):642-50.
22. Vazquez S, Pérez AB, Ruiz D, et al. Serological markers during dengue 3 primary and secondary infections. J Clin Virol. 2005;33(2):132-7.
23. Dondorp AM, Nguyen M, Hoang T, et al. Recommendations for the management of severe malaria and severe dengue in resource-limited settings. Intensive Care Med. 2017;43:1683-5.
24. WHO. (2012). Handbook for Clinical Management of dengue @ World Health Organization 2012. [online] Available from http://www.wpro.who.int/mvp/documents/handbook_for_clinical_management_of_dengue.pdf [Accessed Dec., 2018].
25. Bhamarapravati N. Pathology of dengue infections. In: Gubler DJ, Kuno G (Eds). Dengue and dengue haemorrhagic fever. Wallingford, UK: CAB International; 1997. pp. 115-32.
26. Ngo NT, Cao XT, Kneen R, et al. Acute management of dengue shock syndrome: a randomized double-blind comparison of 4 intravenous fluid regimens in the first hour. Clin Infect Dis. 2001;32:204-13.
27. Wills BA, Dung NM, Loan HT, et al. Comparison of three fluid solutions for resuscitation in dengue shock syndrome. N Engl J Med. 2005;353:877-89. 7
28. Lum L, Abdel-Latif Mel-A, Goh AY, et al. Preventive transfusion in dengue shock syndrome—is it necessary? J Pediatr. 2003;143:682-4.
29. Lye DC, Lee VJ, Sun Y, et al. Lack of efficacy of prophylactic platelet transfusion for severe thrombocytopaenia in adults with acute uncomplicated dengue infection. Clin Infect Dis. 2009;48:1262-5.
30. Dellinger RP, Levy MM, Rhodes A, et al. Surviving sepsis campaign: International guidelines for management of severe sepsis and septic shock. Criti Care Med. 2008;36:296-327.
31. Cam BV, Tuan DT, Fonsmark L, et al. Randomized comparison of oxygen mask treatment vs. nasal continuous positive airway pressure in dengue shock syndrome with acute respiratory failure. J Trop Pediatr. 2002;48(6):335-9.
32. WHO. (2016). Dengue vaccine: WHO position paper—July 2016, 91, 349-364 No 30 Weekly epidemiological record. [online] Available from https://www.who.int/wer/2016/wer9130/en/ [Accessed Dec., 2018].
33. Lee MS, Hwang KP, Chen TC, et al. Clinical characteristics of dengue and dengue hemorrhagic fever in a medical center of southern Taiwan during the 2002 epidemic. J Microbiol Immunol Infect. 2006;39(2):121-9.
34. Lee IK, Liu JW, Yang KD. Clinical and laboratory characteristics and risk factors for fatality in elderly patients with dengue hemorrhagic fever. Am J Trop Med Hyg. 2008;79(2):149-53.
35. Hashmi M, Zainab G, Khan F. Anticipated and unanticipated complications of severe dengue in a primigravida. Indian J Crit Care Med. 2015;19:678-80.
36. Pouliot SH, Xiong X, Harville E, et al. Maternal dengue and pregnancy outcomes: a systematic review. Obstet Gynecol Surv. 2010;65(2):107-18.

CHAPTER 37

Scrub Typhus

Dhruva Chaudhry, Jaikrit Bhutani, Sanya Chaudhry

INTRODUCTION

Scrub typhus, a zoonotic disease, is an acute febrile illness, caused by an *Orientia tsutsugamushi*. It is vectored accidentally to humans by bites of infected chiggers (larval mites) of infected *Leptotrombidium deliense* mites (Trombiculidae family) which normally feed on rodents.[1] Scrub typhus was first reported from Japan in 1899. The World Health Organization has described it amongst the world's most underdiagnosed diseases requiring inpatient admission.[2] This indicates the need of better understanding of epidemiology, transmission, and diagnosis of this potentially fatal illness, beyond what's already known.

EPIDEMIOLOGY

Asia-Pacific region is well known for scrub typhus endemicity and the "tsutsugamushi triangle." It extends from North Japan and far Eastern Russia in north to northern part of Australia in the South and Pakistan and India in the West (Fig. 37.1). Recently, cases from Central Asia, Middle East, and Africa have also been reported which indicate that the geographic distribution and genetic diversity of *O. tsutsugamushi* need further investigation.

The burden of scrub typhus is more in rural Asia, especially in India. About 20% of febrile hospital admissions are diagnosed to have scrub typhus.[3] The exact prevalence and demographic data of scrub infection in India is not available; however, there is recent resurgence of scrub

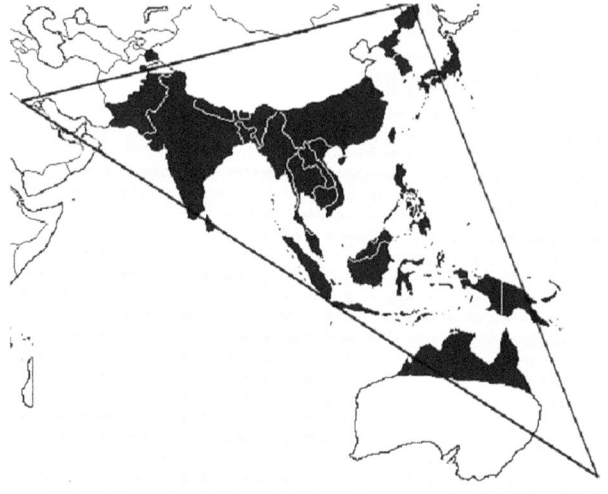

FIGURE 37.1: The tsutsugamushi triangle.

typhus in almost all parts of India unlike the earlier literature which suggested increased prevalence in the foothill areas.[4-7] In India, "postmonsoon spike" in the number of scrub typhus cases has been reported. This is believed to occur due to increased exposure to trombiculid mites during harvesting season as well as the growth of new vegetation, which serves as habitat for this vector.[8]

Despite being most underdiagnosed and under-reported febrile illness, scrub typhus affects one million cases annually, and over one billion people around the world are at risk. The fatality rate of scrub typhus can be as high as 30% if not managed promptly and appropriately.[9]

Section 3: Specific Syndromes

BOX 37.1: Risk factors for developing scrub typhus.[8]

- Low socioeconomic status
- Farmers and field workers
- Age 40–60 years
- July to November months
- Geographic clustering, hilly area inhabitation

Scrub typhus is often missed in routine clinical settings due to atypical clinical features, limited awareness, low index of suspicion, and limited diagnostic modalities. Very often initial presentation of scrub infection closely mimics that of enteric fever. Further, the use of broad-spectrum antibiotics, such as chloramphenicol, earlier as a common treatment for typhoid, and tetracyclines for other infections before specific diagnosis, hindered the accurate detection of scrub infection. This led to the perception, that it is rare in occurrence; however, since the use of beta lactams and fluoroquinolones for the management of typhoid fever, a resurgence of scrub typhus is unmasked.[10]

The risk factors for scrub typhus have been summarized in Box 37.1.

ETIOPATHOGENESIS

Orientia tsutsugamushi is a Gram negative, obligate intracellular bacterium, structurally distinct from other rickettsiae. Lack of cell membrane facilitates its free growth in the cytoplasm of the host eukaryotic cell. The six key serotypes include Karp (which accounts for about 50% of all infections), Kato, Kawasaki, Boryon, Gilliam, and Kuroki. Many new serotypes have also been identified but are still under research.[11] Cross-immunity between different serotypes does not exist. This can cause repeated infection in the same individual and complicates vaccine discovery.[12] The pathophysiology of *O. tsutsugamushi* infection is summarized in Figure 37.2.

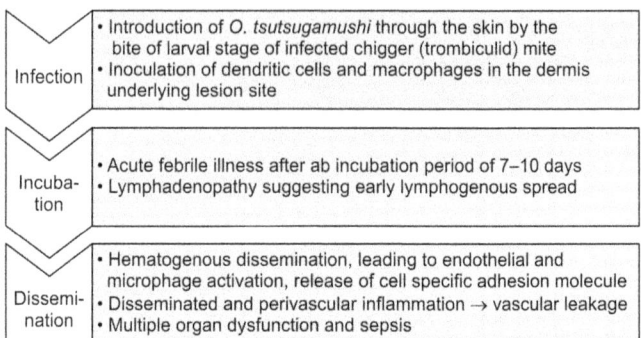

FIGURE 37.2: Pathogenesis of scrub typhus infection.[11]

CLINICAL FEATURES

The clinical manifestations of scrub typhus are myriad and range from mild to severe. Typically, the incubation period of scrub typhus infection ranges from 5–21 days.

Early Manifestations

It starts with localized cutaneous necrosis at the bite site, leading to "eschar" formation. It is often found in areas of groin, genitalia, axilla, and neck.[13] Though characteristic of chigger bite, eschar is only found in only in 50% cases of primary infection, and in very few cases of secondary infection.[14] The "eschar" is visualized easily in Caucasians and East Asians; however, in South Asians and other dark-skinned patients, it is commonly missed on routine examination (Figs. 37.3A to C). This skin lesion is associated with regional lymphadenopathy, followed by development of constitutional symptoms. These include fever, headache, myalgia, generalized lymphadenopathy, cough, gastrointestinal symptoms, rash, transient hearing loss, and conjunctival injection.[15] In a few cases a maculopapular rash may appear after 1 week on trunk and may spread to extremities. Another early but relatively rare clinical sign is hepatosplenomegaly with jaundice.

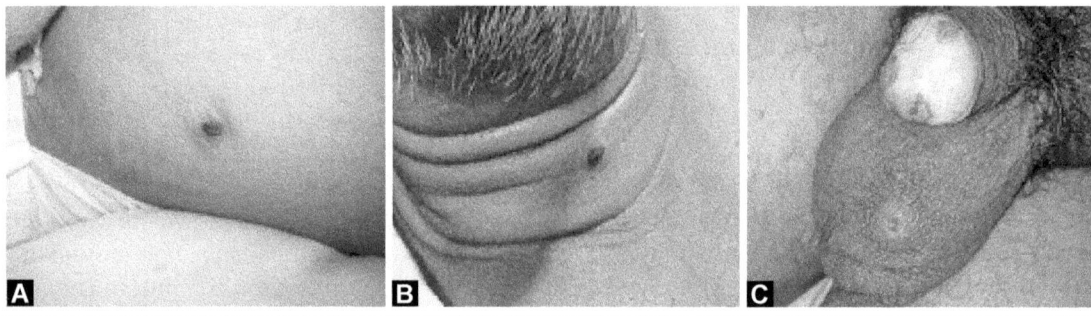

FIGURES 37.3A TO C: Different locations with eschar. (A) Anterior abdominal wall; (B) Neck; (C) Scrotum.

Late Manifestations

The late presentation of scrub typhus is often in the complication phase of disease, which begins after first week of initial febrile illness. The patients who present late often have high morbidity and mortality. The manifestations include atypical interstitial pneumonia, acute respiratory distress syndrome (ARDS), acute kidney injury (AKI), meningoencephalitis, myocarditis, gastrointestinal bleed, jaundice, peripheral gangrene, septic shock, and multiorgan dysfunction syndrome (MODS).[16] The underlying host-determined mechanisms and bacterial virulence responsible for variety of the presentation, such as eschar formation or severe illness, including fatal complications, remain unclear.[17] In severe cases, generalized edema (anasarca) is universal, and its resolution heralds the onset of recovery.

A brief representation of the fever pattern and clinical features is shown in Figure 37.4.

Scrub Typhus Manifestations during Pregnancy[18]

The manifestations of scrub typhus during pregnancy are similar to those in nonpregnant adults; however, a few cases of transplacental and perinatal blood borne spread during labor have been reported.[18] Intrauterine deaths are observed in limited cases, where either infection is fulminant or treatment is delayed.

Intensive Care Unit Manifestations[19]

Majority of patients with scrub typhus infection, who require intensive care unit (ICU) admission, present with one or more complications of this disease. These include complicated pneumonia, ARDS, myocarditis, meningoencephalitis, hepatitis, disseminated intravascular coagulopathy, hemophagocytic syndrome, acute renal shutdown, acute pancreatitis, transient adrenal insufficiency, Guillain-Barre syndrome, polyneuropathy, and transverse myelitis.

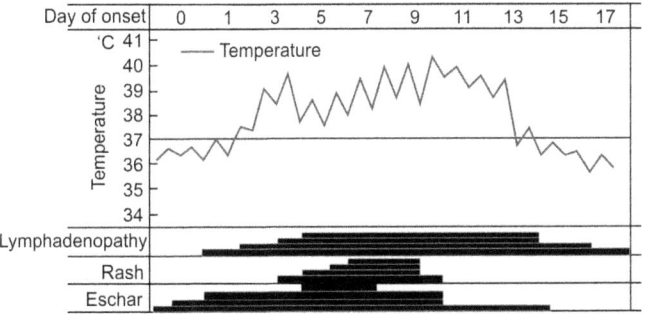

FIGURE 37.4: Natural course of scrub typhus infection.

In addition, MODS associated with sepsis is not uncommon in such patients. In a recent study from India, reporting results from 116 scrub typhus patients admitted in the ICU, 91 patients had dysfunction of three or more organs, and 16 patients (15%) had evidence of dysfunction of six organ systems. Among these patients, 88% required ventilator support, while 11% needed dialysis for AKI. The mortality amongst these patients was 24.1%.[19]

DIAGNOSIS

Early distinction of scrub typhus from other differentials of acute febrile illness is a challenge. Common differentials include other rickettsial infections; viral hemorrhagic fevers, including dengue, leptospirosis, typhoid fever, infectious mononucleosis, malaria; and meningococcal infection. The clinical features of organ dysfunction may vary depending on severity of illness. The exact diagnosis is made by serology and classification of organism by smear or culture depending on the disease.

The key examination finding—"eschar" supports the diagnosis but is found only in few cases. Moreover, other rickettsial diseases may also have eschar formation, and this needs differentiation. Therefore a thorough history, including that of occupation, travel, and insect bite, along with detailed physical examination, with high index of clinical suspicion aids the diagnosis. The monitoring and identification of this disease based purely on clinical examination and history may be challenging, when there is absence of advanced laboratory diagnostic test. Hence, scrub typhus may frequently be missed or misdiagnosed, making it a grave public health issue. Coinfection in patients of scrub typhus with leptospirosis and dengue are reported but are uncommon.[11]

There are a variety of serological tests available for diagnosis of scrub typhus (Box 37.2). The sensitivity and specificity of each test is highly variable as well. These include indirect immunofluorescence assay (IFA), latex agglutination, indirect hemagglutination, indirect immunoperoxidase (IIP) assay, and enzyme-linked immunosorbent assay (ELISA). Due to resource-limited conditions, especially in scrub typhus endemic regions, these tests are available only at select tertiary care centers.

The conventional test for diagnosis of scrub typhus is the Weil-Felix test, which detects cross-reacting antibodies to *Proteus mirabilis* OXK. It is used widely, due to its cost-effectiveness, easy procedure, and prompt results. The antibodies detected by this test, agglutinating immunoglobulin M (IgM) antibodies are detectable in serum of infected patients, as early as 5 days following onset of symptoms. A rising titer greater than four times or a single

BOX 37.2: Serological tests for diagnosis of scrub typhus.

- Indirect immunofluorescence assay
- Latex agglutination test
- Indirect hemagglutination test
- IIP assay
- Enzyme-linked immunosorbent assay

(IIP: Indirect immunoperoxidase)

titer of more than 1:320 to proteus OXK in paired serum is diagnostic of scrub typhus infection. Even though this test lacks sensitivity and specificity, around 50% of patients have a positive test after 14 days of infection.[20] Summary of result of Weil-Felix test in different rickettsial diseases is shown in Table 37.1.

A more sensitive diagnostic test is the IFA which uses fluorescent antihuman antibody to detect specific antibody linked with scrub typhus antigen from patient's serum.[21] IFA has good sensitivity and is currently the gold standard test for the diagnosis of scrub typhus. Limitations of IFA include antigenic variation causing false positivity and high cost. A modification of the standard IFA is the IIP, which incorporates peroxidase in place of fluorescein, eliminating the need of fluorescent microscopy.

A robust alternative in serologic diagnosis of scrub infection is the qualitative ELISA for detection of IgM antibodies against *O. tsutsugamushi*–derived recombinant antigen.[22] The utility of this test is limited by lack of evidence reporting cutoff titers, and it requires further validation.

Recent development of rapid diagnostic tests (RDTs) based on passive red blood cell agglutination method has made bedside quick diagnosis of scrub typhus easier. Two RDT kits are commonly available in the market, supplied by ImmuneMed (ImmuneMed, Rapid ST Immunochromatographic Test), and SD Bioline (SD Bioline Tsutsugamushi Test). They consist of kits with a mixture of cr56, r21, and kr56 of *O. tsutsugamushi* as antigen (0.8 ± 0.08 μg/strip) applied to RDT membrane. These kits detect a complex of antigen–serum antibody–gold conjugated anti-IgM or immunoglobulin G (IgG) against *O. tsutsugamushi*. The ImmuneMed RDT has a superior sensitivity (IgM: 98.6% and IgG: 97.1%) and specificity (IgM: 97.6% and IgG: 97%) as compared to SD Bioline RDT kit (sensitivity IgM: 84.4%, IgG: 85.3%; specificity IgM: 96.3%, IgG: 94.5%).[23] Despite easy procedure and commercial availability, these kits are yet to be validated by guidelines, and for accurate diagnosis of scrub typhus.

The standard cutoffs for all serological tests are yet to be clearly defined in controlled trials. This is due to highly variable sensitivity and specificity of these tests. However, a common consensus is that an equal to or more than fourfold increase in antibodies titer between two consecutive samples is diagnostic of scrub typhus. Literature for diagnosis using single antibody titer is also available, although, the region-specific (scrub typhus endemic and nonendemic) cutoff titer is not yet established. Hence, the clinicians should be aware that results of serological testing are to be interpreted with caution, as serologic diagnosis is only retrospective and cannot guide initial treatment. These tests only corroborate the diagnosis made by clinical history and detailed physical examination.[20]

Polymerase chain reaction (PCR) techniques have also been used for diagnosis of scrub infection. Real-time and nested PCR targeting gene encoding for the 56-kDa antigen of *O. tsutsugamushi* can detect diverse antigenic types of *O. tsutsugamushi*, thus increasing sensitivity and specificity. PCR-based assays are robust at detecting bacteremia irrespective of pre-existing host antibodies in endemic regions thus enable early diagnosis. The sensitivity of a nested PCR assay using buffy coat preparations was 82%, and the specificity was 100% in a study of 135 Korean patients with possible scrub typhus.[24] Similar findings were found in a cohort of Chinese patients using conventional PCR targeting the *16S rRNA* gene.[25] The limitation of these assays is their high cost, and tedious procedure, making them impractical in many areas of scrub endemicity. A confirmatory laboratory diagnosis of scrub typhus could be done with combined antigen or deoxyribonucleic acid and antibody detection testing.

Isolation and culture of *O. tsutsugamushi* are also available but are expensive and require elaborate biosafety level-3 laboratories. Direct immunohistochemical staining of biopsy specimen taken from cutaneous lesions is highly specific and sensitive for diagnosis but is limited by rare presence of such lesions.

A panel of scrub typhus infection, with high diagnostic accuracy, includes following four criteria in Box 37.3.

Table 37.1: Weil-Felix test result in different rickettsial diseases.

Rickettsial disease	OX 19	OX 2	OX K
Epidemic typhus	+++	+	—
Endemic typhus	+++	±	—
Tick-borne spotted fever	++	++	—
Scrub typhus	—	—	++

BOX 37.3: Scrub typhus diagnostic panel.[11]

1. Cell culture isolates
2. Single IgM titer >1:12,800 using IFA
3. Rising IgM IFA titer by four times
4. Positive PCR assay for Orientia tsutsugamushi

The presence of one or more of above criteria indicates high likelihood of scrub typhus infection

(IFA: indirect fluorescent antibody; IgM: immunoglobulin M; PCR: polymerase chain reaction)

Frequently, scrub typhus presents as a systemic illness, involving almost every organ of the body. The findings consistent with scrub infection on investigations, such as hematology, biochemistry, and radiology, have been summarized in Table 37.2 and Figures 37.5 and 37.6.

TREATMENT

The guidelines for appropriate choice of antimicrobial drug and optimal duration of therapy in treatment of scrub typhus are yet to be established, due to lack of clinical trial data. The initiation of treatment should be done as early as possible, based on a presumptive diagnosis. This facilitates meticulous management, with fewer complications, leading to reduction in both morbidity and mortality.

The current drug of choice for treatment is doxycycline 100 mg orally or intravenously twice daily. Chloramphenicol was the first drug to be used for treatment of scrub infection, and is still currently used as an alternative in endemic regions, in doses of 250 to 500 mg orally or intravenously every 6 hours. Most trials comparing the efficacy of doxycycline and chloramphenicol, in terms of time to resolution of fever and incidence of relapse, reported no significant differences between these two drugs.[26] However, these studies had a major limitation as they did not account for the delays in treatment and outcome. Retrospective review of patients with rickettsial disease (n = 92), including those of scrub typhus (n = 34), reported that delayed initiation of doxycycline therapy was independently related with development of systemic complications, including major organ dysfunction [odds ratio (OR) 1.2; confidence interval (CI) 1.0–1.5] and hospitalization >10 days (OR 1.4; CI 1.1–1.9).[15] The appropriate duration of treatment varies from as short as 1 day of doxycycline (400 mg given in two divided doses) to 3 days, up to a maximum of 14 days of doxycycline (200 mg daily). A meta-analysis from Asia comparing efficacy of different antibiotic regimens concluded that treatment with doxycycline resulted in early resolution of symptoms; however, it was associated with more adverse drug reactions, when compared with regimens using azithromycin and chloramphenicol.[27]

Table 37.2: Adjunctive investigations in diagnosis of scrub typhus.[11]

Investigation	Findings
Hemogram	Leukocytosis, thrombocytopenia
Liver function tests	Transaminitis (75–95%), hyperbilirubinemia, raised ALP, hypoalbuminemia
Renal function tests	Elevated serum creatinine and abnormal urinary sediments
Chest skiagram	Unilateral reticulonodular opacities, pleural effusion, hilar lymphadenopathy, unilateral or bilateral nonhomogenous opacities
CT scan chest	Axial interstitial and interlobular septal thickening, centrilobular nodules, ground-glass opacities, mediastinal and hilar lymphadenopathy, and pleural effusion
CT scan abdomen	Splenomegaly with splenic infarct, gallbladder thickening, hepatomegaly, lymphadenopathy, ascites
CT scan head	Periventricular and callosal white matter lesions
MRI brain	Periventricular hyperintensities and ring-enhancing lesions, small cerebral hemorrhages and infarcts
Ultrasound abdomen	Splenomegaly, ascites, and lymphadenopathy
CSF	Lymphocytic pleocytosis, elevated proteins, normal/low sugar and ADA levels less than 10 U/L
Electrocardiogram	Nonspecific ST and T wave changes, tachy- and bradyarrhythmias, and variable degrees of heart block

(ADA: adenosine deaminase; ALP: alkaline phosphatase; CSF: cerebrospinal fluid; CT: computed tomography; MRI: magnetic resonance imaging)

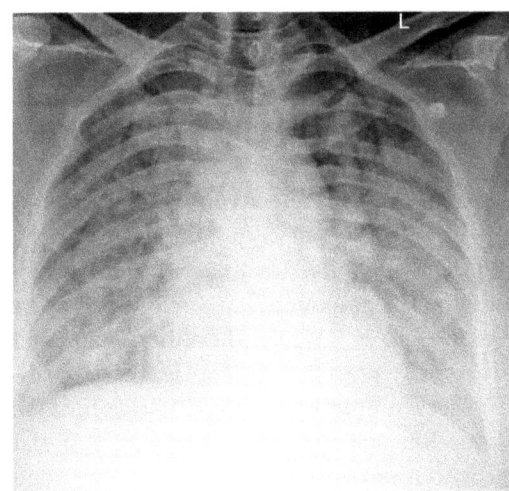

FIGURE 37.5: Chest skiagram showing findings of ARDS. (ARDS: acute respiratory distress syndrome)

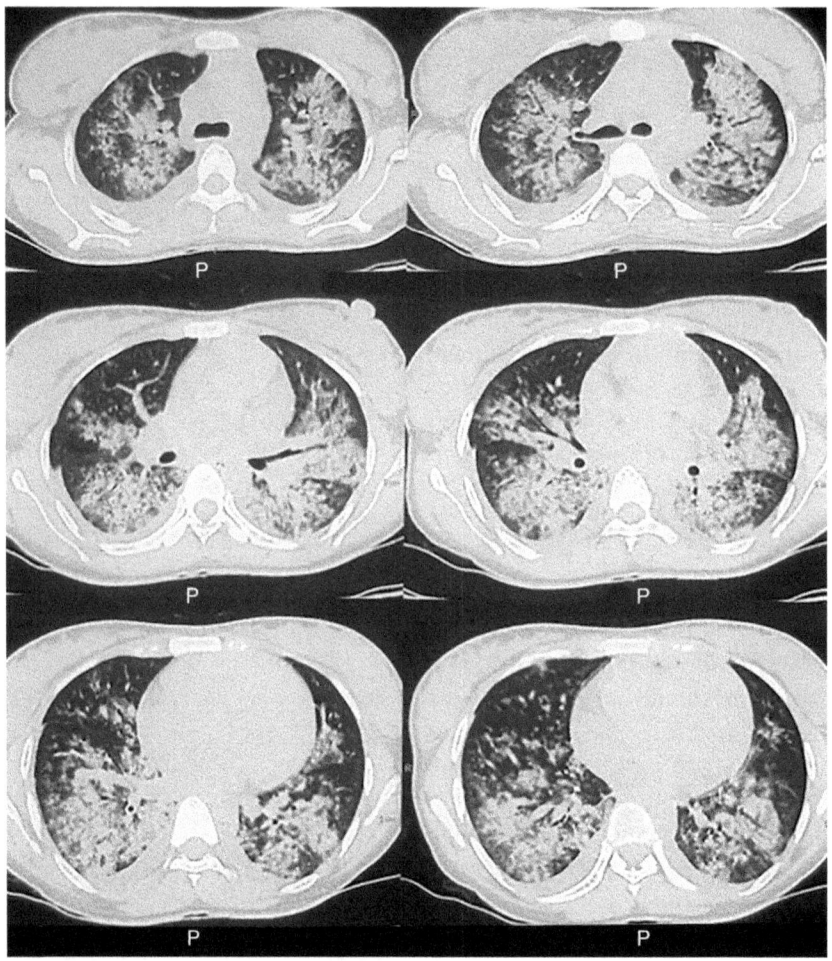

FIGURE 37.6: Images from CT scan chest showing consolidation and ground-glass opacities. (CT: computed tomography)

The data on use of broad-spectrum antibiotics for the treatment of scrub infection is limited. A Cochrane review concluded that use of rifampicin is indicated only in scrub endemic areas, where resistance to doxycycline is suspected. However, more trials are needed to establish the optimal duration of treatment and regimens for treatment of severe infection in endemic areas.[26]

The management of scrub typhus of patients requiring admission in the ICU needs to be more aggressive than other patients diagnosed with scrub infection. As per the guidelines issued by Indian Society of Critical Care Medicine, in all cases of MODS where there is no localization of source, scrub typhus must be considered while deciding choice of treatment. Therefore it is recommended to add doxycycline 200 mg to ceftriaxone as an initial dose, followed by 100 mg bis in daily dose. Defervescence of fever usually takes place within 72 hours of initiation of therapy, and in case it does not settle, an alternate diagnosis must be considered. Along with this, patients are to be observed for encephalopathy, bleeding, seizures, and ARDS. Renal replacement therapy with intermittent hemodialysis or continuous renal replacement therapy may be indicated in the setting of AKI. Specific therapy is initiated once diagnosis is established.[28]

In scrub typhus associated with pregnancy, azithromycin has been shown to be effective. The dose used commonly is 500 mg once daily, and duration of therapy varies from 3 days to 5 days.[18] Early treatment initiation is beneficial in avoiding poor neonatal outcome, defined as stillbirths, preterm birth, or low birth weight and poor maternal outcome as well. Doxycycline (class D) and chloramphenicol (class C) are contraindicated in pregnancy.

PREVENTION

At present, there is no vaccine available for the prevention of scrub typhus. Further, the future research on vaccine development is limited by antigenic heterogeneity of *O. tsutsugamushi*.[12] Thus the only two methods to prevent scrub infection include chemoprophylaxis and mite control.

Chemoprophylaxis is recommended only in individuals from scrub endemic areas. Effective prophylactic therapy includes oral chloramphenicol or tetracycline given once every 5 days for 35 days, or doxycycline 200 mg weekly.[29]

Another effective prophylactic method is mite control. Primarily individuals can begin by avoiding mite-infested areas and should adequately cover lower limbs while entering these areas. Washing exposed sites with soap and water may help remove both attached and unattached chiggers.

Insect repellants, such as *N,N*-diethyl-3-methylbenzamide, permethrin, and benzyl benzoate, are highly effective when applied to both clothing and skin. Endemic and focal areas are treated with chlorinated hydrocarbons, such as lindane, dieldrin, or chlordane, to limit mite spread, although they may cause secondary environmental problems. A paradoxical phenomenon of increased human disease may occur with intensive mite control, as this causes chiggers to lose their preferred and conventional hosts, and instead bite humans.[29]

CONCLUSION

Scrub typhus is an important differential of acute undifferentiated febrile illness with fatal complications, including MODS, ARDS, and sepsis. Due to its geographic variability and resurgence, atypical clinical presentation, limited awareness, low index of clinical suspicion, and limited diagnostic tests, more so in the Indian subcontinent, it is one of most under reported and under-diagnosed conditions. Early clinical recognition with detailed history and physical examination as well as concurrent laboratory testing of this disease may be vital to avert the complications, and thus significantly reduce the associated morbidity and mortality.

REFERENCES

1. Raoult D. 335—Rickettsial infections. In: Goldman L, Schafer AI (Eds). Goldman's cecil medicine, 24th edition. Philadelphia, PA: W.B. Saunders; 2012. pp. 1954-64.
2. World Health Organization. Department of Communicable Diseases. Surveillance and response. In: WHO recommended surveillance standards (vol. 2). Geneva: World Health Organization; 1999.
3. Brown GW, Robinson DM, Huxsoll DL, et al. Scrub typhus: a common cause of illness in indigenous populations. Trans R Soc Trop Med Hyg. 1976;70:444-8.
4. Mahajan SK, Rolain JM, Kashyap R, et al. Scrub typhus in Himalayas. Emerg Infect Dis. 2006;12;1590-2.
5. Varghese GM, Abraham DC, Mathai D, et al. Scrub typhus among hospitalized patients with febrile illness in south India: magnitude and clinical predictors. J Infect. 2006;52:56-60.
6. Mittal V, Gupta N, Battacharya D, et al. Serological evidence of rickettsial infection in Delhi. Indian J Med Res. 2012;135:538-41.
7. Subhalakshmi MV, Madisetty MK, Prasad AK, et al. Outbreak of scrub typhus in Andhra Pradesh—experience at a tertiary care hospital. J Assoc Physician India. 2014;82:490-6.
8. Narvencar KP, Rodrigues S, Nevrekar RP, et al. Scrub typhus in patients reporting with acute febrile illness at a tertiary health care institution in Goa. Indian J Med Res. 2012;136:1020-4.
9. Xu G, Walker DH, Jupiter D, et al. A review of the global epidemiology of scrub typhus. PLoS Negl Trop Dis. 2017;11:e0006062.
10. Chaudhry D, Goyal S. Scrub typhus-resurgence of a forgotten killer. Indian J Anaesth. 2013;57:135-6.
11. Thakur SK, Mahajan SK. Scrub typhus. In: Bhalla A (Ed). Update on tropical fevers. Mumbai: Association of Physicians of India; 2015. pp. 126-35.
12. Kelly DJ, Fuerst PA, Ching WM, et al. Scrub typhus: the geographic distribution of phenotypic and genotypic variants of *Orientia tsutsugamushi*. Clin Infect Dis. 2009;48(Suppl 3):S203-30.
13. Kim DM, Won KJ, Park CY, et al. Distribution of eschars on the body of scrub typhus patients. A prospective study. Am J Trop Med Hyg. 2007;76:806-9.
14. Watt G. Scrub typhus. In: Warrell DA, Cox TM, Firth JD (Eds). Oxford, textbook of medicine, 5th edition. USA: Oxford University Press. 2010. pp. 919-24.
15. Lee N, Ip M, Wong B, et al. Risk factors associated with life threatening rickettsial infections. Am J Trop Med Hyg. 2008;78:973-8.
16. Cowan GO. Rickettsial infections. In: Gordon C (Ed). Manson's tropical diseases, vol. 50, 21st edition. London Saunders Elsevier Science, Health Sciences Division: London, UK; 2003. pp. 891-906.
17. Paris DH, Shelite TR, Day NP, et al. Unresolved problems related to scrub typhus: a seriously neglected life threatening disease. Am J Trop Med Hyg. 2013;89:301-7.
18. Kim SY, Lee JH, Chang YM, et al. Scrub typhus during pregnancy and its treatment: a case series and review of literature. Am J Trop Med Hyg. 2006;75:955-59.
19. Griffith M, Peter JV, Karthik G, et al. Profile of organ dysfunction and predictors of mortality in severe scrub typhus infection requiring intensive care admission. Indian J Crit Care Med. 2014;18:497-502.
20. Koh GC Maude RJ, Paris DH, et al. Diagnosis of scrub typhus. Am J Trop Med Hyg. 2010;82:368-70.
21. Blacksell SD, Bryant NJ, Paris DH. Scrub typhus serological testing with indirect immunofluorescence method as a diagnostic gold standard: a lack of consensus leads to a lot of confusion. Clin Infect Dis. 2007;44:391-401.
22. Inbios International, Inc. Scrub typhus Detect IgM ELISA system. [online] Available from www.Inbios.com.
23. Kim YJ, Park S, Premaratna R, et al. Clinical evaluation of rapid diagnostic test kit for scrub typhus with improved performance. J Korean Med Sci. 2016;31:1190-6.

24. Kim DM, Yun NR, Yang TY, et al. Usefulness of nested PCR for the diagnosis of scrub typhus in clinical practice: a prospective study. Am J Trop Med Hyg. 2006;75:542.
25. Kim CM, Cho MK, Kim DM, et al. Accuracy of conventional PCR targeting the 16S rRNA gene with the Ot-16sRF1 and Ot-16sRR1 primers for diagnosis of scrub typhus: a case-control study. J Clin Microbiol. 2016;54:178.
26. Panpanich R, Garner P. Antibiotics for treating scrub typhus. Cochrane Database Syst Rev. 2000:CD002150.
27. Fang Y, Huang Z, Tu C, et al. Meta analysis of drug treatment for scrub typhus in Asia. Intern Med. 2012;51:2313-20.
28. Singhi S, Chaudhary D, Varghese GM, et al. Tropical fevers: management guidelines. Indian J Crit Care Med. 2014;18: 62-9.
29. Sexton DJ. Scrub typhus: treatment and prevention. [online] Available from https://www.uptodate.com/contents/scrub-typhus-treatment-and-prevention [last accessed September 15, 2018].

CHAPTER 38

Malaria in the Intensive Care Unit

Niteen D Karnik, Priya Bhate, Nupur N Karnik

INTRODUCTION

Malaria is a protozoal infection of the red blood cells (RBCs) transmitted by the bite of the female anopheline mosquito.[1] Five *Plasmodium* species cause malaria in humans—*P. falciparum, P. vivax, P. ovale, P. malariae,* and *P. knowlesi* (monkey malaria). *P. falciparum, P. vivax,* and *P. knowlesi* can cause life-threatening malaria. Severe malaria has a mortality approaching 100% when untreated and is 10–20% with prompt treatment.[1] The World Health Organization (WHO) estimates that 216 million cases of malaria occurred in 2016, of which 90% occurred in Africa, 7% in Southeast Asia, and 2% in the Eastern Mediterranean region.[2] There were 445,000 deaths due to malaria.[2]

PHYSIOLOGY

Life Cycle of the Parasite[3] (Fig. 38.1)

- Sporozoites are inoculated into the bloodstream by an infected female anopheline mosquito.
- Sporozoites invade hepatocytes within an hour.
- Sporozoites divide to from multinucleated schizonts, each containing many merozoites (exoerythrocytic cycle).
- In *P. vivax* and *P. ovale* infections, some sporozoites develop into dormant hypnozoites that can cause relapse.
- After 6–30 days, hepatic schizonts rupture releasing thousands of merozoites into the blood.

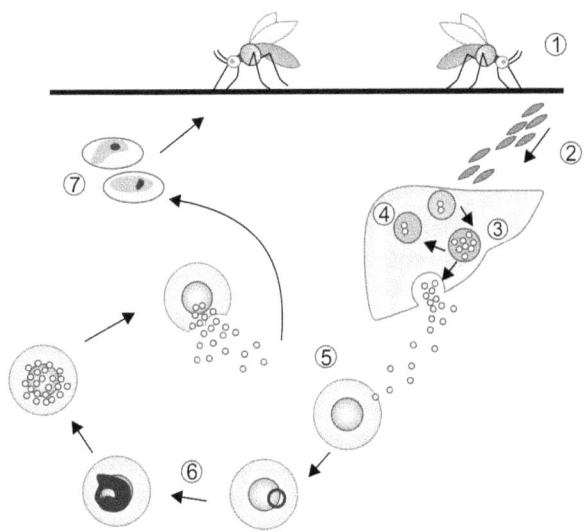

FIGURE 38.1: Life cycle of *Plasmodium*.

- Merozoites invade RBCs and begin the erythrocytic cycle. Merozoites develop into trophozoites and later schizonts. Schizogony occurs in 24 hours (*P. knowlesi*), 48 hours (*P. vivax* and *P. falciparum*), 50 hours (*P. ovale*), or 72 hours (*P. malariae*). Schizonts rupture releasing merozoites into the blood.
- Some merozoites differentiate into gametocytes (sexual forms) which are ingested by mosquitoes during a blood meal. Gametocytes develop into infective sporozoites in the gut of the mosquito and then migrate to the salivary gland.

PATHOGENESIS

Plasmodium falciparum induces the formation of sticky knobs on the surface of RBCs that contain *P. falciparum* erythrocyte membrane protein-1. This protein mediates cytoadherence (attachment of infected RBCs to endothelium).[3] *P. falciparum*-infected RBCs adhere to uninfected RBCs (rosetting) or to other parasitized RBCs (agglutination). Cytoadherence, rosetting, and agglutination cause RBC sequestration and microvascular occlusion.[3] The interaction between endothelium, immune cells, and parasites leads to a cytokine storm causing a systemic inflammatory response (Flowchart 38.1).

Genetic conditions, such as sickle cell trait, hereditary spherocytosis, hemoglobin C and E, thalassemia, pyruvate kinase deficiency, and Duffy negative blood group, confer protection due to reduced parasite invasion and survival in RBCs.[3] Pregnancy is a risk factor for severe malaria.[1] In malaria endemic regions (stable transmission), childhood malaria causes mortality, while multiple subclinical infections lead to immunity in adults. In hypoendemic regions (unstable transmission), severe malaria occurs at all ages.[1]

SEVERE MALARIA

The clinical features of malaria are high-grade fever, chills, and rigors that subside with sweating. If untreated, it progresses to severe malaria which is defined as follows:
- Severe falciparum malaria is defined by the presence of any of the features in Table 38.1, occurring in the absence of an identified alternative cause and presence of *P. falciparum* asexual parasitemia.[1]
- Severe vivax malaria is defined similarly to falciparum malaria but without parasite density thresholds.[1]
- Severe knowlesi malaria is defined similarly to falciparum malaria with[1]
  - *P. knowlesi* hyperparasitemia >100,000/µL
  - Jaundice and parasite density >20,000/µL

Severe malaria causes multiorgan failure. Mortality is low when a single organ fails but increases up to 48.8% with failure of two or more organs.[4]

DIAGNOSIS

Light microscopy and immunochromatographical rapid diagnostic tests (RDTs) can diagnose malaria.[1] Microscopy is the gold standard and detects malaria at a parasite density

FLOWCHART 38.1: Pathogenesis of severe malaria.

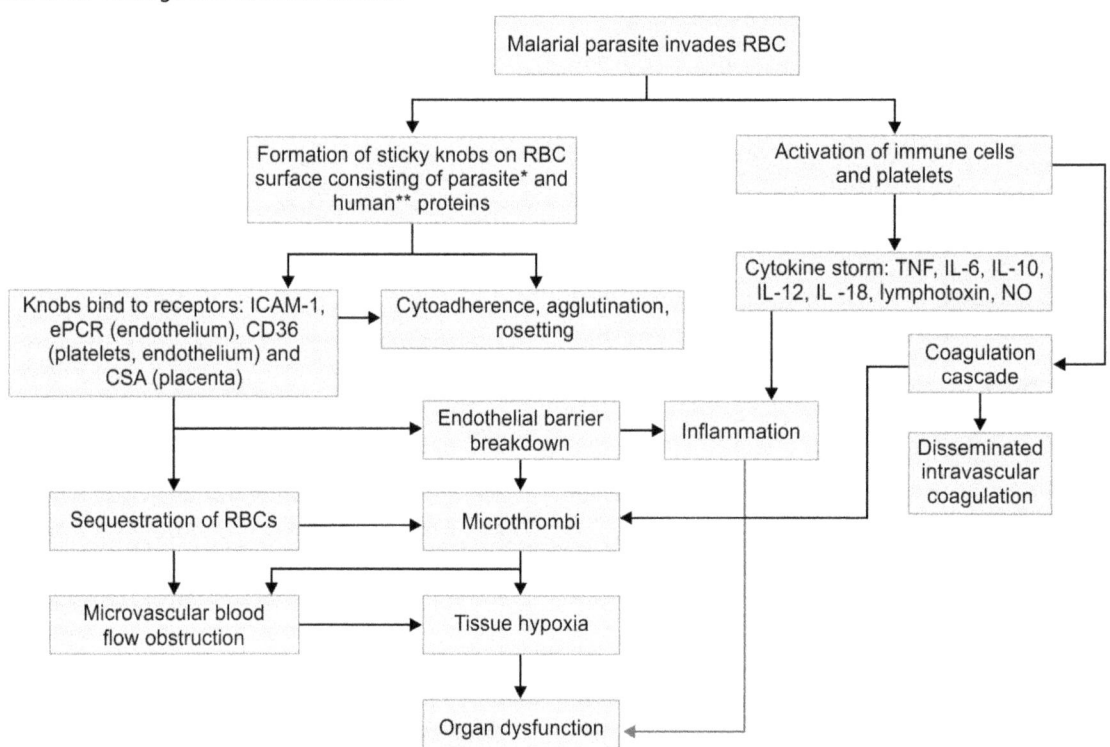

(RBC: red blood cells; CSA: chondroitin sulfate A; PfEMP: *Plasmodium falciparum* erythrocyte membrane protein; ICAM-1: intercellular adhesion molecule 1)
*PfEMP-1, PfEMP-2. **Spectrin, actin, band 4.1.

Table 38.1: World Health Organization criteria (2015) for the diagnosis of severe malaria.[1]

Clinical features	Definition
Impaired consciousness	Glasgow Coma Score <11 in adults or Blantyre Coma Score <3 in children
Prostration	Generalized weakness so that the person is unable to sit, stand, or walk without assistance
Multiple convulsions	>2 episodes in 24 hours
Acidosis	Base deficit of >8 mEq/L, serum bicarbonate >15 mmol/L, or venous plasma lactate ≥5 mmol/L
Hypoglycemia	Blood or plasma glucose <2.2 mmol/L (<40 mg/dL)
Severe malarial anemia	Hemoglobin ≤5 g/dL or hematocrit ≤15% in children less than 12 years of age (<7 g/dL and <20%, respectively, in adults) with a parasite count (number of infected RBCs) >10,000/μL
Renal impairment	Serum creatinine >265 μmol/L or >3 mg/dL or blood urea >20 mmol/L
Jaundice	Serum bilirubin >50 μmol/L or >3 mg/dL with parasite count >100,000/μL
Pulmonary edema	Radiologically confirmed or oxygen saturation <92% on room air with a respiratory rate of >30/min, often with chest indrawing and crepitations on auscultation
Significant bleeding	Includes recurrent or prolonged bleeding from nose, gums, or venepuncture site; hemetemesis or melena
Shock	Compensated shock is capillary refill ≥3 seconds or temperature gradient on leg (mid to proximal limb) but no hypotension. Decompensated shock is defined as systolic blood pressure <70 mm Hg in children and <80 mm Hg in adults with evidence of impaired perfusion (cool peripheries, prolonged capillary refill)
Hyperparasitemia	P. falciparum parasitemia >10%

(RBCs: Red blood cells)

of 50/μL but requires technical skill. Advantages include determining plasmodial species, intraerythrocytic forms, gametocytes, and parasite density. RDTs detect antigens or enzymes that are either genus or species specific. They are rapid, easy and detect malaria at a parasite density of 100/μL. The *P. falciparum*-specific histidine rich protein-2 test detects *P. falciparum* even if blood films are negative due to incomplete antimalarial treatment. RDTs for malarial antigens, such as *P. falciparum*-specific parasite lactate dehydrogenase (Pf-pLDH), pLDH for *P. vivax* and pan *Plasmodium*-specific pLDH (pan-pLDH) are available.[1]

MANAGEMENT

General Principles

Patients with severe malaria rapidly deteriorate. Prompt antimalarial therapy and appropriate supportive management [anticonvulsants, intravenous (IV) glucose and fluids, antipyretics, antibiotics, and blood transfusion] are essential. Neurologic assessment using Blantyre Coma Score (children) or Glasgow Coma Scale (adults) should be done. Vitals, oxygen saturation, capillary refill, and degree of pallor are important clinical parameters. Investigations include full blood count, electrolytes, blood sugars, blood gases, renal function tests, liver function tests, blood grouping, lactate, blood culture, and clotting studies. When not contraindicated, lumbar puncture should be done in patients with altered sensorium to exclude bacterial meningitis. Therapies that are not beneficial include heparin, dexamethasone in cerebral malaria, deferoxamine, aspirin, anti–tumor necrosis factor antibodies, pentoxifylline, prostacyclin, and cyclosporin A.[1]

Antimalarial Treatment: Practice Prescription

Two classes of parenteral drugs are available for severe malaria; artemisinin derivatives (artesunate and artemether) and cinchona alkaloids (quinine and quinidine).[1]

- All adults and children with severe malaria (including infants, lactating and pregnant women in all trimesters) should be treated with parenteral artesunate for at least 24 hours. IV artesunate (2.4 mg/kg body weight in adults and 3 mg/kg body weight in children less than 20 kg) is given at 0, 12, and 24 hours and then once daily. After 24 hours and once oral therapy is tolerated, 3 days of artemisinin-based combination therapy is given. Dose adjustment for renal and hepatic impairment is not needed for artesunate.[1]

Artemisinin-based combination therapy (typical adult dose) available includes:
- Artemether (80 mg) + Lumefantrine (480 mg)
- Artesunate (200 mg) + Amodiaquine (540 mg)
- Artesunate (200 mg) + Mefloquine (440 mg)
- Artesunate (200 mg) + Sulfadoxine-pyrimethamine (1,500/75 mg)
- Dihydroartemisinin + Piperaquine (fixed-dose tablet: 40/320 mg, 36–60 kg: 3 tablets/day, 60–80 kg: 4 tablets/day, >80 kg: 5 tablets/day)

- If IV artesunate is unavailable, intramuscular (IM) artemether (dose: 3.2 mg/kg loading, followed by 1.6 mg/kg daily) is preferred over quinine.[1]
- Quinine was used in the past for severe malaria. The dose (in terms of quinine salt) is IV 20 mg/kg for loading dose, followed by 10 mg/kg IV every 8 hours. If there is no improvement or persistent acute kidney injury (AKI), the dose is reduced after 48 hours to 10 mg/kg every 12 hours. Quinine should be given diluted in 5% dextrose as a slow infusion over 4 hours.[1]

Evidence

In a Prospective randomized controlled trial in African children with the severe falciparum malaria (SEAQUAMAT), 5,425 children (<15 years) with severe falciparum malaria were randomly given parenteral IV artesunate or quinine. There was a 22.5% relative reduction in mortality in the artesunate group (8.5%) as compared to quinine group (10.9%). Coma and convulsions were significantly less in artesunate recipients.[5]

The South East Asian Quinine Artesunate Malaria Trial group studied IV artesunate versus quinine for the treatment of severe falciparum malaria in adult patients of Bangladesh, India, Indonesia, and Myanmar. In this trial, 730 patients received IV artesunate and 731 received IV quinine. Mortality in artesunate recipients was 15% compared with 22% in quinine recipients (absolute risk reduction of 34.7%).[6]

In a systematic review of artesunate for severe malaria, eight randomized control trials (RCTs) in African and Asian countries including 1,664 adults and 5,765 children were analyzed. Compared to quinine, parenteral artesunate reduced mortality by 40% in adults and 25% in children.[7]

Artemether was compared with artesunate and quinine for severe malaria in a systematic review consisting of 18 RCTs. IM artemether was not as effective as IV artesunate in preventing deaths due to malaria in adults. Compared to IV quinine, IM artemether prevented more deaths in adults.[8]

COMPLICATIONS AND MANAGEMENT

Neurological Complications

Cerebral malaria is the most dreaded complication and presents as varying degrees of altered sensorium or seizures. Focal neurological deficits are not common. Cerebral edema and raised ICP (intracranial pressure) are associated with poor prognosis.[9] Neurological outcomes are better in adults but 15% children may develop sequelae, such as visual impairment, spasticity, hemiplegia, and learning disabilities.[10] Hypoglycemia, refractory seizures, and severe anemia are associated with long-term sequelae.[10] Retinal whitening and vessel changes are unique features of cerebral malaria.[11] Retinal hemorrhages, papilledema, and cotton wool spots may be seen. One study showed that malarial retinopathy had a positive predictive value (PPV) of 95% versus a PPV of 77% for parasitemia with exclusion of other causes to diagnose cerebral malaria in any fatal coma.[11] Treatment of fever, seizures, and raised ICP (osmotic therapy and hyperventilation) may be useful.[9] Routine use of anticonvulsants and steroids is not recommended.[12] Postmalaria neurological syndrome is a steroid-responsive rare autoimmune diffuse encephalopathy that presents as confusion, seizures, psychosis, or ataxia within 2 months of acute malaria.[13] Guillain-Barre syndrome is a rare but serious complication[14] which may require mechanical ventilation.

Metabolic Complications

Lactic acidosis occurs due to anaerobic glycolysis as parasitized cells cause microvascular obstruction in tissues, lactate production by the parasite, and impaired lactate metabolism by the liver and kidney.[12] Hypoglycemia is because of impaired hepatic gluconeogenesis and increased glucose consumption by the host and parasite. Hypoglycemia may cause coma and seizures and is common in children, pregnant women, and those receiving quinine.[3]

Hematological Complications

Anemia is caused by increased splenic removal of RBCs, rupture of RBCs due to schizogony and ineffective erythropoeisis.[3] Rapid massive intravascular hemolysis during febrile episodes leads to severe anemia and hemoglobinuria (Blackwater fever).[15] Thrombocytopenia is common. Disseminated intravascular coagulation can occur in severe malaria and carries a grave prognosis.[12] Like other critically ill patients, transfusion is indicated when hemoglobin falls below 7 g/dL.[1] Exchange transfusion may decrease parasitemia by removing infected cells and replacing them with normal cells; however, there is limited evidence supporting it.[1]

Renal Complications

Up to 35% of patients with AKI need early renal replacement therapy.[12] AKI occurs due to:
- Ischemic tubular injury as a result of RBC sequestration in renal microcirculation
- Toxic tubular injury due to intravascular hemolysis and hyperbilirubinemia

- Autoimmune glomerular injury induced by the malarial parasite
- Inflammatory response to malarial antigens or immune complex deposition in glomeruli.[15]

Hepatic and Gastrointestinal Complications

Hemolysis, hepatic dysfunction, and cholestasis cause hyperbilirubinemia. Jaundice without other organ dysfunction has good prognosis but liver dysfunction has a poor prognosis when accompanied by multiorgan dysfunction.[3] Malarial hepatitis may cause acute liver failure presenting with coma, very high bilirubin levels, and hemorrhagic manifestations.[16] Spontaneous rupture of the spleen is a rare but potentially lethal and presents as an acute abdomen. It is most frequently reported with *P. vivax*. Hemodynamic resuscitation and splenectomy is the treatment of choice.[17] Malarial pancreatitis is uncommon[18] and requires supportive management like other causes of pancreatitis.

Pulmonary Complications

Acute respiratory distress syndrome (ARDS) is potentially fatal. It occurs due to cytokine storm, leaky capillaries, or superadded bacterial infections.[12] Low-tidal-volume ventilation and other strategies for ARDS are recommended. Acute pulmonary edema may be precipitated by myocardial dysfunction or fluid overload in severe anemia.[15]

Shock and Bacterial Infections

Shock occurs in up to 10% of patients with severe malaria. Concomitant bacterial sepsis is implicated and should be ruled out. Empirical antibiotics may be given and later de-escalated based on cultures.[12] Salmonella bacteremia is associated with *P. falciparum* in endemic regions and should be treated appropriately if suspected. "Algid malaria" is a term used for hypovolemic shock and septicemia in severe malaria.[15] The Fluid Expansion as Supportive Therapy study was an RCT which showed that fluid boluses could worsen outcomes in African children with severe malaria and impaired perfusion.[19] WHO guidelines do not recommend fluid boluses in children with severe malaria.[1] Vasopressors should be used as recommended for septic shock.[12]

CONCLUSION

Severe malaria is a potentially fatal infection that often causes multiorgan dysfunction and requires intensive care. Prompt diagnosis and treatment is lifesaving.

REFERENCES

1. World Health Organization. Guidelines for the treatment of malaria, 3rd edition. Geneva: WHO Press; 2015. [online] Available from http://www.who.int/malaria/publications/atoz/9789241549127/en/ [last accessed September 10, 2018].
2. World Health Organization. World malaria report 2017. Geneva: World Health Organization; 2017. [online] Available from http://www.who.int/malaria/publications/world_malaria_report/en/ [last accessed September 10, 2018].
3. White NJ, Breman JG. Malaria. In: Kasper DL, Fauci AS, Longo DL, Hauser SL, Jameson JL, Loscalzo J (Eds). Harrison's principles of internal medicine, 19th edition. New York, NY: McGraw-Hill; 2001. pp. 1368-83.
4. Krishnan A, Karnad DR. Severe falciparum malaria: an important cause of multiple organ failure in Indian intensive care unit patients. Crit Care Med. 2003;31:2278-84.
5. Dondorp AM, Fanello CI, Hendriksen IC, et al. Artesunate versus quinine in the treatment of severe falciparum malaria in African children (AQUAMAT): an open-label, randomised trial. Lancet. 2010;376:1647-57.
6. Dondorp AN, Nosten F, Stepniewska K, et al. Artesunate versus quinine for treatment of severe falciparum malaria: a randomised trial. Lancet. 2005;366:717-25.
7. Sinclair D, Donegan S, Isba R, et al. Artesunate versus quinine for treating severe malaria. Cochrane Database Syst Rev. 2012;13:CD005967.
8. Esu E, Effa EE, Opie ON, et al. Artemether for severe malaria. Cochrane Database Syst Rev. 2014;9:CD010678.
9. Seydel KB, Kampondeni SD, Valim C, et al. Brain swelling and death in children with cerebral malaria. N Engl J Med. 2015;372:1126.
10. White NJ, Pukrittayakamee S, Hien TT, et al. Malaria. Lancet. 2014;383:723-35.
11. Beare NAV, Taylor TE, Harding SP, et al. Malarial retinopathy: a newly established diagnostic sign in severe malaria. Am J Trop Med Hyg. 2006;75:790-7.
12. Karnad DR, Nor MBM, Richards GA, et al. Intensive care in severe malaria: report from the task force on tropical diseases by the world federation of societies of intensive and critical care medicine. J Crit Care. 2018;43:356-60.
13. Markley JD, Edmond MB. Post-malaria neurological syndrome: a case report and review of the literature. J Travel Med. 2009;16:424-30.
14. Sokrab TE, Eltahir A, Idris MN, et al. Guillain-Barré syndrome following acute falciparum malaria. Neurology. 2002;59:1281-3.
15. Sarkar PK, Ahluwalia G, Vijayan VK, et al. Critical care aspects of malaria. J Intensive Care Med. 2010;25:93-103.
16. Anand AC, Puri P. Jaundice in malaria. J Gastroenterol Hepatol. 2005;20:1322-32.
17. Severe falciparum malaria. World Health Organization, Communicable Diseases Cluster. Trans R Soc Trop Med Hyg. 2000;94:1-90: https://www.ncbi.nlm.nih.gov/pubmed/11103309.
18. Desai DC, Gupta T, Sirsat RA, et al. Malarial pancreatitis: report of two cases and review of the literature. Am J Gastroenterol. 2001;96:930-2.
19. Maitland K, Kiguli S, Opoka RO, et al. Mortality after fluid bolus in African children with severe infection. N Engl J Med. 2011;364:2483-95.

CHAPTER 39

Tuberculosis in Intensive Care Unit

Pradip Kumar Bhattacharya, Lata Bhattacharya, Nimita Deora

INTRODUCTION

Despite the availability of effective antituberculosis (TB) drugs, mortality in critically ill patients due to TB is high, which is associated with a single identifiable infectious pathogen. In 2016, WHO reported 1 million new TB cases in people living with human immunodeficiency virus (HIV) infection. Other than HIV, conditions that affect immunity and increase likelihood of developing active TB are poor nutrition, diabetes, cancer, chronic obstructive pulmonary disease (COPD), and use of steroids.[1]

Patients, infected with *Mycobacterium tuberculosis* (MTB) admitted to intensive care units (ICUs) with single or multiple organ failure, raise important management issues. Many of them have active infection from drug-sensitive or multidrug-resistant (MDR) mycobacteria. In some patients detection of MTB is an incidental finding, as these patients may have previously failed anti-TB therapy, undiagnosed subclinical disease, or latent infection that manifests under conditions of stress and immunosuppression.

The aim of this chapter is to provide an overview of the reasons and outcome for the ICU admission in TB patients, management in the form of drugs, their various regimens, steroids, organ-specific TB, and HIV coinfection along with required infection control practices.[1]

REASONS AND OUTCOME FOR ICU ADMISSION IN TUBERCULOSIS PATIENTS

Reports from different parts of the world indicate that the poor outcomes of TB result from acute cardiorespiratory failure.[2,3] TB is one of the major issues in sub-Saharan countries with poor health care settings. Acute respiratory distress syndrome (ARDS), acute respiratory failure, septic shock, multiorgan dysfunction, and neurological deterioration are the most common reasons for ICU admission of patients with active TB. Frequent infections associated with active TB are bacterial (e.g. chest infections). Other issues are anti-TB drug toxicity, thromboembolic complications, and pulmonary hemorrhage. One Portuguese study suggested that these patients required mechanical ventilation (66.7%), vasopressors (35.9%), renal replacement therapy (RRT) (7.7%), and extracorporeal membrane oxygenation (ECMO) (5.1%).[4] The mortality in patients with confirmed TB admitted to the ICU can be as high as 68.7%.[5]

It has been shown that the presence of miliary TB, need for mechanical ventilation, and presence of shock are the main determinants of death. Other risk factors for increased mortality are nosocomial pneumonia, multiorgan failure, lung destruction by TB, an Acute Physiologic Assessment and Chronic Health Evaluation II (APACHE II) score more than 20, and duration of symptoms more than 4 weeks.[5]

MANAGEMENT OF PATIENTS WITH TUBERCULOSIS IN THE ICU

Antituberculosis Drugs and Treatment Regimens

The standard treatment of TB as per national and international guidelines includes four drugs,[6,7] which should be given as an intensive phase (2 months therapy with four drugs) followed by a continuation phase (4 months of two drugs, i.e. isoniazid (INH) and rifampicin) (Table 39.1). Treatment is extended up to 9 months in patients with TB of joint or bone, or those with a high risk of relapse (e.g. extensive disease, cavitations, immunosuppression, and sputum culture positive after 8 weeks). It may be extended up to 12 months or longer in patients with tuberculous meningitis (TBM) (Table 39.1).[8]

Early diagnosis (with nucleic acid amplification techniques)[8] and immediate treatment are required even in the absence of positive sputum smear and an infection disease consult to improve survival rate.

Infection with MDR and extensively resistant strains of MTB are associated with high mortality globally.[1] Rapid molecular diagnostic tests (e.g. GeneXpert MTB/RIF assay) provide fast results on strains resistant to rifampicin and other tests such as MeltPro TB/INH for INH.[9] A high degree of suspicion for MDR TB should be considered if the patient originates from a high-risk region, has undergone a treatment course of high-line anti-TB drugs, or fails to respond to standard anti-TB regimens (Table 39.2).[1]

As a rule of thumb, failing regimen should be stopped after sending a sample testing for the presence of MDR TB, and instead of adding any other drugs to the failing regimen, a completely new regimen consisting of four to five second-line anti-TB drugs or drugs to which the pathogen is likely to be susceptible should be started as soon as possible. Here the input of an infectious disease (ID) specialist is important. WHO guidelines for MDR-TB should be followed where possible (Table 39.3).[10]

Starting Treatment for Drug-resistant Tuberculosis

Starting treatment includes at least four second-line drugs like delamanid, bedaquiline, p-aminosalicylic acid, imipenem/cilastatin/meropenem, amoxicillin-clavulanate, and thioacetazone; core drugs like later generation fluoroquinolones, amikacin, capreomycin, kanamycin, ethionamide/prothionamide, cycloserine, linezolid, and clofazimine; and one of the first-line drugs, i.e. pyrazinamide administered over 18 months or more pending culture reports.[1] Treatment success depends on adequate blood levels and minimum pharmacokinetic variability of the regimen chosen, otherwise it will lead to treatment failure and drug resistance. An observational study reported that therapeutic blood levels were achieved only in 30% of critically ill patients when anti-TB drugs were given enterally.[11] Various case reports show inadequate blood levels of anti-TB drugs in patients with RRT and/or ECMO.[12,13] Augmented renal clearance, as well as kidney and liver dysfunction affect drug elimination. In addition, genetic variations in drug metabolism play a role as well.[14,15] It appears pragmatic to at least initially avoid the enteral route and administer anti-TB drugs intravenously to critically ill patients, however this may not be possible currently given the lack of availability of intravenous formulations other than rifampicin. Empirical intravenous fluoroquinolones have been suggested to improve survival of critically ill patients admitted with pulmonary TB.[16] A few studies indicated that higher doses of rifampicin (e.g. 15 mg/kg/day) and addition of a fluoroquinolone (e.g. levofloxacin at 20 mg/kg/day) might be associated with improved survival.[17,18] Therapeutic drug monitoring has been recommended to optimize dosing of anti-TB drugs in critically ill patients.[19,20]

Both rifampicin and INH are responsible for interactions with several drugs commonly administered in critically ill patients. While INH inhibits cytochrome, rifampicin induces its activity. Overall, rifampicin outweighs INH's inhibitory effects. Therapeutic drug monitoring and dose adjustments of other drugs are frequently necessary. Rifampicin may reduce blood levels of selected second-line anti-TB drugs such as moxifloxacin.[21]

Another key challenge is their side effects. Some side effects are INH-induced peripheral neuropathy and ethambutol induced retrobulbar neuritis. See Table 39.1 for detailed description of side effects.

Drug-induced liver injury (DILI) is the most dangerous adverse effect of anti-TB drugs and occurs in almost 3–13% of patients, with increasing incidence with age.[22]

It is recommended to monitor liver tests in patients receiving anti-TB drugs. Symptoms of DILI include derangement of liver enzymes, pain, loss of appetite, dark urine, hypoglycemia, vomiting, etc. Hepatotoxic drugs like rifampicin, INH, and pyrazinamide should be temporarily replaced by an aminoglycoside, levofloxacin or other second-line drugs after an ID consult. It may be possible to go back to a previous regimen once the drug-induced hepatitis has resolved.

Role of Steroids in the Treatment of Tuberculosis

Adrenal insufficiency is a common finding and is caused by an exaggerated proinflammatory response due to tuberculous infiltration or adrenal hemorrhage. Rifampicin causes hypocortisolisms. The incidence of adrenal insufficiency in critically ill patients with TB is unclear. One meta-analysis reported that steroids could reduce mortality for all forms of TB, and the effects could be seen most consistently in patients with an increased disease severity

Table 39.1: Overview of first-line anti-TB drugs.[8]

Drug	Dose	IV form	Contraindications	CSF penetration	Side effects	Comment
Rifampicin	Adults: 10 mg/kg/day (max 600 mg/day) Children: 15–20 mg/kg/day (max 600 mg/day) No dose adjustment in renal failure	Available	Unstable liver disease, known hypersensitivity	10–20%	DILI, vasculitis, nephritis, thrombocytopenia, leukopenia, hemolytic anemia, exfoliative dermatitis	Frequent drug interactions (CYP induction), orange discoloration of body secretions (including urine, tears, sweat), monitoring of liver enzymes and bilirubin recommended
Isoniazid	Adults: 5 mg/kg/day Children: 10 mg/kg/day (max 300 mg/day) No dose adjustment in renal failure	Available (not always accessible)	Unstable liver disease, known hypersensitivity	100%	DILI, peripheral neuropathy, lupus-like syndrome, (hypersensitivity) vasculitis, seizures, altered mental state	Drug interactions (CYP inhibition), combine with pyridoxine [10 (–25) mg/day], clinical monitoring of all patients on isoniazid is essential, monitoring of liver enzymes recommended.
Ethambutol	Adults: 15 mg/kg/day Children: 20–30 mg/kg/day (max 1,200 mg/day) Dose adjustment in renal failure	Available (not always accessible)	Retrobulbar neuritis, known hypersensitivity	25–50%	Retrobulbar neuritis, DILI, thrombocytopenia, leukopenia, myocarditis, pericarditis, altered mental state, exanthema, arthralgia	Visual disturbances often begin with loss of red-green discrimination and then rapidly progress to blindness, patients should be counseled to report any changes in vision. Baseline and monthly visual acuity and color discrimination monitoring should be performed (particular attention should be given to individuals on higher doses or with renal impairment)
Pyrazinamide	Adults: 25 mg/kg/day Children: 35 mg/kg/day (max 2,000 mg/day) Dose adjustment in renal failure	Not available	Unstable liver disease, known hypersensitivity, porphyria	100%	DILI, exanthema, rhabdomyolysis, arthritis	Monitoring of liver enzymes recommended

Source: For drug interaction with food, proton pump inhibitor (PPI), and other medications please refer—Arbex MA, Varella MCL, de Siqueira HR, et al. Antituberculosis drugs: drug interactions, adverse effects, and use in special situations. Part 2: second-line drugs. J Bras Pneumol. 2010;36(5):641-56.

(CSF: cerebrospinal fluid; CYP: cytochrome P450; DILI: drug-induced liver injury; IV: intravenous; TB: tuberculosis)

Table 39.2: Advantages and disadvantages of methods used for diagnosing TB.

Method	How does it work	Advantage	Disadvantage
AFB smear microscopy or pulmonary TB test	A slide is prepared from sputum of suspected TB patient and examined under a microscope	Trained technician is required for microscopy, economical	Less sensitive as at least 5,000 bacilli mL^{-1} are required to be positive
Culture	Growth of bacteria is observed in media containing all essential nutrients	Gold standard	Expensive than microscopy, require enhanced laboratory facilities and equipments, time consuming
Chest X-ray	White patches or abnormal shadow indicates presence of TB	Results are available within hours	Normal chest X-ray cannot exclude extrapulmonary TB
Skin test	Tuberculin (fluid) is injected into the skin	Extensive clinical and published experience	Cannot differentiate between latent TB or active TB
IGRAs	Fresh blood samples are mixed with antigens and controls	Highly specific for MTB, results are available within 24 hours	Blood specimen collecting and running errors can reduce its accuracy
Xpert MTB/RIF assay	Based on nucleic acid amplification test that uses disposable cartridge with the GeneXpert instrument system	Fully automated, rapid detection of MDR TB	It does not replace the need for smear with microscopy for acid fast bacilli
ARMS	In this method, oligonucleotide primer works with PCR	Highly sensitive, rapid detection of mutation	Complex and expensive

(AFB: acid-fast bacilli; MDR: multidrug-resistant; MTB: mycobacterium tuberculosis; RIF: rifampin; PCR: polymerase chain reaction; TB: tuberculosis; ARMS: amplification refractory mutation system; IGRAs: interferon-gamma release assays)

Table 39.3: WHO classification of first- and second-line antituberculosis (TB) drugs and recommended dose.[6]

	Drug group	Antituberculosis drug	Daily dose
First-line drugs	First-line oral agents	Isoniazid Rifampicin Ethambutol Pyrazinamide	5 mg/kg 10 mg/kg 15–25 mg/kg 30 mg/kg
	Injectable/parenteral anti-TB drugs	Streptomycin Kanamycin Amikacin Capreomycin	15 mg/kg 15 mg/kg 15 mg/kg 15 mg/kg
	Fluoroquinolones	Ofloxacin Levofloxacin Moxifloxacin Gatifloxacin	15 mg/kg 15 mg/kg 7.5–10 mg/kg Max 400 mg daily
Second-line drugs	Oral bacteriostatic second-line anti-TB drugs	Ethionamide Prothionamide Cycloserine Terizidone p-aminosalicylic acid p-aminosalicylate sodium	15 mg/kg 15 mg/kg 15 mg/kg 15 mg/kg 150 mg/kg 150 mg/kg
	Anti-TB drugs with limited data on efficacy and/or long-term safety in the treatment of drug resistant TB	Bedaquiline Delamanid Linezolid Clofazimine Amoxicillin/clavulanate High dose isoniazid	400 mg daily/600 mg weekly 200 mg daily 600 mg daily 100 mg daily 875/125 mg (per 12 h) 10–15 mg/kg

such as miliary TB or TB-associated septic shock.²³ However, the role of steroids to improve patient outcome is unclear.

Organ-specific Tuberculosis and Management

Pulmonary Tuberculosis

Tuberculosis primarily affects the liver. It is curable with early diagnosis and treatment. Respiratory failure because of pulmonary TB is relatively low (1.5–5%).²⁴ Immunocompromised patients, small children, people with autoimmune disorder, and patients with diabetes are at higher risk of developing pulmonary TB. An intense proinflammatory reaction at the alveolar capillary membrane increases extravascular lung water, which leads to ventilation/perfusion mismatch and increases the alveolar-arterial (A-a) gradient. Granulomatous infection and obliterative endarteritis patients may develop ARDS. In advanced disease, air spaces are destroyed by caseating granulomas and fibrocavitary lesions. Mortality of patients with ARDS with TB is much higher. However, mortality in patients developing ARDS during antitubercular treatment is lower than in those who present with ARDS at admission. Noninvasive ventilation (NIV) in these patients is not very successful. Principles of invasive ventilation remain the same as applied in other patients with ARDS. Need for mechanical ventilator support is often prolonged.²⁵,²⁶

It occurs in up to two-third of these patients. 13.8% of pulmonary TB patients developed pneumothorax during their admission to the ICU. It happens maximally during mechanical ventilation.²⁷ Pleural adhesions and bronchopleural fistulas are common after drainage of pneumothoraces and pleural effusions. Fibrosis and cavitary lesions develop as long-term sequelae. Hemoptysis is a common complication in tuberculous patients and sometimes it is life-threatening. Endotracheal intubation is necessary along with mechanical ventilation. Tranexamic acid may be used as an adjunct under this circumstance. Bronchoscopy can be used to diagnose and treat pulmonary hemorrhage (e.g. by topical application of epinephrine (adrenaline) 1:10,000 to 1:100,000).²⁸ Pulmonary angiography and embolization are highly effective in bleeding control. Surgical interventions are reserved for unmanageable patients as it is associated with high mortality.

Central Nervous System Tuberculosis

Central nervous system TB includes three categories: (1) meningitis, (2) tuberculous spinal arachnoiditis, and (3) intracranial tuberculoma. It is common in children and immunocompromised patients. It carries very high mortality rates, especially in HIV-positive patients.²⁹ Post-treatment neurological sequelae have been reported in up to 50% of the survivors.¹⁶

Risk factors for central nervous system TB generally include HIV, alcoholism, malnutrition, use of immuno-suppressive agents, and malignancies. Primary symptoms are nonspecific malaise, fever, vomiting, fatigue, headache, and loss of appetite.

Tuberculous meningitis has been classified by the British Medical Research Council as consisting of three stages:
1. *Stage I*: No definite neurological symptoms on admission or in the history before admission, with or without meningismus.
2. *Stage II*: Signs of meningeal irritations with or without slight clouding of consciousness with focal neurological signs such as cranial nerve palsies or hemiparesis.
3. *Stage III*: Severe clouding of consciousness or delirium, convulsions and serious neurological signs such as hemiplegia, paraplegia or involuntary movements.³⁰

High index of suspicion and clinical history are the main clues for diagnosis. The diagnostic tools used to identify CNS TB are:
- Fundoscopy
- Lumbar puncture
- Computed tomography (CT) scan
- Magnetic resonance imaging (MRI).

Increased protein level, decreased glucose level, and lymphocyte predominance (monocytes) are the key findings in cerebrospinal fluid (CSF) analysis. Using GeneXpert and adenosine deaminase (ADA) level in CSF are also recommended as initial diagnostic tests.³¹

In contrast, the CSF examination in HIV-positive patients with meningitis will have lower cell counts, polymorphonuclear cell predominance and normal glucose levels, and it may be confused with cryptococcal meningitis.

Imaging studies of brains with meningitis revealed that nearly 80% had one or more cerebral tuberculoma(s), which develop paradoxically during anti-TB therapy.³²

Nearly all patients with tubercular meningitis experiencing agitation and, more commonly, a decreasing level of consciousness require intensive care because of an altered mental state.

In one study, 75% of critically ill patients with TBM required intubation and mechanical ventilation.³³

British and WHO guidelines recommend timely initiation of anti-TB treatment with first-line drugs including streptomycin.⁶,⁷ Fluoroquinolones have also been found to be helpful.¹⁷

Adjunct therapy in the form of steroids, such as dexamethasone or equivalent doses of prednisolone is recommended,[6,7] as studies suggest that this is associated with improved mortality and functional outcomes.[34]

The duration of steroid therapy is usually 2 months, with weaning off the steroid dose over this period. Large tuberculomas may need to be removed. All general neurointensive care principles need to be followed.

Complications include hydrocephalus, seizures, sodium disturbances [e.g. syndrome of inadequate antidiuretic hormone secretion (SIADH)], and stroke. In nearly 80% of cases, it is a communicating hydrocephalus and must be suspected in all patients with a decreased level of consciousness.

Although conservative management with diuretics (e.g. acetazolamide 100 mg/kg/day) can be attempted, in one-third of cases repeated lumbar drainage or placement of a ventricular catheter is required.[33] For seizure control, valproic acid can be used with caution as it may increase the risk of DILI.[35]

In one study from India including 118 patients with TBM, prophylactic aspirin (150 mg/day) resulted in a 19.1% absolute risk reduction of stroke and a lower mortality (21.7 vs. 43.4%; p = 0.02) compared to a placebo.[36]

Tuberculous Pericarditis

Tuberculous pericarditis is an important complication of TB. Its diagnosis and management are not well defined because of contiguous spread of a lung lesion, hematogenous seedling, rupture of a caseous lymph node into the pericardium. Smear microscopy or molecular testing of tuberculous pericarditis is of limited use and requires that therapy often needs to be initiated without laboratory confirmation.[37]

Steroid treatment for tuberculous pericarditis consists of prednisolone 60 mg/day for 4 weeks followed by 30 mg/day for 4 weeks, 15 mg/day for 2 weeks, and then 5 mg/day for 1 week.

Abdominal Tuberculosis

It mainly affects the gut and peritoneum. Gastrointestinal TB (GITB) mainly results from ingestion of infected sputum when the patient has acute pulmonary TB. The most common sites are the terminal ileum and ileocecal region in 75% of cases.[37] It is predominant in the Indian subcontinent. Patients often present with nonspecific gastrointestinal symptoms and a palpable mass in the right iliac fossa.[38,39] Pathological findings are ulcerations at various parts of the small intestine and duodenum. Presentation is usually in the form of weight loss, abdominal pain, and ascites.

High lymphocyte count, raised ADA levels, and exudate nature of ascitic fluid give a good diagnostic tool. However, CT scan and laparoscopic biopsies are more sensitive diagnostic tests.

Extrapulmonary Tuberculosis

Tuberculosis involving organs other than the lungs is referred to as extrapulmonary. Tuberculous laryngitis can result in airway obstruction. The lower thoracic spine is affected most frequently among other bones and joints. Late presentation may result in cord paralysis. Optalmic involvement can cause blindness. Lymphocutaneous fistulas may be seen.[40]

Miliary or Disseminated Tuberculosis

When mycobacteria spread through the lymph system or blood from the lungs to different parts of the body, it is referred to as disseminated TB. Common symptoms include fever, chills, tiredness, and sweating. It usually affects lungs, but can spread to the liver, spleen, meninges, and kidneys. Its diagnosis can be difficult. Skin lesions (tuberculosis cutis miliaris disseminata) and choroidal tubercles on fundoscopy can give valuable clues in the diagnosis of miliary TB. ICU presentation may be with ARDS and shock.[41]

DIAGNOSIS AND TREATMENT OF TUBERCULOSIS PATIENTS COINFECTED WITH HUMAN IMMUNODEFICIENCY VIRUS

Among HIV-positive patients, the risk of acquiring TB is high. TB accelerates the process of HIV replication and disease progression. TB causes 26% of acquired immune deficiency syndrome (AIDS)-related deaths.[42] The presentation of TB may be atypical at decreased CD4 counts (<200/mm^3) and symptoms are usually absent at CD4 counts of less than 75/mm^3.[43] Anti-TB treatment should be started as soon as TB is diagnosed. Assisted reproductive technology (ART) proved to reduce all causes of mortality.

The WHO recommends initiation of antiretroviral therapy within the first 8 weeks after the start of anti-TB treatment (etravirine, darunavir, and raltegravir trio therapy). Antiretroviral therapy should be initiated within 2 weeks once anti-TB therapy is commenced in patients with a low CD4 count, as these patients are at a particularly high risk of short-term death. Antiretrovirals should be continued without interruption in patients who are already on therapy at the diagnosis of TB.[44]

Mild forms of immune reconstitution inflammatory syndrome (IRIS) with fever and lymph node enlargement develop in one-third of HIV-positive patients with active

Section 3: Specific Syndromes

TB and a CD4 count of less than $50/mm^3$ getting ART. The severity of manifestations will increase once ART is initiated and immunity recovers. Severe forms are rare but can manifest as increasing tuberculomas, worsening of pulmonary gas exchange, and ARDS.

Propensity of IRIS has been correlated with the quantity of bacteremia. No standard treatment for IRIS has been recommended. Management is usually symptomatic and includes steroids in severe cases. Prednisolone is administered at 1.5 mg/kg/day for 2 weeks, followed by 0.75 mg/kg/day for 2 weeks.[45]

INFECTION PREVENTION AND CONTROL MEASURES TO REDUCE TRANSMISSION

Transmission is mainly through airborne droplet nuclei or through ingestion of microorganisms.

Infection control measures (Table 39.4) include negative pressure isolation of patients. These patients should be kept away from non-TB patients in separate rooms or wards. Staff should adhere to strict hand hygiene standards and wear N95 masks and gloves when entering the room. Personal respiratory protection should be used when handling such patients. Care should be taken while performing procedures on infectious cases such as chest X-ray. Closed suction should be used in ventilated patients.

Timing should be adjusted so that minimum contamination and cross infection occurs. Pragmatically, deisolation may be considered after a 2-week course of anti-TB drugs; however, immunosuppressed, diabetic patients, and patients with drug-resistant TB may require a longer period of isolation.[7] Environmental control measures must be added, such as ultraviolet (UV) light to reduce the risk of spreading droplet nuclei in the air (Table 39.4).

CONCLUSION AND SUMMARY

Tuberculosis is a big problem in healthcare settings. An increase in the numbers of critically ill patients with TB has been observed over the past several years with high mortality. Rapid diagnostic tests have been useful in early diagnosis and treatment. Novel drugs are in the

Table 39.4: Key infection control recommendations.[8]

Setting	Environmental control	Respiratory protection control
Intensive care units	• In settings with a high volume of patients with suspected or confirmed TB disease, at least one room should meet requirements for an airborne infection isolation room to be used for such patients • Bacterial filters should be used routinely in breathing circuits of patients with suspected or confirmed TB disease and should filter particles 0.3 μm in size in unloaded and loaded situations with a filter efficiency of ≥95%	• For HCWs, visitors, and others entering the airborne infection isolation room of a patient with suspected or confirmed infectious TB disease, at least N95 disposable respirators should be worn • If the patient has signs or symptoms of infectious TB disease and is suspected of being contagious (positive AFB sputum smear result), consider having the patient wear a surgical or procedure mask, if possible (e.g. if patient is not using a breathing circuit) during transport, in waiting areas, or when others are present. When endotracheal suctioning is performed a closed suction apparatus should be used and a N98 respirator worn
Surgical suites	• If a surgical suite has an OR with an anteroom, that room should be used for TB cases • If surgery is needed, use a room or suite of rooms that meet requirements for airborne infection isolation rooms • If an airborne infection isolation or comparable room is not available for surgery or postoperative recovery, air-cleaning technologies (e.g. HEPA filtration and UVGI) can be used to increase the number of equivalent air change per hour • If the health-care setting has an anteroom, reversible flow rooms (OR or isolation) are not recommended • Bacterial filters should be used routinely in breathing circuits of patients with suspected or confirmed TB disease and should filter particles 0.3 μm in size in an unloaded and loaded situation with a filter efficiency of ≥95%	• For HCWs present during surgery of a patient with suspected or confirmed infectious TB disease, at least N95 disposable respirators, unvalved, should be worn • Standard surgical or procedure masks for HCWs might not have fitting or filtering capacity for adequate protection • If the patient has signs or symptoms of infectious TB disease (positive AFB sputum smear result), consider having the patient wear a surgical or procedure mask, if possible, before and after the procedure • Valved or positive pressure respirators should not be used because they do not protect the sterile surgical field

(AFB: acid-fast bacillus; HCWs: health care workers; HEPA: high-efficiency particulate air; OR: operating room; TB: tuberculosis; UVGI: ultraviolet germicidal irradiation; WHO: World Health Organization)

developmental phase and clinical trials are underway in an attempt to improve the current deficiencies. Infection prevention and control measures play a crucial role in minimizing the risk of TB transmission in healthcare settings. Altered pharmacodynamics and pharmacokinetics in these patients may be a contributing factor to adverse outcomes, although optimal treatment strategies are yet to be defined.

REFERENCES

1. Zumla A, Raviglione M, Hafner R, et al. Tuberculosis. N Engl J Med. 2013;368:745-55.
2. Lin CH, Lin CJ, Kuo YW, et al. Tuberculosis mortality: patient characteristics and causes. BMC Infect Dis. 2014;14:5.
3. Tavares C, Bacelar T, Lins A, et al. Tuberculosis deaths in a tertiary hospital in Goiania, Brazil: a descriptive study. Infez Med. 2013;4:279-86.
4. Duro RP, Dias PF, Ferreira AA, et al. Severe tuberculosis requiring intensive care: a descriptive analysis. Crit Care Res Pract. 2017;2017:1-9.
5. Filiz KA, Levent D, Emel E, et al. Characteristics of active tuberculosis patients requiring intensive care monitoring and factors affecting mortality. Tuber Respir Dis (Seoul). 2016;79:158-64.
6. World Health Organization. (2010). Guidelines for treatment of tuberculosis, fourth edition. [online] Available from http://www.who.int/tb/publications/2010/9789241547833/en/ [Accessed December 2018].
7. National Institute for Health and Care Excellence. (2016). Tuberculosis. [online] Available from https://www.nice.org.uk/guidance/ng 33 [Accessed December 2018].
8. Out A, Hashmi M, Mukhtar AM, et al. The critically ill patient with tuberculosis in intensive care: Clinical presentations, management and infection control. J Critical care. 2018;45:184-96.
9. Wilson ML. Rapid diagnosis of mycobacterium tuberculosis infection and drug susceptibility testing. Arch Pathol Lab Med. 2013;137:812-9.
10. WHO global tuberculosis control report 2010. Summary. Cent Eur J Public Health. 2010;18(4):237.
11. Koegelenberg CF, Nortje A, Lalla U, et al. The pharmacokinetics of enteral anti-TB drugs in patients requiring intensive care. S Afr Med J. 2013;103:394-8.
12. Sin JH, Elshaboury RH, Hurtado RM, et al. Therapeutic drug monitoring of antitubercular agents for disseminated mycobacterium tuberculosis during intermittent haemodialysis and continuous venovenous haemofiltration. J Clin Pharm Ther. 2018;43(2):291-5.
13. Kim HS, Lee ES, Cho YJ. Insufficient serum levels of anti-TB agents during venovenous extracorporeal membrane oxygenation therapy for acute respiratory distress syndrome in a patient with military tuberculosis. ASAIO J. 2014;60:484-6.
14. Weiner M, Burman W, Vernon A, et al. Low isoniazid concentrations and outcome of tuberculosis treatment with once-weekly isoniazid and rifapentine. Am J Respir Crit Care Med. 2003;167:1341-7.
15. Ellard GA. The potential clinical significance of the isoniazid acetylator phenotype in the treatment of pulmonary tuberculosis. Tubercle. 1984;65:211-27.
16. Tseng YT, Chuang YC, Shu CC, et al. Empirical use of fluoroquinolones improves the survival of critically ill patients with tuberculosis mimicking severe pneumonia. Crit Care. 2012;16(5):R207.
17. Ruslami R, Ganiem AR, Dian S, et al. Intensified regimen containing rifampicin and moxifloxacin for tuberculous meningitis: an open-label, randomised controlled phase 2 trial. Lancet Infect Dis. 2013;13:27-35.
18. Te Brake L, Dian S, Ganiem AR, et al. Pharmacokinetic/pharmacodynamics analysis of an intensified regimen containing rifampicin and moxifloxacin for tuberculous meningitis. Int J Antimicrob Agents. 2015;45:496-503.
19. Choi R, Jeong BH, Koh WJ, et al. Recommendations for optimizing tuberculosis treatment: therapeutic drug monitoring, pharmacogenetics, and nutritional status considerations. Ann Lab Med. 2017;37:97-107.
20. Peloquin C. Therapeutic drug monitoring in the treatment of tuberculosis. Drugs. 2002;62:2169-83.
21. Manika K, Chatzika K, Papaioannou M, et al. Rifampicin-moxifloxacin interaction in tuberculosis treatment: a real-life study. Int J Tuberc Lung Dis. 2015;19(11):1383-7.
22. Saukkonen JJ, Powell K, Jereb JA. Monitoring for tuberculosis drug hepatotoxicity: moving from opinion to evidence. Am J Respir Crit Care Med. 2012;185:598-9.
23. Critchley JA, Young F, Orton L, et al. Corticosteroids for prevention of mortality in people with tuberculosis: a systematic review and meta-analysis. Lancet Infect Dis. 2013,13:233-7.
24. Levy H, Kallenbach JM, Feldman C, et al. Acute respiratory failure in active tuberculosis. Crit Care Med. 1987;15:221-5.
25. Penner C, Roberts D, Kunimoto D, et al. Tuberculosis as a primary cause of respiratory failure requiring mechanical ventilation. Am J Respir Crit Care Med. 1995;151:867-72.
26. Banga A, Sharma SK, Mohan A. Acute respiratory distress syndrome in pulmonary tuberculosis. Chest. 2003;124:114S.
27. Erbes R, Oettel K, Raffenberg M, et al. Characteristics and outcome of patients with active pulmonary tuberculosis requiring intensive care. Eur Respir J. 2006;27:1223-8.
28. Jougon J, Ballester M, Delcambre F, et al. Massive hemoptysis: what place for medical and surgical management. Eur J Cardiothorac Surg. 2002;22:345-51.
29. Thwaites GE, Nguyen DB, Nguyen HD, et al. Dexamethasone for the treatment of tuberculous meningitis in adolescents and adults. N Engl J Med. 2004;315:1741-51.
30. Alarcón F, Moreira J, Rivera J, et al. Tuberculous meningitis: do modern diagnostic tools offer better prognosis prediction? Indian J Tuberc. 2013;60:5-14.
31. World Health Organization. (2014). Xpert MTB/RIF implementation manual: technical and operational 'how-to'; practical considerations. [online] Available from http://apps.who.int/iris/bitstream/handle/10665/112469/9789241506700_eng.pdf;jsessionid=25617DC3E6B09EB2E513AD63F4F9FC30?sequence=1 [Accessed December 2018].

32. Wasay M, Kheleani BA, Moolani MK, et al. Brain CT and MRI findings in 100 consecutive patients with intracranial tuberculoma. J Neuroimaging. 2003;13:240-7.
33. Verdon R, Chevret S, Laissy JP, et al. Tuberculous meningitis in adults: review of 48 cases. Clin Infect Dis. 1996;22:982-8.
34. Prasad K, Singh MB, Ryan H. Corticosteroids for managing tuberculous meningitis. Cochrane Database Syst Rev. 2016;4:CD002244.
35. Brancusi F, Farrar J, Heemskerk D. Tuberculous meningitis in adults: a review of a decade of developments focusing on prognostic factors for outcome. Future Microbiol. 2012;7:1101-16.
36. Misra UK, Kalita J, Nair PP. Role of aspirin in tuberculous meningitis: a randomized open label placebo controlled trial. J Neurol Sci. 2010;293:12-7.
37. Reuter H, Burgess L, van Vuuren W, et al. Diagnosing tuberculous pericarditis. QJM. 2006;99:827-39.
38. Mukhopadhyay A, Dey R, Bhattacharya U. Abdominal tuberculosis with an acute abdomen: our clinical experience. J Clin Diagn Res. 2014;8:NC07-9.
39. Mavila R, Kottarath MD, Naseer N, et al. Clinico-pathological profile of abdominal tuberculosis and their treatment response in a tertiary care centre. Int J Res Med Sci. 2016;4:5120-4.
40. Tarcoveanu E, Dimofte G, Bradea C, et al. Peritoneal tuberculosis in laparoscopic era. Acta Chir Belg. 2009;109:65-70.
41. Kethireddy S, Light RB, Mirzanejad Y, et al. Mycobacterium tuberculosis septic shock. Chest. 2013;144:474-82.
42. Getahun H, Gunneberg C, Granich R, et al. HIV infection-associated tuberculosis: the epidemiology and the response. Clin Infect Dis. 2010;50:201-7.
43. Sharma SK, Mohan A, Sharma A. Miliary tuberculosis: a new look at an old foe. J Clin Tuberc Other Mycobact Dis. 2016;3:13-27.
44. WHO. (2017). Guidelines for treatment of drug-susceptible tuberculosis and patient care (2017 update). [online] Available from http://www.who.int/tb/publications/2017/dstb_guidance_2017/en/ [Accessed December 2018].
45. Bosamiya S. The immune reconstitution inflammatory syndrome. Indian J Dermatol. 2011;56:476-9.

CHAPTER 40

Melioidosis

Catherine L Tacon, Thomas A Doyle, Simon Smith

INTRODUCTION

Melioidosis, a disease of both medical and veterinary importance, results from infection with Burkholderia pseudomallei—an environmental, soil dwelling, Gram-negative bacterium found in tropical regions. In humans, clinical manifestations vary widely from subclinical infections detectable only on serology to fulminant and rapidly fatal septic shock and multiorgan failure. Acute presentations include pneumonia, primary bacteremia, skin and soft tissue infections, visceral abscesses, and brainstem encephalitis. However, melioidosis may also present chronically mimicking tuberculosis or as a non-healing skin ulcer. A high index of clinical suspicion and advanced laboratory techniques are required for diagnosis. This alongside appropriate antibiotics and access to intensive care medicine results in a reduced mortality.

EPIDEMIOLOGY

It is estimated that 165,000 cases of melioidosis occur worldwide each year (95% CI: 68,000–412,000) though many of these are undiagnosed due to lack of access to appropriate microbiological techniques.[1] In Northern Australia, annual incidence rates have been over 50 per 100,000 population, and although reported incidence rates in South East Asia are lower, they are increasing.[2,3] The wide range of reported case-fatality rates, ranging from 14% to 70%, reflects differences in host factors, disease site and burden, ability to diagnose, prompt delivery of appropriate antibiotics, and access to sophisticated intensive care medicine.[4] This range of mortality is similarly present in pediatric populations and is dependent on the clinical presentation and presence or absence of bacteremia. In Australia, pediatric melioidosis is relatively uncommon with one series reporting an overall mortality of 7%.[5] In other settings mortality is higher, for example, in a Cambodian case series the overall pediatric mortality was 16.8% increasing to 71.8% in those who were bacteremic.[6]

Geographical Distribution

Although most reported cases are from SE Asia, notably Thailand and Vietnam, and the tropical northern areas of Australia, melioidosis has a much wider geographical distribution which reflects both the tropical climate and soil types required by *Barkholderia pseudomallei*.

Melioidosis is likely endemic to a total of 79 countries across South East and South Asia, Africa and the Americas with cases reported from 45 of these (Fig. 40.1). Many cases are either unrecognized or under-reported due to either a lack of requisite microbiological techniques and/or robust reporting systems in many countries. Also, if not already endemic, many countries have conditions where *B. pseudomallei* could become established if introduced[1] and case reports from countries not previously considered endemic may also represent global dissemination as a result of increased human and animal movements globally.[4]

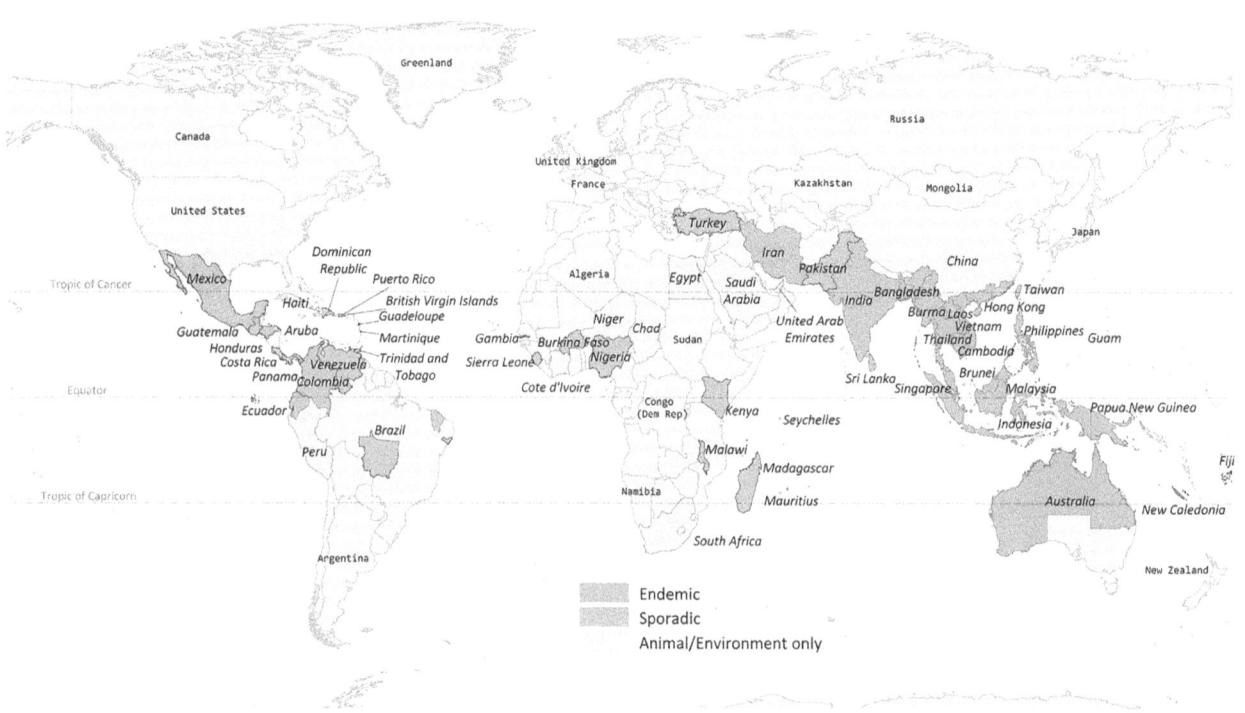

FIGURE 40.1: Global geographical distribution of melioidosis.[7]

Individual Exposure

Melioidosis, an opportunistic disease, is a consequence of an individual's environmental exposure to the soil-dwelling *B. pseudomallei* and the bacterial burden. Therefore, occupations and recreational activities which bring individuals into contact with soil increase the risk of melioidosis, though a clear history of soil exposure is not always present—living or traveling in an endemic area is sufficient for exposure. When there has been a discrete exposure the estimated median time to presentation is 9 days (1-22 days).[8]

Risk Factors for Disease Development (Table 40.1)

Exposure to *B. pseudomallei* usually leads to the development of subclinical disease, either with or without subsequent seroconversion.[4] For those who develop clinical disease several risk factors have been identified. These risk factors are more common in adults (up to 80% have one or more risk factor),[4] than children (16-20% in Australian studies).[5,9]

The most common risk factors for the development of melioidosis are diabetes mellitus (37-60% of patients), hazardous alcohol use (12-39%), renal disease (10-27%), chronic lung disease (12-27%), thalassemia (7%), steroids

Table 40.1: Risk factors for development of melioidosis.

Risk factor	Percentage of patients with risk factor
Diabetes mellitus	37–60%
Hazardous alcohol use	12–39%
Renal disease	10–27%
Chronic lung disease	12–27%
Thalassemia	7%
Steroids or other immunosuppressants	<5%
Malignancy	<5%

or other immunosuppressive therapies (<5%), and cancer (<5%).[4,10] Occupational exposure to surface water has been noted as a risk factor in several countries, including Thailand, Sri Lanka, and Malaysia.[10-12] Other case reports have noted the association of melioidosis with chronic granulomatous disease, mycobacterial disease, dengue hemorrhagic fever, and glucose-6-phosphatase deficiency.[10,12]

The mechanism by which these conditions increase the risk of developing melioidosis is most likely related to an impairment of patients' innate immune function, especially phagocytic cell and neutrophil function.[4,10] Despite the importance of cell-mediated immune response in the defense of disease development, infection with human immunodeficiency virus (HIV) does not appear to be an important risk factor.[4]

Acquisition

Melioidosis demonstrates seasonality in many countries with higher levels of B. pseudomallei present after heavy rains. For example, in endemic regions of Australia, and similarly in NE Thailand, melioidosis is associated with the wet season and in Australia an increase in presentations may be seen following heavy rainfall within a wet season.[4,13] Melioidosis, like other water-related pathogens, may show an increased incidence after extreme weather events such as tsunamis, cyclones, and hurricanes through increased water exposure, skin cuts and abrasions and contact time with infected water or soil.[4,14]

The clinical manifestations of melioidosis may be related to the mode of acquisition and this varies by geographical region. Routes of acquisition include:
- Direct inoculation of skin abrasions and cuts (e.g. rice field workers, lack of footwear, trauma related)
- Inhalation of aerosolized bacteria:
  - This occurs following seasonal heavy rains hence the annual variation of melioidosis within some countries.
  - Other mechanisms such as case reports of helicopter related aerosolization.[15]
- Ingestion of contaminated, unchlorinated water[16]
- Laboratory exposure (rare)[17]
- Human-human and zoonotic infections (rare)[18]
- Biological warfare agent: Listed as a Tier 1 Select agent by the Centre for Disease Control and Prevention—potential agent; not reported.

Recurrence of melioidosis may represent treatment failure (due to inadequate source control or non-adherence to prescribed therapy) or re-infection. Although both exposure and infection result in antibody production these are not sufficient to prevent re-infection by different strains. Finally, following an initial mild or subclinical infection, B. pseudomallei may become latent, re-emerging many years later often in the context of waning host immunity or immunosuppression.[4]

CLINICAL FEATURES

The spectrum of clinical disease caused by B. pseudomallei ranges from localized disease at the site of inoculation with no systemic manifestations (i.e. localized cutaneous infection), to fulminant sepsis and death.[4] It may present acutely (most commonly) or chronically, which is defined as illness that is present for longer than 2 months' duration at the time of presentation (11% of cases).[4]

Pneumonia is the most common presentation of melioidosis and is a feature in over half of presentations,[4,10,19] with secondary pneumonia after an initial focus elsewhere occurring in 10% of cases.[4] Bacteremia rates are variable—from 55% to 74% in different Australian studies,[20,21] with septic shock present in approximately 20% of cases.[4] Presentation with bacteremia without a localized primary site of infection is increasingly recognized.[4]

Besides the primary clinical presentation, it is common for secondary foci of infection to occur, mandating routine imaging to identify internal abscesses. Genitourinary infection is common in Australia, with prostate abscesses occurring in up to 21% of males,[22] but less so in other countries in South East Asia.[4,10,11] These may present with fever, dysuria and suprapubic pain, often with associated diarrhea.[4] In comparison, a higher proportion of liver, spleen, and renal abscesses are seen in Thailand (33-74%), which are often multiple.[23,24] Prostatic abscesses commonly require drainage, whereas other internal abscesses may respond to antibiotic treatment alone.[10]

Osteomyelitis and septic arthritis occur in 6-16% of cases,[11,13] either as the primary site of infection, or secondary to another primary focus, usually pneumonia.[4] Surgical debridement is usually required. Skin and soft tissue infections are also common presentations of melioidosis and although some may present as a localized abscess, other infections can be rapidly progressive, similar to necrotizing fasciitis.[10,11]

Neurological presentations of melioidosis are less common yet are associated with significant morbidity and mortality. Encephalomyelitis accounts for up to 5% of Australian melioidosis cases, although is less common in South East Asia.[4,13] It usually presents with signs of brain stem infection, often with cranial nerve palsies, cerebellar signs, unilateral upper motor limb weakness, or flaccid paralysis.[4,10] Lesions may not be apparent on CT, but require MRI to confirm diagnosis. Most patients with melioidosis encephalomyelitis have no identifiable risk factors and many develop permanent neurological deficits.[4] Primary meningitis and cerebral abscesses are the more common neurological manifestation in South East Asia.[4]

Acute suppurative parotitis occurs at a rate of 30 to 40% in Thai children and is also a common presentation for children in Cambodia, yet has rarely been seen within Australia.[4,10] This may reflect ingestion of B. pseudomallei contaminated unchlorinated water in these regions.[4] It generally has a good prognosis, is less commonly seen in adults and often occurs in children with no defined risk factors.[10]

Other sites of infection reported include mycotic aneurysms, thyroid and scrotal abscesses, and mediastinal infections.[10] Ocular involvement includes orbital cellulitis, corneal ulcers, and subconjunctival abscesses.[10] Cardiac involvement is rare, with pyopericardium the most common manifestation, however case reports of endocarditis and myocardial abscesses also exist.[10]

CLINICAL IMAGES

Figures 40.2 and 40.3 show the chest X-ray and CT images of melioidosis.

DIAGNOSIS

Isolation of B. pseudomallei by culture is the current gold standard for diagnosis, however it may take up to 7 days for culture and confirmation.[4] *B. pseudomallei* grows readily on standard blood culture medium, however the rate of successful diagnosis increases if samples from non-sterile sites (e.g. sputum, ulcer or skin lesion swabs) are placed in Ashdown broth or plated onto Ashdown agar which facilitates the selective growth of the organism.[4]

Serologic testing without culture confirmation is considered inadequate for diagnosis because of the background level of seropositive rates of those living in endemic areas. Its utility in diagnosing melioidosis in an acutely unwell patient is limited. However, positive serology in a symptomatic traveler just returned from an endemic area may support the possibility of melioidosis as a diagnosis.[4]

Several rapid diagnostic tests are currently being evaluated,[25,26] however they are currently less sensitive than blood cultures for detecting B. pseudomallei. Rapid immunofluorescence microscopy of pus, sputum, and urine has been used to aid diagnosis in Thailand, however is not widely available elsewhere.[4]

Due to the high incidence of secondary foci of infection, once diagnosis is confirmed all patients require as a minimum chest X-ray and imaging of the abdomen and pelvis. While computed tomography (CT) of the abdomen and pelvis is the gold standard for post-pubertal males to exclude prostatic abscesses, ultrasound of the abdomen may be an alternative for children and females to reduce radiation exposure.[4]

MANAGEMENT

Treatment of melioidosis consists of an intensive phase with intravenous antibiotics, followed by a prolonged eradication phase with oral antibiotics (Tables 40.2 and 40.3).

Intensive Phase

Intravenous ceftazidime or meropenem is used in the intensive phase. Ceftazidime has been shown in a randomized trial to halve the mortality from melioidosis as compared with the conventional therapy used at the time

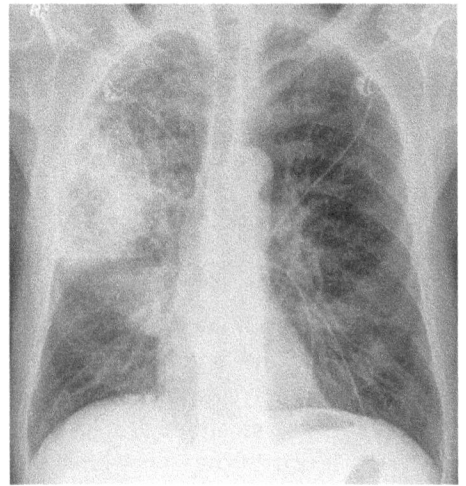

FIGURE 40.2: Chest X ray—right upper lobe pneumonia melioidosis.

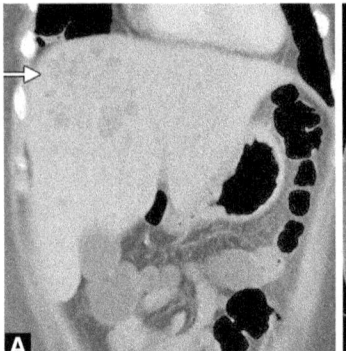 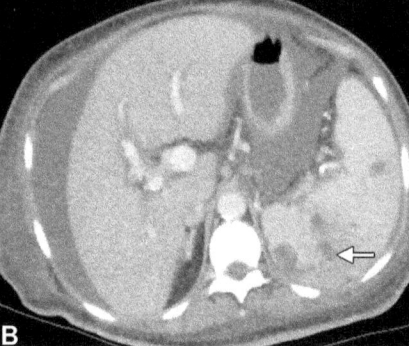 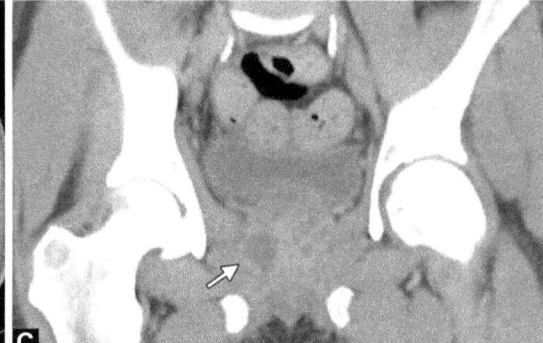

FIGURES 40.3A to C: CT images—melioidosis. (A) Coronal CT image showing a large liver abscess (arrow); (B) Axial CT image showing multiple splenic abscesses (arrow); (C) Coronal CT revealing a large prostatic abscess (arrow).

Table 40.2: Therapy for melioidosis.

Phase	Antibiotic	Dose[a]
Intensive	Meropenem (ICU/critically unwell)	1 g IV 8-hourly [Pediatric: 25 mg/kg (up to 1 g) IV 8-hourly] Or 2 g IV 8-hourly [Pediatric: 50 mg/kg (up to 2 g) IV 8-hourly] for cases with neurological involvement
Intensive	Ceftazidime (ward)	2 g IV 6-hourly [Pediatric: 50 mg/kg (up to 2 g) IV 6-hourly]
Intensive and eradication	Trimethoprim-sulfamethoxazole[b,c]	≥60 kg: 320 + 1600 mg orally 12-hourly 40–60 kg: 240 + 1200 mg orally 12-hourly [Pediatric: 6 + 30 mg/kg up to 240 + 1200 mg orally 12-hourly]
Eradication	Amoxicillin-clavulanate	20/5 mg/kg orally 8-hourly
Eradication	Doxycycline	100 mg orally 12-hourly (Pediatric: Not recommended)

[a] Dose adjust in renal failure
[b] Include trimethoprim-sulfamethoxazole in intensive phase if neurological, skin, soft tissue, bone, joint or prostatic infection
[c] Plus folic acid 5 mg PO daily (Pediatric: 0.1 mg/kg up to 5 mg) while on TMP-SMX

Table 40.3: Duration of antibiotic therapy.[32]

Site of infection	Minimum intravenous intensive phase duration (weeks)[a]	Eradication oral phase duration (months)
Cutaneous infection only	2	3
Bacteremia without focus	2	3
Pneumonia	2–4[b]	3
Prostatic abscess, deep seated collection or septic arthritis	4[c]	3
Osteomyelitis	6	6
Central nervous system infection	8	6
Mycotic aneurysm of other arterial infection	8	6

[a] If blood cultures remain positive at 7 days or slow clinical improvement use clinical judgment to prolong intensive phase duration
[b] 4 weeks if ICU admission or hilar or mediastinal lymphadenopathy >10 mm
[c] Intensive phase duration is timed from the last drainage or tissue specimen growing B. pseudomallei

of the study [chloramphenicol-doxycycline-trimethoprim-sulfamethoxazole (TMP-SMX)];[27] it has been drug of choice for the initial treatment of melioidosis since 1990.[4] Subsequent studies have shown that high dose imipenem is at least as effective as ceftazidime, with observational studies in Australia suggesting meropenem produces better outcomes than ceftazidime in patients with severe melioidosis.[28] Meropenem is therefore recommended for patients with septic shock or requiring admission to intensive care.[4]

The duration of the intensive phase should be a minimum of 10 to 14 days.[4] A longer period should be considered for critically ill patients, or for those with extensive pulmonary disease, deep seated collections, septic arthritis, osteomyelitis, central nervous system infection or arterial infection.[4,13] In Australia, due to the concern of poor adherence to oral eradication therapy a prolonged intensive phase has been adopted, with all patients receiving a minimum of 2 weeks intravenous antibiotics,[13] however the median duration of intensive therapy for patients is now 4 weeks.[4]

Trimethoprim-sulfamethoxazole is added to the regimen during the initial intensive phase in all patients with skin and soft tissue infection, neurological infection, bone or joint infection, and prostatic melioidosis.[4,13] Although Thai studies have shown no mortality benefit from the addition of TMP-SMX to ceftazidime,[29] the excellent tissue penetration of TMP-SMX is the rationale for recommending it as an additional therapy in these conditions.[4] All patients receiving TMP-SMX should routinely be given folic acid 5 mg (child: 0.1 mg/kg up to 5 mg) orally, daily.[13]

Primary or acquired resistance to ceftazidime is rare, but has been documented; resistance to meropenem is yet to have been identified, although decreased susceptibility has been reported.[4,30]

Eradication Phase

Oral eradication therapy after the initial intensive phase is considered necessary to reduce the risk of recurrence of melioidosis. TMP-SMX is considered the eradication antibiotic of choice and should be administered for a minimum of 3 months.[4] A Thai study has shown no benefit in the addition of doxycycline to TMP-SMX alone[31] and primary resistance to TMP-SMX is rare;[4] TMP-SMX is the recommended first line agent for the eradication phase.

Oral doxycycline may be considered an alternative for people who cannot tolerate TMP-SMX, or oral amoxicillin-clavulanate as an alternative to doxycycline in children and pregnancy, however acquired resistance is well documented for both.[4]

Studies have shown the failure of the eradication phase is more likely with poor compliance, more severe disease and a duration of eradication phase of less than 8 weeks; the current recommendation that the eradication phase be at least 3 to 6 months.[4]

Other Therapeutic Aspects

High-level intensive care management has led to a decrease in mortality in patients with severe melioidosis[33] and organ support and management of patients with severe disease should follow standard intensive care practices. The empirical use of granulocyte-colony stimulating factor (G-CSF) in intensive care patients with melioidosis induced septic shock remains controversial. Theoretically G-CSF may counteract the neutrophil functional defects believed to be important in the development of severe disease.[34] Observational data from Darwin, Australia showed a significant improvement in survival with the use of G-CSF, although other improvements in patient management were confounding factors in that series.[34] A further randomized controlled trial in Thailand failed to show a mortality benefit in the administration of G-CSF to patients with severe sepsis caused by suspected melioidosis.[35] Further studies into the use of G-CSF would be beneficial.

Prostatic abscesses usually require drainage, as do other large abscesses, however smaller abscesses, such as those in the liver or spleen usually respond to antibiotic therapy alone.[4] Septic arthritis often requires multiple wash-outs in theater and aggressive debridement of necrotic bone is also commonly required.[4] There is an increasing recognition of mycotic aneurysms, which require urgent surgery and often prosthetic grafts. For patients with prosthetic grafts life-long suppression therapy with TMP-SMX is recommended.[4]

REFERENCES

1. Limmathurotsakul D, Golding N, Dance DAB, et al. Predicted global distribution of *Burkholderia pseudomallei* and burden of melioidosis. Nat Microbiol. 2016;1(1).
2. Limmathurotsakul D, Wongratanacheewin S, Teerawattanasook N, et al. Increasing incidence of human melioidosis in Northeast Thailand. Am J Trop Med Hyg. 2010;82(6):1113-7.
3. Parameswaran U, Baird RW, Ward LM, et al. Melioidosis at Royal Darwin Hospital in the big 2009-2010 wet season: comparison with the preceding 20 years. Med J Aust. 2012;196(5):345-8.
4. Currie BJ. Melioidosis: evolving concepts in epidemiology, pathogenesis, and treatment. Semin Respir Crit Care Med. 2015;36(1):111-25.
5. McLeod C, Morris PS, Bauert PA, et al. Clinical presentation and medical management of melioidosis in children: a 24-year prospective study in the Northern Territory of Australia and review of the literature. Clin Infect Dis. 2015;60(1):21-6.
6. Turner P, Kloprogge S, Miliya T, et al. A retrospective analysis of melioidosis in Cambodian children, 2009-2013. BMC Infectious Diseases. 2016;16(1):688.
7. Melioidosis RCN. Melioidosis Info 2018. [online] Available from: http://www.melioidosis.info/infobox.aspx?pageID=101 [Accessed November 2018].
8. Dan M. Melioidosis in Travelers: Review of the Literature. J Travel Med. 2015;22(6):410-4.
9. Smith S, Stewart JD, Tacon C, et al. Children with melioidosis in Far North Queensland are commonly bacteraemic and have a high case fatality rate. Communicable Diseases Intelligence Quarterly Report. 2017;41(4):E318-e21.
10. Cheng AC, Currie BJ. Melioidosis: epidemiology, pathophysiology, and management. Clin Microbiol Rev. 2005;18(2):383-416.
11. Kingsley PV, Leader M, Nagodawithana NS, et al. Melioidosis in Malaysia: A Review of Case Reports. PLoS Negl Trop Dis. 2016;10(12):e0005182.
12. Corea E, de Silva A, Thevanesam V. Melioidosis in Sri Lanka. Am J Trop Med Hyg. 2018;98(2):607-15.
13. Smith S, Hanson J, Currie B. Melioidosis: An Australian Perspective. "Tropical medicine and infectious disease." Trop Med Infect Dis. 2018;3(1). pii: E27.
14. Merritt AJ, Inglis TJJ. The Role of Climate in the Epidemiology of Melioidosis. Curr Trop Med Rep. 2017;4(4):185-91.
15. Amadasi S, Dal Zoppo S, Bonomini A, et al. A case of melioidosis probably acquired by inhalation of dusts during a helicopter flight in a healthy traveler returning from Singapore. J Travel Med. 2015;22(1):57-60.
16. Currie BJ, Mayo M, Anstey NM, et al. A cluster of melioidosis cases from an endemic region is clonal and is linked to the water supply using molecular typing of Burkholderia pseudomallei isolates. Am J Trop Med Hyg. 2001;65(3):177-9.
17. Green RN, Tuffnell PG. Laboratory acquired melioidosis. Am J Med. 1968;44(4):599-605.
18. Choy JL, Mayo M, Janmaat A, et al. Animal melioidosis in Australia. Acta Tropica. 2000;74(2-3):153-8.
19. Meumann EM, Cheng AC, Ward L, et al. Clinical features and epidemiology of melioidosis pneumonia: results from a 21-year study and review of the literature. Clin Infect Dis. 2012;54(3):362-9.
20. Currie BJ, Ward L, Cheng AC. The epidemiology and clinical spectrum of melioidosis: 540 cases from the 20 year Darwin prospective study. PLoS Negl Trop Dis. 2010;4(11):e900.
21. Stewart JD, Smith S, Binotto E, et al. The epidemiology and clinical features of melioidosis in Far North Queensland: Implications for patient management. PLoS Negl Trop Dis. 2017;11(3):e0005411.
22. Kozlowska J, Smith S, Roberts J, et al. Prostatic Abscess due to Burkholderia pseudomallei: Facilitating Diagnosis to Optimize Management. Am J Trop Med Hyg. 2018;98(1):227-30.
23. Maude RR, Vatcharapreechasakul T, Ariyaprasert P, et al. Prospective observational study of the frequency and features of intra-abdominal abscesses in patients with melioidosis in northeast Thailand. Transactions of the Royal Society of Tropical Medicine and Hygiene. 2012;106(10):629-31.

24. Wibulpolprasert B, Dhiensiri T. Visceral organ abscesses in melioidosis: sonographic findings. JCU. 1999;27(1):29-34.
25. Woods KL, Boutthasavong L, NicFhogartaigh C, et al. Evaluation of a rapid diagnostic test for the detection of Burkholderia pseudomallei in the Lao People's Democratic Republic. J Clin Microbiol. 2018.
26. Peeters M, Chung P, Lin H, et al. Diagnostic accuracy of the InBiOS AMD rapid diagnostic test for the detection of Burkholderia pseudomallei antigen in grown blood culture broth. Eur J Clin Microbiol Infect Dis. 2018;37(6):1169-77.
27. White NJ, Dance DA, Chaowagul W, et al. Halving of mortality of severe melioidosis by ceftazidime. Lancet (London, England). 1989;2(8665):697-701.
28. Cheng AC, Fisher DA, Anstey NM, et al. Outcomes of patients with melioidosis treated with meropenem. Antimicrob Agents Chemother. 2004;48(5):1763-5.
29. Chierakul W, Anunnatsiri S, Chaowagul W, et al. Addition of trimethoprim-sulfamethoxazole to ceftazidime during parenteral treatment of melioidosis is not associated with a long-term outcome benefit. Clin Infect Dis. 2007;45(4):521-3.
30. Sarovich DS, Webb JR, Pitman MC, et al. Raising the Stakes: Loss of efflux pump regulation decreases meropenem susceptibility in Burkholderia pseudomallei. Clin Infect Dis. 2018;67(2):243-50.
31. Chetchotisakd P, Chierakul W, Chaowagul W, et al. Trimethoprim-sulfamethoxazole versus trimethoprim-sulfamethoxazole plus doxycycline as oral eradicative treatment for melioidosis (MERTH): a multicentre, double-blind, non-inferiority, randomised controlled trial. Lancet (London, England). 2014;383(9919):807-14.
32. Pitman MC, Luck T, Marshall CS, et al. Intravenous therapy duration and outcomes in melioidosis: a new treatment paradigm. PLoS Negl Trop Dis. 2015;9(3):e0003586.
33. Stephens DP, Thomas JH, Ward LM, Currie BJ. Melioidosis causing critical illness: A review of 24 years of experience from the Royal Darwin Hospital ICU. Critical Care Med. 2016;44(8):1500-5.
34. Cheng AC, Stephens DP, Anstey NM, Currie BJ. Adjunctive granulocyte colony-stimulating factor for treatment of septic shock due to melioidosis. Clin Infect Dis. 2004;38(1):32-7.
35. Cheng AC, Limmathurotsakul D, Chierakul W, et al. A randomized controlled trial of granulocyte colony-stimulating factor for the treatment of severe sepsis due to melioidosis in Thailand. Clin Infect Dis. 2007;45(3):308-14.

SECTION 4

Organ Support in Critical Care

Outlines

41. Oxygen
42. Positive End-Expiratory Pressure
43. Driving Pressure in Acute Respiratory Distress Syndrome
44. Weaning from Ventilation
45. High-flow Nasal Cannula Respiratory Support
46. Evidence-based Review of Noninvasive Ventilation
47. Extracorporeal Membrane Oxygenation
48. Extracorporeal Carbon Dioxide Removal
49. Continuous Renal Replacement Therapy: An Update
50. Extracorporeal Blood Purification Therapy for Sepsis

CHAPTER 41

Oxygen

Brigitte Hollander, Ross Callum Freebairn

INTRODUCTION

Oxygen is an essential element for mammalian survival.[1] Being used in acute care medicine since 1885, it is almost ubiquitous in the treating the critically ill.[2,3] Current recommended practice comprises the use of the least inspiratory oxygen fraction (FiO_2) associated with an arterial oxygen partial pressure (PaO_2) between 55 mm Hg and 80 mm Hg or an arterial hemoglobin O_2 saturation between 88% and 95%, although in actual clinical practice there is considerable variation.[3-8]

The FiO_2 of air is 0.209, giving a sea level PaO_2 between 150 mm Hg and 160 mm Hg dependent upon humidity.[9] FiO_2 may be increased to as high as 1.0 by oxygen delivery devices.

ROLE OF OXYGEN

The primary role of oxygen is as a metabolic fuel.[9] In adults, normal oxygen consumption is about 250 mL/min, and 90% of oxygen consumption is as the final electron acceptor in the electron transfer chain in the mitochondria, during oxidative phosphorylation.[9] The aerobic process efficiently converts glucose into adenosine triphosphate (ATP), which is used as a cellular fuel. Aerobic oxidative phosphorylation yields 38 ATP per glucose molecule, whereas anaerobic metabolism only yields 2 ATP per glucose molecule. Adequate oxygen delivery to mitochondria facilitates efficient cellular metabolic function.

Pasteur's point: The minimum mitochondrial PaO_2 to achieve aerobic metabolism is 1-4 mm Hg. The oxygen flux (DO_2) is the product of cardiac output (CO) and oxygen content of delivered blood.[3] In normal circumstances, over 98% of oxygen is carried bound to hemoglobin, the remainder being dissolved.

$DO_2 = CO \times [(\text{oxygen saturation } (SaO_2) \times Hb \times 1.39) + (PaO_2 \times 0.03)]$.

Supply of oxygen to the tissues, in adequate amount, maintains aerobic metabolism.[6] In clinical practice, these physiological factors are not routinely measured, and surrogate markers are used to determine sufficient aerobic tissue oxygenation.[6]

Surrogate markers include aerobic and anaerobic markers, aerobic being absolute oxygen levels (PaO_2), or hemoglobin SaO_2, while anaerobic measures include lactate and CO_2 production.[6]

NORMAL PHYSIOLOGICAL ADAPTATIONS

In abnormal health states, physiological adaptations to maintain aerobic cellular metabolism utilize an interplay between the cardiovascular and respiratory systems.

Positive cooperativity, i.e. increased affinity for oxygen (O_2) to bind to hemoglobin protein with the binding of each O_2 molecule, until it is saturated with four O_2 molecules, gives the oxyhemaglobin dissociation curve its sigmoidal shape.

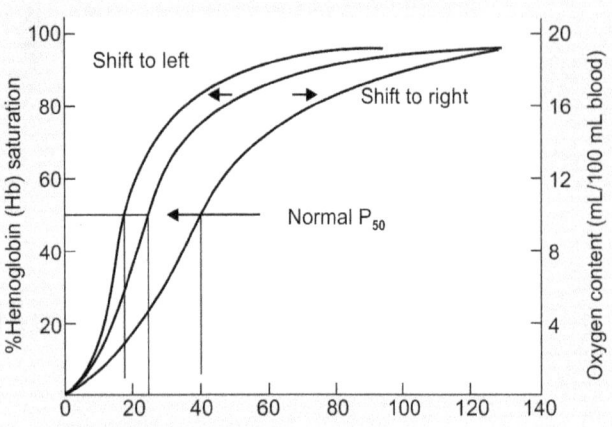

FIGURE 41.1: Oxyhemoglobin dissociation curve.
Source: Askew J, Chacko B, Chan K, et al. BASIC sciences. The scientific basis of intensive care for clinicians, 1st edition. Department of Anaesthesia & Intensive Care; The Chinese University of Hong Kong; 2018.

The shape of the oxyhemoglobin dissociation curve supports the clinical acceptance of a $PaO_2 \geq 60$ mm Hg because this value is on the "precipice" of the steep downslope.[7] Its shape also demonstrates that SaO_2, greater than mid-90s, can also reflect a wide range of high PaO_2 levels (Fig. 41.1).

Certain physiological states change the curve's shape, with a rightward shift increasing oxygen offloading from hemoglobin to the tissues, and a leftward shift decreasing offloading. A rightward shift is induced by increased $PaCO_2$, body temperature, 2,3-diphosphoglycerate, and hydronium ion concentration (decreased pH).

Right or leftward shift of the curve allows the preservation of the tissue DO_2 to maintain aerobic cellular metabolism during abnormal physiological states.

Hypoxemia results in peripheral vasodilation, ameliorating tissue hypoxemia by increasing the tissues blood flow. Hyperoxia results in peripheral vasoconstriction.[10] The pulmonary vasculature response to hypoxia differs from systemic circulation, resulting in pulmonary vasoconstriction. This reduces the perfusion of poorly oxygenated respiratory units, reducing the respiratory shunt, utilizing the most efficient units of the pulmonary system.

OXYGEN AS A DRUG

Medical oxygen is 99.5% O_2 (and 0.4% argon) and is presented completely dehumidified.

Conditioning of oxygen requires mixing (with air) to achieve the desired concentration and humidification.[11]

Supplemental oxygen therapy can be achieved using an external interface (nasal cannulae or face mask) or by advanced ventilatory assistance (endotracheal tube and mechanical ventilation).[3]

OXYGEN CASCADE

Oxygen concentration in the alveoli is determined by the alveolar gas equation, with atmospheric temperature, inspired FiO_2, temperature-dependent humidification, alveolar carbon dioxide, and the respiratory quotient all being determinants. The alveolar gas equation reflects ventilation of atmospheric gas and oxygen delivery to the alveoli.

Alveolar gas equation:
$$PaO_2 = [FiO_2 \times (Patm - PH_2O)] - (PaCO_2/RQ)$$

PaO_2: Partial pressure alveolar oxygen
FiO_2: Fraction inspired oxygen
Patm: Atmospheric pressure
PH_2O: Saturated water vapour pressure, 47 mm Hg at 37°C
$PaCO_2$: Partial pressure arterial CO_2
RQ: Respiratory quotient—in normal lung = 0.8

Atmospheric Pressure

The atmospheric FiO_2 is relatively constant at 0.209 (20.9%), the concentration in moles per unit volume falls with the ambient atmospheric pressure, which in turn is related to the altitude above sea level. Meteorological variations in atmospheric pressure in most environments are inconsequential. In many hospitals, atmospheric pressure approximates sea level, although at higher altitudes (Table 41.1), the reduced atmospheric pressure requires appropriate compensatory strategies.[10,12] While clinicians in higher altitude hospitals are usually aware of the atmospheric pressure, the "cabin pressure" in commercial or aeromedical flights may be underappreciated (Table 41.2). Even at a modest 1,000 m cabin pressure, there is a 10% drop in atmospheric pressure. While minor deficits are easily overcome by increased FiO_2, at high FiO_2, the increase may be insufficient. Pressurizing aircraft substantially reduces the problem. Further readings on the physiological effects of altitude are well covered by other reviews.[13,14]

Fraction of Inspired Oxygen

Closed systems provide supplemental oxygen in a known fraction. Open systems incorporate a low air entrainment, diluting oxygen concentrations reducing the overall inspired fraction. Final inspired fractions are determined by the maximum gas flow, the breathing pattern (including mouth

Table 41.1: The elevation, population, and atmospheric pressures of Asian cities at higher altitudes (various sources).

Country	City	Population	Elevation (m)	Patm air (mm Hg)	Patm O$_2$ (mm Hg)	FiO$_2$ required for sea level PO$_2$
Iran	Tehran	8,847	1,235	658	138	0.24
Mongolia	Ulan Bator	1,372,000	1,284	654	137	0.24
Nepal	Kathmandu	985,000	1,298	653	137	0.24
Nepal	Patan	284,922	1,318	652	136	0.24
Nepal	Pokhara	414,141	1,400	646	135	0.25
Vietnam	Da Lat	305,509	1,500	638	133	0.25
Philippines	Baguio	345,366	1,540	635	133	0.25
India	Srinagar	1,192,792	1,585	632	132	0.25
Pakistan	Quetta	1,001,205	1,680	625	131	0.25
Afghanistan	Kabul	3,678,034	1,807	616	129	0.26
China	Kunming	6,626,000	1,892	610	127	0.26
India	Darjeeling	132,016	2,042	599	125	0.27
Iran	Shahr-e Kord	148,464	2,070	597	125	0.27
India	Shimla	171,817	2,205	588	123	0.27
Pakistan	Skardu	214,848	2,228	586	123	0.27
Yemen	Sana'a	1,937,451	2,253	584	122	0.27
Saudi Arabia	Abha	781,206	2,270	583	122	0.27
China	Xining	1,198,304	2,275	583	122	0.27
Bhutan	Thimbu	114,551	2,320	580	121	0.27
Iran	Fereydunshahr	14,007	2,490	569	119	0.28
China	Kangding	100,000	2,560	564	118	0.28
China	Golmud	205,700	2,809	548	114	0.29
Tibet (CN)	Lhasa	223,001	3,490	506	106	0.31
China	Shigatse	117,000	3,836	486	102	0.33
India	Karzok	1,291	4,570	446	93	0.36

Table 41.2: Commercial aircraft flying altitudes, with the cabin altitude air and partial pressures of oxygen.

	Commercial aircraft	Maximum flying altitude (m)	Cabin altitude (m)	Patm air (mm Hg)	Patm O$_2$ (mm Hg)	FiO$_2$ required for sea level PO$_2$
FAA		13,000	2,400	575	120	0.28
Boeing	B767	12,000	2,100	595	124	0.27
Boeing	787 & 777X	12,000	1,800	616	129	0.26
Airbus	A380	13,000	1,868	611	128	0.26
Depressurization	Maximum allowed cabin altitude in A380		13,000	167	35	0.95

(FAA: Federal Aviation Administration)

Source: http://rgl.faa.gov/Regulatory_and_Guidance_Library%5CrgPolicy.nsf/0/90AA20C2F35901D98625713F0056B1B8?OpenDocument accessed 9/1/19

and nose proportions), the type of delivery device (e.g. face-mask type), and application to the patient's face. Nasal oxygen, previously using low flow rates, can be safely utilized at much higher flows with appropriate humidification and cannula. High-flow nasal cannulae (HFNC) such as Optiflow® (Fisher and Paykel, Auckland, New Zealand) can provide gas flows that match peak inspiratory flows minimizing air entrainment, allowing delivery of known constant FiO_2. HFNC are also capable of providing low level of positive airway pressure,[12] a reduction in dead space through upper airway flushing, and improved mucociliary clearance. Increasing flow, as well as increasing carrier gas oxygen concentration, may optimize inspired oxygen flow; for maximal efficiency, gas flows need to be matched with the peak inspiratory flow (*see* Chapter 45: High-flow Nasal Cannula Respiratory Support). While HFNC increase survival in selected patients and are well tolerated, concerns that the HFNC may mask deterioration and delay intervention exist. It is contraindicated in undrained pneumothorax and is only used with extreme caution in any situation where positive airway pressure is potentially harmful.[3]

Humidification

Room air is partially humidified, and humidification occurs in the normal upper airway. In quiet breathing, 100% relative humidity is achieved by the end of the trachea.[9] Medical oxygen is a dry gas, which in invasive ventilation bypasses the humidifying upper airways resulting in mucosal drying unless the gas is conditioned. Even when using noninvasive techniques, high dry gas flows induce trachea land bronchiole mucosal damage and contribute to patient discomfort.[14,15] Critical illness increases the risk of mucosal damage, with loss of ciliary elevator function that contributes to secretion retention. Mucosal damage is a function of poor humidification, rather than increased FiO_2, and using an appropriate humidification system prevents damage. For nonrebreathing open systems, heat and moisture exchangers have limited effectiveness, while heated water bath humidifiers provide effective humidification even if gas is not rebreathed.[16,17]

The inspired gas will always have 100% relative humidity when it reaches the alveoli, further reducing the PaO_2.

Alveolar Pressure

Oxygenation is increased by increased alveolar pressure. Ventilation assists devices achieve this in a number of ways; first by raising the tidal volume (or driving pressure if using pressure control), second changing the inspiratory expiratory profile to either extend total inspiratory time or increase inspiratory pause time, or both, and finally by increasing the positive end-expiratory pressure (PEEP).

The mean alveolar pressure increases the PaO_2 in the alveoli, so it directly increases the pressure driving oxygen into the pulmonary capillary; each of the above manipulations increases oxygenation by other mechanisms.

- Increasing tidal volume increases minute ventilation and thus lowers alveolar carbon dioxide resulting in increased alveolar oxygen (see alveolar gas equation above).
- Increasing inspiratory time or increasing pause time allows more alveolar filling time, increasing ventilation of alveoli with long-time constants, i.e. those alveoli with high compliance or high resistance, decreasing ventilation perfusion (V/Q) mismatching and reducing the overall shunt fraction.
- Increasing PEEP not only raises mean alveolar pressure but also reopens or prevents the tidal collapse of alveoli, reducing shunt and V/Q mismatch.

Shunt, Dead Space, and *V/Q* Mismatch

The adult lung as a whole receives about 4 L/min alveolar ventilation (*V*) and 5 L/min blood flow (*Q*), $V/Q = 0.8$. The *V/Q* mismatch is a ratio of ventilation: perfusion limited by the two extremes of shunt and dead space. The shunt is wasted perfusion, it is the blood delivered to the pulmonary system that is not ventilated. The dead space is wasted ventilation, it is ventilation delivered to alveoli that are not perfused.

DYSOXIA

Dysoxia from either too much or too little oxygen can both result in host injury in the setting of critical illness. Efforts to avoid injurious ventilator settings, unopposed atelectasis, vasoconstriction, loss of hypoxic ventilatory drive, and free radical injury from high oxygen levels need to balance the putative benefits of "adequate" oxygen delivery.

The alternative risk of marginal hypoxemia is neither well studied nor defined.[18] Recent suspicion that "permissive" hypoxemia while "survivable" may have long-term neurocognitive sequelae and other morbidity needs to be examined further.[18-24] As the tissue DO_2 (or oxygen delivery) is the product of both CO and oxygen content of arterial blood, oxygen delivery to tissue is dependent upon the intimate relationship between the cardiovascular and respiratory systems.[3] High flow, high content, but poorly saturated blood, may ameliorate or even prevent hypoxic damage. Conversely dangers of low PaO_2 may be compounded when other parameters of oxygen delivery such as hemoglobin are compromised.[25] Analysis of the Fuoride and Caring for Children's Teeth (FACCT) study identified that lower PaO_2 in the intensive care unit (ICU) was a significant risk factor for long-term cognitive impairment at a 1-year follow-up, even after adjusting for numerous potential confounders.[21]

Downward titration of oxygen therapy to recommended targets is often given a lower priority, despite evidence that overoxygenation levels may be detrimental.[5] Damage can be as a result of: hyperbaric oxygen, increased inspired oxygen concentrations, increased PaO_2 in the bloodstream or raised tissue oxygen delivery levels.

Hyperbaric Oxygen

Hyperbaric oxygen therapy and its associated toxicity are beyond the scope of this review, but the effects of increased PaO_2 in hyperbaric air, or oxygen-enhanced hyperbaric mixtures, include the other adverse effects listed below.

Increased Inspired Oxygen Concentrations

Dysoxia can occur in the respiratory system. The respiratory tract can be exposed to higher inspired PaO_2 and pathophysiological changes occur, even if arterial partial pressure is not raised. High shunt fractions require higher inspired FiO_2. Alternative strategies to improve oxygenation, and thus to lower the required FiO_2, include raising the mean alveolar pressure through PEEP, tidal volume or inspiratory time, and profile (as discussed above), prone positioning, short-term neuromuscular blockade, and recruitment maneuvers. While pragmatically tempting, the short-term gain in oxygenation from unproven techniques may be unwise. Recent trials of combined recruitment and PEEP titration by compliance intervention resulted in an unexpected increase in mortality.[26]

High inspired PaO_2s can alter the mucous membranes and disrupt ciliary integrity, reactive oxygen species (ROS), and alveolar cellular changes alter surfactant activity and alveoli mechanics.[27-29] In addition, absorptive atelectasis results as a physiological phenomenon with increasing levels of inspiratory oxygen, and increased pulmonary infection has been described with raised FiO_2.[30,31] Changes in mucous membranes denuding cilia in respiratory systems occur as a functioning dry gas, higher flows in respiratory failure and of increased PaO_2.[28,29]

Increased Partial Pressure of Oxygen in the Bloodstream

The third area of dysoxia harm is that of increased PaO_2s in the blood. There are multiple mechanisms by which increased partial pressures can cause harm, the mechanism is largely through overproduction of ROS. These unwanted progeny of hyperoxia play a pivotal role in cellular signaling with manifold effects. When the body's homeostatic balance is disturbed in the critically ill, ROS promote a destructive cycle of tissue injury, characterized by cell damage, cell necrosis, accelerated apoptosis, and inflammation. While symptoms are often prominent in the respiratory system, where PaO_2s are highest, hyperoxia-induced vasoconstriction, altered organ blood flow, alimentary inflammation, necrosis, and other metabolic effects are also important.

Different organ vascular beds respond differently. In healthy lung, oxygen supplementation does not appear to increase global oxygen delivery.[32] Cardiovascular effects include vasoconstriction, which is possibly beneficial during vasodilatory shock, but hemodynamic changes impose risk when organ perfusion such as the coronary supply is impaired. Hyperoxia may considerably decrease CO and increase systemic vascular resistance, but effects differ between patient categories.[32,33] Heart failure patients appear to be the most sensitive, while no hemodynamic effects were seen in septic patients.[33] In contrast, avoiding modest hyperoxia during cardiopulmonary bypass failed to demonstrate any difference in acute kidney injury, markers of organ damage, or length of stay. In severe brain injury, acute hyperoxia significantly improved pressure autoregulation, while increased pulmonary artery and capillary oxygenation reduces pulmonary hypertension.[34]

Observational data suggest that in at least some critically ill, hyperoxia is associated with worse outcomes. Two large retrospective analyses of cardiac arrest outcomes identified that elevated arterial oxygenation was associated with worse outcomes than normoxia.[7,35] Meta-analysis of hyperoxia in a wide variety of clinical scenarios[36,37] also demonstrates overall harm. Adding weight to the argument is numerous strategies that have demonstrably improved arterial oxygenation (e.g. extracorporeal membrane oxygenation, inhaled nitric oxide) have failed to secure any meaningful improvement in clinical outcomes.[38-41] While it is commonly thought that the cellular damage in the critically ill is largely hypoxia driven, it seems that reversal of, or even prevention of this using hyperoxia, does not prevent the damage.

Observational data is fraught with limitations, including association bias. In a randomized interventional trial evaluating controlled oxygen therapy in ventilated patients by Girardi's and colleagues, patients were randomly assigned to receive one of two oxygen regimes.[42] The conservative group received oxygen therapy to maintain PaO_2 between 70 mm Hg and 100 mm Hg or arterial oxyhemoglobin saturation (SpO_2) between 94% and 98%, while the conventional control group were managed according to standard ICU practice, allowing PaO_2 values up to 150 mm Hg or SpO_2 values between 97% and 100%. Among the 434 critically ill patients with an ICU length of stay of 72 hours or longer, the ICU absolute mortality was 8.6% lower in the conservative protocol group compared to the standard group, with similar reductions in shock liver failure and bacteremia. Limitations of the study are that it was single center, it was stopped early following an unplanned interim analysis, and the patients that died within 72 hours were excluded from analysis. These thought-provoking findings require further study to see if this remarkable finding is reproduced. A recently completed Australia and New Zealand study looked at 1,000 patients receiving ventilation in ICU who were randomized to receive either "standard therapy" or "conservative therapy."[43] Similar to Girardi's study, a conservative group had strict protocols to lower the FiO_2 to attain a targeted saturation range, with a standard care control group. The trial has completed enrollment with results of follow-up and analysis expected in early 2019. A pilot study demonstrated that there was separation of saturation between the two groups.[44] While the trial is large, prospective, and randomized, the controlled intervention is limited to the ventilation period in intensive care. The periods immediately prior to and following ventilation, even while in ICU, were not controlled, and many patients would have received high flow oxygen therapy, contaminating any beneficial effect, and raising the potential of a type-two error, despite the large sample size. We await the results.

Raised Tissue Oxygen Delivery Levels

In the critically ill, individual organs may have specific oxygen starvation through reduced blood supply in the presence of normal hemoglobin oxygen content. Increasing content of oxygen to overcome this isolated ischemic hypoxia results in systemic over supply of oxygen, creating the risk of free radical production and subsequent morbidity. Enhancing oxygen delivery, titrated by optimizing CO, oxygen delivery and consumption has been advocated to improve outcomes in sepsis and trauma. Initial reports were promising, but subsequent robustly designed trials demonstrated no benefit and suggested that harm may arise.[20,45-47]

Use of superior vena cava oxygen saturations to titrate resuscitation against systemic oxygen demand was popularized by Rivers in 2001.[48] River's study population of septic shock patients received dobutamine and transfused blood to enhance oxygen delivery, titrated to achieve venous saturations greater than 75%, had an absolute mortality 16% lower than similar patients receiving standard therapy.[48] Three large multicenter randomized controlled trials conducted in three continents to validate the original findings, analyzed separately and together, failed to demonstrate any patient benefit. This suggests that early goal-directed therapy titrated to elevate venous oxygen saturations through increased oxygen delivery, while not harmful, is of no benefit.[49] In pathologies where critical hypoxic ischemia may occur, such as in severe head trauma, optimal oxygen levels remain controversial, but evidence of the putative benefits of enhanced oxygen delivery on outcome is largely lacking.[50]

CONCLUSION

Oxygen is a necessity of life, and delivery to the tissue is a complex and intricate process. As critical illness can interfere with oxygen delivery, supplemental oxygen use is commonly employed. Although most clinical outcomes are still under extensive investigation, careful titration of oxygen supply is warranted in order to secure adequate tissue oxygenation while preventing hyperoxia harm seems wise. There appears to be no evidence that elevated levels of oxygen are systemically useful, and although hypoxemia needs to be avoided, excessive oxygen levels have the potential to be dangerous, and should, through vigilance and care be avoided. Use of techniques other than raised FiO_2 to maintain arterial oxygen in the recommended range should be considered.

REFERENCES

1. McEvoy JW. Excess oxygen in acute illness: adding fuel to the fire. Lancet. 2018;391(10131):1640-2.
2. Chu DK, Kim LH, Young PJ, et al. Mortality and morbidity in acutely ill adults treated with liberal versus conservative oxygen therapy (IOTA): a systematic review and meta-analysis. Lancet. 2018;391(10131):1693-705.
3. McHugh G, Freebairn R. Optimal oxygen therapy in the critically ill patient with respiratory failure. Curr Respir Med Rev. 2010;6(4):229-37.
4. de Graaff AE, Dongelmans DA, Binnekade JM, et al. Clinicians' response to hyperoxia in ventilated patients in a Dutch ICU depends on the level of FiO_2. Intensive Care Med. 2011;37(1):46-51.
5. Young PJ, Beasley RW, Capellier G, et al.; ANZICS Clinical Trials Group and the George Institute for Global Health. Oxygenation targets, monitoring in the critically ill: a point prevalence study of clinical practice in Australia and New Zealand. Crit Care Resusc. 2015;17(3):202-7.
6. Eastwood GM, Reade MC, Peck L, et al. Intensivists' opinion and self-reported practice of oxygen therapy. Anaesth Intensive Care. 2011;39(1):122-6.
7. Kilgannon JH, Jones AE, Shapiro NI, et al. Association between arterial hyperoxia following resuscitation from cardiac arrest and in-hospital mortality. JAMA. 2010;303(21):2165-71.

8. Egi M, Kataoka J, Ito T, et al. Oxygen management in mechanically ventilated patients: a multicenter prospective observational study. J Crit Care. 2018;46:1-5.
9. Lumb AB. Nunn's applied respiratory physiology, 8th edition; Edinburgh; New York: Elsevier; 2017. xii, p. 544.
10. Welsh DG, Jackson WF, Segal SS. Oxygen induces electromechanical coupling in arteriolar smooth muscle cells: a role for L-type Ca^{2+} channels. Am J Physiol. 1998;274(6 Pt 2):H2018-24.
11. BOC. (2016). Compressed Medical Oxygen Medicinal gas, compressed package leaflet: information for the user. [online] Available from http://www.bochealthcare.co.uk/en/images/505550-Patient%20Information%20Leaflet-Compressed%20Oxygen_%28REV4%29%28PRINT%29_tcm409-103365.pdf.
12. Interactive altitude calculators. HYPERLINK "http://Altitude.org" Altitude.org: a high altitude resource. [online] Available from http://www.altitude.org/air_pressure.php.
13. Leissner KB, Mahmood FU. Physiology and pathophysiology at high altitude: considerations for the anesthesiologist. J Anesth. 2009;23(4):543-53.
14. Luks AM. Physiology in medicine: a physiologic approach to prevention and treatment of acute high-altitude illnesses. J Appl Physiol (1985). 2015;118(5):509-19.
15. Chanques G, Constantin JM, Sauter M, et al. Discomfort associated with underhumidified high-flow oxygen therapy in critically ill patients. Intensive Care Med. 2009;35(6):996-1003.
16. Williams R, Rankin N, Smith T, et al. Relationship between the humidity and temperature of inspired gas and the function of the airway mucosa. Crit Care Med. 1996;24(11):1920-9.
17. Sottiaux T, Mignolet G, Damas P, et al. Comparative evaluation of three heat and moisture exchangers during short-term postoperative mechanical ventilation. Chest. 1993;104(1):220-4.
18. Gilbert-Kawai ET, Mitchell K, Martin D, Carlisle J, Grocott MPW. Permissive hypoxaemia versus normoxaemia for mechanically ventilated critically ill patients. Cochrane Database of Systematic Reviews. 2014;2014(5).
19. Hopkins RO, Jackson JC. Long-term neurocognitive function after critical illness. Chest. 2006;130(3):869-78.
20. Hayes MA, Timmins AC, Yau E, et al. Elevation of systemic oxygen delivery in the treatment of critically ill patients. N Engl J Med. 1994;330(24):1717-22.
21. Mikkelsen ME, Christie JD, Lanken PN, et al. The adult respiratory distress syndrome cognitive outcomes study: long-term neuropsychological function in survivors of acute lung injury. Am J Respir Crit Care Med. 2012;185(12):1307-15.
22. Asher SR, Curry P, Sharma D, et al. Survival advantage and PaO_2 threshold in severe traumatic brain injury. J Neurosurg Anesthesiol. 2013;25(2):168-73.
23. Hopkins RO, Weaver LK, Pope D, et al. Neuropsychological sequelae and impaired health status in survivors of severe acute respiratory distress syndrome. Am J Respir Crit Care Med. 1999;160(1):50-6.
24. Tarnow-Mordi W, Stenson B, Kirby A, et al. Outcomes of two trials of oxygen-saturation targets in preterm infants. N Engl J Med. 2016;374(8):749-60.
25. Ramanan M, Fisher N. The association between arterial oxygen tension, hemoglobin concentration, and mortality in mechanically ventilated critically ill patients. Indian J Crit Care Med. 2018;22(7):477-84.
26. Cavalcanti AB, Suzumura ÉA, Laranjeira LN, et al. Effect of lung recruitment and titrated positive end-expiratory pressure (PEEP) vs low PEEP on mortality in patients with acute respiratory distress syndrome—a randomized clinical trial. JAMA. 2017;318(14):1335-45.
27. Zenri H, Rodriquez-Capote K, McCaig L, et al. Hyperoxia exposure impairs surfactant function and metabolism. Crit Care Med. 2004;32(5):1155-60.
28. Rankin HV, Moody AJ, Moate RM, et al. Elevated oxygen fraction reduces cilial abundance in explanted human bronchial tissue. Ultrastruct Pathol. 2007;31(5):339-46.
29. Obara H, Sekimoto M, Iwai S. Alterations to the bronchial and bronchiolar surfaces of adult mice after exposure to high concentrations of oxygen. Thorax. 1979;34(4):479-85.
30. Nußbaum B, Radermacher P, Asfar P, et al. Does hyperoxia enhance susceptibility to secondary pulmonary infection in the ICU?. Crit Care. 2016;20(1):239.
31. Edmark L, Auner U, Enlund M, et al. Oxygen concentration and characteristics of progressive atelectasis formation during anaesthesia. Acta Anaesthesiol Scand. 2011;55(1):75-81.
32. McGuinness SP, Parke RL, Drummond K, et al. A multicenter, randomized, controlled Phase IIb trial of avoidance of hyperoxemia during cardiopulmonary bypass. Anesthesiology. 2016;125(3):465-73.
33. Smit B, Smulders YM, van der Wouden JC, et al. Hemodynamic effects of acute hyperoxia: systematic review and meta-analysis. Crit Care. 2018;22(1):45.
34. Rangel-Castilla L, Lara LR, Gopinath S, et al. Cerebral hemodynamic effects of acute hyperoxia and hyperventilation after severe traumatic brain injury. J Neurotrauma. 2010;27(10):1853-63.
35. Bellomo R, Bailey M, Eastwood GM, et al. Arterial hyperoxia and in-hospital mortality after resuscitation from cardiac arrest. Crit Care. 2011;15(2):R90.
36. You J, Fan X, Bi X, et al. Association between arterial hyperoxia and mortality in critically ill patients: a systematic review and meta-analysis. J Crit Care. 2018;47:260-8.
37. Helmerhorst HJF, Roos-Blom MJ, Van Westerloo DJ, et al. Association between arterial hyperoxia and outcome in subsets of critical illness: a systematic review, meta-analysis, and meta-regression of cohort studies. Crit Care Med. 2015;43(7):1508-19.
38. Taylor RW, Zimmerman JL, Dellinger RP, et al. Low-dose inhaled nitric oxide in patients with acute lung injury: a randomized controlled trial. JAMA. 2004;291(13):1603-9.
39. Adhikari NK, Burns KE, Friedrich JO, et al. Effect of nitric oxide on oxygenation and mortality in acute lung injury: systematic review and meta-analysis. BMJ. 2007;334(7597):779.
40. Zapol WM, Snider MT, Hill JD, et al. Extracorporeal membrane oxygenation in severe acute respiratory failure. A randomized prospective study. JAMA. 1979;242(20):2193-6.
41. Combes A, Hajage D, Capellier G, et al. Extracorporeal membrane oxygenation for severe acute respiratory distress syndrome. N Engl J Med. 2018;378(21):1965-75.

42. Girardis M, Busani S, Damiani E, et al. Effect of conservative vs conventional oxygen therapy on mortality among patients in an intensive care unit: the oxygen-ICU randomized clinical trial. JAMA. 2016;316(15):1583-9.
43. Mackle DM, Bailey MJ, Beasley RW, et al. Protocol summary and statistical analysis plan for the intensive care unit randomised trial comparing two approaches to oxygen therapy (ICU-ROX). Crit Care Resusc. 2018;20(1):22-32.
44. Young PJ, Mackle DM, Bailey MJ, et al. Intensive care unit randomised trial comparing two approaches to oxygen therapy (ICU-ROX): results of the pilot phase. Crit Care Resusc. 2017;19(4):344-54.
45. Yu M, Levy MM, Smith P, et al. Effect of maximizing oxygen delivery on morbidity and mortality rates in critically ill patients: a prospective randomized, controlled study. Crit Care Med. 1993;21(6):830-8.
46. Fleming A, Bishop M, Shoemaker W, et al. Prospective trial of supranormal values as goals of resuscitation in severe trauma. Arch Surg. 1992;127(10):1175-81.
47. Wetterslev J, Meyhoff CS, Jorgensen LN, Gluud C, Lindschou J, Rasmussen LS. The effects of high perioperative inspiratory oxygen fraction for adult surgical patients. The Cochrane database of systematic reviews. 2015(6):Cd008884..
48. Rivers E, Nguyen B, Havstad S, et al. Early goal-directed therapy in the treatment of severe sepsis and septic shock. N Engl J Med. 2001;345(19):1368-77.
49. Rowan KM, Angus DC, Bailey M, et al. Early, goal-directed therapy for septic shock—a patient-level meta-analysis. N Engl J Med. 2017;376(23):2223-34.
50. Lång M, Skrifvars MB, Siironen J, et al. A pilot study of hyperoxemia on neurological injury, inflammation and oxidative stress. Acta Anaesthesiol Scand. 2018;62(6):801-10.

CHAPTER 42

Positive End-Expiratory Pressure

Ross Callum Freebairn, Ravi N Mistry, Michael AJ Park

DEFINITION

Positive end-expiratory pressure (PEEP) is the supra-atmospheric alveolar pressure at end expiration. During positive-pressure ventilation, it is the pressure applied to the breathing circuit in expiratory phase (extrinsic PEEP), or the result of residual alveolar pressure at end expiration (intrinsic PEEP). While not identical to PEEP, continuous positive airway pressure and expiratory positive airway pressure also provide external PEEP. The provision of PEEP increases the end-expiratory lung volume (EELV), reduces alveolar collapse, and increases arterial oxygenation.

HISTORY

Positive end-expiratory pressure was not routinely used in ventilation in the early years, but a form of PEEP was described by Poulton in 1936.[1] The original acute respiratory distress syndrome (ARDS) description by Ashbaugh and colleagues advocated the benefits of PEEP.[2] Initial cautious intervention was with "physiologic PEEP" although Downs's recommendation that PEEP be increased to obtain optimal PaO_2 without hemodynamic compromise led to the use of "super PEEP" as high as 60 cmH_2O to affect the greatest reduction in shunt fraction.[3-6] This led to overdistention of at least some parts of the lungs. The "best PEEP" concept was suggested by Suter et al. in 1975, with "best PEEP" being the lower inflection point (LIP) on the inspiratory compliance curve.[4] Early application of PEEP was thought to prevent ARDS, but initial comparisons of a fixed PEEP to no PEEP in trauma patients did not demonstrate benefit.[7,8] In the 1990s, Lachmann's "Open Lung" approach advocated setting PEEP to keep the lungs fully open at end expiration.[9] While PEEP use in intensive care unit is routine, with harm arising from very low or absent PEEP in lung-protective ventilation strategies in ARDS, methods and indications for titrating higher PEEP, and use in other conditions is less well defined.[7,8,10-12] While recruitment maneuvers are frequently used in combination with PEEP titration, for brevity, this review will examine PEEP titration alone.

GENERAL PHYSIOLOGY

Physiological benefits of PEEP may differ between patients.[13] PEEP raises the peak alveolar (or "plateau") pressure and increases oxygen transfer to the pulmonary capillaries. In addition, PEEP and the end-expiratory compliance determine the EELV, which is the ventilated equivalent of the functional residual capacity (FRC). By raising the end-expiratory pressure, additional PEEP splints opens, recruits, and/or prevents tidal derecruitment of collapsed or collapsible small airways and alveolar units.[14,15] Setting PEEP appropriately is the balance between maintaining alveolar recruitment and small airway patency whilst avoiding alveolar overdistention and cardiovascular compromise.

Positive end-expiratory pressure has a myriad of effects on the cardiovascular, renal, metabolic, and neurologic systems as well as the respiratory system, all of which may influence morbidity and mortality. A relevant example is that the protective effects of PEEP against edema formation shown in some studies contrasts with increased lung edema with increasing PEEP shown in other studies.[16-18] PEEP's protective effect may also be mediated, not by a direct action on the lungs, but by decreased cardiac output or reduced pulmonary blood volume.

Positive end-expiratory pressure precipitates altered respiratory mechanics and pulmonary vascular changes, which changes cardiac output, which in turn results in reactive changes to the cardiocirculatory system. Importantly PEEP alters pulmonary vascular resistance. An optimized lung volume may prevent extra-alveolar vessel tethering in the setting of collapsed parenchyma, or, in contrast, limit overdistension and collapse of intra-alveolar vessels. PEEP modulates performance of left ventricular fibers, increasing contractility, with reduction in left ventricular strain.[19]

The complexity of the effects is such that while surrogate markers may be indicative, patient-centered outcome studies are necessary to demonstrate real benefit of any strategy. It is unlikely that a strategy focused on a single organ system, or physiologic endpoint, will lead to ideal PEEP titration.

POSITIVE END-EXPIRATORY PRESSURE TITRATION

Positive end-expiratory pressure oxygenation tables are commonly used but a variety of alternate strategies to titrate PEEP, have been studied; using carbon dioxide exchange, determining maximum hysteresis or the maximum compliance on the inspiratory and expiratory curve, as well as estimates of the lower inflection point (LIP) or "point of derecruitment" (PDR) and dead space.[20-22] Two recently highlighted concepts—first the driving pressure (ΔP), rather than the plateau pressure, appears to be the most injurious, and second that transalveolar pressures rather than absolute pleural pressure are important in optimizing ventilation, have changed the understanding of PEEP and recruitment.[23-25] In patients with low respiratory compliance, or with spontaneous breathing, differentiating between chest wall, pleural, or lung parenchyma abnormality may alter optimal PEEP settings.[25,26]

Amato et al. recent post hoc analysis of 3,562 subjects with ARDS from nine randomized controlled trials evaluated the relationships between "driving pressure" and mortality.[25] Driving pressure defined as Pplat - PEEP is the denominator of the compliance equation: Compliance = Tidal Volume (V_T)/Driving pressure. Amato's post hoc analysis found an associated increased mortality when driving pressure was >15 cmH$_2$O. It is unfortunate that their "driving pressure" definition incorporates both the component lung and chest wall expansion and could not isolate the "transalveolar driving pressure," which is damaging the lung parenchyma. As earlier studies did not separate the differences in lung and chest wall compliance, this component will need to be re-examined.

These findings have implications for PEEP titration. If increased PEEP produces overdistention, driving pressure will increase with a potential reduced survival; alternatively, if PEEP reopens lung units, compliance will fall and with it the driving pressure.

GAS EXCHANGE: OXYGEN POSITIVE END-EXPIRATORY PRESSURE TABLES

Arterial oxygen or pulse oximetry saturation is a commonly targeted when titrating PEEP for a patient ventilated with ARDS. The Acute Respiratory Distress Syndrome Clinical Network (ARDSnet) protocol (and subsequent trials) titrated PEEP and FiO$_2$ according to a PEEP and FiO$_2$ table, targeting SpO$_2$ (88-95%) or PaO$_2$ (55-80 mm Hg).[27] This was cited as being how PEEP was traditionally adjusted in clinical practice at the study hospitals and was advocated as the best evidence-based practice at the time (Table 42.1).[28]

Table 42.1: Potential methods of PEEP titration proposed with ARDS and other conditions.

Titration principle	Titration method	Examples
Gas exchange	• FiO$_2$ and PEEP tables[27] • End-tidal and arterial CO$_2$ gap[40]	
Pressure–volume curve	Inspiratory curve[4,32,36,48]	• Inspiratory curve compliance • Lower inflection point • Stress index
	• Expiratory curve[12,22,43,44,55]	• Point of derecruitment • Best compliance on expiratory curve • Point of derecruitment
	• Inspiratory and expiratory curve[20]	• Point of maximum hysteresis
Pleural pressure	Esophageal manometry[23,24]	
Lung volume	End-expiratory lung volume[54,57]	
Imaging	Ultrasound, CT, or X-ray[58-61]	

(ARDS: acute respiratory distress syndrome; CT: computed tomography; PEEP: positive end-expiratory pressure)

The tables have a pragmatic appeal to the bedside clinician. They are easy to apply, were used throughout the ARDSnet studies that underpinned the current lung protective strategy, and are now incorporated into protocols and automated systems, such as Intellivent.[27,29,30] Physiological arguments are that in a small group of patients studied, oxygenation-based regimes provided titrated PEEP related to lung recruitability progressively increasing from mild to moderate and severe ARDS, while other methods (compliance, stress index, and esophageal pressure titration) tended to provide PEEP unrelated to recruitability.[31]

Evidence of improved patient-centered outcome supporting the use of FiO_2 tables is scarce. The Assessment of Low tidal Volume and elevated End-expiratory volume to Obviate Lung Injury study comparing one group following the ARDS study PEEP table, with another using a table setting higher PEEP at each FiO_2, showed no difference between the groups (Tables 42.2 and 42.3).[30] Neither the LOV (Lung Open Ventilation) study nor the Expiratory Pressure (Express) Study demonstrated any benefit of using the PEEP table over the alternative.[32,33] A subsequent meta-analysis of these studies suggested the PEEP effect on mortality may be dependent upon severity of ARDS. Mortality was lower with higher PEEP in severe ARDS (34.1% high PEEP vs 39.1% low PEEP), but a nonsignificant trend toward a higher mortality with high PEEP in milder ARDS (27.2% vs 19.4%).[30,34] Two other PEEP comparison studies demonstrated a survival advantage with higher PEEP, but as the higher PEEP group also received a lower tidal volume (V_T, the attributable effect of PEEP was less certain.[35,36]

Subsequent post hoc analysis of the ExPress study and the LOV study also found an increased PaO_2/FiO_2 when PEEP was increased was associated with reduced mortality, while a decrease in PaO_2/FiO_2 after an increase in PEEP was associated with an increase in mortality.[32,33,37] Such PEEP responsive oxygenation association with a lower mortality does not necessarily imply causation. It is noteworthy that the ARDSnet study showed higher tidal volume (TV) also improved early oxygenation, but ultimately was associated with a higher mortality.[27] The same may be true of PEEP. Even if PEEP should be titrated to oxygenation what the optimal level of PEEP is at each FiO_2 remains unclear.

GAS EXCHANGE: CARBON DIOXIDE

For end-tidal CO_2 ($PETCO_2$) to accurately reflect arterial CO_2, not only must lung perfusion and alveoli CO_2 be consistent throughout the lung but V_T must be least three times the 2.2 mL/kg anatomic dead space (V_D).[38] As $PETCO_2/PaCO_2$ ratios are influenced by dead space, potentially capnography could have utility in the titrating best PEEP. Titrating PEEP to achieve the smallest fraction of dead space (V_D/V_T) was described by Suter and then by Fengmei.[4,39] In an experimental model, Murray found that "best PEEP" in ARDS was associated with the smallest $PaCO_2$-$PETCO_2$ gap.[40] Theoretically, an elevated PEEP that produces overdistention will increase the ventilation/perfusion mismatch and will disrupt the steady-state balance between CO_2 production and CO_2 excretion, due to the dual effects on dead space and venous return. Thus there should be a temporary decrease in CO_2 excretion until a new steady state is reached. Clinical studies have had mixed results, and as other ventilation changes (including lowered TVs), confound interpretation.[41] The use of total carbon dioxide excretion (volumetric capnography) for PEEP titration is physiologically enticing, but clinical use has not been well studied.

COMPLIANCE

Titrating PEEP to the highest compliance determined in incremental PEEP titration was described by Suter et al. in 1975.[4] Of the 15 subjects, some were reported to be breathing very low FiO_2, presumably because they had

Table 42.2: PEEP FiO₂ table used in ARDSnet study (and low PEEP for ALVEOLI study).[27]

FiO₂	0.3	0.4	0.4	0.5	0.5	0.6	0.7	0.7	0.7	0.8	0.9	0.9	0.9	1.0
PEEP	5	5	8	8	10	10	10	12	14	14	14	16	18	18–24

(PEEP: Positive end-expiratory pressure; ARDSnet: acute respiratory distress syndrome Clinical Network; ALVEOLI: Assessment of Low tidal Volume and elevated End-expiratory volume to Obviate Lung Injury)

Table 42.3: PEEP FiO₂ table used for high PEEP group in ALVEOLI study.[30]

FiO₂	0.3	0.3	0.3	0.3	0.3	0.4	0.4	0.5	0.5	0.5–0.8	0.9	0.9	1.0	1.0
PEEP	5	8	10	12	14	14	16	16	20	20	22	22	22	24

(ALVEOLI: Assessment of Low tidal Volume and elevated end-expiratory volume to obviate lung injury; PEEP: Positive end-expiratory pressure)

only very mild lung injury. They conducted an incremental PEEP titration from zero end-expiratory pressure to the level at which cardiac output fell. The PEEP corresponding to maximum oxygen delivery also corresponded to the lowest V_D/V_T and highest compliance. Suter's "best PEEP" ranged from 0 cmH$_2$O to 15 cmH$_2$O, but the study used 13–15 mL/kg TVs.

Pintado et al. compared 70 patients with ARDS randomized to receive either the low PEEP/FiO$_2$ table of the ARDSnet (36 patients) or to PEEP titrated to the highest respiratory compliance, using V_T of 6–8 mL/kg ideal body weight, and plateau pressures below 30 cmH$_2$O in both groups.[22] For the compliance group, PEEP was sequentially increased by 2 cmH$_2$O, from 5 cmH$_2$O and with no upper limit, and adjusted once daily. The compliance-guided group had a nonsignificant trend to lower mortality (20.6% compared with 38.9%). The compliance-guided setting of PEEP group also had less organ dysfunction, and better oxygenation. In a physiologic study using an open lung approach and decremental PEEP titration, Fengmei et al. found best PEEP was similar for highest compliance and lowest V_D/V_T.[39] Mercat et al.'s ExPress trial randomized 767 patients to either a low PEEP strategy of 5–9 cmH$_2$O or a maximum PEEP strategy set to reach a plateau pressures of 28–30 cmH$_2$O.[32] There was no difference in mortality, but the plateau pressure titrated group did have better lung function and requires less ventilation. If the higher PEEP produces more recruitment with resultant improved compliance, the driving pressure will decrease, which may improve survival.

The ARDS study randomized over a thousand patients with moderate-to-severe ARDS to either a combined "lung recruitment maneuver and PEEP adjusted to the best respiratory compliance" strategy or a control strategy using low PEEP. Unfortunately the intervention appeared to increase mortality at 28 days.[12] Whether the PEEP titration, the recruitment strategy, or both, caused the harm is not clear, but this finding has curtailed clinical enthusiasm for compliance titrated PEEP.

PRESSURE–VOLUME CURVE: VOLUME

A pressure–volume (PV) curve displays the relationship between pressure and volume during lung inflation and deflation. Traditionally created using a super syringe with constant slow inflation with measurement of plateau pressure at various inflation volumes, PV curves can now be created using automated tools which measure the PV curve with a constant slow pressure increase. Some advanced tools able to measure both inflation and deflation curves.

Suter's description "best PEEP" was the LIP related to the inspiratory compliance curve[4] (Fig. 42.1). The LIP is

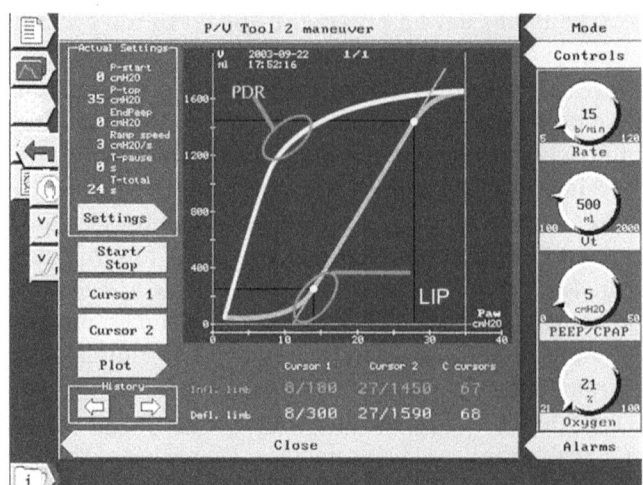

FIGURE 42.1: The inspiratory and expiratory volume curves, the LIP and the PDR, measured on a Hamilton G5® ventilator. (LIP: lower inflection point; PDR: point of derecruitment)

postulated to be the pressure at which numerous alveoli are recruited. Amato proposed that PEEP was ideally set about 2 cmH$_2$O above the LIP.[35]

The inflation limb PV curve is originally used, but hysteresis means the deflation curve has a different shape. Once PEEP is applied, subsequent breathes do not follow original inflation limb but a new curve originating on the deflation limb of the tidal cycle-specific PV curve.[42-44] The LIP described by Suter is a poor indicator of alveolar closure.[4] Creating a PV loop allows placement of the ventilatory cycle onto the deflation limb of the PV envelope of the optimally recruited lung.[42]

The lungs of patients with ARDS are heterogeneous with collapse and recruitment occurring along the entire length of the inflation PV curve.[44] In contrast the expiratory cycle has a greater lung volume than the inspiratory cycle for the same applied pressure. If the pressure at which the lung begins to rapidly deflate can be identified, the PDR and PEEP are set at about this point, alveolar collapse may be prevented.[43] Analysis of the expiratory curve may be able to identify this point.[43,45]

The evaluation of a stepwise reduction in PEEP to find the PDR seems promising in individual titration of PEEP in patients with ARDS.[43] While an attractive concept, practical measurement PV relationship requires sedation and often paralysis, while identifying the LIP or PDR requires mathematical curve fitting[46] (see Fig. 42.1).

The point of maximum hysteresis: It has been postulated the point of maximum difference in volume between the inspiratory and expiratory curve may indicate an ideal ventilation zone. A porcine model comparing setting PEEP

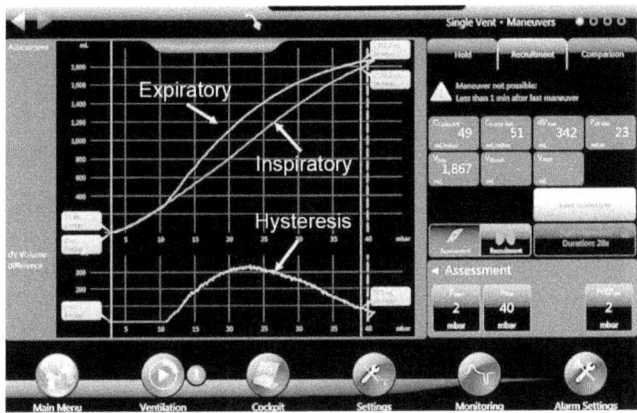

FIGURE 42.2: Point of maximum hysteresis of an inspiratory and expiratory volume loop (measured on an IMT Bellavista® ventilator).

at maximum compliance, LIP or at 90% of the point of maximum hysteresis (PMH) demonstrated that PMH had comparable of favorable lung mechanic and oxygenation parameters.[20] With ventilators now able to generate inspiration and expiration PV curve, the PMH can be calculated. PMH clinical usefulness is yet untested but is promised (Fig. 42.2).

A recent meta-analysis supports that PV-guided PEEP management appears to be associated with a reduction in ARDS mortality, with a number needed to treat of 4.[47] The small number of randomized trials and the confounding influence of TV heterogeneity support the need for further research in this field.[47] The optimal PV loop parameter remains unclear.

STRESS INDEX

The stress index reflects the change in compliance as the lung begins to recruit or becomes overdistended.[48]

A decrease in compliance as the lungs are inflated suggests overdistention and suggests lowering PEEP (or V_T) may be advantageous. An increase in compliance suggests tidal recruitment and the additional recruitment by elevating PEEP may help.

In two small studies evaluating the stress index suggest that the PEEP was lower when titrated using the stress index than with the ARDSnet tables, and that PEEP determined by stress index was similar to that determined by oxygenation but higher than that titrated by compliance and PV curve.[49,50] No definitive outcome studies have been published.

ESOPHAGEAL MANOMETRY

Both the chest wall and lung tissue contribute to the respiratory compliance.[23,24,51] In obesity the chest wall weight lowers chest wall compliance, resulting in increase in pleural pressure, creating the potential for alveolar collapse. In ARDS the decrease in compliance seen can be the result of lung or chest wall changes, or both. Delivering PEEP greater than end-expiratory pleural pressure reduces alveolar collapse. Estimating pleural pressure with esophageal manometry allows more definitive PEEP titration. Talmor randomized 61 subjects with ARDS to receive PEEP adjusted either according to esophageal pressure measurements or according to the ARDSnet "low PEEP" table. The esophageal pressure strategy produced greater oxygenation and compliance. After adjustment for baseline severity score the esophageal-pressure protocol was associated with a lower 28-day mortality, but unchanged 180-day mortality. The Esophageal Pressure-Guided Ventilation 2 (EPVent 2) trial, a large multicenter study looking at 28-day mortality, is due to be completed in September 2018 (ClinicalTrials.gov registration NCT01681225) and should provide some clarification of esophageal manometry's utility.

Esophageal manometry use is fickle and with the current information is not recommended for routine use. Whatever the EPVent 2 study shows, esophageal manometry may be beneficial in selected patients, such as in the morbidly obese or those with raised abdominal pressure, where transalveolar pressures are significantly lower than the measured airway pressures. Grasso highlighted that titrating PEEP using esophageal manometry would have reduced ECMO requirements due to swine flu.[24] Esophageal manometry also allows estimates of pleural pressures in assisted spontaneously breathing where transalveolar pressures may exceed measured airway pressures.[51] In heterogeneous lung disease, such as in ARDS, pleural pressures may not be equally distributed, further complicating interpretation, although utilizing higher PEEP seems to overcome these hazards.[26,52]

LUNG VOLUME

In the ventilated patient with ARDS the lowered compliance and with loss of outward expansion of the thorax, the EELV falls unless additional PEEP is provided. If the EELV could be measured, PEEP could be adjusted to maintain in an optimal EELV. During ventilation, EELV can be measured using a helium dilution technique or using a nitrogen-washout technique.[53] One commercially available ventilator as an integrated modified nitrogen washout tool. Simplistically matching EELV to a healthy FRC seems logical. Unfortunately, as with the other techniques, PEEP-induced increase in EELV might be from the alveolar recruitment but may be because already open alveoli are being overdistended.[15] In disease processes, additional EELV above normal FRC may be required.[54]

While PEEP contributes to improved oxygenation, the increased EELV may not be recruitment of previously nonaerated lung units, but simply, further distension of previously open lung units.[55,56] While EELV alone may not be sufficient to assess PEEP response, identifying recruited volume created by additional PEEP have more relevance. EELV combined with measurement of compliance may be useful.[57]

IMAGING

Computed tomography (CT) imaging has become the gold standard for differentiating alveolar recruitment from overdistention, and titrating PEEP using qualitative improvement in lung fields and quantitatively with measurement of Hounsfield units on CT scan has been advocated.[56,58] The advantage of imaging techniques over other techniques is their ability to assess lung heterogeneity, but risks and resources associated with intrahospital transfer make this a less useful "bedside" tool.[58] Bedside digital chest radiography and ultrasound of the lung have some, possibly complementary, role.[59,60] Ultrasound has no ionizing radiations, is easy to use in trained hands, noninvasive, and can detect recruitment but unfortunately cannot detect overdistention.[61] Visualization may be impaired in the obese or with other chest wall pathologies.

SUMMARY AND RECOMMENDATIONS

- Positive end-expiratory pressure potentially creates both alveolar recruitment and alveolar overdistention, and diverse other physiological changes
- Positive end-expiratory pressure titration should target optimal long-term outcome for patients, not just oxygenation or compliance parameters
- Definitive controlled trials demonstrating benefit of one PEEP strategy over another are lacking
- Evidence from post hoc analysis of trials suggests elevated PEEP in early, or mild, ARDS may be harmful, but elevated PEEP in moderate-to-severe ARDS appear beneficial
- Many clinicians use the PEEP/FiO_2 tables of the ARDSnet or alternatively the best compliance for PEEP titration despite lack of evidence of efficacy
- More advanced methods, such as esophageal manometry, PV loop analysis, stress index, ultrasound, electrical impedance tomography, and EELV, may have a yet to be defined role, but may be of value, even if only for selected patients

REFERENCES

1. Poulton EP. Left-sided heart failure with pulmonary oedema: its treatment with the "pulmonary plus pressure machine". Lancet. 1936;228(5904):981-3.
2. Ashbaugh DG, Bigelow DB, Petty TL, et al. Acute respiratory distress in adults. Lancet. 1967;2(7511):319-23.
3. Albert RK. Least PEEP: primum non nocere. Chest. 1985;87(1):2-4.
4. Suter PM, Fairley B, Isenberg MD. Optimum end-expiratory airway pressure in patients with acute pulmonary failure. N Engl J Med. 1975;292(6):284-9.
5. Downs JB, Klein EF, Jr., Modell JH. The effect of incremental PEEP on PaO_2 in patients with respiratory failure. Anesth Analg. 1973;52(2):210-5.
6. Kirby RR, Downs JB, Civetta JM, et al. High level positive end expiratory pressure (PEEP) in acute respiratory insufficiency. Chest. 1975;67(2):156-63.
7. Pepe PE, Hudson LD, Carrico CJ. Early application of positive end-expiratory pressure in patients at risk for the adult respiratory-distress syndrome. N Engl J Med. 1984;311(5):281-6.
8. Jardin F, Desfond P, Bazin M, et al. Controlled ventilation with best positive end-expiratory pressure (PEEP) and high level PEEP in acute respiratory failure (ARF). Intensive Care Med. 1981;7(4):171-6.
9. Lachmann B. Open up the lung and keep the lung open. Intensive Care Med. 1992;18(6):319-21.
10. Ferguson ND, Frutos-Vivar F, Esteban A, et al. Airway pressures, tidal volumes, and mortality in patients with acute respiratory distress syndrome. Crit Care Med. 2005;33(1):21-30.
11. Algera AG, Pisani L, Bergmans DCJ, et al. RELAx–REstricted versus liberal positive end-expiratory pressure in patients without ARDS: protocol for a randomized controlled trial. Trials. 2018;19(1):272.
12. Cavalcanti AB, Suzumura EA, Laranjeira LN, et al.; Writing Group for the Alveolar Recruitment for Acute Respiratory Distress Syndrome Trial. Effect of lung recruitment and titrated positive end-expiratory pressure (PEEP) vs low PEEP on mortality in patients with acute respiratory distress syndrome: a randomized clinical trial. JAMA. 2017;318(14):1335-45.
13. Kawamura G, Kitamura T, Homma I, et al. Mechanisms underlying the improvement of arterial oxygenation using positive end-expiratory pressure during surgery under sevoflurane anesthesia and propofol anesthesia: a retrospective clinical study. Masui. 2013;62(6):652-9.
14. Halter JM, Steinberg JM, Gatto LA, et al. Effect of positive end-expiratory pressure and tidal volume on lung injury induced by alveolar instability. Crit Care. 2007;11:R20.
15. Mertens M, Tabuchi A, Meissner S, et al. Alveolar dynamics in acute lung injury: heterogeneous distension rather than cyclic opening and collapse. Criti Care Med. 2009;37(9):2604-11.
16. Demling RH, Staub NC, Edmunds Jr LH. Effect of end expiratory airway pressure on accumulation of extravascular lung water. J Appl Physiol. 1975;38(5):907-12.
17. Colmenero-Ruiz M, Fernández-Mondéjar E, Fernández-Sacristán MA, et al. PEEP and low tidal volume ventilation

reduce lung water in porcine pulmonary edema. Am J Respir Crit Care Med. 1997;155(3):964-70.
18. Luecke T, Roth H, Herrmann P, et al. PEEP decreases atelectasis and extravascular lung water but not lung tissue volume in surfactant-washout lung injury. Intensive Care Med. 2003;29(11):2026-33.
19. Ruiz-Bailén M, Cobo-Molinos J, Castillo-Rivera AM, et al. Increasing levels of positive end-expiratory pressure improve the left ventricular strain. J Thorac Imaging. 2017;32(5):333-9.
20. Koefoed-Nielsen J, Andersen G, Barklin A, et al. Maximal hysteresis: a new method to set positive end-expiratory pressure in acute lung injury?. Acta Anaesthesiol Scand. 2008;52(5):641-9.
21. Rodriguez PO, Bonelli I, Setten M, et al. Transpulmonary pressure and gas exchange during decremental PEEP titration in pulmonary ARDS patients. Respir Care. 2013;58(5):754-63.
22. Pintado MC, de Pablo R, Trascasa M, et al. Individualized PEEP setting in subjects with ARDS: a randomized controlled pilot study. Respir Care. 2013;58(9):1416-23.
23. Talmor D, Sarge T, Malhotra A, et al. Mechanical ventilation guided by esophageal pressure in acute lung injury. N Engl J Med. 2008;359(20):2095-104.
24. Grasso S, Terragni P, Birocco A, et al. ECMO criteria for influenza A (H1N1)-associated ARDS: role of transpulmonary pressure. Intensive Care Med. 2012;38(3):395-403.
25. Amato MB, Meade MO, Slutsky AS, et al. Driving pressure and survival in the acute respiratory distress syndrome. N Engl J Med. 2015;372(8):747-55.
26. Morais CCA, Koyama Y, Yoshida T, et al. High positive end-expiratory pressure renders spontaneous effort noninjurious. Am J Respir Crit Care Med. 2018;197(10):1285-96.
27. Brower RG, Matthay MA, Morris A, et al.; Acute Respiratory Distress Syndrome Network. Ventilation with lower tidal volumes as compared with traditional tidal volumes for acute lung injury and the acute respiratory distress syndrome. N Engl J Med. 2000;342(18):1301-8.
28. Kallet RH, Branson RD. Respiratory controversies in the critical care setting. Do the NIH ARDS Clinical Trials Network PEEP/FiO_2 tables provide the best evidence-based guide to balancing PEEP and FiO_2 settings in adults?. Respir Care. 2007;52(4):461-75. Discussion 75-7.
29. Arnal JM, Garnero A, Novonti D, et al. Feasibility study on full closed-loop control ventilation (IntelliVent-ASV) in ICU patients with acute respiratory failure: a prospective observational comparative study. Crit Care. 2013;17(5):R196.
30. Brower RG, Lanken PN, MacIntyre N, et al. Higher versus lower positive end-expiratory pressures in patients with the acute respiratory distress syndrome. N Engl J Med. 2004;351(4):327-36.
31. Chiumello D, Cressoni M, Carlesso E, et al. Bedside selection of positive end-expiratory pressure in mild, moderate, and severe acute respiratory distress syndrome. Crit Care Med. 2014;42(2):252-64.
32. Mercat A, Richard JM, Vielle B, et al. Positive end-expiratory pressure setting in adults with acute lung injury and acute respiratory distress syndrome: a randomized controlled trial. JAMA. 2008;299(6):646-55.
33. Meade MO, Cook DJ, Guyatt GH, et al. Ventilation strategy using low tidal volumes, recruitment maneuvers, and high positive end-expiratory pressure for acute lung injury and acute respiratory distress syndrome: a randomized controlled trial. JAMA. 2008;299(6):637-45.
34. Briel M, Meade M, Mercat A, et al. Higher vs lower positive end-expiratory pressure in patients with acute lung injury and acute respiratory distress syndrome: systematic review and meta-analysis. JAMA. 2010;303(9):865-73.
35. Amato MB, Barbas CS, Medeiros DM, et al. Effect of a protective-ventilation strategy on mortality in the acute respiratory distress syndrome. N Engl J Med. 1998;338(6):347-54.
36. Villar J, Kacmarek RM, Perez-Mendez L, et al. A high positive end-expiratory pressure, low tidal volume ventilatory strategy improves outcome in persistent acute respiratory distress syndrome: a randomized, controlled trial. Crit Care Med. 2006;34(5):1311-8.
37. Goligher EC, Kavanagh BP, Rubenfeld GD, et al. Oxygenation response to positive end-expiratory pressure predicts mortality in acute respiratory distress syndrome. A secondary analysis of the LOVS and ExPress trials. Am J Respir Crit Care Med. 2014;190(1):70-6.
38. Downs JB. $PaCO_2$, $PETCO_2$, and gradient. In: Capnography, 2nd edition. Cambridge, UK: Cambridge University Press; 2011. pp. 225-30.
39. Fengmei G, Jin C, Songqiao L, et al. Dead space fraction changes during PEEP titration following lung recruitment in patients with ARDS. Respir Care. 2012; 57(10):1578-85.
40. Murray IP, Modell JH, Gallagher TJ, et al. Titration of PEEP by the arterial minus end-tidal carbon dioxide gradient. Chest. 1984;85(1):100-4.
41. Tusman G, Bohm SH, Suarez-Sipmann F, et al. Lung recruitment and positive end-expiratory pressure have different effects on CO_2 elimination in healthy and sick lungs. Anesth Analg. 2010;111(4):968-77.
42. Rimensberger PC, Cox PN, Frndova H, et al. The open lung during small tidal volume ventilation: concepts of recruitment and 'optimal' positive end-expiratory pressure. Crit Care Med. 1999;27(9):1946-52.
43. Hickling KG. Best compliance during a decremental, but not incremental, positive end-expiratory pressure trial is related to open-lung positive end-expiratory pressure: a mathematical model of acute respiratory distress syndrome lungs. Am J Respir Crit Care Med. 2001;163(1):69-78.
44. DiRocco JD, Carney DE, Nieman GF. Correlation between alveolar recruitment/derecruitment and inflection points on the pressure-volume curve. Intensive Care Med. 2007;33(7):1204-11.
45. De Robertis E, Servillo G, Pezza M, et al. Derecruitment of the lung induced by stepwise lowering of positive end-expiratory pressure in patients with adult respiratory distress syndrome. Eur J Anaesthesiol. 2003;20(10):794-9.
46. Hickling KG. The pressure-volume curve is greatly modified by recruitment. A mathematical model of ARDS lungs. Am J Respir Crit Care Med. 1998;158(1):194-202.
47. Hata JS, Togashi K, Kumar AB, et al. The effect of the pressure–volume curve for positive end-expiratory pressure titration

on clinical outcomes in acute respiratory distress syndrome: a systematic review. J Intensive Care Med. 2014;29(6):348-56.
48. Hess DR. Respiratory mechanics in mechanically ventilated patients. Respir Care. 2014;59(11):1773-94.
49. Huang Y, Yang Y, Chen Q, et al. Pulmonary acute respiratory distress syndrome: positive end-expiratory pressure titration needs stress index. J Surg Res. 2013;185(1):347-52.
50. Grasso S, Stripoli T, De Michele M, et al. ARDSnet ventilatory protocol and alveolar hyperinflation: role of positive end-expiratory pressure. Am J Respir Crit Care Med. 2007;176(8):761-7.
51. Freebairn R, Hickling K. Spontaneous breathing during mechanical ventilation in ARDS. Crit Care Shock. 2005;8(3):61-6.
52. Yoshida T, Torsani V, Gomes S, et al. Spontaneous effort causes occult pendelluft during mechanical ventilation. Am J Respir Crit Care Med. 2013;188(12):1420-7.
53. Motta-Ribeiro GC, Jandre FC, Wrigge H, Giannella-Neto A. Generalized estimation of the ventilatory distribution from the multiple-breath nitrogen washout. Biomed Eng Online. 2016;15(1):89.
54. Aguirre-Bermeo H, Turella M, Bitondo M, et al. Lung volumes and lung volume recruitment in ARDS: a comparison between supine and prone position. Ann Intensive Care. 2018;8(1):25.
55. Chen L, Chen GQ, Shore K, et al. Implementing a bedside assessment of respiratory mechanics in patients with acute respiratory distress syndrome. Crit Care. 2017;21(1):84.
56. Stahl CA, Moller K, Steinmann D, et al. Determination of 'recruited volume' following a PEEP step is not a measure of lung recruitability. Acta Anaesthesiol Scand. 2015;59(1):35-46.
57. Bikker IG, van Bommel J, Reis Miranda D, et al. End-expiratory lung volume during mechanical ventilation: a comparison with reference values and the effect of positive end-expiratory pressure in intensive care unit patients with different lung conditions. Crit Care. 2008;12(6):R145.
58. Bellani G, Rouby JJ, Constantin JM, et al. Looking closer at acute respiratory distress syndrome: the role of advanced imaging techniques. Curr Opin Crit Care. 2017;23(1):30-7.
59. See KC, Ong V, Tan YL, et al. Chest radiography versus lung ultrasound for identification of acute respiratory distress syndrome: a retrospective observational study. Critical Care. 2018;22(1):203.
60. Warren MA, Zhao Z, Koyama T, et al. Severity scoring of lung oedema on the chest radiograph is associated with clinical outcomes in ARDS. Thorax. 2018;73(9):840-6.
61. Ball L, Vercesi V, Costantino F, et al. Lung imaging: how to get better look inside the lung. Ann Transl Med. 2017;5(14):294.

CHAPTER 43

Driving Pressure in Acute Respiratory Distress Syndrome

Atul Prabhakar Kulkarni, Ruchira W Khasne

INTRODUCTION

Acute respiratory distress syndrome (ARDS) is a life-threatening condition and is associated with substantial morbidity and mortality. A recently published global epidemiologic study reported that ARDS represents 10.4% of total intensive care unit (ICU) admissions and 23.4% of all intubated mechanically ventilated patients.[1] Traditional lung-protective ventilation strategy based on ideal body weight (IBW) and "open lung" approach is associated with less ventilator-induced lung injury (VILI), improved oxygenation, and better outcomes in ARDS. It comprises limiting tidal volume (V_T) and plateau pressure (Pplat) while providing relatively higher positive end-expiratory pressure (PEEP).[2,3] However, it is evident that it does not perform optimally in all ARDS patients. In ARDS the lungs are not stiff as previously described rather have a small aerated portion that is called "baby lung."[4] In any given patient, it is difficult to predict the exact size of the "baby lung" based on IBW.[4]

The impact of V_T on lung injury is better evaluated if it is normalized to respiratory system compliance (Crs) instead of IBW by calculating driving pressure (ΔP) which is quite promising. It is a quotient of V_T and Crs adapted to the size of aerated lung.

The potential importance of ΔP in ventilation strategy was first proposed in 1998 by Amato et al.[5] Recently, a retrospective analysis of previous randomized controlled trials (RCTs) of ventilatory management of ARDS demonstrated that high ΔP is strongly associated with mortality than traditional low V_T lung-protective ventilatory strategy after multivariate analysis. This ratio may be a better indicator of the size of the "baby lung" available for ventilation.[6] However, the use of ΔP has its own limitations and is yet to be subjected to a high-quality RCT to confirm its clinical utility and safety.

WHAT IS AIRWAY DRIVING PRESSURE (ΔP)?

During mechanical ventilation, ΔP across the respiratory system is defined as the pressure delivered by the ventilator to inflate the system. ΔP equals the tidal pressure change between total PEEP ($PEEP_{TOT}$ is the sum of external PEEP and intrinsic PEEP) and end-inspiratory Pplat. The airway ΔP can be a plausible, noninvasive, bedside method and is considered the best surrogate for assessing lung stress and strain in mild and moderate ARDS on mechanical ventilation. It is calculated as Pplat minus PEEP (for patients who are not making inspiratory efforts).[6] Decreasing ΔP is a better way to decrease cyclic or dynamic strain during mechanical ventilation.[7]

ΔP: Pplat - PEEP

Crs = V_T/Pplat - PEEP

Crs = V_T/ΔP

thus

ΔP : V_T/Crs

PHYSIOLOGY OF ΔP

ΔP is a physiological way of adjusting V_T to the "baby lung" or Crs. The relative mortality predictive power of V_T normalized to Crs (i.e. ΔP) performs better compared to V_T normalized to IBW. ΔP represents the best physiologic surrogate to assess the cyclic stress and strain of "baby lung" during each ventilatory cycle.

Stress is defined as pressure developed within the lung to which distending force is applied which indirectly corresponds to transpulmonary pressure (P_{TP}, transpulmonary pressure is the difference between airway pressure and pleural pressure). Pplat is surrogate for lung stress under zero-flow conditions.

Strain is defined as mechanical distortion caused by V_T to ventilate "baby lung." It is the ratio between V_T and baseline gas volume of the "baby lung" and it is called dynamic strain. It is estimated by ΔP which ranges between 0.42 (without any harm) and 2.1 (lethal), induced by V_T 6 mL/kg IBW in a few animal studies.[8] From Figure 43.1, we can see that if the stress index is <1, the pressure volume (PV) curve has a concavity downward implying a decrease in elastance. With stress index of 1, there is no hyperinflation and the line is straight, while an upward concavity (with stress index >1) suggests hyperinflation of the lungs.[9]

Thus safer mechanical ventilation strategy should be based on size of the "baby lung" instead of IBW which is more physiological.[8,10]

ΔP can detect the lung overstress with acceptable accuracy. Chiumello et al. found that patients with high ΔP, as well as high transpulmonary driving pressure (ΔPL), had significantly higher lung stress (dynamic plus static stress). However, lung stress was not related to applied V_T alone. They divided patients into two groups higher and lower ΔP groups and at two different levels of PEEP (5 cmH$_2$O and 15 cmH$_2$O of PEEP). At ΔP of 15 cmH$_2$O the predicted lung stress was 24 cmH$_2$O, a level that has been associated with VILI. Higher ΔP group also had shown higher ΔPL, respiratory system elastance, lung elastance at both levels of PEEP. Further prospective studies are needed to establish the limits of overstress.[10]

EFFECT OF ΔP ON MORTALITY

Recently, Amato et al. performed a retrospective analysis of previously published nine RCTs, which included 3,562 ARDS patients.[6] They concluded that ΔP is a better predictor of mortality than V_T. Further they divided patients into five subsamples of roughly 600 patients each; all with different combinations of PEEP, Pplat, and ΔP. In these subsamples, one parameter remained constant, while the others changed; for example in one test sample, the PEEP remained constant, while the ΔP and Pplat differed. They found that mortality increased with increasing ΔP. Their findings can be summarized as follows:

- At constant PEEP levels when Pplat is rising and threshold of ΔP exceeds 14 cmH$_2$O, the relative risk of mortality is significantly increased.
- Keeping PEEP and ΔP constant but with rising Pplat values, the mortality remains unchanged. Thus higher Pplat is not always risky.
- Protective effect of PEEP (rising PEEP) and its mortality benefit are observed only when it is associated with constant Pplat, and consistently low ΔP. This suggests alveolar recruitment and good respiratory compliance in survivors. Hence, higher PEEP is protective in some but not all patients.
- Lower survival rate is observed among patients with higher ΔP, and higher survival is observed among patients with lower ΔP, independent of concomitant variations in PEEP and Pplat.

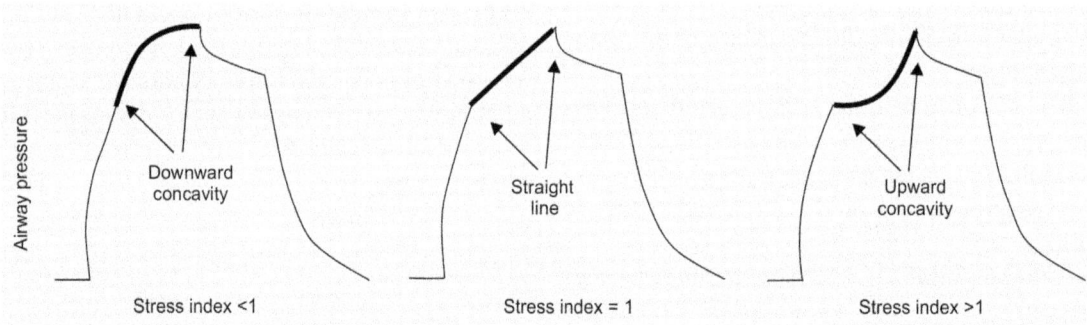

FIGURE 43.1: Stress according to amount of lung inflation.

A systematic review and meta-analysis of seven studies (6,062 patients) demonstrated that higher ΔP is significantly associated with a higher mortality in mechanically ventilated patients with ARDS. The median cutoff of ΔP to differentiate the survivors from nonsurvivors was found to be 13–15 cmH$_2$O.[11]

Guierin et al. retrospectively reviewed data from two large randomized studies, involving 787 ARDS patients. They observed a significant association between ΔP and mortality; there was a 5% increase in the risk of death per each cmH$_2$O increase in ΔP, and a significant mortality reduction when ΔP was lower than 13 cmH$_2$O. However, in contrast to Amato's study, they found that ΔP was not superior to Pplat, V_T, and Crs as a predictor of death, and it shared the same prognostic information as Pplat and Crs.[12]

Large Observational Study to Understand the Global Impact of Severe Acute Respiratory Failure (LUNG SAFE) study involving 2,377 patients in ICUs across 50 countries concluded that higher ΔP (>14 cmH$_2$O) had strong prognostic value in predicting mortality in moderate and severe ARDS patients. They observed that along with ΔP, there were other potentially modifiable and nonmodifiable factors, which play important role in patient outcomes.[13]

Though ΔP has been shown to be a causal factor for mortality, it alone can not lead to mortality. ΔP is dependent on the setting of V_T (signifying the lung strain) and the lung elastance (reflecting the how badly the lung parenchyma is affected).

$$\Delta P = V_T \times E$$

If the V_T, Pplat, and PEEP are set correctly so as to achieve the lung-protective ventilation, setting of ΔP does not offer any further advantage in improving outcomes. We do not need to separately set the ΔP.[14]

MECHANICAL POWER AS APPLIED TO THE RESPIRATORY SYSTEM

Gattinoni et al. describe VILI as caused by a single unified variable as applied to the respiratory system, the mechanical power. They calculated the mechanical power needed to produce a change in the V_T and respiratory rate taking into account the driving pressure ΔP, flow in the system, and PEEP.[15]

$$\text{Power}_{rs} = RR \cdot \left\{ \Delta V^2 \cdot \left[\frac{1}{2} \cdot EL_{rs} + RR \cdot \frac{(1+I:E)}{60 \cdot I:E} \cdot R_{aw} \right] + \Delta V \cdot PEEP \right\}$$

where Power$_{rs}$ is the power applied to the respiratory system, RR is the respiratory rate, ΔV is the change in the V, EL$_{rs}$ is elastance of respiratory system, R$_{aw}$ is airway resistance, ΔP is the driving pressure, and PEEP is the positive end-expiratory pressure.

As evident from the equation, the power needs to be applied to the respiratory system.
- To overcome the airway resistance (which includes the resistive component of airway and equipment RR × 1(+I:E)/60 × (I:E) × R$_{aw}$).
- To overcome the respiratory elastance and distend the lungs [ΔV^2 × (1/2 × EL$_{rs}$)].
- To hold lung open at the end of expiration; ΔP × PEEP (PEEP).

This equation is fairly simple as it describes the contribution of each element as applied to the respiratory system. Application of excessive power through an increase in any of the elements will ultimately lead to the development of VILI.

CONSEQUENCES OF ΔP

Cor pulmonale: In a prospective observational study, 22% of ARDS patients on mechanical ventilation had evidence of cor pulmonale on transesophageal echocardiography. The authors postulated that the presence of intrinsic myocardial dysfunction induced by sepsis would make the patient more susceptible to the development of cor pulmonale. The severity of lung disease with decreased respiratory compliance, high afterload, and pulmonary vascular dysfunction would have further contributed to the development of cor pulmonale.[16] In another study conducted to develop a clinical risk score for acute cor pulmonale, driving pressure (>18 cmH$_2$O) was found to be an independent risk factor for development of cor pulmonale.[17]

Diaphragmatic dysfunction: Goligher et al. in their prospective observational study found that the diaphragmatic thickness, as assessed by ultrasound, at the end of the first week, had an inverse relationship with the driving pressure applied to the respiratory system during the first 3 days of mechanical ventilation and contractile activity.[18]

Postoperative pulmonary complications: A meta-analysis of 17 RCTs, including 2,250 patients, has shown that intraoperative high ΔP and or PEEP manipulation leading to increase in ΔP is associated with higher incidence of postoperative pulmonary complications.

Even in patients with noninjured lungs, it was observed that high ΔP and an increased level of PEEP that led to an increase in ΔP during intraoperative ventilation, raised ΔP, was independently associated with development of pulmonary complications after surgery.[19]

Ferrando et al. compared open lung approach versus standard lung-protective ventilatory strategies and its effects on ΔP on those patients who had undergone major abdominal surgeries without a pre-existing lung disease. ΔP was significantly reduced with improvement in lung compliance in those who received open lung PEEP.[20] Thus the use of intraoperative open lung approach ventilation strategy resulted in better respiratory mechanics, lower ΔP. The authors suggested that open lung approach and individualized PEEP may reduce postoperative pulmonary complications, and further studies are needed to confirm these findings.

Serpa Neto et al. conducted a meta-analysis of pooled patient data ($n = 545$ patients from nine studies) who had refractory hypoxemia and were managed using extracorporeal membrane oxygenation (ECMO). Apart from older age, higher body mass index, and male gender, only higher ΔP during first 3 days of ECMO was associated with increased mortality. Owing to several limitations in the analysis, the authors suggest a need for further studies.[21]

TRANSPULMONARY DRIVING PRESSURE (ΔPL)

Airway pressure alone may be misleading when trying to assess the potential of mechanical ventilation to cause VILI. Effect of chest recoil is ignored by airway pressure. Transpulmonary pressure (P_{TP}) which is the net distending pressure applied to the lung by contraction of the inspiratory muscles or by positive-pressure ventilation differentiates lung compliance from chest wall compliance. It estimates the contribution of lung and chest wall separately to determine respiratory mechanics. It can be a useful guide for PEEP selection and improved respiratory compliance and oxygenation.[22] P_{TP} is measured by performing esophageal manometry during mechanical ventilation.

ΔP = (Pplat − $PEEP_{(TOT)}$)

P_{TP} is the difference between alveolar pressure (P_{alv}) and pleural pressure (P_{pl}):

$P_{TP} = P_{alv} − P_{pl}$

$P_{TP} = P_{alv} − P_{es}$ [(esophageal pressure (P_{es}) is used as a surrogate for P_{pl}]

ΔPL = End-inspiratory transpulmonary pressure − End-expiratory transpulmonary pressure

ΔPL = (Pplat − P_{es} end-insp) − ($PEEP_{TOT}$ − $P_{es\ end-exp}$)

The ΔPL is defined as the difference between Pplat and end-inspiratory esophageal plateau ($P_{es\ end-insp}$) and PEEP (total) and end-expiratory esophageal pressure ($P_{es\ end-exp}$).

It can be obtained by end-inspiratory transpulmonary pressure − end-expiratory transpulmonary pressure.

Measurement of P_{es} is a minimally invasive technique, and it allows accurate respiratory monitoring and assesses physiological effects of mechanical ventilation. Esophageal manometry using dedicated catheters is utilized to determine ΔPL.[23]

In the presence of significant change in chest wall, elastance from normal, due to any of the variables, such as abdominal distension, obesity, chest wall edema, it may affect ΔP, whereas ΔPL eliminates effect of these variables. It may be a better determinant to estimate the risk of VILI and clinical outcome compared to ΔP. A retrospective analysis of 56 patients by Baedorf Kassis et al.[23] observed ΔP and ΔPL at baseline, 5 minutes and 24 hours, and evaluated their relation to 28-day survival. This study concluded that both ΔP and ΔPL were higher in nonsurvivors compared to survivors. In addition, lung elastance and respiratory system elastance were lower in survivors at baseline and decreased over 24 hours. From a physiological point of view, ΔPL represents lung stress and is a better surrogate of lung strain compared to ΔP.[24]

ΔPL measurement requires P_{pl} measurement which is virtually impossible in clinical practice. P_{es} measured by esophageal manometry is a surrogate for P_{pl}, but its validity remains unclear. Esophageal manometry is an old technique, but its use is limited in clinical practice due to variety of factors, such as technical aspects, accuracy in balloon positioning, and precision in signal validation and interpretation of P_{pl} gradient in dependent and nondependent zones. Further studies are required to assess its association with VILI and clinical outcome.[25] The effects of cardiac and pulmonary circulation on P_{pl} alter the outcomes but are not represented by ΔPL. In addition to that, few studies suggested that chest wall compliance is not so widely affected in ARDS patients. Thus ΔP instead of ΔPL may be sufficient in most of the situations.[24]

CLINICAL USE OF ΔP

- At present, ΔP should be used as additional safety measure and not as a substitute for lung-protective ventilatory strategy. The proposed cutoff for ΔP is 13–15 cmH_2O.
- ΔP can be a valuable tool to set PEEP provided the effect of PEEP manipulations on ΔP is taken in to account. In some patients, ΔP may decrease after increasing PEEP. This suggests a decrease in cyclic strain and alveolar recruitment. Likewise, an increase in ΔP suggests a nonrecruitable lung. If ΔP remains above 15 cmH_2O in

spite of optimizing PEEP, further reduction in V_T below 6 mL/kg IBW should be considered.
- In presence of alterations in chest wall compliance and lung elastance ΔPL should be considered.

HOW TO ADJUST VENTILATORY PARAMETERS ACCORDING TO ΔP[7]

- One should follow the traditional ventilatory strategy, with V_T 6–8 mL/kg IBW and moderate PEEP levels, to improve gas exchange.
- Measure the ΔP and apply ventilatory strategy to keep it within safety limit. The proposed cutoff is 13–15 cmH$_2$O.
- If ΔP is <15 cmH$_2$O, follow the same initial ventilatory parameters, provided it improves gas exchange.
- If ΔP is >15 cmH$_2$O, check ventilatory settings first and check if there is possibility of worsening of lung compliance based on severity of ARDS. Limit V_T to 5–6 mL/kg IBW or lower and optimize PEEP to keep ΔP < 15 cmH$_2$O. Simultaneously apply other measures to improve gas exchange, including, manipulation of PEEP, recruitment maneuvers, use of neuromuscular-blocking agents, and prone ventilation while monitoring ΔP.

LIMITATIONS OF ΔP

- ΔP and V_T, Pplat, PEEP: These variables are inter-related in a complex way and are both mathematically and physiologically coupled. Changes in any one variable lead to unpredictable changes in other parameters due to their interdependence, e.g. increase in PEEP may increase Pplat. Along with this, if the Pplat, V_T, and PEEP are set with in the tight ranges of lung-protective ventilation, ΔP does not offer any additional advantage over these indices.[14] It is still debatable which variable has the best predictive performance for mortality.[12,26]
- ΔP and Pplat: Optimum strategy to reduce ΔP is yet not defined, and there are conflicting results on predictive performance of ΔP in comparison to Pplat, e.g. can we accept a high Pplat as long as ΔP remains within acceptable limits?
- ΔP and PEEP: ΔP in isolation gives no or minimal information about lung mechanics. PEEP is still needed to recruit lung and keep it open. ΔP does not clarify the role of PEEP manipulation to prevent further lung collapse, e.g. theoretically to achieve safe level of ΔP of 12 cmH$_2$O can be harmful either with patients requiring high PEEP or inadvertent application of insufficient or extremely low PEEP. ΔP should be referred to the lung and not the respiratory system.[14]
- ΔP and Crs: When ΔP and Crs were analyzed together, neither of them remained statistically significantly associated with patient's outcome. It suggests that both Crs and ΔP convey the same information.
- ΔP and lung stress: Although ΔP accurately detects lung stress, prospective studies are needed to establish the limits of overstress.
- Optimum cutoff of ΔP: The cutoff value of ΔP is yet not defined as there is heterogeneity in the published data. Possibly keeping ΔP below 15 cmH$_2$O should be tested in future trials.[11] This can be achieved by either by reducing V_T (which does not support adequate oxygenation or CO_2 elimination) or increasing Crs (by altering PEEP), either of which may not be possible. Thus how to target ΔP during setting up the ventilation is unclear as of now and is subject to trial and error.
- ΔP and spontaneous breathing: ΔP may not be helpful for patients who are actively breathing and with those with fall in P_{pl} during inspiration as a result of breathing efforts.

CONCLUSION

The concept of ΔP is appealing since it is based on observation of physiological variables. It is easily measured at the bedside and has good biological plausibility as to why it should affect development or progression of VILI. The concept and validation of ΔP has emerged from retrospective studies, and we suggest that they be considered hypothesis generating rather than definitive. There is a complex interplay of various factors related to the mechanical power delivered to the lungs during positive-pressure ventilation, and ΔP is just one of the variables, apart from V_T, PEEP, etc. More prospective studies are needed to clarify the role of ΔP in furthering causation and progression of VILI and its effect on mortality.

REFERENCES

1. Bellani G, Laffey JG, Pham T, et al. Epidemiology, patterns of care, and mortality for patients with acute respiratory distress syndrome in intensive care units in 50 countries. JAMA. 2016;315:788-800.
2. Brower RG, Matthay MA, Morris A, et al.; Acute Respiratory Distress Syndrome Network. Ventilation with lower tidal volumes as compared with traditional tidal volumes for acute lung injury and the acute respiratory distress syndrome. N Engl J Med. 2000;342(18): 1301-8.
3. Ferguson ND, Fan E, Camporota L, et al. The Berlin definition of ARDS: an expanded rationale, justification, and supplementary material. Intensive Care Med. 2012;38(10):1573-82.
4. Gattinoni L, Pesenti A, Avalli L, et al. Pressure-volume curve of total respiratory system in acute respiratory failure. Computed tomographic scan study. Am Rev Respir Dis. 1987;136:730-6.
5. Amato MB, Barbas CS, Medeiros DM, et al. Effect of a protective ventilation strategy on mortality in the acute respiratory distress syndrome. N Engl J Med. 1998;338:347-54.

6. Amato MBP, Meade MO, Slutsky AS, et al. Driving pressure and survival in the acute respiratory distress syndrome. N Engl J Med. 2015;372(8):747-55.
7. Bugedo G, Retamal J, Bruhn A. Driving pressure: a marker of severity, a safety limit, or a goal for mechanical ventilation? Crit Care. 2017;21(1):1-7.
8. Gattinoni L, Marini JJ, Pesenti A, et al. The "baby lung" became an adult. Intensive Care Med. 2016;42(5):663-73.
9. Kulkarni AP, Divatia JV. Ventilator induced lung injury. In: Nayyar V, Peter JV, Kishen R, Srinivas S. (Eds). Critical care update. New Delhi, India: M/s Jaypee Brothers Medical Publishers; 2009. pp. 48-58. ISBN 978-81-8448-972-9.
10. Chiumello D, Carlesso E, Brioni M, et al. Airway driving pressure and lung stress in ARDS patients. Crit Care. 2016;20(1):1-10.
11. Aoyama H, Pettenuzzo T, Aoyama K, et al. Association of driving pressure with mortality among ventilated patients with acute respiratory distress syndrome: a systematic review and meta-analysis. Crit Care Med. 2018;46:300-6.
12. Guierin C, Papazian L, Reignier J, et al. Effect of driving pressure on mortality in ARDS patients during lung protective mechanical ventilation in two randomized controlled trials. Crit Care. 2016;20(1):1-9.
13. Laffey JG, Bellani G, Pham T, et al. Potentially modifiable factors contributing to outcome from acute respiratory distress syndrome: the LUNG SAFE study. Intensive Care Med. 2016;42(12):1865-76.
14. Tonetti T, Vasques F, Rapetti F, et al. Driving pressure and mechanical power: new targets for VILI prevention. Ann Transl Med. 2017;5(14):286.
15. Gattinoni L, Tonetti T, Cressoni M, et al. Ventilator-related causes of lung injury: the mechanical power. Intensive Care Med. 2016;42(10):1567-75.
16. Boissier F, Katsahian S, Razazi K, et al. Prevalence and prognosis of cor pulmonale during protective ventilation for acute respiratory distress syndrome. Intensive Care Med. 2013;39(10):1725-33.
17. Mekontso Dessap A, Boissier F, Charron C, et al. Acute cor pulmonale during protective ventilation for acute respiratory distress syndrome: prevalence, predictors, and clinical impact. Intensive Care Med. 2016;42(5):862-70.
18. Goligher EC, Fan E, Herridge MS, et al. Evolution of diaphragm thickness during mechanical ventilation: impact of inspiratory effort. Am J Respir Crit Care Med. 2015;192(9):1080-8.
19. Neto AS, Hemmes SNT, Barbas CSV, et al. Association between driving pressure and development of postoperative pulmonary complications in patients undergoing mechanical ventilation for general anaesthesia: a meta-analysis of individual patient data. Lancet Respir Med. 2016;4(4):272-80.
20. Ferrando C, Suarez-Sipmann F, Tusman G, et al. Open lung approach versus standard protective strategies: effects on driving pressure and ventilatory efficiency during anesthesia—a pilot, randomized controlled trial. PLoS One. 2017;12(5):1-12.
21. Serpa Neto A, Schmidt M, Azevedo LC, et al. Associations between ventilator settings during extracorporeal membrane oxygenation for refractory hypoxemia and outcome in patients with acute respiratory distress syndrome: a pooled individual patient data analysis: mechanical ventilation during ECMO. Intensive Care Med. 2016;42(11):1672-84.
22. Sahetya SK, Brower RG. The promises and problems of transpulmonary pressure measurements in acute respiratory distress syndrome. Curr Opin Crit Care. 2016;22(1):7-13.
23. Baedorf Kassis E, Loring SH, Talmor D. Mortality and pulmonary mechanics in relation to respiratory system and transpulmonary driving pressures in ARDS. Intensive Care Med. 2016;42(8):1206-13.
24. Henderson WR, Chen L, Amato MBP, et al. Fifty years of research in ARDS: respiratory mechanics in acute respiratory distress syndrome. Am J Respir Crit Care Med. 2017;196(7):822-33.
25. Grieco DL, Chen L, Brochard L. Transpulmonary pressure: importance and limits. Ann Transl Med. 2017;5(14):285.
26. Villar J, Martín-Rodríguez C, Domínguez-Berrot AM, et al. A quantile analysis of plateau and driving pressures: effects on mortality in patients with acute respiratory distress syndrome receiving lung-protective ventilation. Crit Care Med. 2017;45(5):843-50.

CHAPTER 44

Weaning from Ventilation

Ravi N Mistry, Brigitte Hollander, Ross Callum Freebairn

PHYSIOLOGY/SCIENTIFIC RATIONALE/ BIOLOGICAL PLAUSIBILITY

Mechanical ventilation (MV) is the mainstay of support for patients with severe lung disease and a driver of patient complications and health-care costs.[1] MV, which is a necessity of patient care during respiratory failure, is associated with complications that pose time-dependent risks to patients.[2,3] As respiratory function improves, MV needs to be withdrawn at the earliest possible stage balancing the risk and benefit with early or late cessation of MV.

Benefits of the MV in the critically ill are to support, or facilitate, gas exchange, maintain alveolar patency, and unload respiratory muscles. Unfortunately, the harms of MV are myriad. Patient-centered complications include that of ventilator-associated lung injury, side effects of pharmacotherapy used to allow MV, hospital-acquired infection, deconditioning, psychological distress, and mortality. MV is an expensive resource contributing to health-care costs though increases intensive care and hospital length of stay (LOS).[1]

Weaning is the successful separation (or liberation) of the patient from the ventilator. There is a lack of standardized definition and weaning definitions range from being totally free of MV support to just being free of invasive ventilation.[4,5] A 2004 consensus defined prolonged MV as ≥21 consecutive days of MV, for ≥6 h/day.[6]

The end of the weaning process also lacks agreed definitions and is variously defined as first extubation, successful extubation, unassisted breathing for 24 or 72 hours, the first spontaneous breathing trial (SBT) or successful SBT or an ill-defined "successful weaning."[4,7] Transitioning supportive therapy and adjuncts, such as high-flow nasal cannula, to weaning adds further complexity.[7] In contrast, weaning failure has been defined as a failure to discontinue MV or reintubation within 48–72 hours postextubation.[1]

ROUTINE WEANING

Once the need for muscle paralysis, deep sedation, prone positioning, and other complex respiratory interventions are no longer needed, early active weaning should commence.

Generally, once the underlying condition is improving or resolved, the majority of patients can be weaned by simple sequential cessation of neuromuscular-blocking agents, sedation and respiratory support, with wakefulness, spontaneous breathing and extubation following without significant delay. The truly "difficult-to-wean patient" represents one in six of all MV patients in the intensive care unit (ICU), and the required process is complex.[2,8]

The management of the underlying pathology is crucial as it may influence the ability to wean, but beyond the scope of this review. While it is prudent to consider weaning during early recovery, if the precipitant is an ongoing process (i.e. unresolved sepsis), attempts at early weaning may be interrupted by recurrence or by nosocomial complication, and may represent as backward progress in any weaning program.[9] However, the alternative of waiting until complete resolution of the underlying condition will unduly delay recovery and precipitate increased debilitation. The earliest return to spontaneous respiratory effort is important as even short intervals of complete diaphragmatic inactivity during MV may increase diaphragmatic proteolysis and atrophy.[10,11]

Weaning Predictors and Criteria

The patient's capacity to breathe spontaneously needs careful consideration as it is often underestimated. Problematically, neither clinical assessment nor objective assessments are reliable or accurate in assessing readiness to wean. While some patients failing weaning trials have satisfied weaning criteria, up to a third of patients judged by criteria not to be ready to wean can wean successfully. Evidence from studies is difficult to universally apply as nearly half of patients in the defining weaning studies were ventilated because of acute respiratory distress syndrome (ARDS), and many studies were limited to those ventilated for less than 2 weeks.[12]

Previous studies and systematic reviews suggest that weaning protocols be implemented daily which make assessment of weaning predictors to identify patients who may be ready for liberation from MV.[13] The traditional weaning algorithm was based upon moving from controlled modes to assist modes over a relatively short period. The addition of complex modes to the ventilator armamentarium that supports weaning means that the historic criteria are not necessarily relevant and have blurred the line between "ventilation" and "weaning."[14,15] Only five assessment tools were associated with weaning success or failure, with the success of most indices remaining below expectation.[7] A need for a more robust assessment tool remains.
- Negative inspiratory force (maximal inspiratory pressure).
- Minute ventilation.
- Respiratory frequency.
- Tidal volume.
- Frequency-TV ratio (f/TV) *During an SBT a higher ratio reflects a higher number of rapid shallow breaths and >105 was historically a predictor of weaning failure.*

One of the most common tools, the f/TV ratio (or rapid shallow breathing index), has been shown not to convey a survival benefit and did not assist in avoiding tracheostomy or extubation failure.[7] Therefore, we advise caution to the routine application of weaning predictors and instead suggest bedside assessment checklists for clinicians as a possible prompt for weaning.[3,7]

Spontaneous Breathing Trials

Once the determination that weaning is possible, and desirable, the next step is usually an SBT. SBT comprises an assessment of a patient's capacity to breathe and is advocated as the best method to ascertain extubation readiness.[3,7] SBT generally comprises a 30–60 minutes on low levels of pressure support ventilation (PSV) ranging from 0 cmH_2O to 8 cmH_2O (a "minimum level of support" has never been consistently defined), continuous positive airway pressure (CPAP) delivered by the ventilator (or other CPAP device) or using a T-piece attached to the endotracheal tube. A recent Cochrane systematic review confirms earlier reports that there is no difference in overall weaning success or outcomes based on the SBT method, although PSV was more effective than T-tube for successful SBT.[16] Approximately two-third of patients require minimal to no weaning and after the first SBT are extubated without difficulty.[3,8] The remaining one-third requires a more graduated approach of reducing the amount of ventilator support.[2] Both Ezingeard et al. and Cabello et al. found that a PSV trial immediately after a T-piece trial failure was successful in a number of patients, further reducing the "difficult to wean" pool.[17,18] After a failed weaning effort, if evidence for fatigue is apparent, then clinicians should provide 24 hours of rest on full MV before proceeding with the next weaning effort in order to rest the diaphragm.[19] Repeated SBT should be encouraged if the SBT was successful.

Weaning Protocol

The wake-up and breathe protocol is recommended as routine practice. It pairs a daily sedation hold spontaneous awakening trials, with daily SBT and produces better outcomes than historic approaches. The general outline of the standard wake up and wean process is displayed in Figure 44.1 per the Awakening and Breathing Controlled trial.[20]

There is insufficient evidence to evaluate the effectiveness of protocol-directed sedation regimes as results from two randomized controlled trials were conflicting.[21,22] Patients, who are not immediately weaned, need further immediate assessment to identify reversible factors, and then usually undergo either a strategy of progressive reduction of level of assistance, such as PSV, or progressively longer periods of spontaneous breathing, with or without CPAP. There are now a wide variety of alternative modes and strategies, most notably adaptive supportive ventilation (ASV), with apparent equivalence in weaning.[7,23,24]

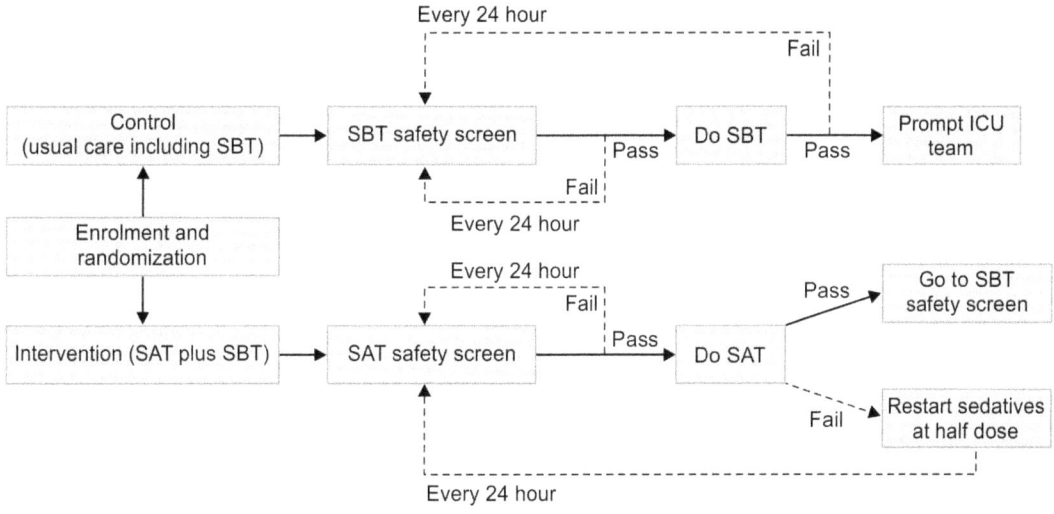

FIGURE 44.1: Treatment protocols.
(ICU: intensive care unit; SAT: spontaneous awakening trial; SBT: spontaneous breathing trial)

BARRIERS AND CHALLENGES TO A SPONTANEOUS BREATHING TRIAL AND WEANING

The factors which are potential barriers to weaning are outlined in Figure 44.2.

Early Challenges

In early severe respiratory failure the value of neuromuscular blockade, and prone positioning (such as in ARDS), means spontaneous breathing cannot not be recommended.[25,26] After this initial period, spontaneous breathing supported by modes, such as ASV, airway pressure release ventilation, bi-phasic inspiratory positive airway pressure, or pressure support, has appeal.[27] In less severe ARDS, and with lung recovery, spontaneous ventilation has potential to improve lung ventilation at lower levels of airway pressure and traditionally has been encouraged as it requires less sedation and improves cardiopulmonary function, possibly by recruiting nonventilated lung units, requiring a shorter duration of ventilatory support. In animals with severe lung injury, spontaneous breathing could worsen lung injury, and muscle paralysis might be more protective for injured lungs by preventing injuriously high transpulmonary pressure and high driving pressure.[27] Inspiratory pressure support provided to match the demand for a higher minute ventilation can lead to large transpulmonary pressure swings and TV that exceed the recommended maximums, both of which are major contributing factors to ventilator-induced lung injury and possibly to weaning failure.[7]

In injured lungs the lungs normal fluid-like behavior is not universally present. With spontaneous breathing the negative pleural pressures generated by diaphragmatic excursion are not uniformly transmitted across lung surfaces, but concentrated in dependent regions (i.e. posteriorly in the supine patient). Locally increased pleural pressure variations cause underdiagnosed regional overstretching in dorsal (dependent) lung regions, accompanying alveolar air shift (pendelluft), from ventral to dorsal parts of the lung. Excessive spontaneous efforts may cause local overstretch because of a significant pendelluft effect. Limiting the transalveolar pressure and tidal volumes generated is important in regard to ventilator-induced lung injury.[28] The cryptic damage, due to high transpulmonary pressures and regional over distension, will postpone successful weaning and increase both morbidity and mortality.

Increased Respiratory Load and Decreased Respiratory Force

Weaning patients have challenges with supranormal minute ventilation, increased airway resistance, decreased pulmonary and or chest wall compliance changes, abnormal intrinsic positive end-expiratory presssure (PEEP), and thus a greater work of breathing.[7] This increased respiratory load will favor failure if the generated respiratory force is unable to overcome it. Reversible factors (such as pulmonary edema and effusions) should be sought and optimization attempted; drainage or diuretics may improve compliance, oxygenation, decrease transpulmonary pressure, and shorten weaning time.[7] Indicators of failure should be

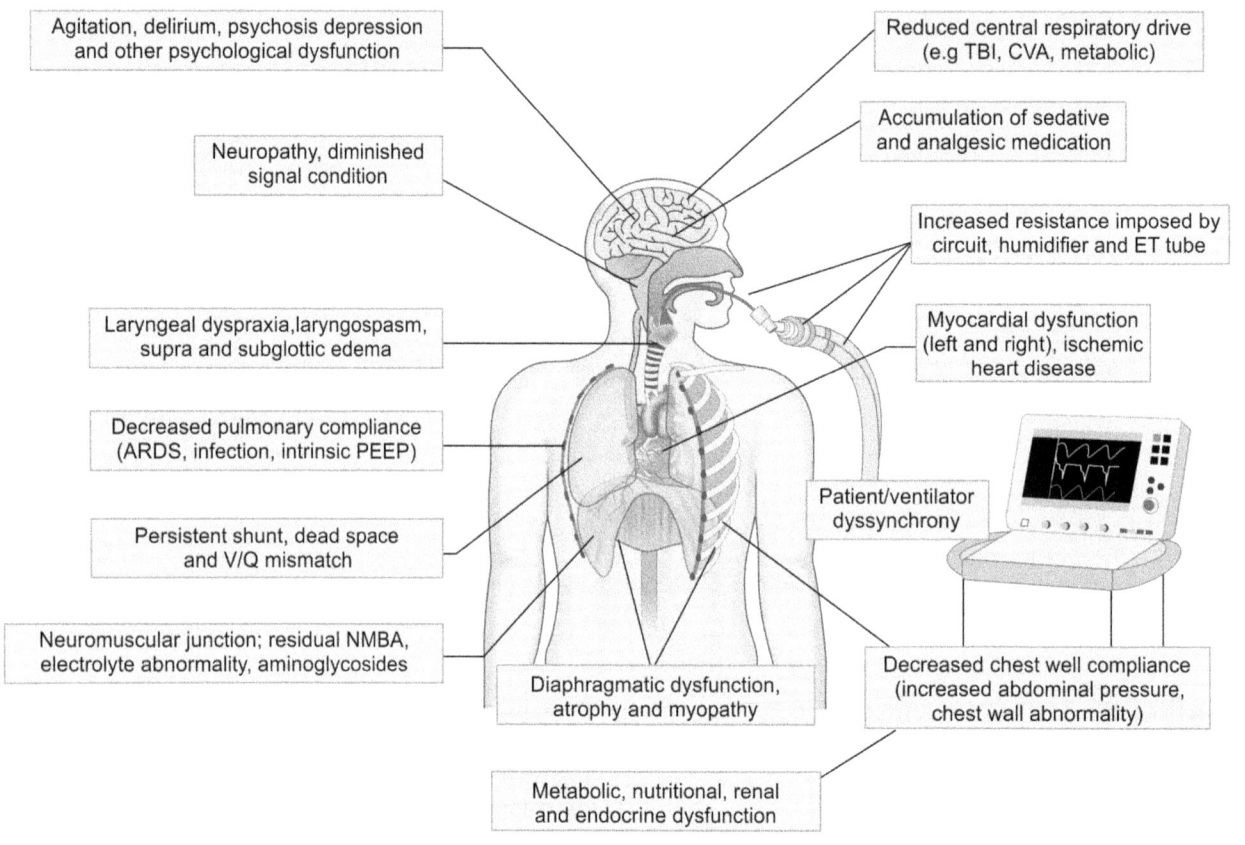

FIGURE 44.2: Barriers to weaning.
(ARDS: acute respiratory distress syndrome; PEEP: positive end-expiratory pressure; ET: endotracheal; CVA: cardiovascular accident; NMBA: neuromuscular blocking agent; TBI: traumatic brain injury)

considered (i.e. work of breathing, cardiopulmonary signs of deterioration), as an initially tolerable load may precipitate failure later in the SBT. After a week of ventilation, one-third of intensive care patients have impaired inspiratory muscle endurance, even after successful weaning. Although inspiratory muscle training improves tidal volumes, there is no increased survival or other benefit.[7,29]

Respiratory Drive

The central respiratory drive is frequently impaired and inappropriate hypoventilation to hypoxemia and/or hypercarbia may ensue with liberation from the ventilator. Though carbon dioxide responsiveness is seldom tested formally, but responsiveness to carbon dioxide assessed from the 100-ms occlusion pressure has been shown to predict weaning.[30]

Excess Sedation and Analgesia

Early sedation depth predicts delayed extubation.[31] Patients may be deeply sedated to facilitate prone positioning and neuromuscular blockade as therapies.[25,26] Kress demonstrated daily interruption of sedative infusions reduced the duration of MV, but protocol-directed sedation is controversial as results from the two randomized controlled trials were conflicting.[20-22]

Shorter MV duration may be assisted by an increased understanding of sedation goals by clinicians and appropriate sedative selection. The increasing use of propofol over midazolam has been associated with a decline in MV duration, tracheostomy rate, and intensive care unit length of stay (ICULOS) and total LOS.[32] The pharmacodynamic side effects of particular sedatives, such as the benzodiazepines, may increase delirium, agitation, and withdrawal and may delay weaning.[33,34]

Cardiac Load

Respiratory failure may be exacerbated by, precipitate and or mask, congestive and right heart failure. Positive pressure reduces pulmonary edema, provides increased alveolar pressures, and reduces left heart afterload. With weaning, spontaneous breathing is re-established, the process reverses and a negative pleural pressure is generated during inspiration.[35] This decrease in intrathoracic pressure increases the systemic venous return pressure gradient, the right ventricular preload, the central blood volume, and subsequently the left ventricular (LV) preload. Per LaPlaces law, the LV transmural gradient is increased and therefore afterload is increased.[36] Consequently, respiratory and cardiac failure may occur, associated with an increased work of breathing and hypoxemia.

Diagnosis and monitoring, augmented by echocardiography, allows titration of treatment by diuretics, vasodilators, and or inotropes. Coronary revascularization may need to be considered. Benefits of a negative fluid balance strategy are suggested by diuretic use tailored to brain natriuretic peptide levels shortening MV duration.[37] The use of a conservative fluid strategy shortened MV in patients with acute lung injury although poor longer term cognitive outcomes are concerning.[38,39]

Muscle Atrophy and Weakness

Early muscle changes are driven by inflammation and disuse, with resultant atrophy from protein degradation.[10,11] Late-phase muscle weakness persists in many despite resolution of lung injury and cessation of ongoing acute inflammation.[40] The effects of critical illness neuromyopathy will be additive to these. Novel therapies suggested for those who cannot exercise include electrical muscle stimulation, but the use in ICU is scarce.[41] Denervation injuries, for which there are no specific therapies, may persist and delay weaning.

Metabolic, Electrolyte, and Endocrine Issues

Metabolic alkalosis is a common disturbance in ICU. It impedes respiratory drive and can be caused by diuretic use, hypernatremia, and hypokalemia, all classically associated with prolonged MV management.[42] Increased serum bicarbonate is associated with increased ICULOS, more days on MV and hospital mortality.[43] Chloride-restricted fluids theoretically could increase metabolic alkalosis, but in a large randomized controlled trial (RCT), chloride restriction did not increase ventilation time.[44,45] Larger studies of "contraction alkalosis" and the effect of medications, such as acetazolamide, on weaning are needed.[46]

Serum calcium, phosphate, magnesium, and potassium deficiency all cause muscle weakness, and early correction of electrolyte abnormality is assistive to successful weaning.[47] Hypothyroidism, hypoadrenalism, and relative or absolute cortisol deficiency also contribute to weaning difficulty. Corticosteroids are used in critical illness for septic shock, specific respiratory pathology, or for other indications, and may also contribute.[48] Corticosteroids- and steroid-based neuromuscular-blocking agents are associated with muscular weakness, but their overall effect on weaning remains unclear.[49]

Psychological Dysfunction

Depression is common with prolonged MV, and weaning failure is twice as common in those with depression.[50] Second-generation antipsychotic and stimulants, such as donepezil, modafinil, and methylphenidate, have been used in difficult-to-wean patients' depression.[7] Whether their effect is through counteracting depression or anxiety or as a direct respiratory stimulus is unclear.

Delirium in the ICU is a common problem and is associated with delayed weaning and higher 6-month mortality.[29,51] Prevention strategies include early exercise and an "**A**wakening and **B**reathing **C**oordination, **D**elirium monitoring management and **E**arly exercise mobility (ABCDE)" bundle approach. Those approached with an ABCDE bundle spent 3 more days breathing without assistance and experienced nearly half the delirium, than patients treated with usual care.[52] Dexmedetomidine is recommended for use in ICU delirium though olanzapine, risperidone, and quetiapine are also used and may have some hemodynamic advantages in the critically ill.[53,54] Haloperidol is commonly used for ICU delirium although evidence is entirely anecdotal.[53] Fatigue and excessive daytime somnolence also delay weaning.[50]

Consent, Compliance, and Comfort

Initiation of weaning is a timely juncture when the objectives of future treatments are considered, as overly optimistic expectations may prevent meaningful discussion surrounding weaning outcomes and or end-of-life decision-making. Long-term outcomes from prolonged MV are worse than generally expected by relatives and physicians.[55] In a recent systematic review of studies reporting outcomes of patients requiring MV for more than 14 days, only half were successfully weaned, one in five were able to return home, and half were dead in 1 year.[56] If the physiological and emotional cost of weaning outweigh the longer term benefits, consideration should be made to stop a futile management strategy (unweanable ventilation) and treat the patient holistically, with palliation of symptoms.

SUMMARY

Weaning in the critically ill varies from a simple "non-event" to an extremely difficult and prolonged process. Whilst attention to the ventilator is important, much attention need to be paid to the adjunct patient cares, including that of sedation, analgesia, nutrition, and psychological support, as well as optimizing global organ function, particularly the cardiac, renal, and neurological systems. There is no magic remedy. A consistent approach, with regular detailed review and attention to housekeeping, is essential to ensure timely extrication of the patient from ventilator dependence.

REFERENCES

1. Webb AR, Angus DC, Finfer S. Oxford textbook of critical care. Oxford: Oxford University Press; 2016.
2. Herridge MS, Tansey CM, Matté A, et al. Functional disability 5 years after acute respiratory distress syndrome. N Engl J Med. 2011;364(14):1293-304.
3. Boles JM, Bion J, Connors A, et al. Weaning from mechanical ventilation. Eur Respir J. 2007;29(5):1033-56.
4. Blackwood B, Clarke M, McAuley DF, et al. How outcomes are defined in clinical trials of mechanically ventilated adults and children. Am J Respir Crit Care Med. 2014;189(8):886-93.
5. Contentin L, Ehrmann S, Giraudeau B. Heterogeneity in the definition of mechanical ventilation duration and ventilator-free days. Am J Respir Crit Care Med. 2014;189(8):998-1002.
6. MacIntyre NR, Epstein SK, Carson S, et al. Management of patients requiring prolonged mechanical ventilation: report of a NAMDRC consensus conference. Chest. 2005;128(6):3937-54.
7. Freebairn R. Weaning in ARDS. In: Acute respiratory distress syndrome. Springer 2017. pp. 133-53. ISBN 978-3-319-41850-6 ISBN 978-3-319-41852-0.
8. Funk GC, Anders S, Breyer MK, et al. Incidence and outcome of weaning from mechanical ventilation according to new categories. Eur Respir J. 2010;35(1):88-94.
9. Ambrosino N, Gabbrielli L. The difficult-to-wean patient. Expert Rev Respir Med. 2010;4(5):685-92.
10. Levine S, Nguyen T, Taylor N, et al. Rapid disuse atrophy of diaphragm fibers in mechanically ventilated humans. N Engl J Med. 2008;358(13):1327-35.
11. Hussain SNA, Mofarrahi M, Sigala I, et al. Mechanical ventilation-induced diaphragm disuse in humans triggers autophagy. Am J Respir Crit Care Med. 2010;182(11):1377-86.
12. Bellani G, Laffey JG, Pham T, et al. Epidemiology, patterns of care, and mortality for patients with acute respiratory distress syndrome in intensive care units in 50 countries. JAMA. 2016;315(8):788-800.
13. Ladeira MT, Vital FM, Andriolo RB, Andriolo BN, Atallah AN, Peccin MS. Pressure support versus T-tube for weaning from mechanical ventilation in adults. The Cochrane database of systematic reviews. 2014(5):CD006056.
14. Okamoto K, Iwamasa H, Dogomori H, Morioka T. Evaluation of conventional weaning criteria in patients with acute respiratory failure. J Anesth. 1990;4(3):213-8.
15. Frutos-Vivar F, Esteban A. Weaning from mechanical ventilation: why are we still looking for alternative methods? Med Intensiva. 2013;37(9):605-17.
16. Ladeira MT, Vital FM, Andriolo RB, et al. Pressure support versus T-tube for weaning from mechanical ventilation in adults. Cochrane Database Syst Rev. 2014;5:CD006056.
17. Cabello B, Thille AW, Roche-Campo F, et al. Physiological comparison of three spontaneous breathing trials in difficult-to-wean patients. Intensive Care Med. 2010;36(7):1171-9.
18. Ezingeard E, Diconne E, Guyomarc'h S, et al. Weaning from mechanical ventilation with pressure support in patients failing a T-tube trial of spontaneous breathing. Intensive Care Med. 2006;32(1):165-9.
19. Laghi F, D'Alfonso N, Tobin MJ. Pattern of recovery from diaphragmatic fatigue over 24 hours. J Appl Physiol. 1995;79(2):539-46.
20. Girard TD, Kress JP, Fuchs BD, et al. Efficacy and safety of a paired sedation and ventilator weaning protocol for mechanically ventilated patients in intensive care (Awakening and Breathing Controlled trial): a randomised controlled trial. Lancet. 2008;371(9607):126-34.
21. Aitken LM, Bucknall T, Kent B, et al. Sedation protocols to reduce duration of mechanical ventilation in the ICU: a Cochrane systematic review. J Adv Nurs. 2016;72(2):261-72.
22. Bucknall TK, Manias E, Presneill JJ. A randomized trial of protocol-directed sedation management for mechanical ventilation in an Australian intensive care unit. Critical Care Med. 2008;36(5):1444-50.
23. Rose L, Schultz MJ, Cardwell CR, et al. Automated versus non-automated weaning for reducing the duration of mechanical ventilation for critically ill adults and children. Cochrane Database Syst Rev. 2014;6:CD009235.
24. McMullen SM, Meade M, Rose L, et al. Partial ventilatory support modalities in acute lung injury and acute respiratory distress syndrome—a systematic review. PLoS One. 2012;7(8):e40190.
25. Guérin C, Reignier J, Richard JC, et al. Prone positioning in severe acute respiratory distress syndrome. N Engl J Med. 2013;368(23):2159-68.
26. Papazian L, Forel JM, Gacouin A, et al. Neuromuscular blockers in early acute respiratory distress syndrome. N Engl J Med. 2010;363(12):1107-16.
27. Yoshida T, Papazian L. When to promote spontaneous respiratory activity in acute respiratory distress patients? Anesthesiology. 2014;120(6):1313-5.
28. Yoshida T, Torsani V, Gomes S, et al. Spontaneous effort causes occult pendelluft during mechanical ventilation. Am J Respir Crit Care Med. 2013;188(12):1420-7.
29. Condessa RL, Brauner JS, Saul AL, et al. Inspiratory muscle training did not accelerate weaning from mechanical ventilation but did improve tidal volume and maximal respiratory pressures: a randomised trial. J Physiother. 2013;59(2):101-7.
30. Montgomery AB, Holle RHO, Neagley SR, et al. Prediction of successful ventilator weaning using airway occlusion pressure and hypercapnic challenge. Chest. 1987;91(4):496-9.
31. Shehabi Y, Bellomo R, Reade MC, et al. Early intensive care sedation predicts long-term mortality in ventilated critically ill patients. Am J Respir Crit Care Med. 2012;186(8):724-31.

32. Jarman AM, Duke GJ, Reade MC, et al. The association between sedation practices and duration of mechanical ventilation in intensive care. Anaesth Intensive Care. 2013;41(3):311-5.
33. Devlin J, Fraser G, Ely EW, et al. Pharmacological management of sedation and delirium in mechanically ventilated ICU patients: remaining evidence gaps and controversies. Semin Respir Crit Care Med. 2013;34(2):201-15.
34. Porhomayon J, El-Solh AA, Adlparvar G, et al. Impact of sedation on cognitive function in mechanically ventilated patients. Lung. 2016;194(1):43-52.
35. Lemaire F, Teboul JL, Cinotti L, et al. Acute left ventricular dysfunction during unsuccessful weaning from mechanical ventilation. Anesthesiology. 1988;69(2):171-9.
36. Pinsky MR. Breathing as exercise: the cardiovascular response to weaning from mechanical variation. In: Applied physiology in intensive care medicine 2: physiological reviews and editorials. Springer 2012. pp. 323-5.
37. Dessap AM, Roche-Campo F, Kouatchet A, et al. Natriuretic peptide-driven fluid management during ventilator weaning: a randomized controlled trial. Am J Respir Crit Care Med. 2012;186(12):1256-63.
38. Dessap AM, Katsahian S, Roche-Campo F, et al. Ventilator-associated pneumonia during weaning from mechanical ventilation: role of fluid management. Chest. 2014;146(1):58-65.
39. Mikkelsen ME, Shull WH, Biester RC, et al. Cognitive, mood and quality of life impairments in a select population of ARDS survivors. Respirology. 2009;14(1):76-82.
40. Files DC, Sanchez MA, Morris PE. A conceptual framework: the early and late phases of skeletal muscle dysfunction in the acute respiratory distress syndrome. Crit Care. 2015;19(1):266.
41. Edwards J, McWilliams D, Thomas M, et al. Electrical muscle stimulation in the intensive care unit: an integrative review. J Intensive Care Soc. 2014;15(2):142-9.
42. Mæhle K, Haug B, Flaatten H, Nielsen EW. Metabolic alkalosis is the most common acid–base disorder in ICU patients. Crit Care. 2014;18(2):420.
43. Libório AB, Noritomi DT, Leite TT, et al. Increased serum bicarbonate in critically ill patients: a retrospective analysis. Intensive Care Med. 2015;41(3):479-86.
44. Krajewski ML, Raghunathan K, Paluszkiewicz SM, et al. Meta-analysis of high- versus low-chloride content in perioperative and critical care fluid resuscitation. Br J Surg. 2015;102(1):24-36.
45. Young P, Bailey M, Beasley R, et al. Effect of a buffered crystalloid solution vs saline on acute kidney injury among patients in the intensive care unit: the SPLIT randomized clinical trial. JAMA. 2015;314(16):1701-10.
46. Mazur JE, Devlin JW, Peters MJ, et al. Single versus multiple doses of acetazolamide for metabolic alkalosis in critically ill medical patients: a randomized, double-blind trial. Crit Care Med. 1999;27(7):1257-61.
47. Barron R, Freebairn R. Electrolyte disorders in the critically ill. Anaesth Intensive Care Med. 2010;11(12):523-8.
48. Peter JV, John P, Graham PL, et al. Corticosteroids in the prevention and treatment of acute respiratory distress syndrome (ARDS) in adults: meta-analysis. BMJ. 2008;336(7651):1006-9.
49. Hermans G, Van den Berghe G. Clinical review: intensive care unit acquired weakness. Crit Care. 2015;19(1):274.
50. Jubran A, Lawm G, Kelly J, et al. Depressive disorders during weaning from prolonged mechanical ventilation. Intensive Care Med. 2010;36(5):828-35.
51. Jeon K, Jeong BH, Ko MG, et al. Impact of delirium on weaning from mechanical ventilation in medical patients. Respirology. 2016;21(2):313-20.
52. Balas MC, Vasilevskis EE, Olsen KM, et al. Effectiveness and safety of the awakening and breathing coordination, delirium monitoring/management, and early exercise/mobility bundle. Crit Care Med. 2014;42(5):1024-36.
53. Reade MC. Optimal sedation for the ventilation of critically ill patients. Curr Respir Med Rev. 2010;6(4):292-9.
54. Shehabi Y, Botha JA, Ernest D, et al. Clinical application, the use of dexmedetomidine in intensive care sedation. Crit Care Shock. 2010;13(2):40-50.
55. Cox CE, Martinu T, Sathy SJ, et al. Expectations and outcomes of prolonged mechanical ventilation. Crit Care Med. 2009;37(11):2888-94.
56. Damuth E, Mitchell JA, Bartock JL, et al. Long-term survival of critically ill patients treated with prolonged mechanical ventilation: a systematic review and meta-analysis. Lancet Respir Med. 2015;3(7):544-53.

CHAPTER 45

High-flow Nasal Cannula Respiratory Support

Jane O' Donnell

INTRODUCTION

Since the 1940s the ubiquitous conventional oxygen therapy (COT) has been in use providing both limited flows and concentrations of unconditioned supplemental oxygen. In reality these cannulas have several inherent limitations.

More than 15 years ago clinicians' saw the introduction of a new form of noninvasive respiratory support now commonly known as nasal high-flow (NHF) therapy. Today this therapy is used throughout hospitals and in the home settings. This therapy was designed for use with in conjunction with specially designed nasal cannula and medical humidifiers. These humidifiers are capable of conditioning the delivered gases, thus fully humidifying (100% saturated with H_2O) and heating these gases to body temperature (37°C). Consequently, the discomfort and drying of upper airway mucosa seen with COT is now offset.

This therapy had first become a standard of care for infants, children, preterm neonates with flows of more than 2 L/min were demonstrated to create a distending pressure akin to nasal continuous positive airway pressure (CPAP); and now it is very much in use for adults.

Therapeutic flows for adults are in the 10–60 L/min range; with an option to independently blend air/O_2 to reliably titrate the FiO_2 delivered between 21–100%. This change in practice has been driven by the number of confirmed clinical benefits seen over conventional respiratory therapy.

There is considerable reliable published evidence which both substantiates the proposed mechanisms of action. The efficacy of this therapy across a variety of clinical applications and settings has been confirmed, however further research is warranted.

This NHF chapter will characterize: Mechanisms of action, therapeutic efficacy, contemporary delivery, and strategies for clinical applications.

NASAL HIGH-FLOW MECHANISMS OF ACTION

The efficacy of this therapy has been demonstrated through the interplay of a series of mechanisms which are distinct to NHF.

Respiratory Support

Many physiological benefits have been demonstrated with the application of NHF therapy, both in healthy volunteers, and those with acute and chronic illness.

The physiological effects of NHF on gas exchange, inspiratory effort, minute ventilation (MV), lung volume, dynamic compliance, transpulmonary pressure, work of breathing and pulmonary homogeneity have been assessed both with standard clinical, and additional advanced measures, such as transesophageal pressure, electrical impedance, respiratory inductance plethysmography, and ultrasound.[1,2]

It is accepted that NHF improves breathing efficiency as demonstrated by an increases in tidal volume and reduction in respiratory rate, at a constant minute volume.[3,4]

Mauri (2016) considered the use of NHF in patients with acute hypoxemic respiratory failure.[1] NHF improved oxygenation; reduced the patient's effort; reduced the MV needed to obtain a physiological $PaCO_2$ level; increased the end-expiratory lung volume; and improved dynamic compliance, transpulmonary pressure, and ventilation homogeneity. These outcomes might confirm the clinical efficacy of NHF therapy.

Itagaki (2014) evaluated levels thoracoabdominal asynchrony using respiratory inductance plethysmography.[2] Thoracoabdominal asynchrony was improved with NHF compared to COT. Additionally, respiratory rate and minute volume were lower with NHF, whilst $PaCO_2$ and tidal volume remained unchanged.

Washout of the Anatomical Dead Space

Nasal high-flow therapy continuously flushes the dead space volume of expired CO_2 (normally present in the nasopharynx) much like tracheal gas insufflation.[5] The CO_2 flushing effect is flow dependent. This effect then optimizes the proportion of the potential MV available for gaseous exchange. More specifically, the turbulence flushes CO_2 from the nasopharynx, augmenting respiratory efficiency by reducing the fraction of inspired CO_2, whilst raising FiO_2. The flushed dead space is then filled with O_2 ready for the next inspiration. It is the mechanism that is often thought to drive both the reductions in respiratory rate and work of breathing often seen.

This effect is correlated with increases in NHF flow as opposed to increases in pressure.[6] Given the fact that NHF is an open system (non-sealed), the volume of dead space flushed cannot be precisely determined.

Delivery of a Dynamic Level of Positive Pressure

A low level dynamic positive pressure effect within the nasopharyngeal and esophageal anatomy has been demonstrated in adults, infants, and neonates.[7-13] This phenomenon has been confirmed both in studies of both healthy and non-healthy participants[7,8] in patients with stable chronic obstructive pulmonary disease (COPD) and idiopathic pulmonary fibrosis (IPF),[9] and post-cardio thoracic surgery.[10-12]

Corley (2011) evaluated both the pressure effect and end-expiratory lung volume using electrical lung impedance tomography.[11] The research found that end-expiratory lung volume was greater with NHF, than with COT; which suggests an association between the NHF pressure effect and enhanced lung volumes.

The pressure generated by NHF therapy is dynamic and it varies across the breath cycle. There is a demonstrated peak at end expiration due to the resistance generated against the incoming flow. During inspiration a low level of pressure exists which provides a small amount of inspiratory assistance which may counterbalance auto-positive end-expiratory pressure (PEEP) (through the aforementioned end-expiration pressure effect). This phenomenon is especially relevant for patients with high levels of intrinsic PEEP, for example, in COPD. The pressure levels seen are variable, NHF is an open (non-sealed) system, and the size of the cannula relative to the nares has an effect as does individual lung compliance.

The pressure recorded during breathing with NHF correlates linearly with the NHF flow rate and is significantly higher when mouths are closed. Parke (2011) observed in adults, that for each increase of 10 L/min flow rate the mean airway pressure increased by 0.69 cm H_2O (p, .01). When subjects breathed with their mouths closed the pressure increased by 0.35 cmH_2O (p, .03).[12]

For infants and neonates, the pressure seen is approximate to that seen with nasal CPAP.[13,14]

Supplemental Oxygen

In some circumstances NHF therapy with air alone is thought to be able to demonstrate beneficial effects, however if supplemental O_2 is required there is the option to titrate it in. For patients with a high inspiratory flow demand COT is often unable to meet the required flow needs, therefore room air is entrained diluting the delivered FiO_2. This entrainment varies breath by breath (as does the inspiratory flow demand) so the actual concentration of delivered O_2 is unknown which could precipitate either a hyperoxic or a hypoxic event. In contrast, and in many cases, NHF has the ability to meet or exceed the inspiratory flow demand therefore less entrainment of room air occurs, as a result the desired FiO_2 is more reliably delivered.[7,15]

In some extreme cases the inspiratory flow demand may even exceed the flow capabilities of NHF, nonetheless NHF still performs better than COT.[16]

Airway Hydration

The conditioning of gases to body temperature 37°C and 100% humidified and delivered by NHF is known to enhance comfort for and tolerance by patients.[17,18] There are a series of other anticipated benefits, some of which are speculative:

- Desiccation of the airways may be avoided, thus supporting both the integrity of mucociliary function, and subsequent secretion clearance.[19]

- Minimizing the bronchoconstriction associated with the delivery of cold, dry gas as delivered per COT.[20]
- Relief of the metabolic burden of conditioning the inspired gas for vulnerable/high-acuity patients.

THERAPEUTIC EFFICACY—CLINICAL OUTCOMES

The therapeutic efficacy of NHF is rapidly evolving, and driven both by the published evidence and the preference of clinicians. This therapy has been described in use in domiciliary settings and throughout the hospital on patients with differing clinical acuities and presentations.

Respiratory Failure

Respiratory Failure Type I

Patients with respiratory failure (whatever the cause) need significant levels of respiratory support in order to avoid escalation. Traditionally, the primary therapy has involved COT, noninvasive ventilation (NIV) and or intubation. In 2010, the first observational study of NHF versus COT was published, NHF was deemed superior for comfort and respiratory rate and SpO_2.[21] NHF has been found to be effective for patients with all severities of respiratory failure. Frat (2015) determined that neither NIV nor NHF decreased the rate of intubation among patients with hypoxemic ARF.[22] In contrast, intubation rates did trend lower with NHF (p = 0.18). NHF use resulted in reduced mortality both within the ICU and up to 90 days. Of note the mortality rates with COT were × 2 NHF (p = 0.046), and with NIV × 2.5 that of the NHF (p = 0.006). For the subgroup with PaO_2: FiO_2 less than 200 mm Hg a significantly lower 28-day intubation rate (p = 0.009). NHF might therefore be considered as a first-line strategy in these patients, conversely NIV should be used cautiously as it may potentially worsen pre-existing lung injury.[23]

Respiratory Failure Type II

There is some evidence to suggest that NHF therapy can support patients with some types of hypercapnic respiratory failure.[24-27] Patients with hypercapnic respiratory failure frequently present and have been historically managed with NIV which is often not well tolerated. Millar (2014) have reported the use of NHF for the successful management of a patient unable to tolerate NIV.[28] Bräunlich (2012) evaluated the use of NHF both in healthy volunteers, and those with COPD, and IPF. Nasal high-flow use was associated with an increased tidal volume in the COPD and IPF groups, whilst respiratory rate and minute volume decreased in all groups.[9]

Immunocompromised

The needs of the immunocompromised patient are complex, with ARF being the most common complication. Careful selection of any intervention is vital NIV has been recommended as a first-line strategy despite the fact that studies have reported no benefit and even deleterious effects related to NIV. Retrospective reports of NHF use for these patients have suggested efficacy, however in a large randomized study NHF was not deemed superior to COT for rates of 28-day mortality.[29]

Postextubation

Effective postextubation respiratory support is vital to avoid reintubation and associated increases in ICU and in-hospital length of stay and mortality. In patients at high risk for reintubation NHF was noninferior to NIV.[30] In patients at low risk for reintubation NHF was superior to COT.[31]

Palliative care/Do-not-intubate

Nasal high-flow is emerging as an effective and ethical alternative to NIV for end of life care. Peters (2013) assessed the efficacy of NHF in patients with a do-not-intubate (DNI) and with hypoxemic respiratory failure.[32] The comorbid conditions of those studied included: pulmonary fibrosis, pneumonia, COPD, cancer, hematologic malignancy, and CHF. The minority (18%) required escalation to NIV and 82% were maintained on NHF.

Procedural Sedation

During invasive interventions hypoxemia is common and supplemental oxygen necessitated. Nasal high-flow has been used to provide a practical solution to both prevent and treat hypoxic events during bronchoscopy,[33] gastroscopy,[34] transesophageal echocardiogram,[35] bronchoalveolar lavage,[36] and during dental surgery.[37]

Peri-intubation

Intubation of the unstable ICU patient is often associated with significant complications. NIV can be applied to preoxygenate these patients however during laryngoscopy it must be removed, thus depriving a patient of O_2. In contrast NHF cannula do not need to be removed and are able to deliver high flows and high concentrations of O_2 throughout the procedure including the apneic period of tracheal intubation. The efficacy of this practice has not been established, robust randomized clinical trials are mandated.

Postoperative

Differing forms of respiratory support have been used to reverse postsurgical respiratory complications. NIV is recommended for the curative and prophylactic management of ARF in postoperative patients in ICU. However, recent studies suggest that NHF may have a role to play.

A large-scale randomized postcardiothoracic study suggested that NHF was equally good as NIV. No significant differences were seen for rates of treatment failure or ICU mortality (p, 0.66).[17]

In a study of post-lung resection patients, similar results were observed in the difference between preoperative and postoperative 6-minute walk test and spirometry between NHF and COT. Length of hospital stay was significantly lower in the NHF group and NHF reduced mortality both in the ICU and up to 90 days.[38]

In a study of postabdominal surgery patients, no differences for postoperative hypoxemia, pulmonary complications or length of hospital stay were found between the two groups studied.[39]

Others

There are many emerging/proposed applications for NHF. We await the conduct of further efficacy studies with appropriate and robust methodologies. The scope of the applications is very broad possibly reflecting the versatility of this therapy, for example, acute pulmonary edema,[40] acute heart failure,[41] and cystic fibrosis.[42]

Contraindications for NHF

The adoption of NHF therapy is now widespread. No absolute NHF contraindications have ever been reported in the literature, consequently the contraindications for NIV may be applied (Box 45.1).[43]

NASAL HIGH-FLOW DELIVERY

There are three options available for the delivery of this therapy:
1. An air/oxygen blender, a heated humidifier, a single heated circuit, and a dedicated nasal cannula. The flow source is the air/oxygen blender, the inspiratory fraction of oxygen (FiO_2) is set from 0.21 to 1.0 in flows of up to 60 L/min. Medical oxygen and air are required. The gas is heated and humidified with a humidifier and delivered through a heated circuit (Fig. 45.1).
2. A specialist ventilator with a high-flow mode, with a heated humidifier, a single heated circuit, and a dedicated nasal cannula. The flow source is the ventilator, the inspiratory fraction of oxygen (FiO_2) is set between 0.21 and 1.0 and flows of up to 60 L/min. Medical oxygen and air is required. The gas is heated and humidified with a humidifier and delivered through a heated circuit.
3. A specialist independent NHF source with an inbuilt heated humidifier, for example AIRVO™ Fisher & Paykel Healthcare, a single heated circuit, and a dedicated nasal cannula. The flow source is the specialist unit, the inspiratory fraction of oxygen (FiO_2) is set from 0.21 to 1.0 with flows up to 60 L/min. Only medical oxygen is required, air is entrained into the flow source. The gas is heated and humidified with an inbuilt humidifier and delivered through a heated circuit. This particular flow source may be used in the home and, or anywhere within a hospital setting (Fig. 45.2).

The specialist nasal cannula (patient interface) are available in a range of sizes (neonates to adults), there is also an option of a tracheostomy interface. These specialist cannulas are designed for maximum comfort and stability. A major difference between NIV and NHF is the interface. NIV interfaces increase anatomical dead space, whereas NHF interfaces decrease dead space (Fig. 45.3).

NASAL HIGH-FLOW STRATEGIES FOR CLINICAL APPLICATIONS

Clinical outcome data for NHF has rapidly emerged, and so too are the reliable recommendations on practical applications of its use. This data combined with the data from the relevant physiological and mechanistic studies can inform clinical decision making around appropriate patient selection.

BOX 45.1: Contraindications to noninvasive ventilation (NIV).

1. Level of consciousness compromised:
   - Unresponsive
   - Agitated
   - Uncooperative
2. Claustrophobia
3. Airway obstruction or unable to be maintained
4. Craniofacial injury or malformation
5. Unstable hemodynamics:
   - Shock
   - Intractable arrhythmia
   - Post-cardiopulmonary resuscitation (CPR)
6. Respiratory and or cardiac arrest either imminent or recent

Source: Jaber (2010)

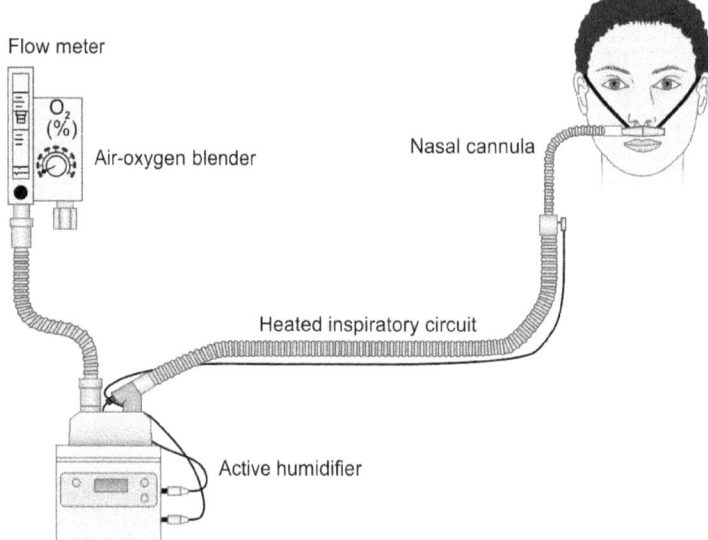

FIGURE 45.1: Delivery of high-flow nasal therapy via an air oxygen blender and heated humidifier. This allows 0.21 to 1.0 FiO_2, and up to 60 L/min flow. The air/oxygen is mixed with a blender, heated and humidified through an active heated humidifier and delivered via a single-limb heated inspiratory circuit [OPT94X cannula, MR850 heated humidifier, RT241 heated delivery tube (Fisher and Paykel Healthcare Ltd, Auckland, New Zealand)].

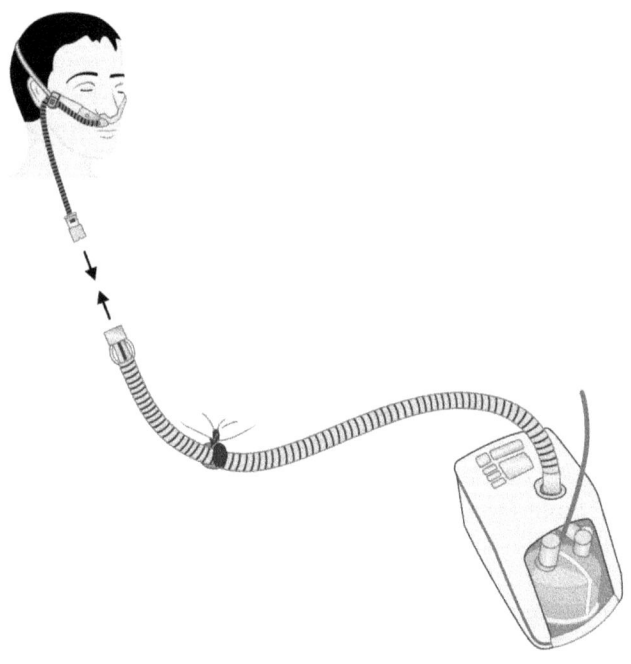

FIGURE 45.2: Delivery of high-flow nasal therapy via an independent flow source with built in humidifier and blender. This allows 0.21 to 1.0 FiO_2, and up to 60 L/min flow. The gas is mixed, heated and humidified through an active heated humidifier and delivered via a single-limb heated inspiratory circuit [OPT94X cannula, AIRVO 2™ flow source, heated delivery tube and chamber 900PT501 (Fisher and Paykel Healthcare Ltd, Auckland, New Zealand)].

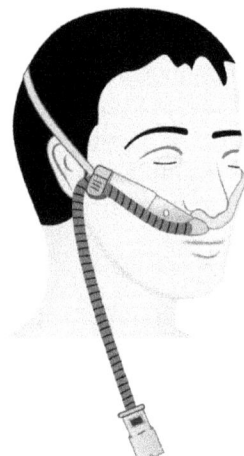

FIGURE 45.3: Adult high-flow nasal cannula interface Optiflow™ [OPT94X cannula (Fisher and Paykel Healthcare Ltd, Auckland, New Zealand)].

Many physiological and mechanistic studies have demonstrated that the beneficial effects demonstrated are related to flow rate. Published studies, involving adults describe starting flow rates of 20, 25, and 35 L/min, but the majority start at 50 L/min.[44] Logic would then suggest that flow should be adjusted first and then FiO_2 titrated to maintain a target oxygenation. Flow rates on commercially available devices differ but range from 5 to 60 L/min.

It would be reasonable to expect that an increase in flow and or FiO_2 or would be expected to improve gaseous exchange, due to the reduced entrainment during inspiration. The requirement to up titrate or conversely down titrate is reliably demonstrated by changes in respiratory physiology particularly respiratory rate. An index known as the ROX index has been validated for use with patients with ARF and pneumonia, the index can identify patients at low risk for NHF failure.[45] The index is defined as the ratio of SpO_2/FiO_2 to respiratory rate.

Escalation/Up Titration in Adults

When aiming to increase SpO_2, up titration of flow is preferable to raising FiO_2. However, if SpO_2 falls substantially below an acceptable target, increases in FiO_2 can potentially raise the PaO_2 more rapidly. Additional increases in flow rate can then be used to maintain targeted SpO_2 while FiO_2 is lowered to nontoxic levels.

Tolerance of continuous NHF for prolonged periods (many days) is high. As with all forms of respiratory support there are limitations and patients on this therapy should be adequately monitored. Just as described with NIV, clinicians' may fail to recognize subtle signs of failure and a need to escalate care, which if delayed has consequences.[46]

De-escalation in Adults

When aiming to deescalate, or wean from NHF it is recommended to wean the FiO_2 first then the flow. A proposed weaning strategy involves first reducing FiO_2 to 40%, then flow in increments of 5 L/min.[44]

RESEARCH FOCUS AREAS

Much of the published research has been conducted within the high acuity arena such as the ICU. Further studies with appropriate and robust methodologies are needed to confirm the efficacy of NHF over other forms of respiratory support in specific populations and conditions in differing settings. This will assist in the development of clinical practice guidelines, and to provide an evidence base to potentially extend the scope of application of this therapy.

REFERENCES

1. Mauri T, Turrini C, Eronia N, et al. Physiologic effects of high-flow nasal cannula in acute hypoxemic respiratory failure. Am J Respir Crit Care Med. 2017;195(9):1207-15.
2. Itagaki T, Okuda N, Tsunano Y, et al. Effect of high-flow nasal cannula on thoraco-abdominal synchrony in adult critically ill patients. Respir Care. 2014;59(1):70-4.
3. Mündel T, Feng S, Tatkov S, et al. Mechanisms of nasal high flow on ventilation during wakefulness and sleep. J Appl Physiol (1985). 2013;114(8):1058-65.
4. Riera J, Pérez P, Cortés J, et al. Effect of high-flow nasal cannula and body position on end-expiratory lung volume: a cohort study using electrical impedance tomography. Respir Care. 2013;58(4):589-96.
5. Spence CJT, Buchmann NA, Jermy MC. Unsteady flow in the nasal cavity with high flow therapy measured by stereoscopic PIV. Exp Fluids. 2011;52(3):569-79.
6. Frizzola M, Miller TL, Rodriguez ME, et al. High-flow nasal cannula: impact on oxygenation and ventilation in an acute lung injury model. Pediatr Pulmonol. 2011;46(1):67-74.
7. Sim MAB, Dean P, Kinsella J, et al. Performance of oxygen delivery devices when the breathing pattern of respiratory failure is simulated. Anaesthesia. 2008;63(9):938-40.
8. Groves N, Tobin A. High flow nasal oxygen generates positive airway pressure in adult volunteers. Aust Crit Care. 2007;20(4):126-31.
9. Bräunlich J, Beyer D, Mai D, et al. Effects of nasal high flow on ventilation in volunteers, COPD and idiopathic pulmonary fibrosis patients. Respiration. 2012;85(4):319-25.
10. Parke R, McGuinness S, Eccleston M. Nasal high-flow therapy delivers low level positive airway pressure. Br J Anaesth. 2009;103(6):886-90.
11. Corley A, Caruana LR, Barnett AG, et al. Oxygen delivery through high-flow nasal cannulae increase end-expiratory lung volume and reduce respiratory rate in post-cardiac surgical patients. Br J Anaesth. 2011;107(6):998-1004.
12. Parke RL, Eccleston ML, McGuinness SP. The effects of flow on airway pressure during nasal high-flow oxygen therapy. Respir Care. 2011;56(8):1151-5.
13. Spence KL, Murphy D, Kilian C, et al. High-flow nasal cannula as a device to provide continuous positive airway pressure in infants. J Perinatol. 2007;27(12):772-5.
14. Saslow JG, Aghai ZH, Nakhla TA, et al. Work of breathing using high-flow nasal cannula in preterm infants. J Perinatol. 2006;26(8):476-80.
15. Wagstaff TAJ, Soni N. Performance of six types of oxygen delivery devices at varying respiratory rates. Anaesthesia. 2007;62(5):492-503.
16. Ritchie JE, Williams AB, Gerard C, et al. Evaluation of humidified nasal high-flow oxygen system, using oxygraphy, capnography and measurement of upper airways pressure. Anesth Intensive Care. 2011:39(6):1103-10.
17. Stéphan F, Barrucand B, Petit P, et al. High-flow nasal oxygen vs noninvasive positive airway pressure in hypoxemic patients after cardiothoracic surgery: a randomized clinical trial. JAMA. 2015;313(23):2331-9.
18. Maggiore SM, Idone FA, Vaschetto R, et al. Nasal high-flow versus Venturi mask oxygen therapy after extubation. Effects on oxygenation, comfort, and clinical outcome. Am J Respir Crit Care Med. 2014;190(3):282-8.
19. Hasani A, Chapman TH, McCool D, et al. Domiciliary humidification improves lung mucociliary clearance in patients with bronchiectasis. Chron Respir Dis. 2008;5(2):81-6.

20. Williams R, Rankin N, Smith T, et al. Relationship between the humidity and temperature of inspired gas and the function of the airway mucosa. Crit Care Med. 1996;24(11):1920-9.
21. Roca O, Riera J, Torres F, et al. High-flow oxygen therapy in acute respiratory failure. Respir Care. 2010;55:408-13.
22. Frat JP, Thille AW, Mercat A, et al. High-flow oxygen through nasal cannula in acute hypoxemic respiratory failure. N Engl J Med. 2015;372(23):2185-96.
23. Frat JP, Coudroy R, Thille AW. Non-invasive ventilation or high-flow oxygen therapy: When to choose one over the other? Respirology. 2018. doi: 10.1111/resp.13435.
24. Bräunlich J, Kohler M, Wirtz H. Nasal high-flow improves ventilation in patients with COPD. Int J Chron Obstruct Pulmon Dis. 2016;11:1077-85.
25. Atwood CW Jr, Camhi S, Little KC, et al. Impact of Heated Humidified High Flow Air via Nasal Cannula on Respiratory Effort in Patients with Chronic Obstructive Pulmonary Disease. J Chron Obstruct Pulmon Dis. 2017;4(4):279-86.
26. Fraser JF, Spooner AJ, Dunster KR, et al. Nasal high flow oxygen therapy in patients with COPD reduces respiratory rate and tissue carbon dioxide while increasing tidal and end-expiratory lung volumes: a randomised crossover trial. Thorax. 2016;71:759-61.
27. Pisani L, Fasano L, Corcione N, et al. Change in pulmonary mechanics and the effect on breathing pattern of high flow oxygen therapy in stable hypercapnic COPD. Thorax. 2017;72:373-5.
28. Millar J, Lutton S, O'Connor P. The use of high-flow nasal oxygen therapy in the management of hypercarbic respiratory failure. Ther Adv Respir Dis. 2014;8(2):63-4.
29. Azoulay E, Lemiale V, Mokart D, et al. Effect of High-Flow Nasal Oxygen vs Standard Oxygen on 28-Day Mortality in Immunocompromised Patients With Acute Respiratory Failure: The HIGH Randomized Clinical Trial. JAMA. 2018. doi: 10.1001/jama.2018.14282.
30. Hernández G, Vaquero C, González P, et al. Effect of postextubation high-flow nasal cannula vs conventional oxygen therapy on reintubation in low-risk patients: a randomized clinical trial. JAMA. 2016;315:1354-61.
31. Hernández G, Vaquero C, Colinas L, et al. Effect of postextubation high-flow nasal cannula vs noninvasive ventilation on reintubation and postextubation respiratory failure in high-risk patients: a randomized clinical trial. JAMA. 2016;316:1565-74.
32. Peters SG, Holets SR, Gay PC. High-flow nasal cannula therapy indo-not-intubate patients with hypoxemic respiratory distress. Respir Care. 2013;58(4):597-600.
33. Lucangelo U, Vassallo FG, Marras E, et al. High-flow nasal interface improves oxygenation in patients undergoing bronchoscopy. Crit Care Res Pract. 2012;2012:506382.
34. La Combe B, Messika J, Fartoukh M, et al. Increased use of high-flow nasal oxygen during bronchoscopy. Eur Respir J. 2016;48(2):590-92.
35. Sakazaki R, Suzuki T, Ikeda N. High-flow nasal cannula oxygen supported-transesophageal echocardiography under sedation in a respiratory compromised patient. J Cardiothorac Vasc Anesth. 2018. pii: S1053-0770(18)30935-2. doi: 10.1053/j.jvca.2018.10.009.
36. Kim EJ, Jung CY, Kim KC. Effectiveness and safety of high-flow nasal cannula oxygen delivery during bronchoalveolar lavage in acute respiratory failure patients. Tuberc Respir Dis (Seoul). 2018;81(4):319-29.
37. Sago T, Harano N, Chogyoji Y, et al. A nasal high-flow system prevents hypoxia in dental patients under intravenous sedation. J Oral Maxillofac Surg. 2015;73(6):1058-64.
38. Ansari BM, Hogan MP, Collier TJ, et al. A randomized controlled trial of high-flow nasal oxygen (Optiflow) as part of an enhanced recovery program after lung resection surgery. Ann Thorac Surg. 2016;101(2):459-46.
39. Futier E, Paugam-Burtz C, Godet T, et al. Effect of early postextubation high-flow nasal cannula vs conventional oxygen therapy on hypoxaemia in patients after major abdominal surgery: a French multicentre randomized controlled trial (OPERA). Intensive Care Med. 2016;42:1888-98.
40. Makdee O, Monsomboon A, Surabenjawong U, et al. High-flow nasal cannula versus conventional oxygen therapy in emergency department patients with cardiogenic pulmonary edema: a randomized controlled trial. Ann Emerg Med. 2017;70:465-72. e2.
41. Carratalá Perales JM, Llorens P, Brouzet B, et al. High-flow therapy via nasal cannula in acute heart failure. Rev Esp Cardiol. 2011;64(8):723-5.
42. Sklar MC, Dres M, Rittayamai N, et al. High-flow nasal oxygen versus noninvasive ventilation in adult patients with cystic fibrosis: a randomized crossover physiological study. Ann Intensive Care. 2018;8(1):85.
43. Jaber S, Chanques G, Jung B. Postoperative noninvasive ventilation. J Anesthesiology. 2010;112(2):453-61.
44. Ischaki E, Pantazopoulos I, Zakynthinos S. Nasal high flow therapy: a novel treatment rather than a more expensive oxygen device. Eur Respir Rev. 2017;26(145). doi: 10.1183/16000617.0028-2017.
45. Roca O, Messika J, Caralt B, et al. Predicting success of high-flow nasal cannula in pneumonia patients with hypoxemic respiratory failure: The utility of the ROX index. J Crit Care. 2016;35:200-5.
46. Kang BJ, Koh Y, Lim CM, et al. Failure of high-flow nasal cannula therapy may delay intubation and increase mortality. Intensive Care Med. 2015;41:623-32.

CHAPTER 46

Evidence-based Review of Noninvasive Ventilation

Abdullah Al Shimemeri

INTRODUCTION

In recent years, the use of noninvasive ventilation for patients suffering from respiratory distress arising from various etiologies has increased many times. Noninvasive ventilation has the advantage that it is less invasive than mechanical ventilation and, hence, poses a lower risk of infections and other complications. It is also better tolerated by most patients. Noninvasive ventilation is the first choice for providing ventilation support in patients with chronic obstructive pulmonary disorder and acute chronic pulmonary edema. In this chapter, we analyze the latest evidence available for the use of noninvasive ventilation in other etiologies as well. We also study data describing the effect of noninvasive ventilation on other parameters of patient health and physiology.

SCIENTIFIC RATIONALE OF NONINVASIVE VENTILATION

Noninvasive ventilation (NIV) is a technique that provides ventilation support through a patient's upper airway through a mask. The use of NIV in medical science can be traced back to the 1930s when it was first described to bring respiratory relief to patients suffering from pulmonary edema, asthma, and pneumonia. Gradually, the use of NIV was extended to patients suffering from post-cardiac arrest and diseases such as neonatal hyaline membrane. By the 1960s, the use of NIV was refined for patients with acute respiratory distress syndrome (ARDS). Currently, NIV is used for patients in all age groups with chronic respiratory disorders, such as chronic obstructive pulmonary disorder (COPD) and obstructive sleep apnea (OSA), where its use has been found beneficial and, hence, extended to the treatment of acute illnesses like pulmonary edema and pneumonia. NIV has fast emerged as an alternative strategy to mechanical ventilation in several different clinical situations due to its flexibility and because it prevents complications associated with mechanical ventilation (Hess, 2013).

Technically, NIV is of two kinds: (1) continuous positive airway pressure (CPAP) and (2) noninvasive positive pressure ventilation (NIPPV). NIV can be applied via two modes: (i) CPAP and (ii) bilevel positive airway pressure (BILEVEL). In the CPAP mode, pressure is set at a single setting that is greater than the atmospheric pressure. This single pressure is applied through the proximal airway for all phases of the respiratory cycle. This pressure is similar to the positive end-expiratory pressure (PEEP) used during mechanical ventilation. CPAP increases the intrathoracic pressure and increases the lung volume. During CPAP, the tidal ventilation is dependent on the respiratory muscles because there is no unloading of the inspiratory muscles. CPAP is most effective in patients with hypoxic respiratory failure. In BILEVEL, two levels of pressure are applied. During initiation of BILEVEL, a set inspiratory positive airway pressure (IPAP) is applied. A pressure support (PS) is also provided during this phase.

The second level of pressure in BILEVEL is the expiratory positive airway pressure (EPAP). This is similar to the PEEP in CPAP. Typically, EPAP and PS are additive and equal to the IPAP. This greater pressure is more effective in unloading the respiratory muscles and, thus, provides complete respiratory support to the patient. BILEVEL is suitable for patients with hypercapnic and hypoxic respiratory failure (Davidson, 2016).

The basic purpose of NIV is to reduce the work of breathing. Application of a positive pressure counteracts the patient's intrinsic PEEP. PS helps the patients in the transpulmonary pressure required during inspiration. This outside help decreases oxygen consumption by the respiratory muscles and overcomes atelectasis. Overall, oxygenation is improved and carbon dioxide is removed more effectively. The application of positive pressure breath also affects the circulatory system and increases the intrathoracic pressure. In patients who are preload-dependent, this may result in hypotension and, thus, should be used with caution. The increase in intrathoracic pressure lowers the cardiac afterload and is beneficial in patients with acute cardiogenic pulmonary edema (ACPE). Thus, clinicians have to be well aware of the changes that may occur due to NIV in accordance with the various patient populations that they may encounter (Piraino, 2016).

CLINICAL EVIDENCE IN SUPPORT OF NONINVASIVE VENTILATION

Noninvasive Ventilation in Hypoxemic Respiratory Failure

There have been many previous reports describing the use of NIV in patients with hypoxemic respiratory failure. Recent studies have also used high-flow nasal cannula (HFNC) therapy in both critically ill and adult patients with hypoxemic respiratory failure. The results have been favorable for the efficacy of HFNC in improving oxygenation and reducing the respiratory rate. The use of NIV or HFNC was associated with a more than 10% reduction in the rates of intubation and also reduced hospital mortality compared with standard oxygen therapy (Jaber, 2016; Carteaux, 2016; Patel, 2016; Liu, 2016).

Noninvasive Ventilation in Cardiogenic Pulmonary Edema

Makdee et al. compared the use of high-flow cannula with conventional oxygen therapy in patients suffering from respiratory failure due to cardiogenic pulmonary edema in emergency department settings. In an open label, randomized controlled trial, they randomly assigned patients to either conventional oxygen or high-flow cannula therapy. The primary outcome of the trial was a respiratory rate of 60 breaths/minute postintervention. The study found that in this patient group suffering from respiratory failure with cardiogenic pulmonary edema, the use of HFNC therapy during the first hour of treatment was effective in decreasing the severity of dyspnea (Makdee, 2017).

Noninvasive Ventilation in Obesity Hypoventilation Syndrome

Obesity hypoventilation syndrome (OHS) is the most common reason for initiating home ventilation. A study by Howard et al. compared BILEVEL and CPAP for the treatment of severe OHS. In a multicenter, parallel, double-blind trial, the authors found that both CPAP and BILEVEL were equally effective in improving ventilation in patients with severe newly diagnosed OHS (Howard, 2017).

In another prospective study by Orfanos et al., stable patients with OHS suffering from OSA were studied for more than two months, first with NIV and then with CPAP. The patients had similar readings of arterial blood gas parameters, quality of sleep, and quality of life. More than 80% of patients favored CPAP over NIV (Orfanos, 2017).

Noninvasive Ventilation in Hypercapnia Respiratory Failure

In COPD patients with chronic hypercapnic respiratory failure, long-term nocturnal use of NIV is controversial. Thus, comparison of the cardiac and pulmonary effects of both low- and high-intensity NIV was done for six weeks in stable COPD patients. The study found that the use of NIV for longer time intervals at high pressure to improve respiration did not have any detrimental effect on different cardiac parameters but improved the quality of life. However, for patients suffering from a pre-existing heart failure, use of high inspiratory pressure was associated with reduced cardiac output (Duiverman, 2017). In another clinical trial to evaluate the role of NIV in patients with cardiac surgery (heart valve replacement), patients were analyzed for functional capacity and length of stay in ICU. Noninvasive ventilation improved the functionality but did not reduce the hospitalization times or length of stay (de Araújo-Filho, 2017).

Use of NIV in Patients in Critical Stages of Cancer

In patients with ARDS arising due to malignancies, NIV is commonly used to provide respiratory relief. The failure of NIV is frequent and is also associated with higher hospital mortality (Neuschwander, 2017). Similar results were obtained by Rathi et al. when NIPPV was used in comparison with invasive mechanical ventilation for acute hypoxemic respiratory failure in critically ill cancer patients as first-line therapy (Rathi, 2017). NIPPV has the best outcomes in patients with renal transplants who have undergone acute hypoxemic respiratory failure after severe pneumonia. In this patient group, the results obtained with HFNC therapy were similar to NIV. Moreover, the use of HFNC resulted in fewer complications and a greater number of days without ventilation support in a period of one month (Tu, 2017).

Evidence for the Use of NIV for ARDS

Data on the use of NIV for ARDS is relatively less. A large-scale international study, LUNGSAFE (Large Observational Study to Understand the Global Impact of Severe Acute Respiratory Failure), examined the utility of the PaO_2/FiO_2 ratio to classify patients receiving NIV and the impact of NIV on outcome. NIV failed in one-third of the patients, resulting in their higher mortality rate. Moreover, NIV was associated with higher ICU mortality than invasive-mechanical ventilation in patients. Thus, the use of NIV in this patient group is cautioned (Bellani, 2017).

Studies on the use of NIV to prevent reintubation have been largely inconclusive. A cohort study was performed to determine the various factors responsible for the failure of NIV. The study found the following factors are associated with failure of NIV and need for reintubation: fluid accumulation of greater than 100 mL/kg; respiratory failure due to pneumonia; heart rate more than 100 bpm 1 hour after starting of NIV; and duration of NIV greater than 96 hours. Among critically ill patients, pneumonia was found to be the only predictive factor found by multivariate analysis for the failure of NIV. Patients who have to be reintubated showed significantly greater hospital mortality compared with patients who were successfully weaned (Thomrongpairoj, 2017). In another study done to measure the quality of life and use of NIV in chronic at-home use patients, Bajema et al. examined the effect of NIV in hot humid environments during moderate to strenuous activities and found that NIV may stress cardiovascular functioning during moderate to high-intensity activities (Bajema, 2017).

PRACTICE PRESCRIPTION

In the past few decades, NIV has been increasingly and successfully used to manage acute and chronic respiratory failures due to various etiologies. NIV is highly recommended and suitable for patients with chronic COPD and has the highest success rate in this population. This is also true for COPD patients who may also become hypercapnic. In this patient group, NIV can result in a reduced need for intubation, reduced in-hospital mortality, reduced length of staying at the hospital, and faster resolution of blood-gas parameters. It also results in fewer complications associated with an artificial airway and invasive ventilation such as ventilator-associated pneumonia (Oga, 2017). In the past few years, the use of NIV for COPD exacerbations has resulted in significant decreases in mortality rates in this patient population. Early application of NIV, before acute distress sets in, is associated with better success rates (Duiverman, 2017). In patients needing ventilator support due to amyotrophic lateral sclerosis (ALS), long-term use NIV may be the key to longer survival and better quality of life for patients. Better results are expected from patients who do not suffer from bulbar impairment due to ALS (Radunovic, 2017). Recent medical guidelines have recommended NIV as the first-line therapeutic approach for the management of all cases of acute hypercapnic respiratory failure whether due to underlying neuromuscular disorders or to other etiologies (Davidson, 2016).

A meta-analysis of clinical trials on NIV in patients with "do-not-intubate" (DNI) directives reveals that patients benefit significantly from the use of NIV for acute respiratory failure (Fig. 46.1). Various studies have shown that such patients had a higher percentage of hospital discharge when NIV was used as ventilator support. For patients with chronic obstructive pulmonary disease and pulmonary edema, the use of NIV was associated with higher survival rates after one year (Wilson, 2018). However, patients with pneumonia and active malignancies fared worse than other patient groups. In patients with acute hypoxemia non-hypercapnic respiratory failure in the ICU, NIV did not decrease mortality rates, but overall hospital mortality was less in patients with successful NIV due to hypoxemia-induced non-hypercapnic respiratory failure (Xu, 2017). NIV patients had a lesser requirement for sedation and painkillers and recorded better scores on the quality of life index compared with standard oxygen therapy. NIV also decreased the rates of endotracheal intubation. The use of NIPPV in patients with DNI directives is controversial because most patients in this category typically have irreversible and terminal disease. Although the use of NIV cannot cure the underlying disease of the patient, it can be used as a form of life support or palliative care. It may provide relief from symptoms of respiratory distress, reduce dyspnea, or reduce the dosage of morphine required by patients with end-stage disease. Most importantly, it allows

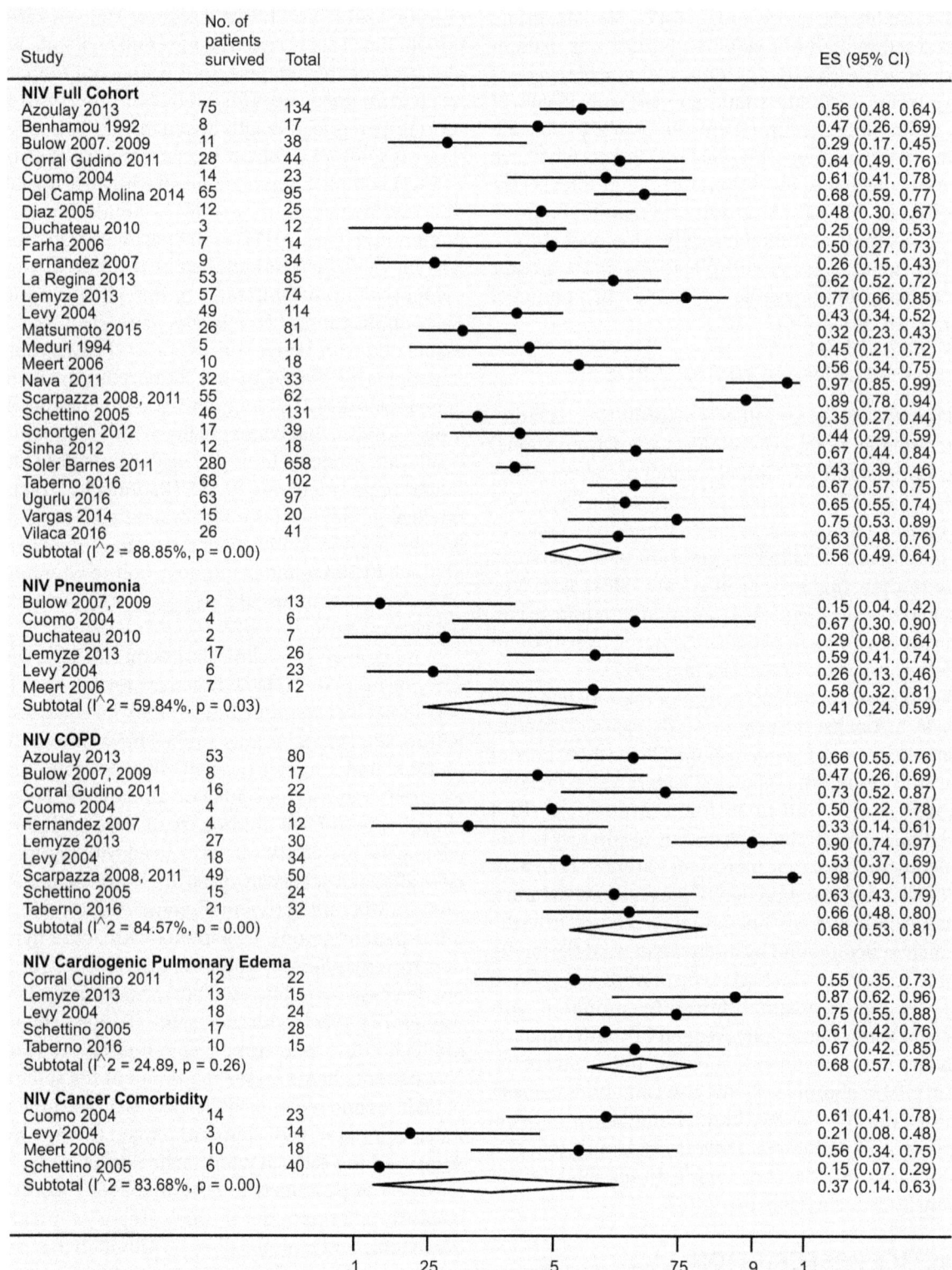

FIGURE 46.1: Patients with "do-not-intubate" (DNI) directives reveals that patients benefit significantly from the use of noninvasive ventilation (NIV) for acute respiratory failure.

Source: Wilson ME, Majzoub AM, Dobler CC, et al. Noninvasive ventilation in patients with do-not-intubate and comfort-measures-only orders: a systematic review and meta-analysis. Crit Care Med. 2018;46:1209-16.

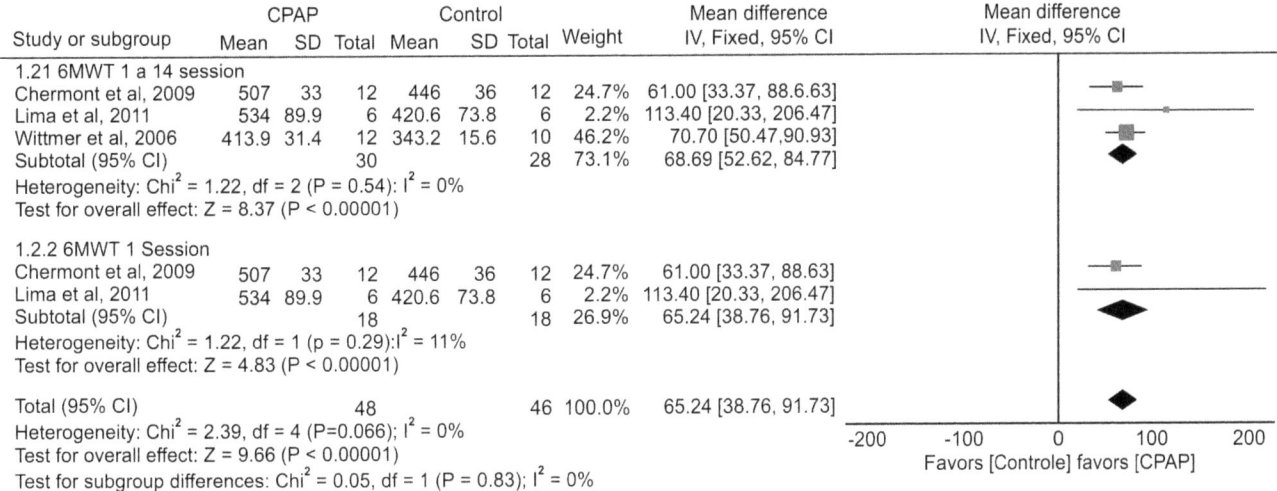

FIGURE 46.2: Patients on noninvasive ventilation (NIV) show an increased tolerance to effort and exercise.

Source: Bittencourt HS, Reis HF, Lima MS, et al. Non-invasive ventilation in patients with heart failure: a systematic review and meta-analysis. Arq Bras Cardiol. 2017;108(2):161-8.

communication between patient and family; hence, NIV is a popular choice for patients with a DNI directive. In some studies of patients who had undergone cardiac surgery, the use of NIV immediately in the postoperative period prophylactically reduced the rate of hypoxemia but was not associated with the reduction in probability of pulmonary complications or the time spent in ICU.

Immunocompromised patients suffering from acute hypoxemic respiratory failure are at increased risk of infection. Thus, this patient group can benefit from NIV because it helps avoid intubation. Immunocompromised patients suffer airway damage during intubation and the risk of ventilator-associated pneumonia and these two problems can be avoided by use of NIV. Studies suggest that if no contraindications to its use are present, NIV can bring down mortality rates and result in fewer intubations in immunocompromised patients with moderate to severe respiratory distress. In general, failure of NIV is higher in this patient group compared with either ACPE or COPD.

Another meta-analysis on trials studying the effect of NIV on patients with heart failure (Bittencourt, 2017) revealed that patients on NIV show an increased tolerance to effort and exercise (Fig. 46.2). However, this should be used with caution as the authors found considerable gaps in the literature as to which parameters of NIV are important for application (Bittencourt, 2017).

SUMMARY

In this chapter, we have presented the latest evidence available on the use of NIV through randomized controlled clinical trials. The chapter includes the use of NIV for respiratory distress arising due to various etiologies. Data from many clinical trials analyzing the various effects of NIV on patient physiology are now available and indicate NIV to be a safe alternative to invasive mechanical ventilation. The risk factors for NIV failure and its contraindications have also been illustrated. There is some evidence to the detrimental effect of high pressure settings on cardiac input of patients with pre-existing heart failure. Moreover, NIV in severe ARDS is associated with higher mortality. Thus, we recommend further and in-depth studies and caution on the use of NIV for these patient groups.

BIBLIOGRAPHY

1. Bajema A, Swinbourne AL, Gray M, et al. Effect of portable non-invasive ventilation & environmental conditions on everyday activities. Respir Physiol Neurobiol. 2017;243:55-9.
2. Bellani G, Laffey JG, Pham T, et al. Noninvasive ventilation of patients with acute respiratory distress syndrome. Insights from the LUNG SAFE study. Am J Respir Crit Care Med. 2017;195(1):67-77.
3. Bittencourt HS, Reis HF, Lima MS, et al. Non-Invasive ventilation in patients with heart failure: a systematic review and meta-analysis. Arq Bras Cardiol. 2017;108(2):161-8.

4. Carteaux G, Millán-Guilarte T, De Prost N, et al. Failure of noninvasive ventilation for de novo acute hypoxemic respiratory failure: Role of tidal volume. Crit Care Med. 2016;44:282-90.
5. Davidson AC, Banham S, Elliott M, et al. BTS Standards of Care Committee Member, British Thoracic Society/Intensive Care Society Acute Hypercapnic Respiratory Failure Guideline Development Group, On behalf of the British Thoracic Society Standards of Care Committee. BTS/ICS guideline for the ventilatory management of acute hypercapnic respiratory failure in adults. Thorax. 2016;71(Suppl 2):ii1-35.
6. de Araújo-Filho AA, de Cerqueira-Neto ML, de Assis Pereira Cacau L, et al. Effect of prophylactic non-invasive mechanical ventilation on functional capacity after heart valve replacement: a clinical trial. Clinics (Sao Paulo). 2017;72(10):618-23.
7. Duiverman ML, Maagh P, Magnet FS, et al. Impact of High-Intensity-NIV on the heart in stable COPD: a randomised cross-over pilot study. Respir Res. 2017;18(1):76.
8. Hess DR. Noninvasive ventilation for acute respiratory failure. Respir Care. 2013;58(6):950-72.
9. Howard ME, Piper AJ, Stevens B, et al. A randomised controlled trial of CPAP versus non-invasive ventilation for initial treatment of obesity hypoventilation syndrome. Thorax. 2017;72(5):437-44.
10. Jaber S, Bellani G, Blanch L, et al. The intensive care medicine research agenda for airways, invasive and noninvasive mechanical ventilation. Intensive Care Med. 2017;43(9):1352-65.
11. Jaber S, Lescot T, Futier E, et al. NIVAS Study Group: Effect of noninvasive ventilation on tracheal reintubation among patients with hypoxemic respiratory failure following abdominal surgery: A randomized clinical trial. JAMA. 2016;315:1345-53.
12. Liu Q, Gao Y, Chen R, et al. Noninvasive ventilation with helmet versus control strategy in patients with acute respiratory failure: A systematic review and meta-analysis of controlled studies. Crit Care. 2016;20:265.
13. Luo Z, Cao Z. Risk factors for noninvasive ventilation failure in patients with acute cardiogenic pulmonary edema: A prospective, observational cohort study. J Crit Care. 2017;40:277-8. Makdee O, Monsomboon A, Surabenjawong U, et al. High-Flow Nasal Cannula Versus Conventional Oxygen Therapy in Emergency Department Patients With Cardiogenic Pulmonary Edema: A Randomized Controlled Trial. Ann Emerg Med. 2017;70(4):465-72.
14. Neuschwander A, Lemiale V, Darmon M, et al. Noninvasive ventilation during acute respiratory distress syndrome in patients with cancer: Trends in use and outcome. J Crit Care. 2017;38:295-9.
15. Oga T, Taniguchi H, Kita H, et al. Comparison of Different Disease-Specific Health-Related Quality of Life Measurements in Patients with Long-Term Noninvasive Ventilation. Can Respir J. 2017;(2017):8295079.
16. Orfanos S, Jaffuel D, Perrin C, et al. Switch of noninvasive ventilation (NIV) to continuous positive airway pressure (CPAP) in patients with obesity hypoventilation syndrome: a pilot study. BMC Pulm Med. 2017;17(1):50.
17. Patel BK, Wolfe KS, Pohlman AS, et al. Effect of noninvasive ventilation delivered by helmet vs face mask on the rate of endotracheal intubation in patients with acute respiratory distress syndrome: A randomized clinical trial. JAMA. 2016;315:2435-41.
18. Piraino T. 2016 Year in Review: Noninvasive Ventilation. Respir Care. 2017;62(5):623-8.
19. Radunovic A, Annane D, Rafiq MK, et al. Mechanical ventilation for amyotrophic lateral sclerosis/motor neuron disease. Cochrane Database Syst Rev. 2017;10:CD004427.
20. Thomrongpairoj P, Tongyoo S, Tragulmongkol W, et al. Factors predicting failure of noninvasive ventilation assist for preventing reintubation among medical critically ill patients. J Crit Care. 2017;38:177-81.
21. Wilson ME, Majzoub AM, Dobler CC, et al. Noninvasive Ventilation in Patients With Do-Not-Intubate and Comfort-Measures-Only Orders: A Systematic Review and Meta-Analysis. Crit Care Med. 2018;46:1209-16.
22. Xu XP, Zhang XC, Hu SL, et al. Noninvasive Ventilation in Acute Hypoxemic Nonhypercapnic Respiratory Failure: A Systematic Review and Meta-Analysis. Crit Care Med. 2017;45(7).

CHAPTER 47

Extracorporeal Membrane Oxygenation

Lyndal Russell, Ross Callum Freebairn, Ravindranath Tiruvoipati

INTRODUCTION

Extracorporeal membrane oxygenation (ECMO) is a form of cardiorespiratory support where blood is pumped from the venous circulation, through a membrane oxygenator and returned to a major vein or artery. Indications for ECMO include severe but potentially reversible cardiorespiratory failure unresponsive to conventional therapies, where the risk of death or severe disability from the condition outweighs the risk of death or severe disability from ECMO. This chapter focuses on ECMO in adult patients.

Extracorporeal therapies can potentially provide three distinct types of support:
1. Hemodynamic support by augmenting cardiac output [with venoarterial ECMO (VA-ECMO)]
2. Oxygenation
3. Carbon dioxide removal (*see* Chapter 48).

EVIDENCE

Extracorporeal membrane oxygenation was first described in the early 1970s but after initial studies failed to demonstrate reduced mortality, with a high complication rate and cost, enthusiasm waned.[1,2] Following a clinical renaissance during the late 2000's following the CESAR[3] trial, fuelled in part by the H1N1 influenza pandemic, there has been a sustained growth in ECMO use over the past decade in multiple patient cohorts.[3-7] Research in the area is prolific, a recent systematic search performed on venovenous (VV) extracorporeal membrane oxygenation for refractory acute respiratory distress alone returned a total of 1,423 published studies.[8] Unfortunately 43% of these studies included fewer than 50 patients, and there are few firm evidence-based recommendations.[8]

The first randomized control trial of ECMO, performed by the National Institutes of Health in patients with acute respiratory distress syndrome (ARDS), recorded a survival rate of only 10% in both groups.[2] This 1979 study used only VA-ECMO and equipment that is now outdated. As effective lung protective strategies were not used prior to, while on ECMO or at all in the control group the relevance of this obsolescent data to modern practice is dubious.

The 2009 **C**onventional ventilator support versus **E**xtracorporeal membrane oxygenation for **S**evere **A**dult **R**espiratory failure (CESAR) trial was a UK multicenter randomized study with a single ECMO center.[3] Patients were randomized to either a "consideration for ECMO" arm or conventional ventilation. At 6 months more patients treated in the intervention arm (63%) were alive without severe disability compared to those patients in the conventional arm (43%). There are confounding issues with the CESAR study. The first was that in the "consideration for ECMO" arm only 75% received ECMO. The remaining 25% managed by conventional low-volume low-pressure ventilation without ECMO, had a very low mortality (18%). The second issue was more patients in the interventional arm received low-volume low-pressure ventilation (93%) than the control group (70%).[3] The overall bias these factors have created is unknown.

The latest large, multicenter, prospective randomized trial, the EOLIA study, enrolled patients with severe ARDS.[9] The 60-day mortality of those in the ECMO arm was not significantly different from those in the conventional mechanical ventilation arm.[9] The trial was curtailed early (after 249 patients) after an interim analysis fulfilled a futility rule. A secondary analysis suggests that the end point of "death or treatment failure" showed a significant survival benefit. As 28% of the conservative arm patients received rescue ECMO and the mortality following any ECMO use is not different from those receiving only conventional ventilation, the validity of this analysis is disputed.[10] Overall, EOLIA did show that routine ECMO in severe ARDS is not superior to "rescue" ECMO.[11]

Despite lack of prospective studies of VA-ECMO, the use of VA-ECMO during cardiopulmonary resuscitation (CPR) episodes increased over 10-fold over the 12 year period. Advances in provision of ECMO care have not produced improved risk-adjusted survival.[5,12] Neurological outcome is dependent upon the time until ECMO implementation, with a 40-minute maximum downtime being proposed as the threshold for a good recovery.[13] Patient selection is vital but the narrow time windows to gauge appropriateness of ECMO in individual patients creates controversy and time pressure.[14]

PRACTICE

Extracorporeal membrane oxygenation has multiple indications including various causes of respiratory and cardiovascular failure, and utilises variations in techniques with widely differing outcomes in different patient cohorts.[5,12,15]

Modes of ECMO: The location of where the blood drained from the patient and where the oxygen-rich blood is returned defines the ECMO mode. Blood drained from and returned to the vena cava is termed VV, whereas blood drained from the vena cava and returned to a peripheral artery (most commonly the femoral artery) is termed peripheral VA-ECMO. Central VA-ECMO is where blood is drained from the right atrium (RA) and returned to the ascending aorta.

Configurations

The two most commonly used modes are VV and VA, but there are many hybrid configurations that are also available.

Venovenous ECMO is indicated for patients with isolated respiratory failure. Blood is drained by an access cannula in the inferior vena cava around the level of the liver by a blood pump through a membrane oxygenator and returned to the patient at the level of the junction of the IVC and RA. While not providing direct cardiac support, the delivery of oxygenated blood to the pulmonary vasculature during VV-ECMO reduces hypoxic pulmonary vasoconstriction potentially reducing pulmonary hypertension. This may also improve left and right ventricle interdependence.

Venoarterial ECMO is used for isolated cardiac or cardiorespiratory failure. Peripheral VA-ECMO involves draining blood from the IVC/RA junction by a pump to a membrane oxygenator where oxygen is added and carbon dioxide is removed. The blood is returned to the patient via a central artery (femoral or iliac) retrograde up the aorta. VA-ECMO is used to support a failing heart, and as such there is still transpulmonary blood flow with the native heart ejecting blood. The interface between native cardiac ejection and retrograde VA-ECMO flow occurs between the arch and descending aorta such that the upper body and brain are supplied by native cardiac output and the lower body is perfused by the ECMO circuit. A potential complication of peripheral VA-ECMO, Harlequin syndrome, occurs when cardiac function improves but the lungs are not able to adequately oxygenate and decarboxylate the blood. This results in the ejection of hypoxic blood from the native heart resulting in differential oxygen saturation between the upper body (supplied by native cardiac ejection) and the lower body (supplied by the ECMO circuit).

In contrast, central VA-ECMO is usually utilized after cardiopulmonary bypass surgery. Blood is drained via the RA and returned via the ascending aorta.

Circuit

An ECMO circuit consists of access and return cannula, tubing, a blood pump, a membrane oxygenator and a heat exchange unit (Fig. 47.1).

Cannulas: Blood is drained from the patient via an access /drainage cannula attached by tubing to a membrane oxygenator by way of a blood pump. Here carbon dioxide is removed and oxygen is added to the blood prior to being returned to the patient via a return cannula. Choosing the size of cannula depends on the blood vessel diameter as well as the mode of ECMO. ECMO cannulas are of three main types: drainage, return, and backflow. *Drainage cannula* for VV and peripheral VA-ECMO range from 21 Fr to 29 Fr, with drainage holes along the distal 10–15 cm of the cannula to enable better drainage at lower negative pressures. *Return cannula* are single stage cannula with blood returning to the patient's circulation via the tip.[16] Arterial return cannulas are typically 15–21 Fr and venous return cannulas are usually between 19 Fr and 25 Fr.[16,17] *Backflow cannula* (usually 7–9 Fr) are inserted to prevent ischemia occurring distally to the femoral arterial cannulation site in peripheral VA-ECMO.

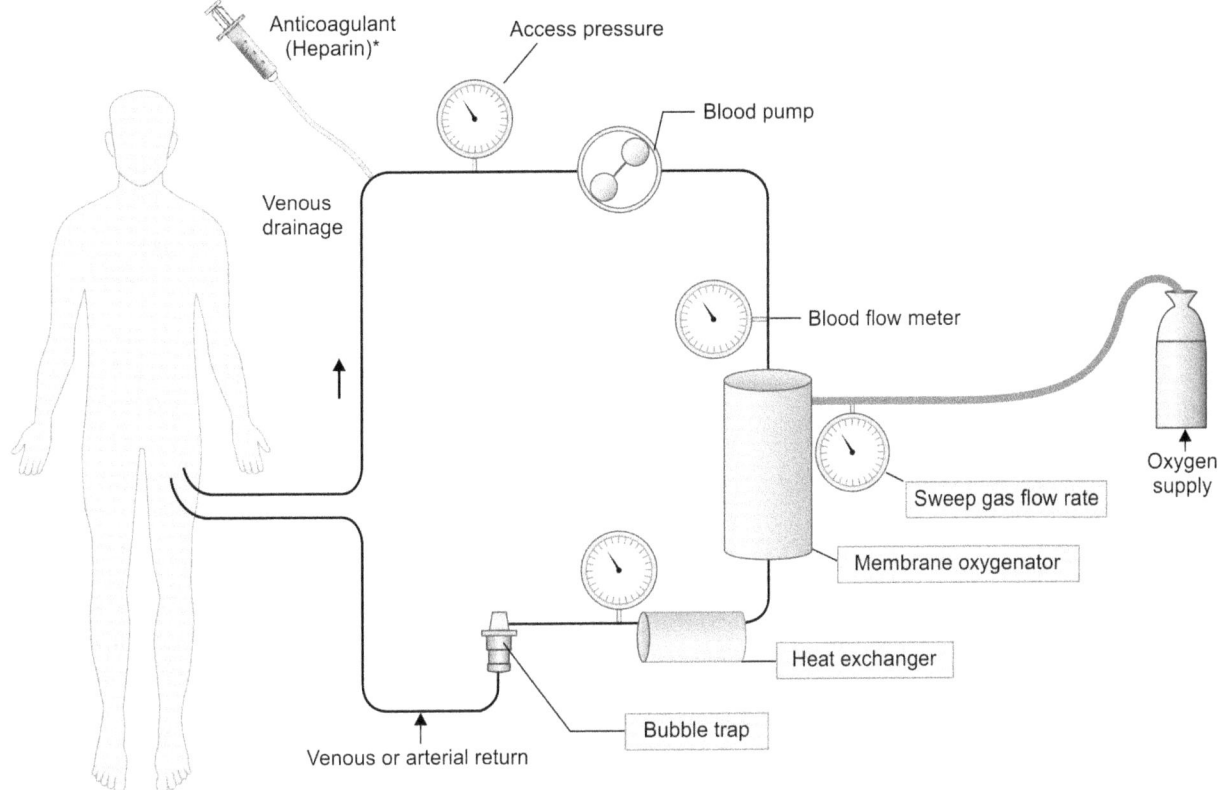

FIGURE 47.1: A simple extracorporeal membrane oxygenation circuit.
*Some systems administer the anticoagulant systematically, others directly to the circuit.

One of the recent advances in VV-ECMO is a dual-lumen, single cannula that is inserted into the superior vena cava (SVC) via the internal jugular vein. The walls are wire-reinforced and have drainage side holes for both SVC and inferior vena cava (IVC). The reinfusion is by a single hole directed toward tricuspid valve to reduce recirculation.

Tubing: ECMO circuit tubing is made from a polyvinylchloride based plastic compound. ECMO circuits can vary from simple to complex and may include a variety of blood flow and pressure monitors, continuous oxyhemoglobin saturation monitors, circuit access sites, and a bridge connecting the venous access and arterial infusion limbs of the circuit.[18] The tubing of the ECMO circuit may be coated with a biocompatible lining to reduce the systemic inflammatory response, risk of bleeding and thrombosis, although no coating to date has been shown to eliminate this reaction completely.[19]

Blood pump: ECMO pumps can be categorized as positive displacement, such as the modified roller pumps, and rotary, including the most commonly used centrifugal pump. Flow generated by the pump is preload dependent and afterload sensitive. Determinants of pump preload and the ability to achieve the desired blood flow rate include the volume status of the patient, venous tone, the position of the venous drainage cannula and the radius and length of the venous cannula/tubing. The determinants of pump afterload include systemic vascular resistance, the performance of the oxygenator in addition to the diameter, and length of the return tubing.

Oxygenator: The membrane oxygenator adds oxygen and removes carbon dioxide from the blood. The surface area of the oxygenator and blood path mixing determine the oxygenation capacity of the oxygenators. Modern ECMO practice generally use hollow fiber polymethylpentene (PMP) membrane oxygenators which are extremely efficient at gas exchange and demonstrate minimal plasma leakage with relatively low resistance to blood flow, making them easy to prime; and are well suited for use with centrifugal blood pumps.[20] Some of the new generation oxygenators also contain an integrated heat exchange device, making it possible to precisely control body temperature without the need for additional components.[18]

In the PMP membrane oxygenators, the deoxygenated venous blood is channeled around the polymethylpentene hollow fibers while sweep gas (fresh gas flow of air, oxygen enriched air, or pure oxygen) passes through them. Oxygen and carbon dioxide diffuse between the sweep gas and the blood driven by the partial pressure gradient across the membrane.

Oxygenation via the membrane lung is a function of:[21]
- Blood flow rate
- The gas exchange device
- FiO_2 of the membrane oxygenator
- Oxygen-carrying capacity of the blood (hemoglobin concentration)
- Degree of recirculation.

Decarboxylation is dependent on:
- Membrane surface area and properties
- Blood pCO_2
- Membrane lung gas flow (sweep gas flow).

Monitoring the ECMO Circuit

Monitoring of the ECMO circuit needs to be done regularly. The circuit must be inspected for clots in the tubing, membrane oxygenator and pump. Monitoring of blood gases and pressures upstream and downstream of the membrane oxygenator will help in assessing the function of this device. The pre-membrane pressure is measured at the venous inlet of the oxygenator and the post-membrane pressure is measured at the oxygenator outlet. The pre- and post-membrane pressures should be recorded regularly, at least every 6 hours. An acceptable transmembrane pressure is 8 mm Hg times the ECMO blood flow rate in liters per minute. Increasing transmembrane pressure is an early warning sign of oxygenator failure due to thrombus formation. Conversely, an concomitant increase in upstream and downstream oxygenator pressures without a change in pump rotations may indicate kinking of the arterial cannula.

Indications and Contraindications

Indications for ECMO can be divided into two groups: cardiac (VA-ECMO) and respiratory (VV-ECMO).[7,23]

Venovenous ECMO indications are potentially reversible respiratory failure where oxygenation cannot be maintained, or pH <7.2 despite—(1) optimal lung protective ventilation; (2) trial of a recruitment maneuver; (3) trial of adjunctive therapy (e.g. prone positioning, inhaled nitric oxide, neuromuscular blockade); (4) optimal treatment of the underlying cause; and (5) exclusion of reversible pathology (e.g. pleural effusion, fluid overload).

The Extracorporeal Life Support Organization (ELSO) Guidelines for ECMO for adult patients with respiratory failure recommend VV-ECMO be considered into the following circumstances:[24]

Table 47.1: Mortality risk in hypoxic respiratory failure.[24]

	50% mortality risk	80% mortality risk
PaO_2/FiO_2	<150 on FiO_2 >0.9	<100 on FiO_2 >0.9
		and/or
Murray score	2–3	3–4
AOI score	60	>80

(AOI: age-adjusted oxygenation index; PaO_2/FiO_2: arterial partial pressure of oxygen to fraction of inspired oxygen ration)

- In hypoxic respiratory failure, ECMO should be considered when the risk of mortality is 50% or greater and is indicated when the risk of mortality is greater than 80% using the Murray score or AOI score (Table 47.1)
- Carbon dioxide retention on mechanical ventilation despite a plateau pressure more than 30 cmH_2O
- Severe air leak syndromes
- Ventilatory support as a bridge to lung transplantation.

Other indications include smoke inhalation, status asthmaticus, airway obstruction, alveolar proteinosis, pulmonary contusion, massive hemoptysis or pulmonary hemorrhage.[25]

Several predictive scores to determine the patients with ARDS most likely to benefit from ECMO have been developed and tested.[28] The disparate indications for ECMO, the variation in techniques and large patient heterogeneity limit their general applicability.[29] Without further validation and development these scores have limited roles in clinical practice because of their relatively poor performance.[29,30]

Venoarterial ECMO may be indicated in severe, potentially reversible causes of cardiogenic shock refractory to conventional treatment where pharmacologic hemodynamic support is likely to worsen cardiac injury and there has been—(1) optimal treatment of underlying cause; (2) optimal fluid management; (3) appropriate use of vasoactive support; and (4) exclusion of reversible pathologies.

Venoarterial ECMO should be considered in:
- Cardiac/circulatory failure/refractory cardiogenic shock[7,14,23] (e.g. acute myocardial infarction, myocarditis, peripartum cardiomyopathy, drug overdose/toxicity with profound cardiac depression)
- Massive pulmonary embolism
- Cardiac arrest[26]
- Refractory ventricular arrhythmia
- Failure to wean from cardiopulmonary bypass after cardiac surgery
- As a bridge to either cardiac or lung transplantation or placement of a ventricular assist device.[27]

Contraindications may include:[23-25]
- All forms of ECMO:
  - Progressive and non-recoverable disease and not suitable for transplantation
  - Severe neurologic injury or intracerebral bleeding
  - Advanced age
  - Major pharmacologic immunosuppression (absolute neutrophil count <400/mm^3)
- Venoarterial ECMO:
  - Unrepaired aortic dissection
  - Severe aortic valve regurgitation
- Venovenous ECMO:
  - Severe cardiac failure
  - Cardiac arrest
  - Severe pulmonary hypertension (mean pulmonary artery pressure >50 mm Hg)
  - Mechanical ventilation at high settings including:
    - FiO_2 more than 0.9 for more than or equal to 7 days
    - Plateau pressure more than 30 cmH_2O for more than or equal to 7 days.

Ventilatory Support

Ventilation support during ECMO support has two objectives—first, to ensure adequate oxygenation and decarboxylation and second, to minimize further ventilator-induced lung injury by employing a low-volume, limited pressure ventilation strategy, which conventional ventilation management alone may not be able to achieve.[31]

Recommended strategies include airway pressure release ventilation (APRV) with positive end-expiratory pressure (PEEP) 10-15, plateau pressure less than 25 cm H_2O, driving pressure less than 15 and FiO_2 less than 0.4 thereby promoting "lung rest".[11] A lung protective strategy is recommended for potential ECMO patients prior to ECMO but are not always applied.[3,32,33] Prospective studies limiting driving pressure on ECMO have yet to be undertaken but "ultraprotective" ventilation using tidal volumes below 4 mL/kg ideal body weight (IBW) combined with ECMO or extracorporeal carbon dioxide removal ($ECCO_2R$) have been used successfully.[34,35] Higher PEEP both prior to and during ECMO may be advantageous and is commonly used.[9,33,36] Tracheostomy to facilitate reduced requirements for sedation, enable physiotherapy and rehabilitation to commence should be considered. Airway toileting can be achieved using serial bronchoscopy via endotracheal intubation or tracheostomy.

Patients requiring VA-ECMO primarily for cardiac support typically have a shorter duration of mechanical ventilation and consideration could be given for extubating and spontaneous ventilation even while on ECMO.[31]

Other adjunctive strategies to ventilation including neuromuscular blockade and prone positioning must be considered.[31] Extreme care with positioning because of the limited respiratory and cardiac reserve is obviously important, but use of prone positioning as an adjunctive support for patients on ECMO has been used with very few adverse hemodynamic episodes or other complications.[37] Prone positioning during VV-ECMO appears to be safe and reliable when performed in a recognized ECMO center with appropriately trained staff.[38]

Timing

Timing of institution of ECMO is paramount to the overall outcome of the patient. In VV-ECMO, one of the goals of management is to prevent ventilator-associated lung injury and in VA-ECMO, to prevent the use of unnecessary high dose of vasoactive drug support with ensuing multiorgan failure. The exact trigger point to institute VV- and VA-ECMO is contentious.[11]

Sedation

Commonly, patients are heavily sedated at ECMO initiation to facilitate cannulation and minimise the risk of vascular and embolic complications. Further, cannulation usually requires echocardiographic guidance which may be transthoracic echocardiography. Sedation is achieved in a similar way to a non-ECMO patient with a sedative (commonly propofol or midazolam) and an opioid (commonly fentanyl or morphine) infusion.[39] It is important to appreciate that some sedatives and opioids are adsorbed by the ECMO circuit necessitating higher than usual doses of the drugs.[40]

Neurological complications occur in about 13% of all ECMO patients, more frequently in VA-ECMO.[41] The ability to examine neurology without sedation is important, but must be balanced against the risk of ventilator-associated lung injury with spontaneous ventilation, risk of removing cannula or other devices, or interfering with circuit flow in the case of coughing or dyssynchrony.[34,41,42]

Anticoagulation

The ECMO circuit presents an artificial non-endothelial surface to blood, inciting an inflammatory response that may result in a prothrombotic state.[43] Unless contraindicated systemic anticoagulation to reduce oxygenator and circuit clotting is used, commonly achieved with a bolus and titrated infusion of unfractionated heparin. Consensus on anticoagulation targets is lacking.[43] Institution specific targets can include activated partial thromboplastin time

(APTT), activated clotting time (ACT), anti-Xa levels, or thromboelastography (TEG). In the absence of bleeding, an APTT of 50–70 seconds or an ACT of 180–200 seconds is generally considered adequate.[44] Anticoagulation may need to be ceased in the setting of significant bleeding while on ECMO.

Adjunctive Organ Support

While ECMO successfully manages patients with cardiac and/or respiratory failure, once patients develop renal failure during ECMO, further multiorgan dysfunction is likely, including hepatic and hematological complications, resulting in increased mortality.[45] When multiple organ support modalities are used together, organ crosstalk between the native and artificial organs dramatically increases the complexity. Whether early implementation of other organ support such as renal replacement therapy helps in organ recovery and overall survival is still a matter of open debate.[46]

Weaning of Support

Weaning from extracorporeal support differs between VV- and VA-ECMO. In VV-ECMO, weaning is achieved by reducing the sweep gas/fresh gas flow and achieving oxygenation and ventilation through the native lungs. Reduction in extracorporeal blood flow is not required. Once the native lungs provide adequate oxygenation and ventilation via a protective ventilator strategy decannulation from VV-ECMO can be contemplated.

Weaning from VA-ECMO involves a "weaning trial". Prior to attempting a VA-ECMO weaning trial, the patient should have a mean arterial pressure more than 60 mmHg on no or low-dose vasoactive agents and a pulsatile arterial waveform maintained for at least 24 hours and when pulmonary blood oxygenation is not compromised. Clinical, hemodynamic, and echocardiographic parameters are used to assess success of a weaning trial for consideration of liberation from VA-ECMO. During such a trial, ECMO blood flows are sequentially reduced to 66% then 33% and/or to a minimum of 1–1.5 L/min. Doppler echocardiography is performed at each ECMO flow level. Successful weaning from VA-ECMO can be predicted by three parameters: left ventricular ejection fraction (LVEF) more than 20–25%, aortic time-velocity integral (VTI) more than or equal to 10 cm and lateral mitral valve annulus peak systolic velocity (TDSa) more than or equal to 6 cm/s.[47]

Decannulation in VV-ECMO can be done at the bedside with digital pressure to the cannulated vein on removal of the device. In contrast, VA-ECMO decannulation is usually performed in a surgical theater with surgical closure of the cannulated artery.

Organizational Aspects

Extracorporeal membrane oxygenation use may vary widely across health systems.[14] Attempts at codifying the use of this rapidly expanding technology have lead the International ECMO Network to publish position paper for the organization of ECMO programs for acute respiratory failure in adult patients which has been endorsed by ELSO.[48] A multidisciplinary team of experts to guide institutional use of ECMO and the care of patients receiving it have been recommended.[14] Ultimately, concentration of the most complex care at high-volume centers with advanced cardiac capabilities may be a way to significantly improve the care of this patient population.[14,48] Paradoxically a recent North American audit found increased in-hospital mortality in high-volume institutions and in patients transferred to tertiary centers. Whether this represents selection bias or transfer from another facility warrants investigation.[49]

CONCLUSION AND RECOMMENDATIONS

Extracorporeal membrane oxygenation has evolved substantially and there has been progressively increasing use in the last decade. Although recently reported practice has a low attributable mortality, patient selection and operator expertise clearly influence these outcomes. Optimizing ventilation and adjunctive supports, such as prone positioning and neuromuscular paralysis prior to consideration of extracorporeal support, consideration of the reversibility of the precipitating condition, and the other comorbidities are key to treatment success. Debate continues over the threshold for, and timing of, interventions, the use of additional extracorporeal organ support, as well as the optimal endpoints for oxygenation, decarboxylation or perfusion. Recent evidence does not provide additional support for earlier intervention, and there continues to be an urgent need for robust evidence of benefit for this potentially helpful but complicated, resource dependent intervention. Improved understanding of both the potential clinical applications and the optimal techniques for performing ECMO will guide improved clinical practice in this area, while limiting redundant use.

REFERENCES

1. Hill JD, Fallat R, Cohn K, et al. Clinical cardiopulmonary dynamics during prolonged extracorporeal circulation for acute respiratory insufficiency. Trans Am Soc Artif Intern Organs. 1971;17(1):355-61.

2. Zapol WM, Snider MT, Hill JD, et al. Extracorporeal membrane oxygenation in severe acute respiratory failure. A randomized prospective study. JAMA. 1979;242(20):2193-6.
3. Peek M, Mugford M, Tiruvoipati R, et al. Efficacy and economic assessment of conventional ventilatory support versus extracorporeal membrane oxygenation for severe adult respiratory failure (CESAR): a multicentre randomised controlled trial. Lancet. 2009;374(9698):1351-63.
4. Chen GL, Qiao YR, Ma JH, et al. Extracorporeal cardiopulmonary resuscitation in children of Asia Pacific: A retrospective analysis of Extracorporeal Life Support Organization Registry. Chin Med J. 2018;131(12):1436-43.
5. Richardson ASC, Schmidt M, Bailey M, et al. ECMO Cardio-Pulmonary Resuscitation (ECPR), trends in survival from an international multicentre cohort study over 12-years. Resuscitation. 2017;112:34-40.
6. Extracorporeal Life Support Organization. (2018). ECLS Registry Report International Summary: Extracorporeal Life Support Organization. [online] Available from https://www.elso.org/Registry/Statistics/InternationalSummary.aspx [Accessed December 2018].
7. Ouweneel DM, Schotborgh JV, Limpens J, et al. Extracorporeal life support during cardiac arrest and cardiogenic shock: a systematic review and meta-analysis. Intens Care Med. 2016;42(12):1922-34.
8. Vaquer S, de Haro C, Peruga P, et al. Systematic review and meta-analysis of complications and mortality of veno-venous extracorporeal membrane oxygenation for refractory acute respiratory distress syndrome. Ann Intens Care. 2017;7(1).
9. Combes A, Hajage D, Capellier G, et al. Extracorporeal membrane oxygenation for severe acute respiratory distress syndrome. N Engl J Med. 2018;378(21):1965-75.
10. Shanholtz C, Reed RM, Brower RG. ECMO for severe acute respiratory distress syndrome. N Engl J Med. 2018;379(11):1090.
11. Hardin CC, Hibbert K. ECMO for severe ARDS. N Engl J Med. 2018;378(21):2032-4.
12. Sun T, Guy A, Sidhu A, et al. Veno-arterial extracorporeal membrane oxygenation (VA-ECMO) for emergency cardiac support. J Crit Care. 2018;44:31-8.
13. Yukawa T, Kashiura M, Sugiyama K, et al. Neurological outcomes and duration from cardiac arrest to the initiation of extracorporeal membrane oxygenation in patients with out-of-hospital cardiac arrest: a retrospective study. Scand J Trauma Resusc Emerg Med. 2017;25:95.
14. Abrams D, Garan AR, Abdelbary A, et al. Position paper for the organization of ECMO programs for cardiac failure in adults. Intens Care Med. 2018;44(6):717-29.
15. El Sibai R, Bachir R, El Sayed M. Outcomes in cardiogenic shock patients with extracorporeal membrane oxygenation use: A matched cohort study in hospitals across the United States. BioMed Res Int. 2018;2018.
16. Kohler K, Valchanov K, Nias G, et al. ECMO cannula review. Perfusion. 2013;28(2):114-24.
17. Fukuhara S, Takeda K, Garan AR, et al. Contemporary mechanical circulatory support therapy for postcardiotomy shock. Gen Thorac Cardiovasc Surg. 2016;64(4):183-91.
18. Lequier L, Horton SB, McMullan DM, et al. Extracorporeal membrane oxygenation circuitry. Pediatr Crit Care Med. 2013;14(5 Suppl 1):S7-12.
19. McMullan DM, Emmert JA, Permut LC, et al. Minimizing bleeding associated with mechanical circulatory support following pediatric heart surgery. Eur J Cardiothorac Surg. 2011;39(3):392-7.
20. Horton S, Thuys C, Bennett M, et al. Experience with the Jostra Rotaflow and QuadroxD oxygenator for ECMO. Perfusion. 2004;19(1):17-23.
21. Schmidt M, Tachon G, Devilliers C, et al. Blood oxygenation and decarboxylation determinants during venovenous ECMO for respiratory failure in adults. Intens Care Med. 2013;39(5):838-46.
22. Romano TG, Mendes PV, Park M, et al. Extracorporeal respiratory support in adult patients. J Bras Pneumol. 2017;43(1):60-70.
23. Extracorporeal Life Support Organization. (2013). ELSO Guidelines for Adult Cardiac Failure 2013. [online] Available from: https://www.elso.org/Portals/0/IGD/Archive/FileManager/76ef78eabcusersshyerdocumentselsoguidelinesforadultcardiacfailure1.3.pdf [Accessed December 2018].
24. Extracorporeal Life Support Organization. (2017). ELSO Guidelines for Adult Respiratory Failure. [online] Available from: https://www.elso.org/Portals/0/ELSO%20Guidelines%20For%20Adult%20Respiratory%20Failure%201_4.pdf [Accessed December 2018].
25. Platts DG, Sedgwick JF, Burstow DJ, et al. The role of echocardiography in the management of patients supported by extracorporeal membrane oxygenation. J Am Soc Echocardiogr. 2012;25(2):131-41.
26. Debaty G, Babaz V, Durand M, et al. Prognostic factors for extracorporeal cardiopulmonary resuscitation recipients following out-of-hospital refractory cardiac arrest. A systematic review and meta-analysis. Resuscitation. 2017;112:1-10.
27. Hakim AH, Ahmad U, McCurry KR, et al. Contemporary outcomes of extracorporeal membrane oxygenation used as bridge to lung transplantation. Ann Thorac Surg. 2018;106(1):192-8.
28. Hilder M, Herbstreit F, Adamzik M, et al. Comparison of mortality prediction models in acute respiratory distress syndrome undergoing extracorporeal membrane oxygenation and development of a novel prediction score: The prediction of Survival on ECMO Therapy-Score (PRESET-Score). Crit Care. 2017;21:301.
29. Enger TB, Müller T. Predictive tools in VVECMO patients: Handicap or benefit for clinical practice? J Thorac Dis. 2018;10(3):1347-51.
30. Brunet J, Valette X, Buklas D, et al. Predicting survival after extracorporeal membrane oxygenation for ARDS: An external validation of RESP and PRESERVE scores. Resp Care. 2017;62(7):912-9.
31. Parekh M, Abrams D, Brodie D, et al. Extracorporeal membrane oxygenation for ards: Optimization of lung protective ventilation. Resp Care. 2018;63(9):1180-8.
32. Freebairn R, McHugh G, Hickling K. Extracorporeal membrane oxygenation for ARDS due to 2009 influenza A(H1N1). JAMA. 2010;303(10):941-2.

33. Schmidt M, Stewart C, Bailey M, et al. Mechanical ventilation management during extracorporeal membrane oxygenation for acute respiratory distress syndrome: A retrospective international multicenter study. Crit Care Med. 2015;43(3):654-64.
34. Schmidt M, Pellegrino V, Combes A, et al. Mechanical ventilation during extracorporeal membrane oxygenation. Crit Care. 2014;18(1).
35. Amato MB, Meade MO, Slutsky AS, et al. Driving pressure and survival in the acute respiratory distress syndrome. N Engl J Med. 2015;372(8):747-55.
36. Grasso S, Terragni P, Birocco A, et al. ECMO criteria for influenza A (H1N1)-associated ARDS: role of transpulmonary pressure. Intens Care Med. 2012;38(3):395-403.
37. Culbreth RE, Goodfellow LT. Complications of prone positioning during extracorporeal membrane oxygenation for respiratory failure: a systematic review. Resp Care. 2016;61(2):249-54.
38. Lucchini A, De Felippis C, Pelucchi G, et al. Application of prone position in hypoxaemic patients supported by veno-venous ECMO. Intensive Crit Care Nurs. 2018;48:61-8.
39. DeGrado JR, Hohlfelder B, Ritchie BM, et al. Evaluation of sedatives, analgesics, and neuromuscular blocking agents in adults receiving extracorporeal membrane oxygenation. J Crit Care. 2017;37:1-6.
40. Wildschut ED, Ahsman MJ, Allegaert K, et al. Determinants of drug absorption in different ECMO circuits. Intensive Care Med. 2010;36(12):2109-16.
41. Sutter R, Tisljar K, Marsch S. Acute neurologic complications during extracorporeal membrane oxygenation: a systematic review. Critical Care Medicine. 2018;46(9):1506-13.
42. Crotti S, Bottino N, Spinelli E. Spontaneous breathing during veno-venous extracorporeal membrane oxygenation. J Thorac Dis. 2018;10:S661-S9.
43. Esper SA, Welsby IJ, Subramaniam K, et al. Adult extracorporeal membrane oxygenation: an international survey of transfusion and anticoagulation techniques. Vox Sanguinis. 2017;112(5):443-52.
44. Marasco SF, Lukas G, McDonald M, et al. Review of ECMO (extra corporeal membrane oxygenation) support in critically ill adult patients. Heart Lung Circ. 2008;17 Suppl 4:S41-7.
45. Devasagayaraj R, Cavarocchi NC, Hirose H. Does acute kidney injury affect survival in adults with acute respiratory distress syndrome requiring extracorporeal membrane oxygenation? Perfusion (United Kingdom). 2018;33(5):375-82.
46. Husain-Syed F, Ricci Z, Brodie D, et al. Extracorporeal organ support (ECOS) in critical illness and acute kidney injury: from native to artificial organ crosstalk. Intensive Care Med. 2018;44(9):1447-59.
47. Aissaoui N, Luyt CE, Leprince P, et al. Predictors of successful extracorporeal membrane oxygenation (ECMO) weaning after assistance for refractory cardiogenic shock. Intensive Care Med. 2011;37(11):1738-45.
48. Combes A, Brodie D, Bartlett R, et al. Position paper for the organization of extracorporeal membrane oxygenation programs for acute respiratory failure in adult patients. Am J Respir Crit Care Med. 2014;190(5):488-96.
49. Bailey KL, Downey P, Sanaiha Y, et al. National trends in volume-outcome relationships for extracorporeal membrane oxygenation. J Surg Res. 2018;231:421-7.

CHAPTER 48

Extracorporeal Carbon Dioxide Removal

Valencia Lim, Matthew Edward Cove

INTRODUCTION

The potential of extracorporeal carbon dioxide removal ($ECCO_2R$) devices to supplement or replace pulmonary ventilation was first demonstrated by Ted Kolobow and his team in 1977.[1] As the name implies, these devices remove carbon dioxide directly from the bloodstream and provide a strategy to manage hypercapnia which, for example, develops during low tidal volume ventilation in patients with acute respiratory distress syndrome (ARDS).[2] Since 1977, the technology has changed significantly, and commercial low-flow $ECCO_2R$ devices are now available for use in intensive care units familiar with managing dialysis equipment. In this chapter, we will review the principles of $ECCO_2R$ technology and how its use has the potential to benefit different groups of critically ill patients.

PRINCIPLES OF EXTRACORPOREAL CARBON DIOXIDE REMOVAL

Extracorporeal carbon dioxide removal devices remove carbon dioxide through an extracorporeal circuit consisting of four main components: a drainage cannula (central vein or artery), a pump, a membrane lung and a return cannula (venous) (Fig 48.1). The "membrane lung" facilitates gas exchange and is connected to a flow of air or oxygen, which acts as a "sweep gas", creating a gradient favouring carbon dioxide diffusion out of the blood; a principle similar to that of hemodialysis.

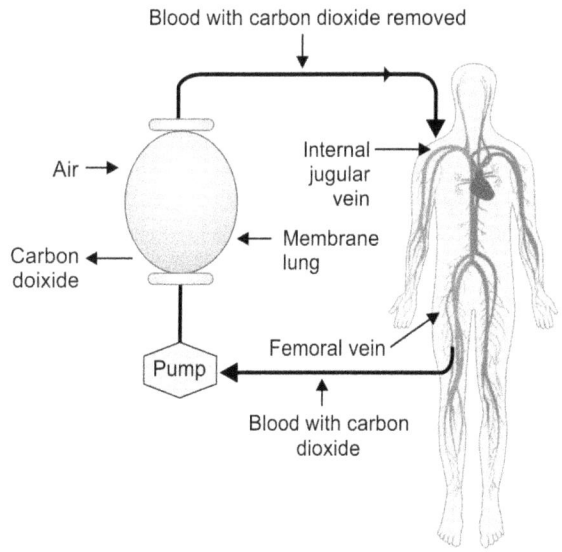

FIGURE 48.1: Essential components of extracorporeal carbon dioxide removal circuit.

Modern "membrane lungs" are composed of efficient hollow fibers which contain many micropores. These create a blood–gas interface where gas exchange occurs. An important development was the use of poly-4-methyl-1-pentene (PMP) to construct the hollow fibers, because PMP resists plasma leak through the micropores.[3] Factors that determine the efficiency of gas exchange include: the diffusion gradient, membrane-blood contact time, and membrane diffusion characteristics. Therefore, the fibers are arranged into a complex lattice because this increases contact surface area (1–3 m²) and encourages mixing subjacent to the hollow fiber. In addition, heparin is often covalently bound to the fiber surface, enhancing biocompatibility and reducing circuit thrombosis.[3]

Transport Physiology of Carbon Dioxide

In many ways, an $ECCO_2R$ circuit resembles an extracorporeal membrane oxygenation (ECMO) circuit, sometimes causing confusion in distinguishing the two technologies. The principle difference is that ECMO aims to achieve both oxygenation and carbon dioxide removal, whereas $ECCO_2R$ only aims to remove carbon dioxide. Important differences in the way oxygen and carbon dioxide are transported in the bloodstream means ECMO requires a much higher blood flow rate than $ECCO_2R$.

Carbon dioxide is mainly transported as dissolved bicarbonate. A liter of venous blood with a PCO_2 of 5kPa, and bicarbonate level of 25 mmol/L, carries approximately 500 mL of carbon dioxide. Since the rate of carbon dioxide production is approximately 250 mL/min for an average adult at rest, a blood flow of less than 1 L/min is sufficient to remove most of the metabolically produced carbon dioxide, provided the device is efficient.

In contrast, oxygen is transported bound to hemoglobin, a process that exhibits saturation kinetics, i.e. once hemoglobin is saturated with oxygen, it cannot carry any more. As a result, a liter of blood with normal hemoglobin levels is only capable of transporting 40–60 mL of oxygen. In order to satisfy the metabolic oxygen demands of an average adult at rest, typically 250 mL/min, ECMO devices need to provide a blood flow rate in the range of 5L/min.[3]

Cannulation Strategies in $ECCO_2R$ (Arteriovenous versus Venovenous)

Since lower blood flow rates are required for $ECCO_2R$, there is greater flexibility in the choice of cannulation strategy. Two broad strategies have been used: arteriovenous (AV-$ECCO_2R$) and venovenous (VV-$ECCO_2R$). In AV-$ECCO_2R$, the drainage cannula is placed in a large artery and the return cannula is sited in a central vein, allowing the pressure gradient between the arterial and venous system to drive blood flow, creating a pumpless system. AV-$ECCO_2R$ effectively creates an extravascular bed requiring a compensatory increase in cardiac output, and is consequently not suitable for patients with circulatory shock.

In VV-$ECCO_2R$, both drainage and return cannulas are placed in central veins, allowing the use of double lumen cannulas in a single vein, resembling dialysis catheters.[2,3] Typically, the cannulas are wire-reinforced and coated with heparin to maintain flow, minimize blood trauma and reduce clotting. There are currently four commercially available $ECCO_2R$ devices which are approved for use in Europe, but not all are Food and Drug Administration (FDA) approved yet (Table 48.1).

Table 48.1: Commercially available extracorporeal carbon dioxide removal ($ECCO_2R$) devices.

Device	Description
Pump-assisted lung protection (PALP) (Maquet, Rastatt, Germany)	Designed as variation which can be used with Maquet's CARDIOHELP™ console, a portable heart–lung support system. It uses a smaller membrane lung and lower blood flows than the full extracorporeal membrane oxygenation (ECMO) configuration
iLAActivve™ (Novalung, Germany)	Uses a small diagonal pump and operational console. Since it has a blood flow range of 0.5–4.5 L/min, it can provide $ECCO_2R$ or ECMO
Hemolung™ system (Alung Technologies, Pittsburgh, USA)	Designed for carbon dioxide removal and is used with Alung's 15.5F wire reinforced double lumen catheter. It can remove up to 90 mL/min of carbon dioxide using low blood flow rates (350–550 mL/min)
Prismalung™ (Baxter, Illinois, US)	Uses the Prismaflex continuous renal replacement therapy console to pump blood through a decarboxylation membrane. It can be mounted with, or without a dialysis filter in series, and removes 40–60 mL/min of carbon dioxide, using blood flow rates of 400 mL/min or less[19]
Abylcap™ (Bellco, Medtronic)	Similar to the Prismalung, a roller pump which is part of continuous renal replacement therapy console is used to remove approximately 50 mL/min of carbon dioxide with blood flow rates of 400 mL/min or less

$ECCO_2R$ IN CLINICAL PRACTICE

Role of $ECCO_2R$ in ARDS

Gattinoni and colleagues first used $ECCO_2R$ to support patients with ARDS in the 1980's.[4,5] These observational studies reported impressive ARDS survival rates compared to the high ARDS mortality at the time. Encouraged by these, and other observations,[3] the efficacy of VV-$ECCO_2R$ was studied in a randomized controlled trial by Morris et al. in the early 1990s.[6] In this trial, 40 patients with severe ARDS were randomized to receive low frequency protective ventilation, supported by $ECCO_2R$, versus conventional therapy. Although the study showed no benefit, it is noteworthy that patients receiving $ECCO_2R$ received what we would now consider harmful ventilation. The mean tidal volume exceeded 8 mL/kg actual body weight

(8.9 mL/kg in ECCO$_2$R group vs. 10.2 mL/kg in control group) and mean peak inspiratory airway pressures were high (55 in therapy group vs. 56 in control group). The fact that plateau pressures were not reported, and that tidal volumes were described in terms of actual body weight, highlights how little was understood about ARDS ventilation at the time. Furthermore, the ECCO$_2$R technology available had a high complication rate and was stopped early in 37% of patients (7 out of 19) due to bleeding or clotting complications.

After Morris's study, the landmark ARDS net study was completed, showing that a mean tidal volume of about 6 mL/kg ideal body weight, targeting a plateau pressure less than 30 cmH$_2$O, reduced mortality by nearly 25%.[7] However, about 15% of these patients developed hypercapnia.[8] More recently, Terragni et al. observed that tidal volumes even lower than conventional ARDS net volumes resulted in more rapid resolution of pulmonary inflammatory markers in severe ARDS, but also led to hypercapnia.[9] Hypercapnia can harm the injured lung through impaired epithelial repair and supressed immune responses, as well as worsening right heart failure and causing hemodynamic instability.[10] This suggests ECCO$_2$R could play an important role in supporting lung protective ventilation by mitigating the resultant hypercapnia.

The Xtravent trial set out to evaluate the effect of "ultra-low" tidal volumes (3 mL/kg ideal body weight) supported by AV-ECCO$_2$R in a randomized controlled trial.[11] Unfortunately, the study was stopped early due to slow patient recruitment, resulting in a small sample size of 80 patients. As a result, the trial was not statistically powered to demonstrate significant difference in the primary outcome of ventilator-free days, but a post hoc analysis demonstrated shorter duration of mechanical ventilation in the group treated with ECCO$_2$R. The primary recruitment challenge was the use of AV-ECCO$_2$R, since many patients with ARDS were excluded on the basis on unstable hemodynamics.

A systemic review of 14 studies (including the trials by Bien et al.[11] and Morris et al.[6]) concluded that ECCO$_2$R facilitates lower tidal volume ventilation and increases ventilator free days in patients with severe ARDS.[12] The need for more robust, adequately powered trials to assess mortality has fuelled two new trials, which are currently in progress: SUPERNOVA and REST. SUPERNOVA (ClinicalTrials.gov NCT02282657) is a European multicenter study which aims to prospectively evaluate the safety and feasibility of reducing tidal volume to 4 mL/kg with the use of ECCO$_2$R in patients with moderate ARDS. The REST study (ClinicalTrials.gov NCT02654327) is a multicenter randomized controlled trial in the UK that aims to determine whether low tidal volume ventilation supported by VV-ECCO$_2$R improves outcomes and is cost effective compared to current standard of care in patients with hypoxemic respiratory failure. A summary of key ECCO$_2$R studies in ARDS can be found in Table 48.2.

Role of ECCO$_2$R in Chronic Obstructive Pulmonary Disease

As ECCO$_2$R devices become safer and easier to use, there has been increased interest in their use to manage hypercapnic respiratory failure in patients with chronic obstructive pulmonary disease (COPD). When patients with COPD receive invasive mechanical ventilation, it can be challenging to wean them off ventilator support.[16] By addressing the primary issue of hypercapnia, ECCO$_2$R provides an attractive alternative to mechanical ventilation when noninvasive ventilation has failed. One of the earliest studies to investigate this showed that the use of AV-ECCO$_2$R avoided intubation in 90% of patients with acute exacerbations of COPD.[15] However, it was not a randomized controlled trial as the comparison group was a matched control group.

Pilot studies conducted by Burki et al.[16] and Abrams et al. in 2013[17] showed that VV-ECCO$_2$R avoided invasive mechanical ventilation in COPD patients as well as facilitating extubation and weaning of noninvasive ventilation. Burki et al. showed that low-flow VV-ECCO$_2$R with Hemolung™ avoided intubation in all patients who were at high risk of requiring intubation (n = 7), allowed weaning of noninvasive ventilation in 2 patients and facilitated extubation in 3 of 11 intubated patients.[16] In a pilot study involving 5 intubated COPD patients, Abrams et al. used more conventional VV-ECCO$_2$R blood flow rates to show the efficacy of ECCOR in reducing time to extubation (mean duration to extubation was 4 hours, range 1.5–21.5 hours).[17]

More recently, Del Sobo et al. conducted a matched cohort study with matched historical controls.[18] They treated 25 COPD patients with noninvasive ventilation and low-flow VV-ECCO$_2$R (blood flow rates <400 mL/min) and showed a reduced need for intubation (12% in study group vs. 33% in control group receiving only noninvasive ventilation). Perhaps one of the major drawbacks of ECCO$_2$R use continues to be high complication rates, especially when high blood flow rates are used. In the relatively recent ÉCLAIR study, Brune et al. reported significant bleeding complications in 36% (9 out of 25 patients) when VV-ECCO$_2$R with a mean blood flow rate of 1.3 L/min was used to avoid intubation in patients with COPD.[19] There is a need for larger randomized controlled trials to evaluate the risk–benefit balance of ECCO$_2$R use in COPD before its routine use can be considered.[20]

Table 48.2: Relevant clinical studies of extracorporeal carbon dioxide removal ($ECCO_2R$) use in acute respiratory distress syndrome (ARDS).

	Study type	$ECCO_2R$ technique	Results
Terragni et al.[11]	Prospective study	Venovenous extracorporeal carbon dioxide removal (VV-$ECCO_2R$) with membrane lung via 14Fr catheter with blood flow of 191–422 mL/kg	• 10 patients with Pplat* between 28 cm H_2O and 20 cm H_2O placed on $ECCO_2R$ with reduction in tidal volume from 6.3 ± 0.2 mL/kg to 4.2 ± 0.3 mL/kg per body weight. Pplat* decreased from 29.1 ± 1.2 to 25.0 ± 1.2 cm H_2O ($p < 0.001$) • Showed reduction in pulmonary cytokines ($p < 0.01$) after 72 hours of ventilation. No patient-related complications; membrane clotting in 3 patients
Fanelli et al.[15]	Prospective study	VV-$ECCO_2R$ via 15.5 Fr catheter with blood flow of 435 mL/min	• 15 patients with moderate ARDS, ventilated at 4 mL/kg, $ECCO_2R$ started when pH <7.25 and pCO_2 > 60 mm Hg. • $ECCO_2R$ was effective in correcting pH and pCO_2 • Proning and ECMO were necessary in four and two patients, respectively for severe hypoxemia. Two adverse events; intravascular hemolysis and femoral catheter kinking
Bein et al.[11]	RCT¶	Arteriovenous extracorporeal carbon dioxide removal (AV-$ECCO_2R$ via 15 Fr arterial cannula and 17Fr venous cannula) with mean blood low of 1.3 L/min	• 79 patients with moderate/severe ARDS evaluated after 24-hours stabilization period with higher positive end-expiratory pressure, randomized to $ECCO_2R$ with ~3 mL/kg predicted body weight (PBW) ventilation or control with ~6 mL/kg PBW • No significant differences in ventilator free days at day 28 (10 vs. 9 days, $p = 0.78$) or day 60 (33 vs. 29, $p = 0.47$). Post hoc analysis showed shorter duration of ventilation in patients with P/F ratio ≤150 • Main adverse event was higher blood transfusion requirements
Morris et al.[6]	RCT¶	VV-$ECCO_2R$	• 40 patients with severe ARDS were evaluated. 21 patients were randomized to receive low frequency protective ventilation plus $ECCO_2R$, 19 patients received conventional therapy • No difference in mortality, mean PIP† airway pressures were high and tidal volume large in both groups. Plateau pressures were not reported • Systemic bleeding occurred in all patients in the treatment groups
SUPERNOVA (NCT02282657§)	RCT¶ (in progress)	VV-$ECCO_2R$	Aims to prospectively evaluate the safety and feasibility of reducing tidal volume to 4 mL/kg with the use of $ECCO_2R$ in 100 patients with moderate ARDS
REST (NCT02654327§)	RCT¶ (in progress)	VV-$ECCO_2R$	Aims to determine whether low tidal volume ventilation with venovenous extracorporeal carbon dioxide removal (VV-$ECCO_2R$) improves outcome and is cost effective compared to current standard of care
U-PROTECT (NCT02252094§)	RCT¶ (in progress)	VV-$ECCO_2R$	Aims to evaluate the use of ultra-protective ventilation (with very low tidal volumes) in combination with $ECCO_2R$ in patients with severe ARDS

*Plateau pressure, †Peak inspiratory pressure, ¶Randomized controlled trial, §Clinicaltrials.gov registration number
Source: Morelli et al.[2]

Role of $ECCO_2R$ as a Bridge to Lung Transplant

Patients awaiting lung transplant often develop respiratory failure with refractory hypercapnia. In this setting ECMO may be considered as a bridge to lung transplant, but long-term ECMO still has a high complication and mortality rate, and is therefore not an ideal long-term bridging measure. Low-flow $ECCO_2R$ has a lower complication rate and might be a suitable alternative. In 2006 Fisher et al.[21] reported the use of low-flow AV-$ECCO_2R$ as a bridge to transplant. 12 patients with refractory hypercapnia were treated, 10 were successfully transplanted, and 8 remained alive at

1 year. More recently, Schellongowshi et al.[22] evaluated the use of ECCO$_2$R (both AV-ECCO$_2$R and VV-ECCO$_2$R) in 20 patients with hypercapnic respiratory failure. 19 patients were successfully transplanted, 1 one-year survival was 72%, and complications (bleeding or arterial thrombosis) only occurred in 5 patients. Increasingly, observational studies of ECCO$_2$R demonstrate efficacy in managing respiratory failure in patients awaiting transplant, as a result ECCO$_2$R has been recognized in major guidelines as a useful bridging to transplant therapy.

ECCO$_2$R Complications

The main complications of ECCO$_2$R can be classified into patient-related or circuit-related, and differ slightly between AV-ECCO$_2$R and VV-ECCO$_2$R. The complications affecting both strategies include circuit clotting, membrane malfunction, catheter displacement, localized bleeding, and systemic bleeding (Table 48.3). AV-ECCO$_2$R has the additional complication of limb ischemia due to obstruction of arterial flow distal to the arterial cannula.

Furthermore, since ECCO$_2$R does not provide meaningful oxygenation, its use may be associated with worsening oxygenation. Gattinoni et al.[23] cites a combination of physiological processes that account for this. First, the use of lower tidal volumes supported by ECCO$_2$R reduces tidal recruitment and increases gravitational atelectasis (where low end inspiratory pressures cause collapse). Consequently, it is important to consider an open lung ventilation strategy when using ultra-low tidal volumes supported by ECCO$_2$R. Second, when the ECCO$_2$R sweep gas is pure oxygen, rather than air, nitrogen wash-out of the blood occurs. This results in alveolar nitrogen washout, leading to absorption atelectasis. To prevent this, the FiO$_2$ of the sweep gas should not exceed the FiO$_2$ set on the ventilator.

GUIDELINES FOR ECCO$_2$R USE

The availability of a variety of commercial ECCO$_2$R devices and emerging evidence supporting their use has resulted in several leading bodies developing recommendations for the clinical use of ECCO$_2$R. In April 2016, the new British Thoracic Society (BTS) guidelines for ventilator management of acute hypercapnic respiratory failure in adults gave ECCO$_2$R use a level 2 recommendation in patients with persistent severe hypercapnic respiratory acidosis (pH <7.15) when lung protective ventilation is being used, and also recommended ECCO$_2$R as a bridge to lung transplant.[24] In addition, the guidelines highlighted that the use of VV-ECCO$_2$R in patients with acute exacerbations of COPD and a suboptimal response to non-invasive ventilation is not recommended based on existing evidence, citing that high ECCO$_2$R complication rates outweighed uncertain benefits.

In the same year, the National Institute for Health and Care Excellence (NICE) published guidelines for the use of ECCO$_2$R in acute respiratory failure. Like the BTS guidelines, NICE recommend that ECCO$_2$R only be used in patients with reversible respiratory failure, or in patients awaiting lung transplant. In recognition that ECCO$_2$R experience is limited, the NICE guidelines highlight that ECCO$_2$R should only by used by trained specialists given the limited evidence on efficacy and potential for complications.[25]

CONCLUSION

Extracorporeal carbon dioxide removal facilitates low tidal volume ventilation in ARDS by avoiding the ill effects of hypercapnia. The use of ECCO$_2$R in COPD exacerbations promises to avoid invasive mechanical ventilation, but needs to be robustly investigated with newer low-flow ECCO$_2$R technologies that have lower complication rates. ECCO$_2$R has also been recognized as an effective bridge to lung transplantation. Technological improvements continue to make ECCO$_2$R devices simpler to use, more efficient and more biocompatible, allowing for lower blood flow rates and less anticoagulation. At present, ECCO$_2$R can be considered in selected patients with severe ARDS and

Table 48.3: Comparison of arteriovenous extracorporeal carbon dioxide (AV-ECCO$_2$R) and veno-venous extracorporeal carbon dioxide removal (VV-ECCO$_2$R).

	AV-ECCO$_2$R	VV-ECCO$_2$R
Vascular access	Percutaneous arterial (13–15F) and venous (15–17F) cannula	Percutaneous double lumen venous cannula (15.5–24F)
Approximate circuit priming volume	350 mL	500 mL
Approximate flow rates	1–2 L/min	Low-flow 0.3–0.5 L/min or conventional 0.5–1.5 L/min
Complications	• Bleeding (local > systemic) • Lower limb ischemia • Compartment syndrome • Catheter displacement • Cannula thrombosis • Aneurysm	• Bleeding (systemic > local) • Pump malfunction • Membrane/filter clotting • Catheter displacement

hypercapnic respiratory failure; but clinical use should be restricted to physicians with expertise in its application. As the technology improves and more robust clinical trials are conducted, $ECCO_2R$ may eventually find a place in routine intensive care practice.

REFERENCES

1. Kolobow T, Gattinoni L, Tomlinson TA, et al. Control of breathing using an extracorporeal membrane lung. Anesthesiology. 1977;46:138-41.
2. Andrea M, Lorenzo DS, Antonio P, et al. Extracorporeal carbon dioxide removal ($ECCO_2R$) in patients with acute respiratory failure. Intensive Care Med. 2017;43(4):519-30.
3. Cove ME, MacLaren G, Federspiel WJ, et al. Bench to bedside review: Extracorporeal carbon dioxide removal, past present and future. Crit Care. 2012;16(5):232.
4. Gattinoni L, Pesenti A, Mascheroni D, et al. Low-frequency positive-pressure ventilation with extracorporeal CO_2 removal in severe acute respiratory failure. JAMA. 1986;256:881-6.
5. Gattinoni L, Kolobow T, Tomlinson T, et al. Low-frequency positive pressure ventilation with extracorporeal carbon dioxide removal ($LFPPV-ECCO_2R$): an experimental study. Anesth Analg. 1978;57:470-7.
6. Morris AH, Wallace CJ, Menlove RL, et al. Randomized clinical trial of pressure-controlled inverse ratio ventilation and extracorporeal CO_2 removal for adult respiratory distress syndrome. Am J Respir Crit Care Med. 1994;149(2 Pt 1):295-305.
7. Brower RG, Mattay MA, Morria A, et al. Ventilation with lower tidal volumes as compared with traditional tidal volumes for acute lung injury and the acute respiratory distress syndrome. NEJM. 2000;342(18):1301-8.
8. Kregenow DA, Rubenfeld GD, Hudson LD, et al. Hypercapnic acidosis and mortality in acute lung injury. Crit Care Med. 2006;34:1-7.
9. Terragni PP, Del Sorbo L, Mascia L, et al. Tidal volume lower than 6 m/kg enhances lung protection: role of extracorporeal carbon dioxide removal. Anesthesiology. 2009;111(4):826-35.
10. Curley G, Laffey JG, Kavanagh BP, et al. Bench to bedside review: Carbon dioxide. Crit Care. 2010;14(2):220.
11. Bein T, Weber-Carstens S, Goldmann A, et al. Lower tidal volume strategy (≈3 ml/kg) combined with extracorporeal CO2 removal versus 'conventional' protective ventilation (6 ml/kg) in severe ARDS: the prospective randomized Xtravent-study. Intensive Care Med. 2013;39(5):847-56.
12. Fitzgerald M, Millar J, Blackwood B, et al. Extracorporeal carbon dioxide removal for patients with acute respiratory failure secondary to the acute respiratory distress syndrome: a systematic review. Crit Care. 2014;18:222
13. Fanelli V, Ranieri MV, Mancebo J, et al. Feasibility and safety of low-flow extracorporeal carbon dioxide removal to facilitate ultra-protective ventilation in patients with moderate acute respiratory distress syndrome. Crit Care. 2016;20:36.
14. Esteban A, Alia I, Ibañez J, et al. Modes of mechanical ventilation and weaning: A national survey of Spanish hospitals. Chest. 1994;106(4):1188-93.
15. Kluge S, Braune SA, Engel M, et al. Avoiding invasive mechanical ventilation by extracorporeal carbon dioxide removal in patients failing noninvasive ventilation. Intensive Care Med. 2012;38(10):1632-9.
16. Burki NK, Mani RK, Herth FJF, et al. A novel extracorporeal CO_2 removal system: results of a pilot study of hypercapnic respiratory failure in patients with COPD. Chest. 2013;143(3):678-86.
17. Abrams DC, Brenner K, Burkart KM, et al. Pilot study of extracorporeal carbon dioxide removal to facilitate extubation and ambulation in exacerbations of chronic obstructive pulmonary disease. Ann Am Thorac Soc. 2013;10:307-14
18. Del Sorbo L, Pisani L, Filippini C, et al. Extracorporeal Co2 removal in hypercapnic patients at risk of noninvasive ventilation failure: a matched cohort study with historical control. Crit Care Med. 2015;43:120-7.
19. Braune S, Sieweke A, Brettner F, et al. The feasibility and safety of extracorporeal carbon dioxide removal to avoid intubation in patients with COPD unresponsive to noninvasive ventilation for acute hypercapnic respiratory failure (ECLAIR study): multicentre case–control study. Intensive Care Med. 2016;42(9):1437-44.
20. Sklar MC, Beloncle F, Katsios CM, et al. Extracorporeal carbon dioxide removal in patients with chronic obstructive pulmonary disease: a systematic review. Intensive care medicine. 2015;41(10):1752-62.
21. Fischer S, Simon AR, Welte T, et al. Bridge to lung transplantation with the novel pumpless interventional lung assist device NovaLung. J Thorac Cardiovasc Surg. 2006;131(3):719-23.
22. Schellongowski P, Riss K, Staudinger T, et al. Extracorporeal CO_2 removal as bridge to lung transplantation in life-threatening hypercapnia. Transpl Int. 2015;28(3):297-304.
23. Gattinoni L. Ultra-protective ventilation and hypoxemia. Crit Care. 2016;20(1):130.
24. Davidson AC, Banham S, Elliott M, et al. BTS/ICS guideline for the ventilatory management of acute hypercapnic respiratory failure in adults. Thorax. 2016;71 Suppl2:ii1-ii35.
25. National Institute for Health and Care Excellence (NICE). (2016). Extracorporeal carbon dioxide removal for acute respiratory failure. Interventional Procedures Guidance [IPG64]. [online] Available from https://www.nice.org.uk/guidance/ipg564 [Accessed November 2018].

CHAPTER 49

Continuous Renal Replacement Therapy: An Update

Nattachai Srisawat, Nuttha Lumlertgul, Sadudee Peerapornratana

INTRODUCTION

Acute kidney injury (AKI) is an independent risk factor for increased mortality in critically ill patients. In severe AKI, renal replacement therapy (RRT) could confer benefits by removal of uremic and putative toxins, achieving volume and solute control, correcting electrolyte imbalances, and may help remove cytokines and provide nutritional supplements. It is still unestablished regarding the optimal time, early versus standard, and the reliable parameter for decision to initiate RRT in severe AKI. Adequate continuous renal replacement therapy (CRRT) dosage is also very important to control metabolic waste product which normally eliminate by native kidney. In this article, we aim to review the latest update knowledge of CRRT, focusing on optimal timing for CRRT initiation and optimal dosage to be prescribed.

OPTIMAL TIMING OF CONTINUOUS RENAL REPLACEMENT THERAPY

Concept of Early RRT

Optimal time to initiate RRT has eluded physicians for years[1] with no unifying solution as yet.[2,3] Proposed mechanism behind the potential benefits of early RRT includes early removal of uremic toxins and better fluid balance.[4] Due to the fact that fluid overload is associated with poor clinical outcome.[5] Early RRT may improve immunomodulation in infected patients by the convective removal of small and medium-sized toxins such as endotoxin and cytokines, eliminate carbon dioxide in patients with respiratory failure, reduce the increased intracranial pressure in patients with acute brain injuries, and to prevent complications from AKI, such as arrhythmia caused by electrolyte disorders. If the initiation of RRT is delayed, the waste products might be accumulated, which is described by the increased urea breaking down in plasma to cyanate. Urea can promote the carbamylation of serum and tissue proteins, such as hemoglobin, albumin, and other proteins and cause uremia.

However, RRT is not a benign procedure. There are potential complications, i.e. risk of vascular access complication, hemodynamic instabilities, risk of delay renal recovery, and the high cost of treatment[6] (Fig. 49.1). Traditional or conventional indications for RRT include volume overload, metabolic acidosis, hyperkalemia that patients do not respond to drug therapy, overt uremia (uremic encephalopathy and uremic pericarditis), overdose toxicity, or intoxication with a dialyzable toxin. However, apart from symptoms, clinical manifestations, and blood test results relating to potentially life-threatening problems, there is no clear conclusion about the timing and the criteria of initiation of RRT.

How to Define Early RRT

It is difficult to determine the moment when AKI occurs unless there is an explicit risk factor, such as receiving radiocontrast agents, heart surgery. Consequently, various criteria for early and late commencement of RRT are established. In the past, blood urea nitrogen (BUN)

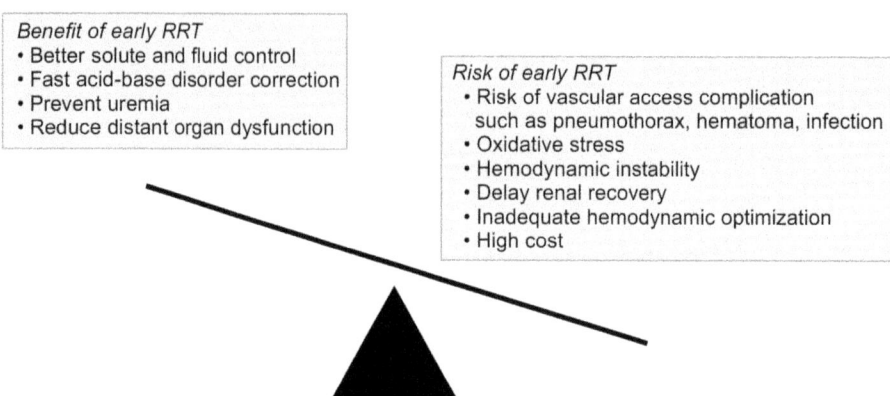

FIGURE 49.1: Risk and benefit of early renal replacement therapy (RRT).

and creatinine were divided into high and low levels to represent that patients with high level were likely to face more serious and prolonged AKI. The limitation is that BUN and creatinine are not toxic per se, but they represent that if the kidney function is reduced, other uremic toxins are likely to be in high level and cause symptoms. In addition, BUN and creatinine in the body, measured in milligram per deciliter, are varied by other confounding factors not related to kidney function, such as body fluid levels (hydration status), gastrointestinal bleeding, decomposition and composition of muscle, nutrition, and etc. Observational studies and randomized controlled trial (RCT) by Bouman et al. found that the group of early initiation of RRT (early RRT) and the group of standard indication for RRT (standard RRT) showed an average BUN at 47 and 104 mg/dL.[7] In addition the studies by Jamale et al. found that the early RRT and the standard RRT had average BUN at 71 and 101 mg/dL, respectively.[8] In both studies there was no difference in mortality rate. As a result, BUN was not a good indicator for the initiation of RRT.

Later, admission-based time such as time from hospital admission to RRT initiation or time from intensive care unit (ICU) admission to RRT initiation was introduced as a criterion for the early initiation of RRT. Of note, there would be different selection policies of ICU admission at each hospital. It seems the more appropriate based time should be time from AKI diagnosis to RRT initiation. Bagshaw et al. stratified time from ICU admission into early (<2 days), delayed (2-5 days), and late (>5 days). Late RRT was associated with greater crude (72.8% vs. 62.3% vs. 59%, P <.001) and covariate-adjusted mortality (OR, 1.95; 95% CI, 1.30-2.92; P = .001).[9]

Subsequent study found fluid accumulation is associated with mortality and non-recovery of kidney function in critically ill adults with AKI. Fluid overload was defined as more than a 10% increase in body weight relative to baseline. This fluid overload might be the potential indication for RRT initiation to avoid the uneventful from AKI[10] (Fig. 49.2).

According to the Acute Renal Failure Trial Network Study (ATN),[11] and the Randomized Evaluation of Normal versus Augmented Level Replacement Therapy (RENAL) Trial,[12] the median number of days on initiation of renal replacement therapy after ICU admission was 6.7 and 2.1 days, respectively. However, after comparing the time from diagnosis of AKI to RRT initiation of these two studies, it was found that there was no difference.

Of note, the definition for separation of early RRT from late or delayed RRT might produce misleading information. Late or delayed RRT might be understood that RRT will be delayed until complications occur, while early or accelerated RRT might be understood as unnecessarily urgent for initiation of RRT. Therefore, the terms of preemptive RRT and standard RRT, performing RRT when there is no and there is traditional or conventional indication for RRT, respectively have been proposed.

Evidence Base of Comparative Studies of Timing of RRT Initiation (Table 49.1)

Observational studies should be interpreted with caution because there are many confounding factors. In addition, most study participants did not include patients with AKI who did not receive RRT into analysis, which it might be that some patients could spontaneously recover kidney function. If patients recovering kidney function and patients receiving late RRT were combined, its average mortality rate may not be different from that of patients receiving early RRT. There was considerable heterogeneity between studies in terms of definition of AKI, definition of timing of initiation of RRT, selection of patients for trials and modalities of RRT. Most studies were retrospective studies conducted in a single hospital, there was not enough population and they were poor quality studies.

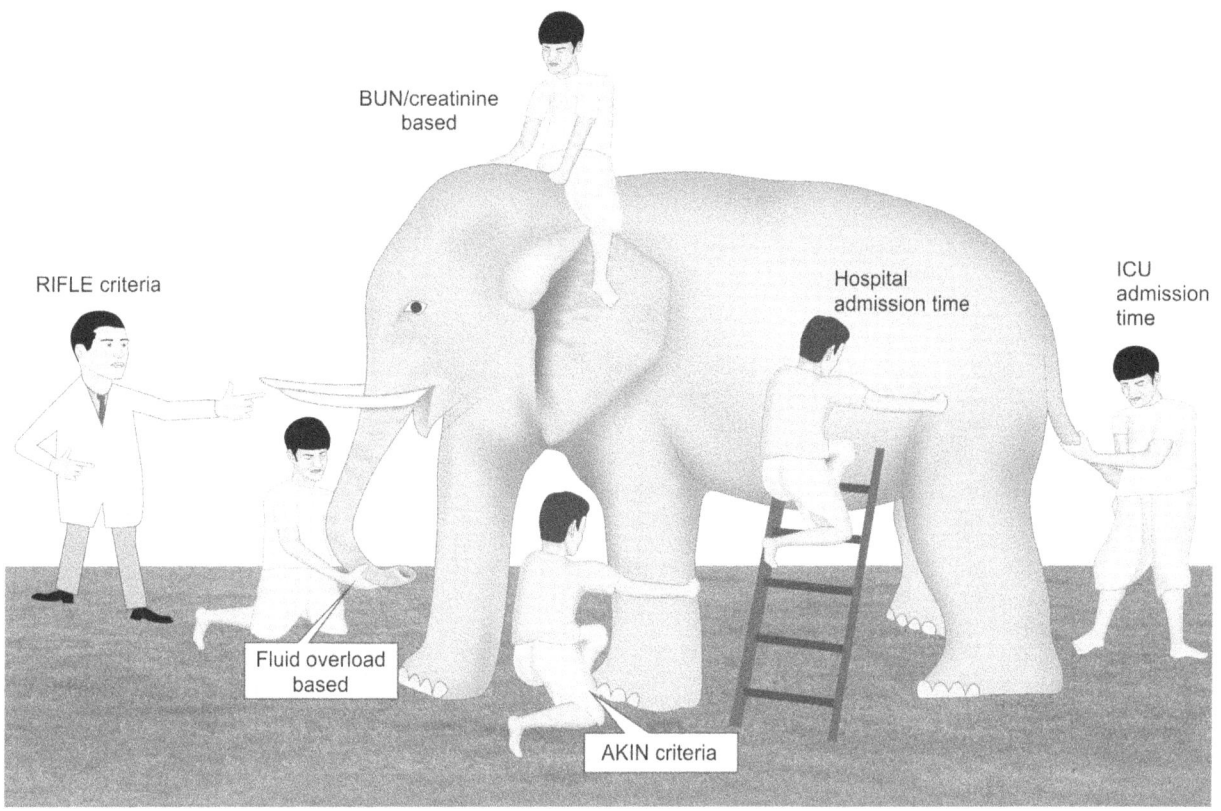

FIGURE 49.2: Parameters using for defining early initiation of renal replacement therapy.
(BUN: blood urea nitrogen; RIFLE: Risk, Injury, Failure, Loss of kidney function and End-stage kidney diseases; AKIN: acute kidney injury network; ICU: intensive care unit)

Table 49.1: Comparison the differences of recently completed and ongoing randomized trials evaluating the optimal timing of n terms renal replacement therapy initiation.

	STARRT-AKI (pilot)[13]	ELAIN[15]	AKIKI[14]	IDEAL-ICU[16]	STARRT-AKI (main)[17]	EARLY-RRT[20]	FST[21]
Country	Canada	Germany	France	France	Various nations	Thailand	Thailand
Number of ICU	12	1	31	24	>60	1	5
Number of patient	100	231	620	864*	2866*	60	118
Demographic features	Total surgical patients/ internal medicine patients (6% surgical patients)	Total surgical patients/ internal medicine patients (94.8% surgical patients, 47% patients with heart disease)	Total surgical patients/ internal medicine patients	Total surgical patients/ internal medicine patients (79.7% internal medicine patients)	Total surgical patients/ internal medicine patients (septic shock)	Total surgical patients/ internal medicine patients	Total surgical patients/ internal medicine patients
Sepsis (%)	54	21	67	TBA	TBA	73	55
CKD (%)	N/A	41	10	TBA	TBA	0	0
Absolute risk reduction	N/A	18	15	10	6	N/A	N/A

Contd...

Contd...

	STARRT-AKI (pilot)[13]	ELAIN[15]	AKIKI[14]	IDEAL-ICU[16]	STARRT-AKI (main)[17]	EARLY-RRT[20]	FST[21]
SOFA score	13	16	10.9	TBA	TBA	9.3	12
Mechanical ventilation (%)	93	88	87	TBA	TBA	100	49
Vasopressors (%)	85	88	85	TBA	TBA	97.5	46
Intervention Early RRT	KDIGO stage 2 (within 12 hours) Median 7.4 (IQR 6.1–9.6) hours	KDIGO stage 2 (within 8 hours) Median 6 (IQR 4–7) hours	KDIGO stage 3 (within 6 hours) Median 2 (IQR 1–3) hours	KDIGO stage 3 (within 12 hours)	KDIGO stage 2 (within 12 hours)	Plasma NGAL ≥400 ng/mL and initiate CRRT within 6 hours	FST positive and initiate CRRT within 6 hours
Control Standard RRT	Follow traditional or conventional indications (more than 12 hours) Median 31.6 (IQR 22.8–59.5) hours	KDIGO stage 3 (within 12 hours) Median 25.5 (IQR 18.8–40.3) hours	Follow traditional or conventional indications Median 57 (IQR 25–83) hours	48–60 hours after trial recruitment or when there is an indication	Follow traditional or conventional indications (more than 12 hours)	Plasma NGAL ≥400 ng/mL and initiate CRRT according to traditional or conventional indications	ST positive and initiate CRRT according to traditional or conventional indications
Creatinine at the initiation of RRT Early vs. standard [Mean (SD)]	3.2 (0.7) vs. 2.8 (0.7)	1.9 (0.6) vs. 2.4 (1.0)	3.3 (1.4) vs. 5.3 (2.3)	TBA	TBA	2.6 (0.8) vs. 2.2 (0.8)	2 (2,3) vs. 2.5 (2,3)
% RRT of standard RRT group	75	91	51	TBA	TBA	40	75
Modes of RRT	CRRT 69% HD 31%	CVVHDF 100%	CRRT 30% HD 55%	According to Physician's discretion	Physician's discretion	CRRT 100%	CRRT 100%
Primary outcome Early vs. Delayed	Mortality rate at 90 days 38% vs. 37%	Mortality rate at 90 days 39.3% vs. 54.7%	Mortality rate at 60 days 48.5% vs 49.7%	Mortality rate at 90 days TBA	Mortality rate at 90 days TBA	Mortality rate at 28 days 50% vs. 45%	Mortality rate at 28 days 62.1% vs. 58.3%
Fragility index	N/A	3	18	TBA	TBA	N/A	N/A

* sample size from calculation.
(CKD: chronic kidney disease; CRRT: continuous renal replacement therapy; CVVHDF: continuous venovenous hemodiafiltration; FST: furosemide stress test HD: hemodialysis; ICU: intensive care unit; IQR: interquartile range; N/A: not available; KDIGO: kidney disease improving global outcomes; RRT: renal replacement therapy; SOFA: sequential organ failure assessment; TBA: To be announced)

Clinical Trials Using Conventional Markers

Before 2015, the comparative studies of timing of RRT initiation study were small-scale studies and BUN or Cr were used as indications. However, in recent studies, phase of AKI was used as a criterion for initiation of RRT.

Since 2015, three RCTs were published, i.e. Standard vs. Accelerated initiation of Renal Replacement Therapy in Acute Kidney Injury (STARRT-AKI) pilot study,[13] Artificial Kidney Initiation in Kidney Injury (AKIKI) trial,[14] and Effect of Early vs. Delayed initiation of Renal Replacement Therapy on Mortality in Critically Ill Patients with Acute Kidney Injury (ELAIN) trial.[15] At present, two large-scale RCTs are being conducted, i.e. Initiation of Dialysis Early Versus delayed in Intensive Care Unit (IDEAL-

ICU) (clinicaltrials.gov NCT1682590)[16] and STARRT-AKI (clinicaltrials.gov NCT02568722).[17] It is expected that they will be completed by 2020. The detail of each study is summarized in Table 49.1.

STARRT-AKI was a multinational RCT and preliminary research findings were reported by Wald et al. In the study, 101 patients diagnosed with acute kidney injury stage 2, together with serum neutrophil gelatinase-associated lipocalin (NGAL) more than 400 ng/mL, were enrolled. After the patients participated in the study, in the early RRT group the average time to RRT initiation was 7.4 hours, but in three patients (6%) RRT was initiated after 12 hours. It is noticeable that in the standard RRT group, 75% of patients had the indications of RRT and the average time to RRT initiation was 31.6 hours (24 hours difference from the early RRT group); 25% of the patients could recover kidney function and six patients died before the initiation of RRT.

AKIKI study was a multicenter RCT in critically ill patients and 620 internal medicine and surgical patients were included. In early RRT group, RRT was initiated within 6 hours after diagnosis of AKI stage 3; while in standard RRT group, RRT was initiated when there were traditional or conventional indications. The result showed no difference in mortality rate at 60 days (48.5% compared with 49.7%, P = 0.79). It was found that only 51% of standard RRT patients required RRT, compared to 98% of early RRT patients. The difference of the average time to RRT initiation in the two groups was 57 hours. It was found that in standard RRT group, RRT-free days were greater (19 days compared with 17 days, P< 0.001), vascular access-related sepsis was lower (5% compared with 10%, P = 0.03) and hypophosphate rate was lower (15% compared with 22%, P = 0.03), as well as spontaneous voiding rate was higher than that of the early RRT group. There were no significant differences between the two groups on other outcomes, i.e. number of days on mechanical ventilation, number of days spent in the ICU, number of days spent in the hospital, and dialysis event rates at 60 days. Post-hoc analysis showed that the group of patients, who did not receive RRT, had lowest mortality rate (37.1%), followed by the early RRT group (48.5%) and the standard RRT group (61.8%), respectively. However, when control variable was severity of illness, no difference in mortality rate was found.

ELAIN study was a RCT of 231 critically ill patients in a single Germany institution. NGAL greater than or equal to 150 ng/mL was also a criterion for patient enrollment for the trial. The early RRT group received RRT when AKI was in stage 2, while the standard RRT group started RRT when AKI was in stage 3. 94.8% of patients were admitted into surgical wards and 47% of patients had heart disease. The patients in ELAIN study had a chronic renal failure stage 3 at 40% compared with 10% in AKIKI study. The study found that at 90 days the patients in the early RRT group significantly had a lower mortality rate when compared with the standard RRT group (39.3% compared with 53.6%, P = 0.03). In addition, they had higher recovery rate of kidney function (53.6% compared with 38.7%, P = 0.02, but there was no statistically significant difference when the patients who died within 90 days were excluded). Moreover, the early RRT group had lower number of days spent receiving RRT (9 days compared with 25 days, P = 0.04), lower number of days spent in the hospital (51 days compared with 82 days, P< 0.001), and lower circulating interleukin-6 (IL-6) and interleukin-8 (IL-8). After 24 hours of RRT, there was no difference in severity of illness score, number of days spent in the ICU or dialysis event rates at 90 days.

Both trials are important studies and help guide on the initiation of RRT. The procedure of both trials is well-designed randomized trials. However, both studies were still underpowered to show the survival benefit of early RRT because there are many factors resulting in the treatment of the critically ill patients. When taking the population characteristics into consideration, the patients in ELAIN study were mostly postoperative patients, but AKIKI patients were mostly general internal medicine patients. In addition, the patients in the standard RRT group in ELAIN study were patients with AKI stage 3, which was equivalent to the patients in the early RRT group in AKIKI study. As for the trial enrollment criteria, AKIKI study excluded patients with fluid overload and non-responders to pharmacological treatment; while ELAIN study included them. Therefore, the average amount of fluid accumulation of 6 liters could be found at the predicted time in the body of the patients in the early RRT group of ELAIN study, who had postoperative AKI, and some patients had a volume overload so that when the early initiation of RRT was implemented, they received the benefit from controlling fluid balance, which was a life-threatening condition in critically ill patients.

ELAIN study had an advantage over AKIKI study since the same practice of RRT, i.e. continuous venovenous hemodiafiltration (CVVHDF) was applied in ELAIN study. While in AKIKI study, 55% of patients received intermittent hemodialysis because 85% of patients required vasopressors. Intermittent hemodialysis for RRT might affect the stability of vital signs in patients. However, there were three reasons that should be taken into consideration from ELAIN study. Firstly, the basic characteristics of patients in ELAIN study, in the standard RRT group, the number of patients with glomerular filtration rate less than 60 mL/kg/min, and the number of patients undergoing liver transplantation was higher than that of the early RRT group. Their plasma NGAL was also higher than that of the early RRT group, even though the difference was not statistically significant. Consequently, the worse outcome in the standard RRT group might be explained as a result of these things. Secondly, fragility index is 3, which means if only three more patients in the early RRT group die or only three more patients in the standard RRT group survive, there will be no difference in the mortality rate of both groups. Lastly, it looks suspicious that only 25-hour difference in the initiation of RRT can reduce the mortality rate up to 15%, which may be an overstatement.

The use of information from these two studies should be done with extreme caution. ELAIN study showed that the initiation of RRT from AKI stage 2 can reduce mortality rate higher than the initiation in AKI stage 3. On the other hand, AKIKI study found that even patients had AKI stage 3, 49% of them could recover their kidney function, similar to the finding from STARRT-AKI (pilot study) that 1 in 4 patients could recover their kidney function. Therefore, physicians can apply the watchful waiting approach as the strategy for initiation of RRT when there is an indication and fully provide supportive care including medication since some patients eventually do not require RRT.

Wald et al. performed a pool meta-analysis of a collection of results from recent RCTs including two recent studies.[14,15] With a total of 1,343 patients, they found that the early RRT group had a mortality rate 37.5% when compared with the standard RRT 41.8% (RR 0.77, 95% CI 0.43, 1.27) with no significant difference of mortality.[18]

Clinical Trials Using Novel AKI Biomarkers

There is evidence that biomarkers assess better prognosis in patients with AKI than BUN or creatinine and can be used to predict the recovery from AKI.[19] It is interesting that these biomarkers may help identify patients who benefit from the early initiation of RRT or identify patients who can recover kidney function (non-progressors). ELAIN study defined serum NGAL of more than or equal to 150 ng/mL and STARRT-AKI defined serum NGAL of more than or equal to 400 ng/mL as one of the criteria for patient enrollment for the trial. It is noticeable that in ELAIN study, serum NGAL in the early RRT group is likely to be lower than that in the standard RRT (490 compared with 619 ng/mL), although it is not statistically significant.

We recently conducted two RCTs to test the role of plasma NGAL and furosemide stress test (FST) in identifying the high risk AKI patients who will get the most benefit from early RRT. The first study was the *EARLY-RRT* study which was the study using plusicomprised of triage trial and interventional trial running subsequently. As a using plasma NGAL guiding for triage to RRT.[20] We measured plasma NGAL at the enrollment time. 40 patients with plasma NGAL more than or equal to 400 ng/mL (high pNGAL group) were randomized to "early" (within 6 hours) or "standard" group. Patients with pNGAL less than 400 ng/mL (n =20) were defined as low pNGAL group. We found that plasma NGAL selected AKI patients with more severity of illness and worse clinical outcome. However, in high pNGAL group, early RRT did not result in different 28-day mortality from the standard group. The median numbers of day free from mechanical ventilation were significantly higher in the early RRT group. Of note, no one in the low pNGAL group received RRT, and 40% in standard group (high pNGAL group) received RRT. The early RRT group had a greater chance of stopping RRT (90% compared with 0%), had more free days of mechanical ventilation and number of days after ICU discharge was higher than that of standard RRT group.

The second study was FST trial,[21] the FST has been shown to predict the need for RRT and therefore could be used to exclude low-risk patients from enrollment in trials of RRT timing. Therefore, we conducted the multicenter pilot study to determine whether FST could be used to screen patients at high risk for RRT and to determine the feasibility of incorporating FST into a trial of early initiation of RRT. FST was performed using intravenous furosemide (1 mg/kg in furosemide-naive patients or 1.5 mg/kg in previous furosemide users). FST-nonresponsive patients (urine output less than 200 mL in 2 hours) were then randomized to early (initiation within 6 hours) or standard (initiation by urgent indication) RRT. We found that only 6/44 (13.6%) FST-responsive patients ultimately received RRT while 47/60 (78.3%) non-responders randomized to standard RRT either received RRT or died (P <0.001). Among 118 FST-nonresponsive patients, 98.3% in the early RRT arm and 75% in the standard RRT arm received RRT. The adherence to the protocol was 94.8% and 100% in the early and standard RRT group, respectively. We observed no differences in 28-day mortality (62.1 versus 58.3%, P = 0.68), 7-day fluid balance, or RRT dependence at day 28. However, hypophosphatemia occurred more frequently in the early RRT arm (P = 0.002). Again, both studies are still under power to test the survival benefit of early RRT.

Therefore, it is possible to use biomarkers to identify high risk groups and give clue to initiate RRT, which there may be new studies clarifying these issues in the future.

Another concept getting more attention lately is a consideration of the unequal adaptability of the body to the pathophysiology of each patient's illness due to pre-existing disease, age, previous renal function, and etc. (capacity), together with severity of illness and the body's demand for resources (demand), such as sepsis and the number of organ dysfunction. If a patient is very old and suffering multiple organ failure, i.e. he has very little physical capacity, but has high demand for kidney function, he may benefit from the early initiation of RRT. On the contrary, if the patient is young, strong, does not suffer from pre-existing disease, and his AKI can be quickly treated by supportive care, the RRT can be initiated when there is an indication. This concept is supported by a prospective observational study. Park et al. found that when patients aged 65 years or over were divided into the group of initiation of RRT when the output urine was more than 0.24 mL/kg/hour in 6 hours (the early RRT group) and the group of initiation of RRT when the output urine was less than 0.24 mL/kg/hour (the late RRT group), the early initiation of RRT significantly reduced mortality rate from 70% to 58%. It is noticeable that the patients in this study are very old person.[3] Unlike the study by Jamale in patients with community-acquired AKI, the average age of the patients was 42 years and the mortality rates in both groups were only 12% and 21%.[2] As a result, for initiation of RRT, the personalized RRT should be performed by taking the basic characteristics of each patient and the severity of AKI into consideration for determining how much the reduction of organ function can be compensated by bodily capabilities (Table 49.2).

SUMMARY

Until now there is no clear consensus for early RRT initiation in AKI patients who do not have absolute indication. In 2016, two large randomized studies, i.e. the AKIKI trial and ELAIN trial were published. However, the results of these studies were different. We are still waiting for the result from the upcoming large RCT. In the meantime, novel AKI biomarkers might be other parameters to help physician in selection the suitable patients for early RRT initiation (Flowchart 49.1).

Table 49.2: Proposed concept of initiation of renal replacement therapy (RRT) by taking severity of illness (demand) and body condition of each patient (capacity) into consideration.

Personalized renal replacement therapy		Capacity	
		Low	High
Demand	Low	According to Physician's discretion	Standard initiation of RRT
	High	Early initiation of RRT	According to Physician's discretion

FLOWCHART 49.1: Proposed algorithm for initiation renal replacement therapy in critically ill patients with acute kidney injury.

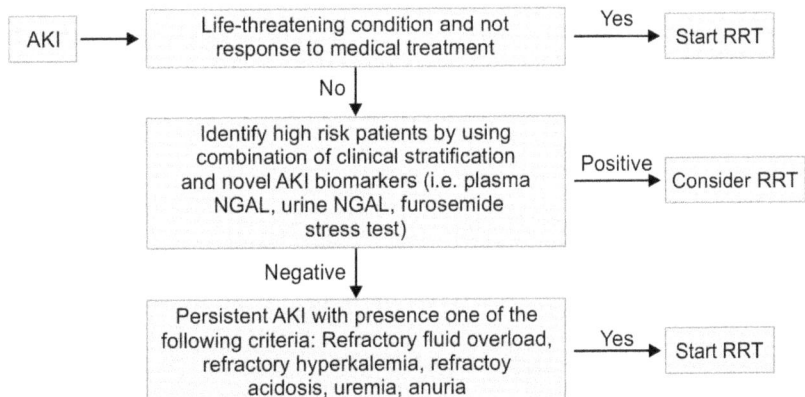

(AKI: acute kidney injury; NGAL: neutrophil gelatinase-associated lipocalcin; RRT: renal replacement therapy)

REFERENCES

1. Seabra VF, Balk EM, Liangos O, et al. Timing of renal replacement therapy initiation in acute renal failure: a meta-analysis. Am J Kidney Dis. 2008;52(2):272-84.
2. Karvellas CJ, Farhat MR, Sajjad I, et al. A comparison of early versus late initiation of renal replacement therapy in critically ill patients with acute kidney injury: a systematic review and meta-analysis. Crit Care. 2011;15(1):R72.
3. Kellum JA, Mehta RL, Levin A, et al. Development of a clinical research agenda for acute kidney injury using an international, interdisciplinary, three-step modified Delphi process. Clin J Am Soc Nephrol. 2008;3(3):887-94.
4. Peng Y, Yuan Z, Li H. Removal of inflammatory cytokines and endotoxin by veno-venous continuous renal replacement therapy for burned patients with sepsis. Burns. 2005;31(5):623-8.
5. Mehta RL, Bouchard J. Controversies in acute kidney injury: effects of fluid overload on outcome. Contrib Nephrol. 2011;174:200-11.
6. Srisawat N, Lawsin L, Uchino S, et al. BEST Kidney Investigators. Cost of acute renal replacement therapy in the intensive care unit: results from The Beginning and Ending Supportive Therapy for the Kidney (BEST Kidney) study. Crit Care. 2010;14(2):R46.
7. Bouman CS, Oudemans-Van Straaten HM, Tijssen JG, et al. Effects of early high-volume continuous venovenous hemofiltration on survival and recovery of renal function in intensive care patients with acute renal failure: a prospective, randomized trial. Crit Care Med. 2002;30(10):2205-11.
8. Jamale TE, Hase NK, Kulkarni M, et al. Earlier-start versus usual-start dialysis in patients with community-acquired Acute Kidney Injury: a randomized controlled trial. Am J Kidney Dis. 2013;62(6):1116-21.
9. Bagshaw SM, Uchino S, Bellomo R, et al. Beginning and Ending Supportive Therapy for the Kidney (BEST Kidney) Investigators. Timing of renal replacement therapy and clinical outcomes in critically ill patients with severe acute kidney injury. J Crit Care. 2009;24(1):129-40.
10. Bouchard J, Soroko SB, Chertow GM, et al. Program to Improve Care in Acute Renal Disease (PICARD) Study Group. Fluid accumulation, survival and recovery of kidney function in critically ill patients with acute kidney injury. Kidney Int. 2009;76(4):422-7.
11. Palevsky PM, Zhang JH, O'Connor TZ, et al. Intensity of renal support in critically ill patients with Acute Kidney Injury. N Eng J Med. 2008;359(1):7-20.
12. RENAL Replacement Therapy Study Investigators, Bellomo R, Cass A, et al. Intensity of continuous renal-replacement therapy in critically ill patients. N Engl J Med. 2009;361(17):1627-38.
13. Wald R, Adhikari NK, Smith OM, et al. Comparison of standard and accelerated initiation of renal replacement therapy in Acute Kidney Injury. Kidney Int. 2015;88(4):897-904.
14. Gaudry S, Hajage D, Schortgen F, et al. Initiation strategies for renal-replacement therapy in the intensive care unit. N Eng J Med. 2016;375(2):122-33.
15. Zarbock A, Kellum JA, Schmidt C, et al. Effect of early vs delayed initiation of renal replacement therapy on mortality in critically ill patients with acute kidney injury: The ELAIN Randomized Clinical Trial. J Am Med Assoc. 2016;315(20):2190-9.
16. Barbar SD, Binquet C, Monchi M, et al. Impact on mortality of the timing of renal replacement therapy in patients with severe Acute Kidney Injury in septic shock: the IDEAL-ICU study (initiation of dialysis early versus delayed in the intensive care unit): study protocol for a randomized controlled trial. Trials. 2014;15:270.
17. Smith OM, Wald R, Adhikari NK, et al. Standard versus accelerated initiation of renal replacement therapy in Acute Kidney Injury (STARRT-AKI): study protocol for a randomized controlled trial. Trials. 2013;14:320.
18. Bagshaw SM, Wald R. Strategies for the optimal timing to start renal replacement therapy in critically ill patients with acute kidney injury. Kidney Int. 2017;91(5):1022-32.
19. Srisawat N, Murugan R, Lee M, et al. Genetic and Inflammatory Markers of Sepsis (GenIMS) Study Investigators. Plasma neutrophil gelatinase-associated lipocalin predicts recovery from acute kidney injury following community-acquired pneumonia. Kidney Int. 2011;80(5):545-52.
20. Srisawat N, Laoveeravat P, Limphunudom P, et al. The effect of early renal replacement therapy guided by plasma neutrophil gelatinase associated lipocalin on outcome of acute kidney injury: A feasibility study. J Crit Care. 2018;43:36-41.
21. Lumlertgul N, Peerapornratana S, Trakarnvanich T, et al. FST Study Group. Early versus standard initiation of renal replacement therapy in furosemide stress test non-responsive acute kidney injury patients (the FST trial). Crit Care. 2018;22(1):101.

Extracorporeal Blood Purification Therapy for Sepsis

Nattachai Srisawat

INTRODUCTION

Extracorporeal blood purification (ECBP) has been widely used during the past 30 years, initiating from the treatment of patients with end-stage renal disease (ESRD) with hemodialysis technique. The advancement in terms of the equipment and techniques related to blood purification as well as a better understanding and an increased body of knowledge about the mechanism of the solute clearance and fluid removal have led to an adaptation of the new techniques based on the principles of acute dialysis. Apart from being used in renal replacement therapy (RRT), this knowledge can be applied and used in the treatment of other organs such as in liver support therapy, respiratory support, and cardiac support. Moreover, the techniques employed in continuous renal replacement therapy (CRRT) can also be used to remove inflammatory mediators in patients with septic shock and multiple organ dysfunction syndrome (MODS).

The main objective of this chapter is to compile the body of knowledge related to the techniques used in ECBP in sepsis.

EXTRACORPOREAL BLOOD PURIFICATION FOR SEPSIS

Sepsis is frequently found and is the major cause of death in an intensive care unit. The average mortality rate is 30% and can be increased to 50% if septic shock is involved. For sepsis, the use of bactericidal antibiotics and fluid administration are considered as a standard medical therapy (SMT). With sepsis, however, not only is there bacteria that can negatively affect the body, but inflammatory mediators or bacterial toxins can also have a direct effect on the function of the major organs, such as the heart, lung, kidneys and the livers, causing circulatory failure, and hemodynamic instability.

The principle of an ECBP therapy is that it is an adjunctive therapy that helps remove inflammatory mediators or bacterial toxins from blood circulation. It is an adjunctive therapy to SMT at present. There are several techniques to remove these inflammatory mediators including high-volume hemofiltration (HVHF), cascade hemofiltration, hemoadsorption (hemoperfusion), plasmapheresis, coupled plasma filtration adsorption (CPFA), and high cutoff (HCO) hemodialysis.

This chapter will discuss the principles and theories related to the use of ECBP in sepsis, following by current techniques in use and clinical evidences.

Principles of Blood Purification[1]

It is commonly known that a systemic inflammatory response occurring during sepsis and septic shock can cause immunologic instability. When this becomes uncontrollable, it can lead to a multiorgan failure syndrome (Fig. 50.1 and Table 50.1). Currently, there are four main theories trying to describe the mechanism of how ECBP can help with sepsis as follows:

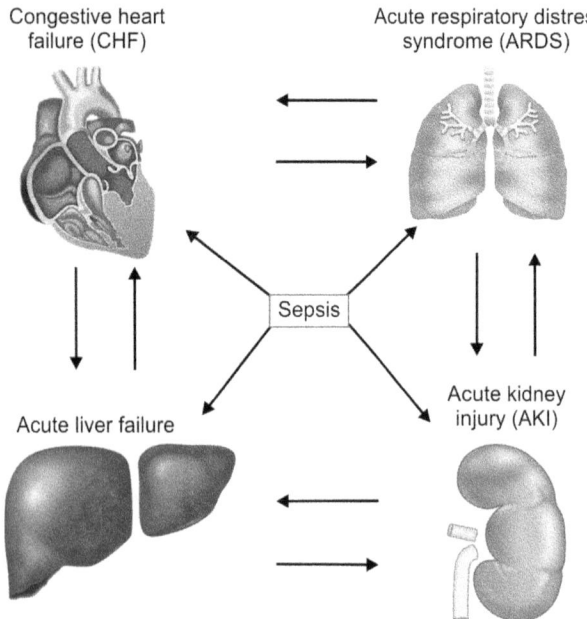

FIGURE 50.1: Illustrating the role of extracorporeal blood purification in the treatment of multiple organ dysfunction syndrome namely performing isolated ultrafiltration for congestive heart failure, CO_2 removal blood purification for the treatment of acute respiratory distress syndrome, liver dialysis for liver failure, and continuous renal replacement therapy (CRRT) for the treatment of acute kidney injury.

1. *Peak concentration hypothesis or "Ronco concept"*: The mechanism of sepsis involves the production of proinflammatory cytokines and anti-inflammatory cytokines (shortly called a compensated anti-inflammatory response syndrome or CARS). This can occur in a serial manner, that is, proinflammatory cytokines are generated first, following by anti-inflammatory cytokines. This is called the serial sepsis theory. It can also occur in a parallel manner, that is, both pro- and anti-inflammatory cytokines are generated simultaneously. At present, there is still no consensus on which is the principle theory.
   Ronco and Bellomo postulated the "peak concentration hypothesis" suggesting that both proinflammatory and anti-inflammatory mediators should be removed by any methods so as to cut the "peak" of these mediators in blood circulation in order to restore the situation of immunohomeostasis, that is, an immune-modulatory effect in the tissue level.[2]
2. *Threshold immunomodulation hypothesis or "Honore' concept"*: This theory proposes that when the removal of cytokines in blood circulation occurs, other cytokines in the tissue level will be released into the circulation in order to create the balance point between the cytokines in blood circulation and tissues. This theory can explain the phenomenon why blood purification therapy in sepsis patients, possibly decrease the mortality rate in the patients without any reduction of inflammatory cytokines detected.
3. *Mediator delivery hypothesis or "Alexander concept"*: According to this theory, not only HVHF is used to remove various mediators, but it also involves a large input of incoming fluids (3–5 L/h) into the body, causing the lymphatic flow to increase 20–40 times. This results in an increase of mediators and cytokines lymphatic drag from the tissue level to blood circulation.[3]
4. *Cytokinetic hypothesis*: Peng and colleagues believes that blood purification has an effect on inflammatory cells as it enhances the performances of monocytes, neutrophils, and lymphocytes after removal pro- and anti-inflammatory cytokines. There has been evidence in animal study which showed more inflammatory cells infiltrating around the infectious sites. This result in a better clearance of bacteria.

Extracorporeal Blood Purification Technique in Sepsis

High-volume Hemofiltration

High-volume hemofiltration is a modality of blood purification therapy that is most easily adapted and was widespread in the past. HVHF is in fact an increase of dose of CRRT (the UF rate of more than 35 mL/kg/h or 60 L/day in a patient of 70 kg) in order to increase the convection. The findings from an animal experiment pointed out that the use of HVHF to treat sepsis could yield the best result for the survival rate if used from the initial stage of sepsis. The HVHF of 100 mL/kg/h was used in experimental animals while that of averagely 40 mL/kg/h was used in patients with septic shock/severe sepsis. It was found that HVHF helped improve the hemodynamics, decreased the need of vasopressor,[4-7] and tended to increase the survival rate of the patients.[5-9]

Clinical evidence: The latest data was derived from the IVOIRE study (h**I**gh **VO**lume in **I**ntensive ca**RE**), a multicenter randomized controlled study in France targeting the treatment of septic patients with AKI based on the Risk, Injury, and Failure and Loss and End-stage Kidney (RIFLE) criteria. In this study, the 480 patients were randomized to treat with CVVH at the dose of 35 mL/kg/h compare with the dose of 70 mL/kg/h for 96 hours, and evaluate the survival rate on the 28th, 60th, and 90th day after ICU admission.

Table 50.1: A summary of the studies on the use of high-volume hemofiltration in patients with septic shock.[1]

Study	Design	N	Clinical setting	Dose mL/kg/h	Improved hemodynamic with HVHF	Improved survival with HVHF	P value (survival)
Honore' et al. 2000	Prospective Cohort, uncontrolled	20	Refractory septic shock	115	Yes	Yes 28-day survival: (expected) uncontrolled to 45% (observed)	<0.05
Cole et al. 2001	Randomized, cross over	11	Septic shock with multiple organ failure	6,000 mL/h	Yes	Not assessed	N/A
Joannes-Boyau et al. 2004	Prospective Cohort, uncontrolled	24	Septic shock	40–60	Yes	Yes 28-day survival: 30% (expected) to 54% (observed)	<0.075
Laurent et al. 2005	RCT	61	Resuscitated cardiac arrest	200	Yes	Yes 6-month survival: 21–45%	0.026
Jiang et al. 2005	RCT	37	Severe acute pancreatitis	4,000 mL/h	Yes	Yes 14-day survival: 68.4–94.4%	<0.01
Ratanarat et al. 2005	Prospective Cohort, uncontrolled	15	Severe sepsis	85 (pulse HVHF)	Yes	Yes 28-day survival: 30% (expected) to 53% (observed)	N/A
Piccinni et al. 2006	Retrospective, uncontrolled	80	Septic shock	45	Yes	Yes 28-day survival: 27.5–55%	0.005
Cornejo et al. 2006	Prospective Cohort, uncontrolled	20	Refractory septic shock	100	Yes	Yes Hospital survival: 37% (expected) to 60% (observed)	<0.03
Boussekey et al. 2008	RCT	20	Septic shock	65	Yes	No	0.65
Zhu et al. 2009	Retrospective	63	Severe acute pancreatitis	60–80	No	Yes 28-day survival: 65.5–91.2%	0.014
IVOIRE study, 2013	RCT	150	Septic shock	70	No	No 28-day mortality HVHF 37.9% vs SVHF 40.8%	0.94

(HVHF: high-volume hemofiltration; RCT: randomized controlled trial)

Names of adsorbers	manufacturers	Types of sorbents	Substances to be adsorped
PMX	Toray, Japan	PMX covalently bound to polypropylene-polystyrene fiber	Endotoxin
oXiris	Baxter, USA	AN69, PEI, heparin grafting	Endotoxin, cytokines
HA330	Jafron, China	Neutral resin	Cytokines
MG350	Biosun, China	Neutral resin	Cytokines
CPFA	Bellco, Italy	PES plasma filter, hydrophobic resin cartridge, high-flux hemofilter	Cytokines
Cytosorb	Cytosorbents, USA	Polystyrenedivinyl benzene copolymer beads with biocompatible polyvinylpyrrolidone coating	Cytokines
LPS adsorber	Alteco, Sweden	Synthetic polypeptide bound to porous polyethylene disks	Endotoxin

Table 50.2: A list of adsorbers, manufacturers, and the types of sorbents available at present.

(PMX: polymyxin; CPFA: coupled plasma filtration absorption; LPS: lipopolysaccharide; PEI: polyethylenimine; PES; polyethersulfone)

The findings, however, show that no significant differences in the mortality rate were found.[10]

Hemoadsorption

Hemoadsorption is a technique utilizing a sorbent to adsorp undesirable substances using the quality of hydrophobic interactions, ionic attraction, hydrogen bonding, and the van der Waals forces.[11] The interesting aspect of hemoadsorption is its ability to adsorb substances with high molecular weight that cannot generally be filtered through a common high-flux filter. At present, there are certain filters with the ability to adsorb endotoxin, proinflammatory cytokines, and anti-inflammatory cytokines as shown in Table 50.2. This chapter will mainly discuss the polymyxin hemoperfusion technique as it is the technique with abundant clinical data and the longest clinical use.

Polymyxin B Hemoperfusion, PMX-HP (Toraymyxin®)

Polymyxin B is a bactericidal antibiotic used against Gram-negative bacteria and it can neutralize endotoxin (lipopolysaccharide) by directly binding with endotoxin. This antibiotic cannot be administered through IV as it will become toxic for the kidneys and the nervous system. Polymyxin-B is bound with synthetic to form polymyxin B-immobilized fiber which possesses an ability to be a hemoperfusion column that can adsorb endotoxin, but without its bactericidal quality or its systemic effect until it becomes toxic for the kidneys and the nervous system (Fig. 50.2).

In Japan, there is a widespread use of PMX-HP because since 1994, the Pharmaceuticals and Medical Devices Agency of Japan has approved the use of it in patients with all three conditions as follows:

1. With endotoxemia or having indication to be infected with Gram-negative bacteria.
2. Having evidence of having systemic inflammatory response syndrome (SIRS).
3. Patients with septic shock who need to be treated with vasopressor.

PMX-HP Techniques

PMX-HP employs the same circuit as normal hemodialysis, with the use of a double lumen dialysis catheter like in hemodialysis. During the process, there is no need for any dialysate solution or replacement fluid. Two sessions of PMX-HP are needed, with the duration of 2 hours per session. During the PMX-HP process, it is advisable that 3,000 unit of heparin is employed as anticoagulant, with the rate of 20 unit/kg/h. However, even with contraindication against the use of anticoagulant, PMX-HP can still be performed. After the treatment, if the condition of the patient is still not better, it is possible to consider increasing the duration per session or increasing the number of session for PMX-HP process for particular patient. Figure 50.3 illustrates the PMX-HP circuit.

Clinical evidence: A meta-analysis examining the use of PMX-HP in the treatment of sepsis patients was conducted by compiling 16 comparative studies done on 1,040 patients (nine out of these studies were RCT), and 16 pre-post studies on 385 patients, 83 of which using hemoperfusion with PMX-F together with a SMT, with the blood flow rate of 50–150 mL/min through venovenous access for 2 hours/session, for 1–2 times. It was found that the patients receiving PMX-F had a lower rate of endotoxin, increased mean arterial pressure (MAP) (26%), could decrease the use of dopamine/dobutamine, and had a significant increase of

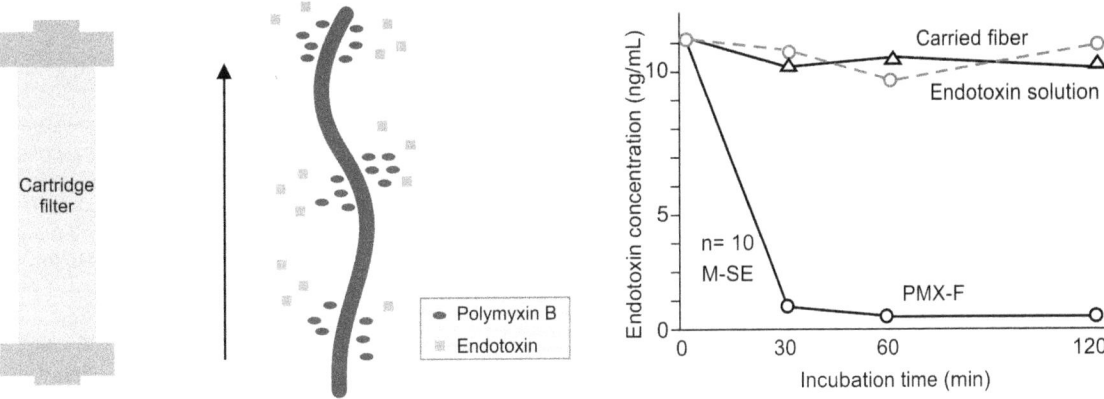

FIGURE 50.2: Illustrating an adsorber with polymyxin B coated on the surface, enabling it to have no systemic side effect as polymyxin B will directly bind with endotoxin.

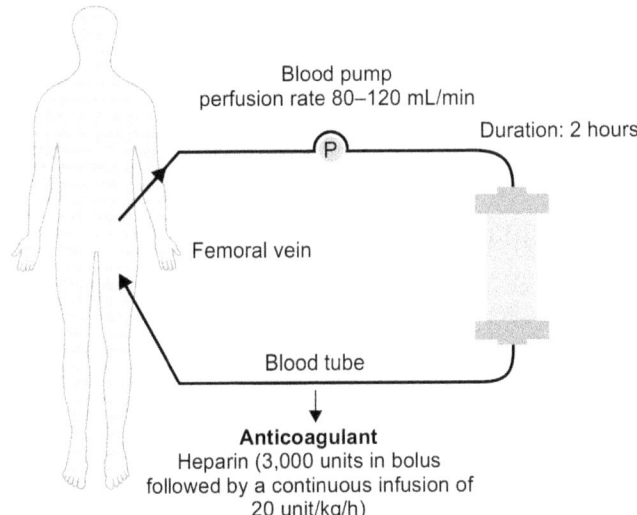

FIGURE 50.3: Illustrating the PM-HP circuit in which the blood is directly passed through PMX filter without any fluid input or output from the patients' body.

oxygenation (PaO_2/FiO_2). When including only the studies that reported the mortality rate on the 28th and 30th day done on 704 patients were compared, it was found that the treatment with PMX-F could decrease the mortality rate with statistical significance compared with SMT (relative risk 0.5; 95% confidence interval 0.43–0.68).

Two RCT studies done in Europe by Vincent and colleagues[12] together with the EUPHAS[13] study (Early Use of Polymyxin B Hemoperfusion in Abdominal Septic Shock) done on postoperative patients with severe sepsis/septic shock from abdominal infection found that PMX-HP could increase cardiac output and oxygen delivery index, decrease the treatment using CRRT 80 MAP, decrease the use of vasopressor, increase oxygenation (PaO_2/FiO_2 ratio), and decrease the mortality rate on the 28th day (32%) when compared with the use of standard medical therapy (SMT) (53%) [adjusted hazard ratio (HR) 0.36; 95% confidence interval 0.16–0.80].[13] Still, a concerning that the EUPHAS trial was terminated too early, and as a result, under power to conclude the benefit of decreasing of the mortality rate. The interesting point is that, in this study, PMX-HP was initiated quite early, that is, within 6 hours after operations. Moreover, the study was conducted on patients who tended to have a high level of endotoxin and with the sources of infection that could be well controlled. Because of this, if the findings from this study are to be applied to patients with severe sepsis/septic shock resulting from other causes, it is still very crucial to consider clinical context and its high cost.

According to the latest study referred to as ABDOMIX by Payen and colleagues[14] conducted in 18 hospitals throughout France, no significant differences in the mortality rate on the 28th day were found in the patients treated with PMX-HP compared with the controlled group. Of note, there were only 81 of 119 patients (69.8%) who received 2 PMX-HP sessions in ABDOMIX study. Both EUPHAS study, and ABDOMIX study did not use EAA level to guide PMX-HP initiation. The latest meta-analysis by Fujii et al. included 6 trials, 857 participants, could not show the benefit of PMX-HP on 28-day mortality and organ dysfunction scores. Again, most of the included studies did not use endotoxin level to guide intervention (Table 50.3).[15-17]

We conducted a randomized controlled trial in patients with EAA level more than or equal to 0.6 to explore the effect of PMX-HP on immune cell (monocyte and neutrophil). Patients in the PMX-HP group received a 2-hour PMX-HP treatment plus standard treatment for 2 consecutive days. Patients in the non-PMX-HP group received only standard treatment. The primary outcome

Studies	Vincent JL et al. (2005)[12]	EUPHAS study (2009)[13]	Iwagami et al. (2014)[15]	Iwagami et al. (2016)[16]	ABDOMIX study (2015)[14]
Population	Severe sepsis and septic shock after surgery due to abdominal cavity infection	Severe sepsis and septic shock requiring emergency surgery due to intra-abdominal cavity infection	Abdominal septic shock triggered by lower-gastrointestinal tract perforation	Septic shock requiring CRRT	Severe sepsis and septic shock requiring emergency surgery due to intra-abdominal cavity infection
Types of studies	RCT	RCT	Retrospective	Retrospective	RCT
Number of patients	36	64	1,080	2,230	232
PMX initiation timing	Within 24~48 hours after surgery	Within 24 hours after surgery	Day 0 or day 1 after operation	At the timing of CRRT initiation	Within 12 hours after surgery
Number of PMX-HP Sessions	1	2	1 or 2	1 or 2	2
Findings					
28-day mortality (%)	P = NS	P = 0.01	P = NS	P = 0.003	P = NS
• PMX treated	29 (n = 17)	32 (n = 34)	17 (n = 590)	41 (n = 1,115)	40 (n = 119)
• Control	28 (n = 19)	53 (n = 30)	16 (n = 590)	47 (n = 1,115)	27 (n = 113)

(CRRT: continuous renal replacement therapy; NS: nonsignificant; PMX-HP: polymyxiin hemoperfusion; RCT: randomized controlled trial)

compared the groups on median change in mHLA-DR expression between day 3 and baseline. 59 patients were randomized to PMX-HP (n = 29) and non-PMX-HP (n = 30) groups. At baseline, mHLA-DR expression, CD11b, neutrophil chemotaxis, and clinical parameters were comparable between groups. The median change in mHLA-DR expression between day 3 and baseline was higher in PMX-HP patients than in patients receiving standard therapy alone, P = 0.027. The mean change in CD11b between day 3 and baseline was significantly lower in PMX-HP than in non-PMX-HP, P = 0.002. There were no significant changes from baseline in neutrophil chemotaxis, presepsin, CVS SOFA scores, vasopressor doses, or EAA level between groups. On day 28 after enrollment, mortality, ICU-free days, ventilator-free days, dialysis dependence status, renal recovery, serum creatinine, vasopressor-free days, and MAKE 28 were comparable between groups.[18]

Currently, there is the largest multicenter randomized trial, Evaluating the Use of Polymyxin B Hemoperfusion in a Randomized controlled trial of Adults Treated for Endotoxemia and Septic shock (EUPHRATES), which finished trial in 2017, but yet unpublished. This study aimed to prove the concept of using a biomarker, EAA, to identify the patients who will receive the most benefit form PMX-HP treatment.[19]

REFERENCES

1. Rimmele T, Kellum JA. Clinical review: blood purification for sepsis. Crit Care. 2011;15:205.
2. Ronco C, Bonello M, Bordoni V, et al. Extracorporeal therapies in non-renal disease: treatment of sepsis and the peak concentration hypothesis. Blood Purif. 2004;22(1):164-74.
3. Di Carlo JV, Alexander SR. Hemofiltration for cytokine-driven illnesses: the mediator delivery hypothesis. Int J Artif Organs .2005;28:777-86.
4. Cole L, Bellomo R, Journois D, et al. High-volume haemofiltration in human septic shock. Intensive Care Med. 2001;27(6):978-86.
5. Honore PM, Jamez J, Wauthier M, et al. Prospective evaluation of short-term, high-volume isovolemic hemofiltration on the hemodynamic course and outcome in patients with intractable circulatory failure resulting from septic shock. Crit Care Med. 2000;28(11):3581-7.
6. Ratanarat R, Brendolan A, Piccinni P, et al. Pulse high-volume haemofiltration for treatment of severe sepsis: effects on hemodynamics and survival. Crit Care. 2005;9(4):R294-302.
7. Joannes-Boyau O, Rapaport S, Bazin R, et al. Impact of high volume hemofiltration on hemodynamic disturbance and outcome during septic shock. ASAIO J. 2004;50(1):102-9.
8. Oudemans-van Straaten HM, Bosman RJ, van der Spoel JI, et al. Outcome of critically ill patients treated with intermittent high-volume haemofiltration: a prospective cohort analysis. Intensive Care Med. 1999;25(8):814-21.
9. Laurent I, Adrie C, Vinsonneau C, et al. High-volume hemofiltration after out-of-hospital cardiac arrest: a randomized study. J Am Coll Cardiol. 2005; 2;46(3):432-7.

10. Joannes-Boyau O, Honoré PM, Perez P, et al. High-volume versus standard-volume haemofiltration forseptic shock patients with acute kidney injury (IVOIRE study): a multicenter randomized controlled trial. Intensive Care Med. 2013;39(9):1535-46.
11. Laleman W, Wilmer A, Evenepoel P, et al. Effect of the molecular adsorbent recirculating system and Prometheus devices on systemic haemodynamics and vasoactive agents in patients with acute-on-chronic alcoholic liver failure. Crit Care. 2006;10(4):R108.
12. Vincent JL, Laterre PF, Cohen J, et al. A pilot-controlled study of a polymyxin B-immobilized hemoperfusion cartridge in patients with severe sepsis secondary to intra-abdominal infection. Shock. 2005;23(5):400-5.
13. Cruz DN, Antonelli M, Fumagalli R, et al. Early use of polymyxin B hemoperfusion in abdominal septic shock: the EUPHAS randomized controlled trial. JAMA 2009;301(23):2445-52.
14. Payen DM, Guilhot J, Launey Y, et al. ABDOMIX Group. Early use of polymyxin B hemoperfusion in patients with septic shock due to peritonitis: a multicenter randomized control trial. Intensive Care Med. 2015;41(6):975-84.
15. Iwagami M, Yasunaga H, Doi K, et al. Postoperative polymyxin B hemoperfusion and mortality in patients with abdominal septic shock: a propensity-matched analysis. Crit Care Med. 2014;42(5):1187-93.
16. Iwagami M, Yasunaga H, Noiri E, et al. Potential survival benefit of polymyxin b hemoperfusion in septic shock patients on continuous renal replacement therapy: A Propensity-Matched Analysis. Blood Purif. 2016;42(1):9-17.
17. Fujii T, Ganeko R, Kataoka Y, et al. Polymyxin B-immobilized hemoperfusion and mortality in critically ill adult patients with sepsis/septic shock: a systematic review with meta-analysis and trial sequential analysis. Intensive Care Med. 2018;44(2):167-78.
18. Srisawat N, Tungsanga S, Lumlertgul N, et al. The effect of polymyxin hemoperfusion on modulation of human leukocyte antigen DR in severe sepsis patients. Crit Care. 2018;22:279.
19. Klein DJ, Foster D, Schorr CA, et al. The EUPHRATES trial (Evaluating the Use of Polymyxin B Hemoperfusion in a Randomized controlled trial of Adults Treated for Endotoxemia and Septic shock): Study protocol for a randomized controlled trial. Trials. 2014;15:218.

Index

Page numbers followed by *b* refer to box, *f* refer to figure, *fc* refer to flowchart, and *t* refer to table

A

Abdomen
    computed tomography 152
        angiography of 153
    plain X-ray of 152
    ultrasound 267
Ablett classification 246*t*
Abrus precatorius 224
Accidental falls 57
Acephate 191
Acetaminophen 130, 132, 220, 259
    suspension 140
    toxicity 206
Acetate 181
Acetazolamide 180, 181
Acetic acid 167
Acetylcholine 192
Acetylcholinesterase 192, 195*f*, 196*f*
    anionic site of 196*f*
    inhibitor 190, 209
Acetylcysteine 206
Acetylsalicylic acid 258
Acid 207
    base
        abnormalities 83
        imbalances 260
    endogenous 181
    exogenous 181
    fast bacillus 279, 282
Acidosis 178, 273
Aconitum napellus 219
Acquired immunodeficiency syndrome 281
Activated clotting time 342
Activated partial thromboplastin time 341
Acute Renal Failure Trial Network Study 352
Acute respiratory syndrome, severe 240
Adenosine
    deaminase 267
    triphosphate 295
Adequate oxygen delivery 298
Adrenaline 97, 280
Adult respiratory failure, severe 337
Aedes aegypti mosquito 125, 256
Aeromonas hydrophilia 173
Age-adjusted oxygenation index score 340
Agglutination test, microscopic 253
Agitation 51, 192, 215
    moderate-to-severe 209
Air oxygen blender and heated humidifier 328*f*
Airway 168, 194
    disruption 109
    driving pressure 311
    hydration 325
    management 169
    obstruction 108, 327
    pressure 314, 341
Akinetic hypertonic syndrome 220
Albumin 181
    dialysis, single-pass 135
Alcohol 157, 207
    abuse, chronic 30
    dehydrogenase 206
    misuse 55
    use, hazardous 286
Alkaline phosphatase 267
Alkalosis, contraction 321
Alpha-2 adrenergic agonists 248
Alpha-methyldopa 213
Aluminum hydroxide gel 140
Alveolar
    function 109
    gas equation 296
    pressure 298
Amanita phalloides 130
    poisoning 134
Amantadine hydrochloride 226
American College of Cardiology Guidelines 9
American Heart Association 9, 86
American Thoracic Society 29
Amikacin 279
Amino acids 23
Aminoglycosides 43, 46, 253
Aminophylline 97
Aminotransferases 131
Amiodarone 86, 87
Amodiaquine 273
Amoxicillin 253, 279, 289
Amphetamines 211
Amplification refractory mutation system 279
Amrinone 213
Analgesia 320
    patient-controlled 51
Anaphylaxis 185
    encompass, treatment of 219
Anemia 83, 274
    severe malarial 273
Aneroid sphygmomanometers 3
Aneurysms 7
Angel's trumpet 223
Angioedema 185
Angiography, intravenous contrast for 152
Angiotensin converting enzyme inhibitors 12
Anion gap 180*f*
    acidosis
        normal 180, 181
        raised 180, 181*t*
    method 179
Anopheline mosquito 271
Antiarrhythmic agents 86
Antibiotic 45*f*, 97, 215, 248, 253, 273
    allergy 44
    broad-spectrum 268
    prophylaxis 45
    protocol 170
    therapy 290
        duration of 289*t*
    treatment 253, 287
    use of 160
Antibodies, pathogenic 125
Anticholinergic 96
    antidote 210
    syndrome 209
    toxicity, diagnosis of 208
    toxidrome 208, 208*f*
Anticoagulation 11, 104, 154, 341
    strategy 88
Anticonvulsant 273
Antidepressants, tricyclic 206-208
Antiepileptic 247
    agents 247
Antihistamines 187, 208
Antimalarial treatment 273
Antimicrobial therapy, delayed 30
Antimigraine agents 215
Antineuronal nuclear antibody-1 127
Antiplatelet
    agents 10
    drugs 212
Antipsychotics 208
Antipyretics 273
Antiretroviral therapy 281
Antisnake venom 201
    administration 202
    scarcity of 199
Antithrombotic therapy 92
Antituberculosis
    drug 276, 277, 279
    treatment 276, 281
Antiviral
    agents, classes of 235
    prophylaxis 236
    resistance 236
Anxiety 192
Aortic dissection 112
    acute 19
    unrepaired 341
Aortic injury 109, 112, 112*b*, 114
    diagnosis of 112
Aortic intervention 152
Aortic knuckle, obliteration of 112
Aortic valve regurgitation, severe 341

Aortopulmonary window, loss of 112
Apixaban 14
Apnea 65
Arboviral infection 127
Arboviral viruses 125
Arrhythmia
　cardiac 72
　intractable 327
Artemether 273
Arterial applanation tonometry 4
Arterial disease, peripheral 11
Arterial infection 289
Arterial oxyhemoglobin saturation 299
Arterial pressure
　trace 7f
　mean 4, 6, 7, 7f, 362
Arteriovenous extracorporeal carbon dioxide removal 348, 349t
Artesunate 273
Arthralgia 257
Arthropod vectors 125
Ascites 281
Aspartate transaminase 157
Aspartic acid 181
Aspiration
　embolectomy 154
　pneumonia 60
　signs of 121
Aspirin 9-11, 92, 258
Asthma 12, 88, 96, 98, 211
　exacerbation 211
　prevalence of 96
Atelectasis 72, 109
Atherosclerotic disease 152
Atlanta classification 156
Atmospheric pressure 296
Atrial fibrillation 83, 84, 84f, 85, 86, 88, 89
　classification of 84, 85t
　diagnosis of 84
　etiopathology 83
　evidence 85
　impact of 84
　long-standing persistent 85
　management of 85, 89fc
　new-onset 84, 89
　permanent 85
　persistent 85
　pre-existing 84
　risk factors for 83b
Atrioventricular canal 19f
Atropa belladonna 222
Atropine 195, 208, 211
　sulfate 213, 214
　therapy 213
Australian and New Zealand Intensive Care Society 65
Autoimmune encephalitis, treatment of 128
Autonomic dysfunction 246, 247
　control of 247, 249
　manifestation of 246
Auto-positive end-expiratory pressure 325
Autumn crocus 224
Azathioprine 157
Azithromycin 43, 140

B

Baby lung 311, 312
Backflow cannula 338
Baclofen 211
　intrathecal 248

Bacteremia 28, 30, 173, 285, 289
Bacteria 23
　Gram-negative 43, 160
　Gram-positive 43, 160
　multidrug-resistant 42
Balthazar-Ranson CT scoring system 158t
Barbiturate 211
　coma 123
Barkholderia pseudomallei 285
Basic life support 216
Basilar fractures 117
Bee sting 204
　classification of manifestations of 205t
　envenomation, Mueller grading of 205t
Behavioral pain scale 48
Benzodiazepines 49, 52, 55, 194, 206, 212, 226, 247, 248
　doses of 213
　infusions of 247
Beta-adrenergic blocking agents 11
Beta-agonists 96, 97
Beta-blocker 86, 247
　withdrawal of 83
Beta-coronavirus 240
Beta-lactam 45
　antibiotics 45
Bicarbonate 179, 181
Bicuculline 211
Bifidobacteria 141
Bile acid 140
　absorption 138
Biliary sludge 157
Black widow spider envenomation 219
Blackwater fever 274
Bleeding 26
　gastrointestinal 265
　intracranial 218
　severe 261
　significant 273
　signs of 254
Blood
　biochemistry 211
　brain barrier 248
　flow rate 340
　gas, arterial 92, 102
　group 167
　level 208
　pressure 3, 4, 70, 185, 188, 254
　　high 3
　　intermittent noninvasive 3
　　invasive 4, 134
　　low 3, 185
　pressure measurement
　　automated 4
　　manual noninvasive 3
　　noninvasive continuous 4
　pressure monitoring
　　invasive 4, 7
　　methods of 3
　　noninvasive 3
　pump 339
　purification, principles of 359
　sugar 134
　　levels 123
　　random 167
　transfusion 260, 273
　urea nitrogen 28, 351, 353
　vessels, dilation of 186
Bloodstream 299
Blunt thoracic

　injury 108
　trauma 83
Body mass index 24, 31
Bone, long 114
Botulinum 213
Botulism 213, 214
Bowel
　hypoperfusion of 147
　ischemia 91
　sounds 146
Bradycardia 186, 192, 209, 210
Brain 209
　damage 77
　death 63-65, 70, 73, 206, 210
　　biological plausibility of 64
　　development of 69
　　donation after 69, 71
　　higher 65
　injury
　　primary 117, 121
　　secondary 118, 121, 123
　　severe 51
　parenchyma 122
　primarily affecting 252
Brainstem 246
　encephalitis 285
　ischemia 72
　reflexes 119, 210
Breast adenocarcinoma 128
Breathing 194
　coordination 60, 321
　evaluation 168
　shortness of 87
　trials, spontaneous 318, 319
Breathlessness 9
Bretylium tosylate 213
Bristol stool chart 137
British Thoracic Society 349
Bromocriptine 226
Bronchodilator therapies
　inhaled 96
　intravenous 97
Bronchopleural fistula 111
Bronchorrhea 192
Bronchoscopy 111
Bronchospasm 185, 192, 211
Bronchospastic airways disease, severe 12
B-type natriuretic peptide 103
Budd-Chiari syndrome, acute 134
Bundle branch block 84
Bungarus caeruleus 199
Burkholderia pseudomallei 285-288
Burn 23, 165, 170, 245
　chemical 167
　classification of 165
　contact 167
　depth of 166
　electrical 167
　flame 167
　friction 167
　injury 167
　management, acute 169
　pathophysiology of 165
　physical appearance of 166t
　radiation 166
　silencer 167
　surface area, assessment of 168
　type, assessment of 166t
　wound assessment 166
Butyrylcholinesterase 192, 193

C

Cabin pressure 296
Cadaveric organ donation 70
Calcium 182
    channel blockers 14, 86
Cancer 28
    critical stages of 332
Candida albicans 140, 160
Capreomycin 279
Carbamate 196, 197, 207
    poisoning 196
Carbamazepine 207
Carbapenems 253
Carbohydrate 219
    malabsorption 138
Carbon dioxide 305, 346
    removal 337
    retention 340
    transport physiology of 346
Carbon monoxide 216
Carboxyhemoglobin concentrations 216
Cardiac arrest 75, 216, 247, 340, 341
    high risk of 76
    response 78
Cardiac disease 152
Cardiac failure 340, 341
Cardiac function
    impaired 186
    poor 72
Cardiac injury 109, 112
    direct 109
    repair of 113
Cardiac load 320
Cardiac massage, open 113
Cardiac tamponade 108, 121
    relief of 113
Cardiac tissue 87
Cardiac troponin 92
Cardiogenic shock 21, 91, 94
    diagnosis 91
    etiology 91
    management 92
    pathophysiology 92
Cardiopulmonary resuscitation 75-77
    therapy 75
Cardiorespiratory support, withdrawal of 70
Cardiovascular
    accident 320
    disease 235
    management 133
    system 72, 135, 225
Cascabela thevetia 220
Cascade hemofiltration 359
Castor bean 224
Catabolic state, chronic 99
Catecholamine 97, 247
Catheter
    embolectomy 105
    occlusion 26
Ceftazidime 288, 289
    intravenous 288
Ceftriaxone 43, 253
Cellular dysfunction 206
Cellulitis 172
Central nervous system 58, 71, 135, 192*t*, 208
    infection 58, 289
    monitoring 134
    receptor stimulation 192
    risk factors for 280
    tuberculosis 280

Cephalic tetanus 246
Cephalosporins 253
Cerebral
    blood flow 63
    contusions, focal 118
    edema 121, 133
        management of 133
    herniation, signs of 121
    malaria 274
    perfusion pressure 7, 117
    vasospasm 118
Cerebrospinal fluid 117, 125, 127, 178, 267, 278
    drainage 122
Charcoal aspiration 207
Cherry red skin 216
Chest
    computed tomography 31
    decompression, manual 99
    infections 276
    injury 114
        mechanisms and 110*fc*
    pain 87
        sympathomimetic-induced 212
    skiagram 267
    trauma 108
        managing 109
        penetrating 114
        severe 109
    wall 109
        impedance 87
        injury 109
        trauma 112
    X-ray 112*b*, 127, 254, 288*f*
Chlamydia pneumoniae 29
Chloramphenicol 247, 253, 267
Chloride 181
    channel disturbances 181
    effect 181
    ion 183
Chlormephos 191
Chlorpheniramine 202
Chlorpyrifos 190, 191
    methyl 191
Cholangitis 159
Cholecystitis 159
Cholecystokinin 145
Cholinergic crisis 210
Cholinergic system 209
Cholinergic toxidrome 192, 209
Chondroitin sulfate A 272
Chronic obstructive pulmonary
    disease 25, 31, 32, 96, 276, 325, 347
        exacerbation 28
    disorder 331
Circulatory death, donation after 69, 71
Circulatory failure 340
Citrus 225
Claustrophobia 327
Clavulanate 279, 289
Clindamycin 247
Clinical leptospirosis guidelines 253*b*
Clofazimine 279
Clonidine 195
Clopidogrel 9, 10
Clostridium botulinum 213
Clostridium difficile 42
    infection 138
Clostridium perfringens 42, 140

Clostridium tetani 245
    germinates 246
    spores 245
Coagulopathy 130, 133, 219
    disease-related 88
Cobra 199
Cocaine 130, 211
Codeine 214
Colchicum autumnale 224
Colonization 44
Coma 77, 192
    medication-induced 55
Combination therapy 86
Compartment syndrome, abdominal 158
Complete blood count 92, 167
Computed tomography 120, 267, 304
    angiography 139, 154
    contrast enhanced 159
    guided percutaneous aspiration 159
    imaging 308
    pulmonary angiogram 103, 104*f*
    scan
        abdomen 267
        chest 267
        head 267
    severity index 158*t*
Confusion 52, 192, 215
Conium maculatum 223
Consciousness
    level of 127
    long-term 57
Continuous positive airway pressure 318, 324, 331
Contusions 118
Conventional oxygen therapy 324
Cor pulmonale 313
Coronary artery
    bypass graft surgery 92
    occlusion 18*f*
Coronary syndrome
    acute 7, 9
    non-ST elevation acute 10
Coronaviruses 240
Cough 102, 252
    medicines 215
Coupled plasma filtration absorption 362, 359
Cranial nerve 66, 209
Craniectomy, decompressive 123
C-reactive protein 182
Creatine phosphokinase 211
Creatinine 167
Critical care
    pain observation tool 48
    unit 16
Critically ill score, nutrition risk in 25, 149
Crystalloids, isotonic 123
Curb-65 score 29
Cutaneous infection, localized 287
Cute malaria 274
Cyanide 206
    antidotes 216
    intoxication 216
    poisoning 215, 217
        diagnosis of 216
        signs of 216
        treatment of 216
    toxidrome 215
    transforming 216
Cyanophos 191
Cycloserine 273, 279
Cytochrome 278
    oxidase 216

Cytokines 234
Cytomegalovirus 127, 130

D

Dabigatran 14
Daboia russelii 199
Dantrolene 226
Dapsone 207
Darunavir 281
Datura aureua 223
Datura stramonium 208, 222
D-dimer 103, 153
De novo dementia, development of 61
Death
    camas 221
    circulatory 70
Deep venous thrombosis 101, 103
Dehydration 59
Delamanid 279
Delirium 52, 54, 55, 57*fc*, 208
    clinical features of 55*t*
    development of 52*t*
    diagnosis of 55
    duration of 56
    hallmark of 55
    management of 59
    moderate-to-severe 209
    monitoring 321
        tools 55
    postoperative 55, 56, 60
    risk factors for 55*t*
    subtypes of 54
    syndrome 50
    system interview 55
    three subtypes of 54
    tools, assessment of 56*t*
    treatment of 58
Delivery hypothesis, mediator 360
Dementia 28
    worsening of preexisting 61
Dengue 125, 252, 256, 257, 261, 265
    classification of 257*f*
    disease
        antiviral treatment for 259
        phase of 259
    illness, clinical course of 257*f*
    infection, serological markers of 259*f*
    risk of developing 256, 286
    serology 261
    severe 256, 258
    shock 258*f*
        syndrome 257*f*
    vaccine 261
        initiative 256
    virus 256
    warning signs 257
Dengvaxia 261
Deoxyribonucleic acid 45, 225
Depression, cardiac 340
Dexmedetomidine 49, 50
    role of 59
Dextrose 207
Diabetes
    insipidus 65, 72, 73
    mellitus 28, 173, 286
Diagnostic coronary angiography 9
Diaphoresis 209, 211, 215, 226
Diaphragmatic injury, plain radiography of 114*f*
Diarrhea 127, 137, 138, 142, 181, 185, 192, 210, 252
    antibiotic associated 140
    causes of 137
    classification of 137
    Clostridium difficile 44, 139
    enteral feeding associated 140
    exudative 138
    life-threatening 139
    management of 141, 142*fc*
    mechanism of 138
    non-life-threatening 138, 140
    secretary 138
Diastolic arterial pressure 4
Diazepam 211, 213, 248
Diazinon 191
Dichlofenthion 191
Dichlorvos 191
Dicrotophos 191
Digestive system, physiology of 137
Digitalis alkaloid toxicity 206
Digitalis lanata 220
Digoxin 88
    binding antibodies 206
    solution 140
Dihydroartemisinin 273
Dihydroergotamine 213
Diltiazem 86
Dimethoate 191
Dipeptidyl-peptidase-like protien-6 127
Diphenhydramine 213
Disseminated intravascular coagulation 258
Distinct toxic actions 218
Distress, gastrointestinal 210
Dizziness 192
Dobutamine 93
Docosahexaenoic acid 123
Donation, system for 73
Donor management 72
Dopamine 93
    agonist 226
    antagonists 147
    reduces 226
Doppler echocardiography 17
Doppler techniques 16, 17
Doxycycline 253, 289
    efficacy of 267
Drainage cannula 338
Dronedarone 86
Droperidol 212
Drug 140
    overdose 340
        miscellaneous 220
    reactions 44
    resistant tuberculosis, starting treatment for 277
Dry heat 167
Duke's criteria, modified 21
Dynamic response testing 5
Dysarthria 226
Dyselectrolytemia 137
Dyskinesia 226
Dysoxia 298, 299
Dyspnea 102
Dysrhythmia 209
    cardiac 219
Dysuria 287

E

Echis carinatus 199
Echocardiography 16, 21
    cardiac 16
Eclampsia 261
Eicosapentaenoic acid 123
Ejection fraction, preserved 84
Electrical cardioversion 87
Electrocardiogram 267
Electrocardiography 84*f*, 85
    criteria 84*b*
Electroencephalogram 67
Electrolyte 260
    abnormalities 83
    correction of 85
Elevated end-expiratory volume 305
Embolectomy, surgical 105, 106
Embolic stroke, risk of 88
Emerging therapies 134
Emesis 192, 207, 210
Emphysema, presence of 31
Encephalitis 58, 125, 126
    autoimmune 125-128
    clinical definition of 126
    evidence 126
    infectious 125
    mortality of 126
    pathophysiology 125
    prevalence of 126
Encephalopathy 130, 210
    hepatic 135
    hypertensive 58
End-diastolic pressure 91
End-expiratory lung volume 303
Endocarditis, management of 20
Endocrine disorders 58
Endogenous rhodanese 217
Endoscopic repair techniques 114
Endoscopic retrograde cholangiopancreatography 162
Endothelium 272
Endotracheal tubes 58
Endovascular thrombolysis 153, 154
Enoxaparin 13
Enteral nutrition 144, 148, 148*fc*, 161
    early 123
    timing of 161
Enterobacteriaceae 160
Enterovirus infection 127
Enzyme-linked immunosorbent assay 241, 253, 259, 265
Ephedra alkaloids 211
Ephedrine 211
Epicardial artery, major 18
Epilepsy, post-traumatic 123
Epinephrine 187, 215
    administration 186*b*
    bolus intravenous administration of 187
    topical application of 280
Epithelial cells 233
Epstein-Barr virus 127, 130
Erythema 185
Erythromycin 140, 147, 149, 247
Escharotomy 169
Escherichia coli 29, 138, 160
Esophageal manometry 307
Esophagus 146
    deviation of 112
Estrogen 157
Ethambutol 278, 279
Ethionamide 279
Ethylene glycol 181
    toxicity 206
Etravirine 281

Euphorbia 225
European Society of Intensive Care Medicine 137
Exacerbations, acute 31
Excite peripheral neuromuscular junctions 218
Expiratory positive airway pressure 332
Expiratory volume curves 306f
Extended spectrum beta-lactamase 43
External ventricular drain 122
Extracorporeal blood purification 359, 360f
    technique 360
    therapy 359
Extracorporeal carbon dioxide removal 345, 348t
    circuit 345f
    devices 345, 346t
    facilitates 349
    potential of 345
    principles of 345
Extracorporeal life support
    organization 340
    system 94
Extracorporeal membrane oxygenation 25, 31, 299, 314, 337, 338, 346
    circuit 339f, 340
    modes of 338
Extravascular lung water index 30
Eye response 119
Eyelids
    closed 119
    open 119

F
Face mask 296
Facial burn 166
Falciparum malaria, severe 272, 274
False acacia 224
False hellebore 221
Fasciitis 172
Fasciotomy 169
Fast flush test 5, 5f, 6f
Fatigue 192
Fatty acids, short-chain 141
Fatty diarrhea 141
Febrile 158
    acute respiratory illness 241
    illness 263, 265
Fecal oral viral transmission 130
Fentanyl 49
Fenthion 191
Fever 287
    hemorrhagic 252
    treatment of 274
Firecracker burn 167
Flaccid paralysis 287
Flail chest 108
Flavivirus 125, 256
Flecainide 87
Fluconazole suspension 140
Fluid
    and electrolyte abnormalities 60
    collections 158
    effect of 182
    extravasation of 185, 186
    intravenous 187, 273
    overload 26, 83
    replacement 259
    resuscitation 104, 169
    therapy 159, 187, 259
Flu-like illnesses, moderate 238
Flumazenil 211
Fluoroquinolones 45, 279
Fomepizole 206
Fondaparinux 13
Food allergy and anaphylaxis network consensus clinical definition of anaphylaxis 185b
Formaldehyde 181
Fosamine 191
Fournier's gangrene 172
Foxgloves 219, 220
Fractures 77
    first rib 112
    ribs 114
    second rib 112
Fresh frozen plasma 194, 201, 260
Full blood count 176
Fungal
    infection 26
    organism 160
Furosemide stress test 354

G
Gamblegram 178, 179f
Gamma-aminobutyric acid 49, 127
Gamma-glutamyl transferase 252
Gangrene 172, 245
    peripheral 265
Gas
    embolism 9
    exchange 30, 304, 305
        device 340
Gastric
    antrum 146f
        ultrasonography of 146
    aspiration, intermittent 145
    decompression 139
    dysmotility 147
    emptying 207
        delayed 144
        physiology of 144
    feeding 161
    lavage 194, 207, 213
    motility
        assessment of 145
        disorder 144
    reservoir function 144
    residual volume 144, 145, 148
    scintigraphy 145
    stasis 144
        pathophysiology of 145
Gastrinoma 138
Gastroenteritis 219
Gastrointestinal
    complication 275
    decontamination 207
    motility 144
        disturbances 144
    perforation 159
    systems 185
Gastroparesis 144
Gatifloxacin 279
Gelatin 181
General supportive therapy 194
Genetic mutations 138
Giant hogweed 225
Glasgow coma scale 70, 119t, 120
Glucagon like peptide-1 145
Glucose
    control 260
    intravenous 273
Glufosinate 190
Glutamate dehydrogenase 140
Glutamic acid decarboxylase 127
Glutamine supplementation, use of 162
Glycemic control 93
Glycolate 181
Glycopeptide 43, 46
Glycoprotein antigens hemagglutinin 233
Glycopyrrolate 208, 210
Glycopyrronium bromide 214
Glycosides 87
Glyphosate 190
Granulocyte-colony stimulating factor 290
Griffith's point 151
Ground-glass opacities 268f
Guanethidine 213
Guillain-Barre syndrome 209, 252, 265, 274
Gunshot wounds 108
Gut hormones 140

H
H1N1 influenza A
    complications of 235
    virus 234, 235
H5N1 avian influenza 236
Haemophilus influenzae 41, 234, 240
Hallucinogenic plants 219
Haloperidol 59, 60, 213
Hampton's hump 102f
Harris-Benedict and Ireton-Jones equations 24
Head injuries 113, 114
Headache 192, 252
Health care 240
    cost 57, 61
    facilities 233
    systems 116
    workers 233, 282
Heart
    block 86
    disease
        coronary 32
        ischemic 83
        structural 87
    failure 17, 83, 84, 86, 87
        absence of 206
        acute decompensated 91
        congestive 12, 360f
        severe 86
    primarily affecting 252
    rate 6, 7, 157
        reduce 86
    sound, fourth 102
    subcostal of 18f
Heat stroke 130
HELLP syndrome 134, 261
Hematocrit, onterpretation of 260b
Hematoma
    epidural 117, 117f, 119
    expansion 123
Hemoadsorption 359, 362
Hemoconcentration 153
Hemodialysis 354
Hemodynamic
    instability, severe 103fc
    management 93, 123
    monitoring system 4
    support 104, 202
Hemofiltration 195
    high volume 359-361, 361t
Hemoglobin
    C 272

concentration 340
  E 272
  transformation of 217
Hemoglobinuria 274
Hemogram 267
Hemolysis 134
  elevated liver enzymes 261
Hemoperfusion 195, 359
Hemoperitoneum 121
Hemoptysis 102
Hemorrhage 91, 109, 252
  abdominal 113
  adrenal 277
  catastrophic 109
  control of 113
  internal 77
  intracerebral 117, 119
  intraventricular 118, 120
  severe 258
  subarachnoid 117, 118f, 119
Hemorrhoids 200
Hemothorax 112, 121
Hemotoxic syndrome 200
Heparin 9, 12, 92
  low-dose 226
  unfractionated 104
Hepatic encephalopathy, grading of 131b
Hepatic failure 153
  fulminant 71, 130
  ischemic 132
Hepatic injury
  recognition of 132
  severe 130
Hepatitis
  A 130
  autoimmune 131, 134
  B 130, 134
  C 71
  D 130
  E 130
  ischemic 130
  malarial 275
Hepatocyte transplantation 134
Hepatosteatosis 26
Heracleum mantegazzianum 225
Hernia
  external 152
  internal 152
Heroin 214
Herpes simplex 132, 134
  virus 126, 127, 130
High flow nasal
  cannula
    oxygen therapy 98
    respiratory support 324
  therapy, delivery of 328f
High illness severity score 31
Homovanillic acid 181
Horse flies 186
Hospital elder life program 60
Host cell necrosis 233
Human
  coronaviruses 238
  disease 233
  hepatocytes 135
  immunodeficiency virus 70, 71, 157, 276, 281, 287
    infection 71
  tetanus immunoglobulin 248
  to-human transmission 238
  vaccine development 242

Humidification 298
Hybrid sphygmomanometers 4
Hydrocarbons 207
Hydrocodone 214
Hydrofluoric acid 167
Hydrogen ion 179
  concentration 183, 183t
Hydroxocobalamin 206, 216, 217
Hydroxyphenyllactic acid 181
Hymenoptera stings 186
Hyperbaric oxygen 176, 299
Hypercalcemia 157
Hypercapnia 31
  chronic 31
  prevention of 109
  respiratory failure 98, 332
Hypercarbia, severe 30
Hyperemia 133
  zone of 165
Hyperglycemia 26, 28, 118
  causes of 260
  control 260
Hyperkalemia 201, 260
Hypernatremia 72
  development of 73
Hyperosmolar agents 140
Hyperparasitemia 273
Hyperreflexia 215
Hypertension 32, 192, 211, 212
  intracranial 122
Hyperthermia 211, 212, 215, 226
  sympathomimetic-induced 211
Hyperthyroidism 91
Hypertriglyceridemia 157
Hyperventilation, short-term 133
Hypoadrenalism 321
Hypoalbuminemia 141
Hypocortisolisms 277
Hypoglycemia 58, 273, 274
Hypokalemia 260
Hypomania 215
Hyponatremia 118, 260
Hypotension 12, 55, 72, 83, 120, 121, 158, 185, 192, 210
  after snakebite 219
  persistent 91
  profound 213
  severe 213
Hypothermia 72
Hypothesis, cytokinetic 360
Hypothyroidism 91, 321
Hypovolemia 73, 122, 152
Hypoxemia 9, 83, 102, 111
Hypoxemic respiratory failure 332
Hypoxia 55, 85, 120, 121
Hypoxic respiratory failure 340t
  management of 98
Hysteresis, point of maximum 307, 307f

I

Ibuprofen 140, 258
Ibutilide 87
Ileostomy, high output 181
Illegal street drugs 211
Immune reconstitution inflammatory syndrome 281
Immunization 247, 261
Immunoglobulin 127
  intravenous 127, 128, 176
  M 267

Immunoperoxidase assay, indirect 265, 266
Immunosuppression 277
Immunotherapy 128fc
Inadequate antidiuretic hormone secretion, syndrome of 281
Indian cobra 199
Indian krait 199
Indirect fluorescent antibody 267
Indwelling catheters 55
  inadvertent removal of 60
Infarcts 121
Infection 71, 91
  bacterial 157, 275
  control measures 282
  granulomatous 280
  hospital-acquired 61
  lower risk of 122
  multidrug-resistant 30
  mumps 157
  prevention of 242
  primary 264
  removal of source of 246
  risk factors for 251
  site of 289
  treatment of 242
  viruses 157
Infectious disease 45, 128, 277
Infectious Disease Society of America 29
Inferior vena cava 20, 339
Inflection point, lower 303, 306
Influenza 233
  A 233
    H7N9 234
    viruses 233, 235
  B 233
  D 233
  mild cases of 234
  viral infections 233, 234
  virus 233, 235, 236
Injury
  craniofacial 327
  diaphragmatic 114
  diffuse axonal 117, 118, 118f
  gastrointestinal 137
  hepatocellular 26
  inhalation 169
  intra-abdominal 114
  ischemic 151
Inotropic therapy 260
Inspiratory positive airway pressure 331
Inspiratory volume curves 306f
Inspired oxygen, fraction of 25, 157
Intensive care 128
  delirium screening checklist 52, 55, 56
  intervention 83
  unit 3, 23, 28, 42, 44, 48, 50t, 52, 54-56, 58, 69, 83, 88, 89, 137, 144, 156, 233, 254, 282, 299, 311, 317, 319, 352-354
  management 122, 123, 133
  polyneuromyopathy 99
  populations 83
  risk of 97
Intercellular adhesion molecule 272
Interferon 234
  gamma release assays 279
International normalized ratio 131, 135
Intestinal
  ischemia, pathophysiology of 151
  obstruction 159

Intestine
    infection of 152
    inflammation of 152
Intra-aortic balloon
    counter 93
    pump 91-93, 188
Intracellular pathogens 42
Intracranial pressure 7, 64, 274
    management 122
    monitoring 122, 134
    raised 118
Intrathoracic pressures, elevated 98
Intravenous therapies, doses of 97t
Intubation, complications of 31
Iron 207
Ischemia 118, 151
    acute mesenteric 154
    coronary 212
    end-organ 72
    intestinal 151
    starts, warm 70
    treatment of 85
Ischemic syndromes, acute 13
Isolation 55
Isoniazid 130, 278, 279
    high dose 279
    solution 140

J

Japanese encephalitis 125
Jaundice 252, 254, 265, 273
Jejunal feeding 161
Jellyfish stings 186
Jimson weed 222

K

Kanamycin 279
Ketamine 49, 97
Ketoacidosis 181
    diabetic 153
Kidney
    disease 354
        chronic 354
        end-stage 353
    injury
        acute 7, 133, 200, 211, 265, 351, 354, 357, 357fc
        network, acute 353
        treatment of acute 360
        primarily affecting 252
        recipients 69
King cobra 218
Klebsiella pneumonia 160
Klebsiella sepsis 253
Knockdown toxidrome 214
Knowlesi malaria, severe 272
Korotkoff technique 3
Krait 199
    bite 199, 205
Krebs cycle intermediates 181
Kussmaul's breathing 258

L

Labetalol overdose 213
Lachmann's open lung approach 303
Lacrimation 210
Lactate 181, 183
    dehydrogenase 157
Lactic acidosis 181, 216, 274

Lactobacilli 141
Lactulose solution 140
Laparotomy 154
Larval mites 263
Laryngeal spasm 213
Latex agglutination 265
Left main stem bronchus, depression of 112
Left ventricular
    assist devices 94
    diastolic dysfunction, abnormal 19
    ejection fraction 18
    end diastolic pressure 20
    hypertrophy 84
    outflow tract 18f
Legionella 42
Leptospirosis 251, 252, 253, 253b, 255, 265
    epidemiology 251
    infection 251
    intensive care management of 251
    risk factors 251
    treatment for 252
Leptotrombidium deliense 263
Lethal cardiac complications 211
Lethal multisystem disease 251
Leucine-rich glioma inactivated-1 127
Leukocyte count 131
Leukocytosis 152
Leukopenia 261
Levofloxacin 279
Levosimendan 93
Life-threatening multisystem disease, severe 252
Light sedation 51
Limbic encephalitis 127
Line sepsis 26
Linezolid 279
Lipid emulsions 194
Lipopolysaccharide 362
Listeria 125
Lithium 182, 207
Liver 130, 209
    abscess, large 288f
    disease
        chronic 131, 286
        pre-existing 130
    enzymes, elevated 132, 134
    failure 134
        acute 130, 130b, 132, 132t, 133t, 134t, 135, 135t
        management of acute 132
    function 131, 240
        tests 92, 267
    graft function 73
    injury 132
        acute 132
        drug induced 277, 278
        primarily affecting 252
    transplantation 135
        emergency 135b
        surgery 135
        team 71
        timing of 134
Local tissue necrosis 219
Lomotil 209
Lorazepam 49, 60, 213, 248
Low tidal volume, assessment of 305
Low-molecular-weight heparin 13
LRINEC score 175t
Lumefantrine 273
Lund and Browder chart 168f

Lung 186
    alveoli stimulate, viral particles in 240
    and liver transplantation 71
    biopsy 30
    cancer, small cell 128
    function 30
    infection 206
    inflation 312f
    injury 211, 305
        hypoxic 240
        ventilator-induced 311
    primarily affecting 252
    recruitment maneuver 306
    volume 307, 324
Lymphoma 128

M

Macrolides 253
Magnesium 97, 138, 140, 182
    sulfate 247, 248
Magnetic resonance
    angiography 152
    cholangiopancreatography 159
    imaging 159, 176, 267
        brain 267
Malaria 252, 265, 271
    in intensive care unit 271
    severe 272, 273t, 275
Malathion 191
Malnutrition 60, 137
Massive hemothorax 108
Massive pulmonary embolism 340
McConnell's signs 102
Mechanical respiratory failure 109
Mechanical ventilation 55, 98, 121, 317
    duration of 56
Mediastinal infections 288
Mediastinum, widened 112
Medical oxygen 296
Mefloquine 208, 273
Melioidosis 285, 287, 288f
    epidemiology 285
    geographical distribution 285
    global geographical distribution of 286f
    risk factors for development of 286t
    suspected 290
    therapy for 289t
    treatment of 288
Membrane lung 345
    gas flow 340
Meningitis 280
Meningococcal infection 265
Meningoencephalitis 125, 265
Mephedrone 211
Meropenem 288, 289
Mesenteric arterial
    embolism 152
    thrombosis 152
Mesenteric artery
    inferior 151
    superior 151
Mesenteric ischemia 44, 139, 151, 152, 159
    etiology of 152
Mesenteric venous thrombosis 152
Metabolic
    acidemia 178
    acidosis 72, 178, 179, 182, 247
        management of 182
        presence of 152

alkalosis 321
bone disease 26
complications 274
disorders 58
Metaraminol 188
Metastatic cancer 70
Methamphetamine 211
Methanol 181
Methemoglobin 217
Methicillin-resistant *Staphylococcus aureus* 43, 176
Methyldopa, severe 213
Methylxanthines 97
Metoclopramide 147, 149
Microlithiasis 157
Microprocessor 4, 6
Midazolam 49, 213, 248
Middle east respiratory syndrome 240, 241
coronavirus 239, 239*f*
Migrating motor complex 144
Miliary 281
Mimic multiorgan failure 206
Minoxidil causes 213
Minute ventilation 324
Miosed pupils, small 210
Miosis 192, 210
Mitochondria 23
Mitral regurgitation 20*f*
Mitral valve 20*f*
Molecular adsorbent recirculating system 135
Molecular weight heparin, low 104
Monkey malaria 271
Monocrotophos 191
Mononucleosis, infectious 265
Monro-Kellie doctrine 118, 119*f*
Morbid obesity 235
Morphine 9, 48, 49
Morris's study 347
Mosquito-borne viral disease 256
Motilin agonists 147
Motor diarrhea 138
Motor dysfunction, primary 145
Motor limb weakness, upper 287
Motor vehicle accidents 108
Movement disorder 127
Moxifloxacin 279
Mucosal inflammation 219
Multiorgan dysfunction 276
syndrome 265
Multiorgan failure 31, 130, 206, 218, 219, 259, 276
Multisystem injury, severe 113
Murray score 340
Muscarinic
receptor stimulation 192
symptoms, list of 192*t*
Muscle
atrophy 321
cramps 192
relaxants 247
rigidity consists 226
weakness, nicotinic effects of 210
Mushroom poisoning 130
Myalgia 257
Myasthenia gravis 214
Mycobacteria 276
Mycobacterium tuberculosis 276, 279
Mycoplasma 42
pneumoniae 29, 157
Mycotic aneurysm 288, 289
Mydriasis 192, 215

Myelin oligodentrocyte glycoprotein 127
Myocardial contractility 93
Myocardial infarction 10, 44, 83, 212
acute 9, 10, 14, 91, 340
long-term evaluation, survival of 12
non-ST segment elevation 10
ST-segment elevation 9
Myocardial ischemia 84, 212
Myocarditis 265, 340
Myoclonus 215
Myositis 172
Myotonia 127

N

N-acetylcysteine, role of 134
Naja naja 199
Naloxone 207, 214
Narcolepsy medications 211
Narcotics 55
Nasal cannulae 296
Nasal high-flow
delivery 327
mechanisms of action 324
strategies 327
therapy 324
National Institute for Health and Care Excellence 349
National Institute of Allergy and Infectious diseases 185*b*
Natriuretic peptides 92, 219
Neck 264*f*
trauma 207
Necrotic collection, acute 156, 158
Necrotizing fasciitis 172, 175
risk indicator for 175
Neostigmine 214
Neuroendocrine stress response 260
Neurofilament light polypeptide 123
Neuroleptic malignant syndrome 220, 226
Neuromuscular blocking
agent 122, 320
drugs 214
Neuromuscular junction 192
Neuronal apoptosis 118
Neurons, autonomic 245
Neuroparalytic syndrome 199
Neuropsychiatric disorders 209
Neurotoxicity 219
Neurotransmitter acetylcholine 208
Neurovascular tissues 117
Neutropenia 139
Neutropenic enterocolitis 139
Neutrophil
function 286
gelatinase-associated lipocalcin 355, 357
Nicotinic receptor stimulation 192, 209
Nitazoxanide 236
Nitrates 10
Nitric oxide, inhaled 299
Nitrofurantoin 130
N-methyl-D-aspartate 49
receptor 126, 127
Nonacetaminophen 130
Nondepolarizing neuromuscular blocking drugs 214
Nondihydropyridine calcium-channel antagonists 86
Noninvasive ventilation
evidence-based review of 331

scientific rationale of 331
support of 332
Nonocclusive mesenteric ischemia 152
Nonpharmacological therapy 58
Nonprotein toxins 219
Nonrespiratory disease 30
Nonthermal burn 166, 167
Nontoxic stable derivatives 216
Nonvalvular atrial fibrillation 85
Noradrenaline 72
Norepinephrine 93, 215
Normocapnia 122
Nosocomial pneumonia 60, 276
Novel avian influenza A H7N9 234
Noxious newts 218
Nucleic acid amplification techniques 277
NUTRIC score 25*t*
Nutrients, types of 162
Nutrition 123, 170

O

Obesity 30, 83
hypoventilation syndrome 332
Obidoxime 196
Occlusive mesenteric ischemia 139
Ofloxacin 279
Ohm's law 6
Olanzapine 59, 60, 212
Omethoate 191
Opioid 48, 49, 49*t*, 207
analgesics 214
antagonist 214
toxidrome 214
Opportunistic organisms 242
Oral amoxicillin-clavulanate 289
Oral anticoagulants 13
Oral chloramphenicol 269
Oral doxycycline 289
Oral eradication therapy 289
Oral nutrition, timing of 161
Oral thrombin inhibitor 14
Organ donation 69 70, 70*f*, 71, 71*t*
and community 73
conversations 71
Organ donors 69
Organ dysfunction 58, 81, 157*t*, 235, 267
syndrome, multiple 359, 360*f*
Organ failure 77
assessment, sequential 25, 354
end-stage 69
single 206
Organ function, failed 206
Organ hypoperfusion 73
Organ transplantation 69
Organ warm ischemia 69
Organophosphate 207, 211
encephalopathy, delayed 193
poisoning 190
Organophosphorus compounds 191
basic chemical structure of 191*f*
binding of 195*f*
classification of 191*t*
Organophosphorus
hydrolases 195
induced delayed polyneuropathy 193
pesticides, classification of 191*t*
poisoning 192, 192*t*
Orientia tsutsugamushi 263, 264, 266, 269
Osmotic diarrhea 138

Osmotic therapy 122
Osteomyelitis 287, 289
Otorrhea 117
Ovarian teratoma 128
Oxalate 181
    plants 225
Oxalic acid 181
Oxime 195
    phosphate compound 196
Oxycodone 214
Oxygen 9, 216, 295, 300
    arterial partial pressure of 340
    carrying capacity of blood 340
    cascade 296
    concentrations, inspired 299
    fraction, inspiratory 295
    inspiratory fraction of 327
    partial pressure of 157, 295, 297t, 299
    positive end-expiratory pressure tables 304
    role of 295
    supplementation 121
    therapy 9, 98
Oxygenation 337
    failure of 30
Oxyhemoglobin dissociation curve 296f

P

Pain 48, 50, 50t, 55
    abdominal 152, 185, 252, 281
    management 59, 170
    severe 77
P-aminosalicylate sodium 279
P-aminosalicylic acid 279
Pancreas 209
    pseudocysts of 156
Pancreatic
    divisum 157
    fistula 181
    necrosis 158
    polypeptide 145
    pseudocyst 158
Pancreatitis
    acute 156, 157, 160, 160t
    chronic 157
    complications of 158, 158t
    interstitial edematous 158
    management of 159
    necrotizing 156, 158
    types of 158
Paracetamol 130, 259
    overdose 130
    poisoning 135
Paradoxical septal motion 17f
Paraldehyde 181
Paralysis 51, 192
    types of 209
Paraneoplastic disorders 128
Paraoxonase 191
Parasites 272
    life cycle of 271
Parasympathetic nervous system 208
Parathion 191
Paratracheal stripe, widened 112
Parenchymal necrosis 158
Parenteral nutrition 149, 161
    total 26, 139, 148, 161
Parkland formula 169
    modified 169
Parotitis, acute suppurative 287

Paroxysmal atrial fibrillation 85
Parvovirus 130
Pasteur's point 295
Patient-ventilator
    asynchrony 51
    dyssynchrony 122
Peak concentration hypothesis 360
Peak expiratory function 185
Pediatric diseases 212
Pelvis 114
Penetrating injuries 117
Penicillin 246, 253
    allergy 44
    intravenous 253
Pentoxifylline 273
Percutaneous coronary intervention 9, 92
Pericardial effusion 20
Perimesencephalic cisterns 120
Peripancreatic fluid collection, acute 156, 158
Pesticidal plants 217
Petroleum products 207
Pharmacological cardioversion 87
Phenobarbital 207
Phentolamine 213
Phenylephrine 215
Phenytoin 130
Pheochromocytoma 138
Phorate 191
Phosphate 138, 181
Phosphodiesterase inhibitors 213
Phosphorothioate 191
PICCO monitor 6f
Piloerection 211
Piperaquine 273
Plant
    poisoning victims 219
    toxidromes 219, 220t
Plasma 178
    exchange 128
    lactate concentration 216
    leak, severe 258
Plasmapheresis 359
    high volume 135
Plasmodium 271-273, 275
    falciparum
        asexual parasitemia 272
        erythrocyte membrane protein 272
        infected 272
    knowlesi 271, 272
    life cycle of 271f
    malariae 271
    ovale 271
    vivax 271, 275
Platelet
    count syndrome, low 132, 134
    transfusion of 260
Pleocytosis 125
Pleural injury 109
Pleuritic chest pain 102
Pneumomediastinum 111
Pneumonia 28, 109, 146, 241, 285, 287, 289
    community-acquired 28, 42
    hospital-acquired 28, 29
    melioidosis, right upper lobe 288f
    severity index 29
    ventilator-associated 29, 44
Pneumopericardium 111
Pneumoperitoneum 111
Pneumothoraces 109, 111

Pneumothorax 26, 108, 111, 211
Poison 207
    hemlock 223
Poisonous products 217
Polyethersulfone 362
Polyethylenimine 362
Polymerase chain reaction 126, 235, 252, 253, 266, 267, 279
Polymyxin 362
    hemoperfusion 362, 364, 364t
Polyneuropathy 265
Poor perfusion, signs of 185
Porcine hepatocytes 135
Positive end-expiratory pressure 93, 98, 98f, 111, 298, 303-305, 311, 319, 320, 331
    noninvasive 331
    oxygenation 304
    titration 304
Postmalaria neurological syndrome 274
Postmonsoon spike 263
Postpyloric feeding 149
Potassium
    chloride 140
    supplements 260
Potential donor 70
    identification 69
Potential organ donor 73
Potential recipient requirements 70
Potential serotonin syndrome 215
Pralidoxime 195, 211
    binding of 196f
    structure of 195f
Prasugrel 11
Prazosin 204
Pregnancy 261
    acute fatty liver of 132, 134
    test 209
Premature neonates 71
Pressure
    intra-abdominal 157
    volume curve 306
Procoagulant enzymes 219
Prokinetic agents 140, 147, 149
Propafenone 87
Prophylactic antibiotics 45
Prophylaxis 123
Propionic acid 213
Propofol 49, 50, 249
    infusion syndrome, development of 50
Propoxyphene 214
Propylthiouracil 130
Prostacyclin 273
Prostatic abscess 289, 288f, 290
Protein 181, 123
    acute-phase 181
    intake 26
    intestinal 138
Proteus mirabilis 265
Prothionamide 279
Protozoal infection 271
Pseudomonas aeruginosa 29, 160, 166
Psychoactive drugs, use of 55
Psychological dysfunction 321
Psychosis 127
Pulmonary artery
    catheter 83, 93
    right main 104f
Pulmonary complications 133, 275
    postoperative 313

Pulmonary congestion 84
Pulmonary contusions 109, 110f
Pulmonary edema 12, 72, 247, 273
    cardiogenic 332
Pulmonary embolism 44, 92, 261
    acute 101, 103fc
    catheter directed therapy for 106
    classification of 101, 101t
    clinical features 102
    investigations 102
    low probability of 103
    signs of 102t
    symptoms of 102t
    treatment 104
Pulmonary hemorrhage 276, 280
    syndrome, severe 254
Pulmonary hilar injuries 113
Pulmonary infection, evidence of 97
Pulmonary parenchymal
    disease 241
    injury 109
Pulmonary tuberculosis 280
Pulmonary vascular
    dysfunction 30
    permeability indices 30
Pupil constriction predominate 209
Pupillary dilatation 211
Pyrazinamide 278, 279
Pyrimethamine 273
Pyroglutamic acid 181

Q

QRS complex, wide 85f
QT interval prolongation 211
Quality improvement techniques 60
Quetiapine 59, 60
Quinine 207
Quinolphos 191

R

Radical injury 118
Raltegravir trio therapy 281
Randomized controlled trial 161, 311, 321, 352,
    361, 364
Ranson signs of severity 157b
Rapid diagnostic tests 266
Rapid sequence intubation 121
Rash 252
Red blood cells 271-273
Refeeding syndrome 26
Refractory
    cardiogenic shock 340
    intracranial hypertension 123
    seizures 274
    shock state 87
    ventricular arrhythmia 340
Reintubation 60
Remifentanil 49
Renal disease 286
    end-stage 359
Renal failure 153, 181, 226, 252, 254, 255
Renal function tests 267
Renal impairment 273
Renal insufficiency 217
Renal replacement therapy 133, 351, 352f, 353f, 353t,
    354, 357, 357fc, 357t, 359
    continuous 351, 354, 359, 360, 364
    delayed initiation of 354
    early initiation of 354
    personalized 357

Renal tubular acidosis 181
Renin-angiotensin aldosterone system 93, 151
Repetitive nerve, normal 209
Reserpine 213
Respiration 119
Respiratory
    acidosis 111
    alkalosis, compensatory 217
    arrest 76
    depression 209
    distress syndrome
        acute 28, 30, 159, 234, 240, 252, 265, 267f,
            275, 276, 303, 304, 311, 318, 320, 331,
            337, 345, 348t
        clinical network, acute 304, 305
    drive 320
    embarrassment and hypoxia 109
    failure 99, 109, 192, 216, 254, 326
        acute 255, 276, 334f
        early 209
    muscles 209
    paralysis 209
    pathogen antimicrobials 73
    rate 28
    support 104, 324
    system 72, 313
    tract infections 96
Resuscitation
    cardiopulmonary 77
    hemodynamic 275
    post-cardiopulmonary 327
Resuscitative thoracotomy 113, 113b
Rhinorrhea 117
Rhodanase 217
Rhododendron 221
Rhythm-control 87
    strategy 87
Rib fracture management 109
Ribonucleic acid 233
    single-stranded 238
Richmond agitation-sedation scale 48
Ricinus communis 224
Rickettsial disease 266, 266t, 267
Rickettsial infection 252, 265
Rifampicin 277-279
Rifampin 279
Right bundle branch block 102
Right ventricular 103
    dysfunction 92
Ringer's lactate 160
    plus 160
        hydroxyethyl starch 160
Risperidone 213
Rivaroxaban 14
Road traffic accident 116
Robinia pseudoacacia 224
Rosary pea 224
Rotterdam score 120t
Rumack-Matthew nomogram 220
Russell's viper 199, 201
Ryle's tube 60

S

Saccharomyces boulardii 141
Salbutamol 97
Salicylate 181, 207
    toxicity, management of 217
    toxidrome 217
Saline administration 181
Salivation 192, 210

Salmonella bacteremia 275
Sanguinary snakes 217
Sarafotoxins 219
Sarin 209
Saw-scaled viper 199
Scald burn 167
Scopolamine 208
Scorpion
    antivenom 204
    sting 218
        clinical grading of 203t
        envenomation 202
        fatalities of 202f
        management of 204fc
Scrotal abscesses 288
Scrotum 264f
Scrub infection 264
Scrub typhus 263, 265, 266, 268, 269
    affects 263
    burdens of 263
    diagnosis of 265, 266b, 267t
    diagnostic panel 267b
    early distinction of 265
    endemicity 263
    infection 264, 265
        natural course of 265f
        pathogenesis of 264f
    management of 268
    manifestations during pregnancy 265
    risk factors for developing 264b
Sea snakes 199
Second heart sound, accentuated pulmonic
    component of 102
Sedation 48, 341
    agitation scale 48
    daily interruption of 51
Sedatives, use of 52
Seizures 58, 216
    control of 212
    treatment of 274
Sepsis 23, 55, 83, 359, 360
    campaign, surviving 261
    treatment of 85
Septic
    abortions 245
    arthritis 287, 289, 290
    shock 265, 276, 361t
        manage 261
Serological tests 266b
Serotonergic drugs 215
    multiple 215
Serotonin syndrome 215
Serotoninergic toxidrome 215
Serum 208
    amylase 153
    creatinine 92
        kinase level 209
    electrolyte 92, 167
    glutamic
        oxaloacetic transaminase 159
        pyruvic transaminase 159
    lactate level 152
Severe acute pancreatitis study, audit of 161
Severe disease 252
    signs of 251
Severe malaria, pathogenesis of 272fc
Shock 83, 153, 158, 253, 273
    cardiogenic 91b
    causes of 87
    compensated 258

decompensated 258
distributive 185
hypotensive 258
hypovolemic 21, 185
infection 275
management of 21
obstructive 21
Sialic acid 233
Sickle cell trait 272
Sinus
  bradycardia 213
  rhythm 87
  tachycardia 211
Six organ systems, dysfunction of 265
Skin 165
  decontamination 194
  grafting 169
  infection 285
  lesion 281
    swabs 288
Skull fractures 117
Sleep
  apnea, obstructive 331
  deprivation 55
  hygiene 58
Small bowel, proximal 145
Smooth muscle 209
  contraction 186
Snake
  envenomation 199
  venom 199, 218
Snakebite 205, 245
  envenomation, management of 201
  management of 200*fc*
  related acute kidney injury 219
  victims 219
Sodium
  bicarbonate 183, 195, 206
    role of 183
  ion 183
  loss 181
  nitrite 217
  thiosulfate 216, 217
Soft tissue infection 285
  necrotizing 172, 173, 175, 176*fc*
Sorbents, types of 362
Sotalol 86
Spasms 127
Spherocytosis, hereditary 272
Splenic abscesses, multiple 288*f*
Spurge 225
Sputum 288
Standard medical therapy 359, 363
Staphylococcal infections 125
Staphylococcus
  aureus 29, 139, 160, 166, 172, 234, 240
  epidermidis 160
Stasis, zone of 165
Status epilepticus 51, 127
Steam burn 167
Steatorrhea 141
Steroid 97, 286
  glucocorticoid 187
  role of 277
  treatment 281
  use of 276
Stewart's strong ion difference 181
Stiffness 127
Stinging scorpions 217

Stomach 146
  ultrasonography of 146*f*
Streamlining antimicrobial therapy 43
Streptococcus 240
  pneumoniae 29, 42, 234, 240
Streptokinase 105
Streptomycin 279
Stress
  index 307
  induced cardiac syndromes 18
  ulcer prophylaxis 93
Stridor 185
Stroke 7, 32, 87, 281
  volume 7, 20
Strychnine-sensitive glycine receptor 127
Subcutaneous emphysema 111
Subdural hematoma 117, 118*f*, 119
Substance abuse 58
Succinic acid 181
Sucking chest wound 111
Sulfadoxine 273
Sulfate 138, 181
Superior mesenteric artery, thrombosis of 153*f*
Superior vena cava 339
Suprapubic pain 287
Surrogate 72
  decision maker 76
  role of 76
Sweating 210
Sweep gas 345
  flow 340
Swelling syndrome, progressive 199
Sympathetic nervous system 151
Sympathomimetic toxidrome 211, 212*f*
Sympathoplegia toxidrome 213
Symptomatology 208, 209
Syphilis 125
System vascular resistance 7
Systemic capillary leak syndrome 200
Systemic inflammatory response 118
  syndrome 156, 362
  features of 157*b*
Systolic blood pressure 4, 28, 91, 121
Systolic pressure, normal 258

T

Tabernanthe iboga 222
Tachyarrhythmia
  induced cardiomyopathy 88
  tolerate 84
Tachycardia 102, 131, 158, 192, 208, 211, 215, 226, 247
Tachypnea 102, 131, 158
Takotsubo syndrome 18, 19*f*
Tamponade 20*fc*
Taxus baccata 222
Temephos 191
Tension pneumothorax 108, 121
Terizidone 279
Tetanus 245
  biological plausibility 245
  clinical features of 245
  diagnosis of 246
  evidence base 248
  generalized 246
  immunoglobulins 248
  localized 246
  natural history of 245
  neonatal 246

pathogenesis of 245
severity of 246*t*
toxin 247
toxoid 248
treatment of 246, 247
Tetracycline 247, 269
  toxicity 132
Tetraethyl pyrophosphate 190
Thalassemia 272, 286
Theophylline 207
Therapeutic hypothermia 51, 123
Thermal burn 166, 167
Thermal inhalation injury 169
Thiamine 207
  deficiency 26
Thoracic aorta 20*f*, 113
Thoracic injury 108, 114
  multiple 110*f*
Thoracic surgery 83
Thoracic trauma 108, 111
  pathophysiology of 109*t*
Thoracostomy
  formal 111
  tube 111
Thoracotomy, resuscitative 113*b*
Thrombocytopenia 10, 219, 252
Thromboembolism 93
Thrombolysis, half dose 106
Thrombotic disorders 152
Thymoma 128
Thyroid 288
Ticagrelor 11
Tick-borne spotted fever 266
Tissue
  hypoxia 91
  oxygen delivery levels, raised 300
Toxic alcohols 206
Toxicity 214
Toxidrome 206, 207, 209, 215
  management of 207
Toxin 207, 217, 219
Tracheobronchial injuries 111
Tracheostomy 109, 169, 247
Tramadol overdose 215
Transalveolar driving pressure 304
Transesophageal echocardiography 17, 20*f*
Transient bacteremia, hematogenous spread of 174*f*
Transjugular intrahepatic portosystemic shunt 134
Transoesophageal echocardiography 88
Transplantation system 73
Transpulmonary pressure 324
Transthoracic echocardiography 16, 20*f*
Transverse myelitis 265
Trauma 23, 83, 157
  penetrating 111, 157
    abdominal 113
  with intercostal catheter 111*f*
Traumatic aortic injury 112
Traumatic brain injury 58, 116, 118*f*, 119, 123, 320
  and mortality 119*t*
  causes of 116*f*, 117*f*
  classification of 120*t*
  pathophysiology of 117
  severity of 119
Traumatic subarachnoid hemorrhage 120
Tremor 215
Triethylphosphate 190
Trimethoprim-sulfamethoxazole 289

Trizophos 191
Trombiculidae family 263
Troponin 103
Tsutsugamushi triangle 263, 263f
Tuberculoma, intracranial 280
Tuberculosis 276, 278, 279, 282
  abdominal 281
  cutis miliaris disseminata 281
  diagnosis of 281
  disseminated 281
  extrapulmonary 281
  gastrointestinal 281
  in intensive care unit 276
  management of 276
  organ-specific 280
  patients coinfected, treatment of 281
  treatment of 277
Tuberculous
  meningitis 277, 280
  pericarditis 281
  spinal arachnoiditis 280
Tumor 58
  necrosis factor 234
Typhoid 252
  fever 265
Typhus
  endemic 266
  epidemic 266

U

Ulcers 245, 288
  chronic 173
  pressure 60
Ultrasound, abdominal 159
Ultraviolet germicidal irradiation 282
Unbound toxin 246
  neutralization of 247
Upper abdominal pain 159
Upper respiratory tract 235
Urates 181
Urinary
  catheters 60
  retention 208
  tract infections, catheter related 44
Urination 192, 210
Urine output, normal 254

V

Vaccination 29
Vaccine 242
Vaginal bleeding, causes of 261
Valproate 130, 132
Valproic acid 157
  solution 140
Valvular disease, severe 19
Valvular regurgitation 7
Vancomycin 46
  resistant *Enterococcus* 43
Varicella zoster virus 127, 130
Vascular
  disease, peripheral 173
  ileus 145
  injury 109
  intrathoracic structures 108
  stenting 154
Vasculotoxic syndrome 200
Vasoconstrictor catecholamine 72
Vasoplegic shock 21
Vasopressor therapy 260
Vecuronium bromide 214
Venoarterial extracorporeal membrane oxygenation 337, 340, 341
Venom neurotoxins block 218
Venomous scorpion stings, endemic distribution of 203f
Venous thromboembolism 101
  prophylaxis 123
Venovenous extracorporeal
  carbon dioxide removal 348, 349
  membrane oxygenation 338, 341
Venovenous hemodiafiltration, continuous 354, 355
Venovenous hemofiltration, continuous 134
Ventilation
  esophageal pressure-guided 307
  improvement of 242
  invasive 98
  noninvasive 30, 98, 109, 255, 261, 280, 326, 327b, 331, 332, 334f, 335f
  perfusion scan 103
  positive-pressure 99
  pressure support 318
Ventilator support 169, 341

Ventricular enlargement trial, survival and 12
Verapamil 86
Veratrum 221
Vessels, abdominal 152
Vibrio vulnificus 173
Viper venoms 218, 219
Viperidae 199
Viral hepatitis 131, 252
Viral pneumonia 234
Viremia 125
Virus 23, 240, 256
Viscera, abdominal 114
Visceral abscesses 285
Vivax malaria, severe 272
Volatile anesthetic agents 50
Volume clamp method 4
Volvulus 159
Vomiting 185, 192, 252
Vorapaxar 11
Voriconazole suspension 140

W

Water accidents 9
Water hemlock 223
Weil-Felix test 266t
Wells' score 103t, 104
Wernicke's encephalopathy 58
West Nile encephalitis 125
Westermark's sign 102f
White blood cell 157
Whole blood clotting test, twenty-minute 201
Wild carrot and parsley 223
Wilson's disease 130, 134
Wound
  assessment 166
  care 248

Y

Yellow oleander 220

Z

Zigadenus 221
Ziprasidone 59, 60, 213
Zoonotic disease 263
Zoonotic infection 251

EU GSPR Authorised Reprsentative
Logos Europe, 9 rue Nicolas Poussin
1700, La Rochelle, France
Phone: +33 (0) 6 67 93 73 78
E-mail: contact@logoseurope.eu